DISEASES OF MARINE ANIMALS

DISEASES OF MARINE ANIMALS

Editor

OTTO KINNE

Biologische Anstalt Helgoland
Hamburg, Federal Republic of Germany

VOLUME I

General Aspects, Protozoa to Gastropoda

A Wiley – Interscience Publication

1980

JOHN WILEY & SONS

Chichester · New York · Brisbane · Toronto

British Library Cataloguing in Publication Data

Diseases of marine animals.
  Vol. 1: General aspects, protozoa to
  gastropoda
  1. Marine fauna – Diseases
  I. Kinne, Otto
    591.2   SF997.5.M/   79-40580

    ISBN 0 471 99584 3

Typeset by Preface Ltd., Salisbury, Wiltshire
Printed in Great Britain by The Pitman Press, Bath.

FOREWORD

'Diseases of Marine Animals' is a derivative of 'Marine Ecology – A Comprehensive, Integrated Treatise on Life in Oceans and Coastal Waters', edited by myself and published by John Wiley & Sons Ltd. (London/Chichester). Originally, I had planned to include a chapter on 'Diseases of Plants' and another on 'Diseases of Animals' in Volume III (Cultivation). However, after the reviewers had completed their syntheses, it became apparent that size, emphasis and importance of the latter account would disrupt the concept of Volume III. Publisher, editor and contributors have, therefore, decided to omit the review on plant diseases and to publish the information available on animal diseases in a separate treatise.

The treatise 'Diseases of Marine Animals' consists of four volumes. **Volume I** contains the following chapters:

Chapter 1: Introduction to the Treatise and to Volume I
Chapter 2: Diseases of Marine Animals: General Aspects
Chapter 3: Diseases of Protozoa
Chapter 4: Diseases of Mesozoa
Chapter 5: Diseases of Cnidaria
Chapter 6: Diseases of Cnidaria
Chapter 7: Diseases of Ctenophora
Chapter 8: Diseases of Tentaculata
Chapter 9: Diseases of Sipunculida, Priapulida and Echiurida
Chapter 10: Diseases of Platyhelminthes
Chapter 11: Diseases of Nemertea
Chapter 12: Diseases of Mollusca: Gastropoda.

We consider disease primarily as an ecological phenomenon. Volumes I to IV demonstrate that knowledge on the diseases of marine animals provides new leads for solving a variety of ecological and evolutionary problems and contributes significantly to the understanding of the diseases of terrestrial animals, including man. Many biologists have failed to recognize, or neglected to take into account, disease as a basic denominator of organismic coexistence.

The potential impact of diseases has received insufficient attention in most attempts to analyze, comprehend or model ecosystems. Biological oceanographers, fisheries scientists and marine ecologists have often focused their views exclusively on the role played by hydrological factors for organismic distributions in space and time, food-web interrelations, productivity and related holistic ecosystem properties.

The treatise is intended for all those professionally interested in the marine environment—be it its comprehension, utilization, management or protection. It addresses especially researchers, teachers and students in the fields of pathology, parasitology, ecology, fisheries biology, and aquaculture.

Much of what is known on the diseases of marine animals stems from species which (i) are of commercial interest; (ii) live near the coast or are otherwise easily accessible; (iii) are often used in cultivation and laboratory experiments. As in other fields of biology, such selection tends to affect, if not to distort, the overall picture. More basic research is necessary, also on organisms without apparent commercial significance and less readily available for collection and experimentation, before we can present a more complete, balanced and objective account of the diseases of marine animals.

Investing a considerable amount of work and determination, as well as revealing a remarkable synthesizing potential, Dr. Gerhard Lauckner of the Biologische Anstalt Helgoland has expanded the originally rather limited chapter to the most comprehensive compilation of our knowledge on the diseases of marine animals yet available. Except for the introductory chapters, he is the sole author of all forthcoming contributions to this treatise.

The publisher's support and cooperation is deeply appreciated. I am very grateful for having been allowed to proceed with my plans without any restrictions in regard to scope, organization, space or time. Monica Blake and Helga Witt have been most efficient and careful helpers in all matters of literature research.

O. KINNE

Hamburg, July 3, 1978

CONTENTS
OF
VOLUME I

viii

xii

CONTRIBUTORS
TO
VOLUME I

KINNE, O., *Biologische Anstalt Helgoland (Zentrale), Palmaille 9, 2000 Hamburg 50, Federal Republic of Germany.*

LAUCKNER, G., *Biologische Anstalt Helgoland (Litoralstation), 2282 List/Sylt, Federal Republic of Germany.*

GENERAL ASPECTS, PROTOZOA TO GASTROPODA

1. INTRODUCTION TO THE TREATISE AND TO VOLUME I

O. KINNE

SCOPE OF THE TREATISE

As has already been stated in the foreword, 'Diseases of Marine Animals' was originally planned as a contribution to 'Marine Ecology', Volume III 'Cultivation', which reviews our present capacity for supporting, and experimenting with, marine organisms under environmental and nutritional conditions which are, to a considerable degree, controlled.

However, a comprehensive, critical treatment of all essential information on the diseases of marine animals demands attention in its own right. Such assessment is not only important for successful cultivation and experimentation: it contains a multitude of detail and elucidates essential principles pertaining to the fields of general pathology, parasitology, ecology, evolution, fisheries and human health. The very large body of information available, as well as the interdisciplinary significance of the subject and its bearing on all major fields of biology and medicine, have prompted us to extend the original concept to a four-volume treatise of which we present here Volume I. The work on Volumes II to IV has largely been completed, and we expect the whole treatise to be published in the near future.

While diseases have their roots in a variety of circumstances—genetic background, nutrition, stress, injury, or coexisting organisms (p. 16)—the scope of the treatise is limited to diseases caused by coexisting organisms (agents), i.e. to biotic diseases, as well as to proliferative disorders (tumours) and to structural abnormalities. 'Diseases of Marine Animals' attempts to review all essential information available on the pertinent diseases of the major taxonomic groups of marine animals. It is the product of seven years of literature studies and brings together, for the first time, a host of data scattered over a wide array of scientific journals and books. Largely based on original-source information, the treatise corrects numerous misquotations and distortions of facts which have, over the years, found entrance into the scientific literature and which have subsequently been requoted time and again—falsifying the resulting picture of the state-of-the-art.

Diseases affect basic phenomena of life in oceans and coastal waters: for example, life span, life cycle, abundance, distribution, metabolic performance, nutritional requirements, growth, reproduction, competition, evolution, as well as organismic tolerances to natural and man-made environmental stress. In short, diseases are a major denominator of population dynamics. The significance of diseases for present-day ecosystems, as well as for long-term evolutionary dynamics, is referred to and discussed in most chapters of this treatise.

Although the information at hand on the diseases of marine animals is in many cases fragmentary and often inadequate, we sincerely hope that this treatise will help to emphasize to marine scientists the importance of the relationships between disease agent and host and their capacity for affecting, directing or even controlling the flow patterns of energy and matter in marine ecosystems. Hardly any individual animal in oceans and coastal waters is completely free of agents which can potentially cause a disease, and all major taxonomic animal groups have been shown to comprise representatives which can act either as agent or host, or both.

Research on animal diseases has been of major and long-standing concern to numerous aquafarmers and pet-fish breeders. Among the aquatic animals studied thus far, oysters, mussels, decapod crustaceans and teleost fishes have received most attention. Investigations on the diseases of marine fishes, and for that matter of several invertebrates, have been stimulated by limnological studies. In many cases, the diseases of freshwater-living animals are better known than those of their marine counterparts which are often less accessible and more difficult to maintain under culture conditions. Where desirable and pertinent, we have, therefore, included information on the diseases of limnic animals.

ORGANIZATION OF THE TREATISE

'Diseases of Marine Animals' is organized around the two partners, or antagonists, involved in a biotic disease: agent and host. The disease agent (pathogen) benefits from its host—another, different organism which tends to be affected negatively by the presence of the agent. Agent benefits include procurement of energy, matter, protection or habitat space; they involve behavioural, physiological, biochemical and genetic aspects of both agent and host. Negative effects in the host are caused, for example, by the release of metabolic agent products, by agent competition for life-supporting processes and substances, and by modification of essential functional and structural host properties.

The organization of the treatise follows the major groups of potential host animals. These are considered in the usual sequence, i.e. beginning with the Protozoa and ending with the Vertebrata.* Within each major host group, disease agents are reviewed according to the following general key: Viruses, Bacteria, Fungi, Protozoa, Mesozoa, Porifera, Cnidaria, Platyhelminthes, Aschelminthes, Mollusca, Annelida, Arthropoda and Pisces. Wherever available, pertinent information has been included on the physiology and ecology of both host and agent, with special emphasis on life-cycle dynamics. Unfortunately, the taxonomy of disease agents is incomplete or confusing in many cases. A rich harvest awaits systematically inclined pathologists.

Volume IV also contains information on applied aspects. Special attention is devoted to: (i) The prevention and treatment of diseases in research cultivation and in commercial cultivation (aquaculture), and—though less intensively practicable—in the field (biological control of intermediate hosts); and (ii) the significance of the diseases of marine animals for human health.

*The groups of hosts and agents treated do not necessarily represent comparable systematic units, nor do they in all cases reflect the newest systematic concepts. Organisational simplicity and readability of the text have been of primary concern to us—sometimes overruling purely systematic considerations.

INTRODUCTION TO VOLUME I

In addition to this introductory chapter, Volume I contains a chapter on general aspects of the diseases of marine animals—biotic diseases, proliferative disorders and structural abnormalities—and ten chapters on the pertinent diseases of major animal groups ranging from the Protozoa to the Gastropoda.

Volume I witnesses that our present knowledge on the diseases of the host groups reviewed is very incomplete. There is a remarkable scarcity of informational hardware. Much of what we know today is based on incidental observations and casual reports. There is great need for well-planned in-depth research. For example, the absence of information on virus-, bacteria- or fungi-caused diseases in many of the host groups treated seems to mirror lack of pertinent investigations rather than the non-existence of microbial disease-agent activities.

In the future, we can expect important new insights into the diseases of the host groups reviewed in this volume. Of no or limited economical importance, most of the animals concerned await thorough investigation. Even high losses due to disease and hence the practical need for etiological studies have had little impact on the research thus far conducted. In contrast, commercial interests have directed considerable funds and efforts into analyzing disease phenomena in bivalves, decapod crustaceans and teleost fishes–host groups treated in subsequent volumes.

Comments on Chapter 2: Diseases of Marine Animals: General Aspects

Chapter 2 attempts to elucidate basic perspectives and to outline unifying principles pertaining to the facts and interpretations presented in Volumes I to IV of this treatise. The chapter focusses on the ecological significance of diseases; evolutionary aspects of agent–host interactions; the general types and groups of marine disease agents; the contrasting roles of agent and host (agent virulence versus host defence); as well as on disease diagnosis, prevention and therapy. It ends with a glossary of important terms.

The ecological significance of biotic diseases has received little attention from most marine scientists—whether concerned with biological oceanography, experimental ecology or ecosystem modelling. This is unfortunate because disease is an important ecological principle. No marine organism seems to be completely free of potential disease agents and all systematic animal groups contain members which can act as agent or host.

In principle, organisms on earth exist either in the free-living state, characterized by predominantly multilateral interrelations, or in the state of symbiosis, characterized by predominantly bilateral interrelations. Biotic diseases, as well as many proliferative disorders and structural abnormalities, result from interactions among symbiotes. Wherever the ecological balance between symbiotes is significantly modified, disease may result. The equilibrium can shift due to variations in environment or nutrition as well as to otherwise induced changes in the partners' ecological potential.

The seas abound with symbioses and these have many faces. Depending on the essential effects exerted, as well as the flow or exchange of energy and matter among symbiotes, four basic types of symbioses are distinguished: phoresis, commensalism, parasitism and mutualism. In most cases, only parasitic symbioses qualify as potential causes of biotic diseases. Ecologically, symbioses add a new dimension to the limitations of a single organism. By combining different, heterospecific characteristics of discrete units of life—individuals—a symbiosis combines, complements and economizes their requirements and chances for energy procurement. Mutualistic symbiotes tend to internalize the recycling of essential life-supporting substances, i.e. to maximize resource exploitation and to minimize the escape of utilizable energy and matter to the ambient environment.

In parasitic symbioses, disease (a demonstrable, negative deviation from the normal state of an organism) prevails where the equilibrium between the two partners involved—agent (parasite) and host—shifts significantly in favour of the former. In addition to changes in environment or nutrition, such shifting can be brought about by increase in agent number or impact, by a diminution in host defence, or both. In terms of the above considerations, disease and health represent different, dynamic states of organismic existence which mirror the result of the contrasting roles played by agent and host.

Major evolutionary prerequisites for the development of a symbiosis comprise spatial, chronological, biochemical and strategical compatibilities between potential symbiotes. The evolutionary strategies of agent and host are based on limited-conflict principles. On this basis, the agent tends to adjust increasingly to specific host characteristics, thus attaining progressive specificity at the expense of versatility.

A basic theme of Chapter 2 concerns the contrasting and conflicting forces of agent virulence and host defence. Virulence refers to the disease-producing potential of the agent; its important components are contact making, establishment, reproduction, and distribution of the agent. Host defence refers to the potential of the host for counteracting agent virulence; it comprises behavioural, mechanico-chemical and immunity mechanisms. The latter are based on a variety of cellular activities which are harmonized with the host's own characteristics, but suppress, neutralize or eliminate foreign materials, living or non-living. The processes involved in non-genetic immunity are visualized to be homologues of those involved in non-genetic adaptation to environmental factors such as temperature. In both cases, ontogenetic adjustments are induced which result in a relative increase in the capacity of the individual concerned to survive, reproduce or compete. The adjustments require time to develop and reinforcement for continued effectiveness; they persist beyond the circumstances which induced them.

Disease diagnosis, prevention and therapy in marine animals have remained almost virgin fields. Much more research is necessary before the marine biologist has an instrumentarium at hand which is comparable to that available in veterinary and human medicine. Nevertheless, the growing body of knowledge on the diseases of marine animals provides new perspectives and will increasingly affect our concepts and understanding of the diseases of domestic animals and man.

Comments on Chapter 3: Diseases of Protozoa

The number of known Protozoa is still increasing and most of the marine representatives have not yet been studied in sufficient detail. In order to present a comprehensive state-of-the-art account we have therefore included pertinent data on non-marine protozoans. Presumably, there exists considerable parallelism between disease phenomena in marine and limnic Protozoa.

The majority of disease agents affecting marine Protozoa belong to the following four groups: viruses, bacteria, fungi and other protozoans. In relatively few cases, also larval trematodes and nematodes have been shown to act as parasites—the former in flagellates, the latter in rhizopods. Based on the information at hand, bacteria and other protozoans rank highest as disease-causing agents. Although virus-like particles have been reported from several protozoans, clear cases of virus-caused diseases have still to be provided. However, several protozoans are vectors of virus diseases of higher animals, including man. Among the fungi, the Chytridiales play a dominant role. Fungal infections of the nucleus appear to be lethal. Since sporozoans are exclusively parasites, all parasitic agents of sporozoans qualify as hyperparasites.

Most endobiotes of protozoans depend metabolically on their host. However, as in other animal groups, a clear distinction between parasites, commensals and mutualists is often difficult. The major reasons for this are: (i) insufficient knowledge on the metabolic interrelationships between the symbiotes concerned; (ii) the dependence of these interrelationships on environmental circumstances; (iii) equilibrium shifts due to variations in the ecological potentials of agent and host.

Although demonstrated in several marine Protozoa, structural abnormalities require more attention before definite generalizations are possible. Among freshwater protozoans, giant individuals, nuclear aberrations, and distortions of the contractile vacuole have been documented in *Paramecium caudatum*, and 'monsters' in *Tetrahymena pyriformis*.

The symbioses between Protozoa and their different partners represent simple biosystems which offer unique possibilities for studying and analyzing such phenomena as biological exclusion, quantitative aspects of agent–host interaction and epizootiology.

In an annex to Chapter 3, we have considered some Protophyta hosts for the following reasons: (i) In the unicells, proper distinction between animal and plant members is not always possible; some unicells exhibit primarily animal-like or primarily plant-like characteristics, depending on prevailing environmental or nutritional conditions. (ii) Some agents known to cause diseases in Protophyta are similar to organisms acting as pathogens in marine invertebrates and may be expected to inhabit unicellular animals. (iii) For comprehending history, dynamics and ecological significance of a disease of Protozoa, comparative knowledge of related diseases in the Protophyta may reveal important clues. (iv) Protophyta may act as vectors of agents causing diseases in invertebrates and vertebrates, including man.

In *Platymonas* sp. evidence has been obtained for the first time in marine algae for the presence of intranuclear virus-like particles. The particles resemble a herpes-type virus infecting the oyster *Crassostrea virginica*. A number of other virus diseases are known from algae, both prokaryotic and eukaryotic. Several marine Protophyta have been shown to be attacked by bacteria, fungi and protozoans.

Comments on Chapter 4: Diseases of Mesozoa

Our literature studies have revealed no reports on the presence of disease-causing agents in marine Mesozoa. However, dicyemids exhibit a number of structural abnormalities, such as increased cell numbers, 'double monsters', and vermiform or giant larvae. The causes for such abnormalities are not known.

Comments on Chapter 5: Diseases of Porifera

Sponges possess effective defence mechanisms, especially for counteracting microbial agents. In addition to whole-cell defence mechanisms, cell-product mechanisms are available which can inactivate pathogens such as bacteria. Several authors have reported the presence of antimicrobial substances.

The symbiotes commonly observed in sponges comprise bacteria, fungi, protozoans, protophytes and a large variety of metazoans. While viruses have not yet been reported to cause disease in Porifera, bacteria, fungi and protozoans appear to represent the major potential disease agents. Especially fungi may cause diseases of epizootic proportions. The parasites and diseases thus far known are practically restricted to calcareous and hexactinellid sponges. However, the etiology of sponge diseases is insufficiently investigated.

In several marine sponges, populations of mutualistic bacteria have been shown to attain considerable biomass values. Presumably, these bacterial symbiotes are of nutritional significance for the host sponge. In addition to extracellular bacterial mutualists, sponges such as *Verongia aerophoba* and *V. cavernicola* have been shown to occasionally entertain intranuclear symbiotes. The role of these symbiotes remains to be analyzed.

The mass mortalities of sponges ascribed to fungus infections may be related to environmental circumstances such as high salinities. During the peak of the epizootics near the Bahamas, presumably fungus-infected individuals rotted completely within one week. The relations between potential fungus agents and their host sponges require critical investigation. The present evidence is insufficient for drawing definite conclusions.

Protophyta appear to classify primarily as mutualists. While the occurrence of algae such as Cyanophyceae in sponge tissues has been known for a century, the interrelations between symbiote and host still await analysis in regard to potential metabolic cooperation or pathogenicity.

The metazoan symbiotes of Porifera include cnidarians, rotifers, molluscs, annelids, copepods, amphipods, cirripeds, mysidaceans, decapods, arachnids and pantopods, as well as fishes. In general, the metazoans appear to utilize the sponges' cavities as living quarters and mostly appear to play a role as commensals (lodgers). However, the trophic relations between these symbiotes and their host are inadequately investigated. In some cases the symbiotes have been shown or suspected to cause 'inconveniences' such as irritation or occlusion of water passages, in others to display histophagic activities.

Sponges can respond to intruders by overgrowth, formation of fibrous layers or by activating repair mechanisms. Except for modifications in skeletal and spicule growth, no information is available on tumours and other structural abnormalities.

Comments on Chapter 6: Diseases of Cnidaria

Common symbiotes of marine Cnidaria include bacteria, fungi, protozoans, sponges, other cnidarians, larval trematodes and cestodes, molluscs, crustaceans, larval pantopods and fishes. Of these, the following groups qualify as most important disease agents: protozoans, cnidarians, molluscs and crustaceans.

Although viruses and bacteria are assumed to be capable of causing disease in cnidarians, none of the diseases known can be ascribed with certainty to viral or bacterial agents. Certain fungi penetrate the calcareous skeletons of corals, but definite evidence of fungi-caused diseases has not come to the reviewer's attention.

Protozoans seem to be of major importance as potential disease agents. However, the reports available on protozoan-caused diseases of Cnidaria refer primarily to hydrozoans. Here, protozoan pathogens may exhibit high degrees of virulence and even assume control over abundance and distribution of host populations. It must be emphasized though that most of the pertinent information is restricted to limnic forms.

Some sponges—especially members of the genus *Cliona*—can penetrate dead coral as well as skeletal portions of denuded living coral. While they have not been shown to attack living coral tissue, sponges may cause considerable destruction of skeletal material and thus interfere with coral growth. Cnidarian agents parasitize scyphozoans and, especially, hydrozoans. Among the other potential metazoan pathogens, trematodes, cestodes, copepods and amphipods (particularly *Hyperia galba*) may attack scyphozoans and hydrozoans. Scyphozoans have also been affected by isopods, decapods and several fishes; hydrozoans by molluscs and pantopods. Metazoan agents which may attack anthozoans include—in addition to poriferans—larval trematodes, molluscs, annelids, many copepods, as well as some cirripeds, amphipods, mysidaceans, decapods and pantopods. No metazoan-caused disease has yet been demonstrated in cubozoans.

While there exists some vague, circumstantial evidence for the presence of tumours and structural abnormalities in scyphozoans, hydrozoans and anthozoans, definite facts have not been established and in-depth research has still to be conducted. Due to their simple morphology and the fact that at least several of them can be kept under controlled laboratory conditions without much effort, cnidarians constitute potentially excellent material for analytical studies on proliferative disorders and structural abnormalities.

While the Cnidaria appear to largely lack behavioural and mechanical mechanisms of host defence, there is some evidence for biochemical defence responses. Several cnidarians have been shown to produce antimicrobial substances, and a few authors have claimed the presence of antibody-like compounds. In view of their obvious vulnerability (limited motility, soft body boundaries), internal defence mechanisms may be postulated to play the dominant role in the strategy of cnidarians for counteracting potential disease agents.

Comments on Chapter 7: Diseases of Ctenophora

No disease due to viruses and bacteria has thus far been reported in ctenophores. However, laboratory observations, as well as comparative theoretical considerations, suggest that micro-organisms may potentially play a significant role as disease agents in this interesting group of marine animals. Among the protozoans, foettingeriid ciliates (*Pericaryon cesticola*) have been shown to coexist with and apparently parasitize *Cestus veneris*.

While cnidarians, other ctenophores, trematodes, cestodes, nematodes and amphipods have been found as symbiotes on or in ctenophores, the most important disease-causing agents recorded thus far belong to the Trematoda, Cestoda, Nematoda and Amphipoda. Among the latter, *Hyperoche mediterranea* and *H. medusarum* are very common. Apparently, these opportunistic hyperiids are predominantly facultative endoparasites during their early development, but live as ectoparasites or in the free-living state during later phases of their ontogeny.

While structural abnormalities of the locomotory apparatus of *Pleurobrachia pileus* have been reported from the North Sea, causes and consequences of proliferative disorders (tumours) and of structural abnormalities remain unknown.

Comments on Chapter 8: Diseases of Tentaculata

Very little is known about the diseases of Tentaculata, i.e. the Phoronida, Bryozoa and Brachiopoda.

An unidentified gregarine, a ciliate and unidentified trematode metacercariae are the only agents thus far reported from the Phoronida. The gregarines occurred attached to intestinal epithelium of members of three *Phoronis* species. The ciliate *Heterocineta phoronopsidis* fed on epithelial cells of *Phoronopsis viridis* tentacles. The trematode metacercaria parasitized the lophophoral coelom of *Phoronis psammophila*.

In Bryozoa, microsporidans, undetermined organisms ('brown' and 'vermiform' bodies), trematode metacercariae and polychaetes (*Serpula oblita*) have been observed. The identity and potential role as disease agent of most of the organisms involved remains to be investigated.

In the Brachiopoda, only larval trematodes have been shown to act as true parasites. The nature of associations between the amphipod *Aristias neglectus* and the brachiopods *Terebratulina caputserpentis* and *Macandrewia cranium* requires analysis.

Neither microbial agents nor proliferative disorders have become known from tentaculates. However, antineoplastic substances occur in *Nugula nerita, Amathia convoluta* and *Thalamaporella gothica*. In a few bryozoans, monster zooids and double polypids have been reported.

Although no definite information is available on host defence, structural barriers, phagocytosis, encapsulation and cell-product mechanisms may be assumed to be of significance.

Comments on Chapter 9: Diseases of Sipunculida, Priapulida and Echiurida

The symbiotes found associated with the sipunculids, priapulids and echiurids examined belong to the Bacteria, Protozoa (flagellates, sporozoans, ciliates), Trematoda, Cestoda, Mollusca and Copepoda. The information available on etiological aspects is largely restricted to Sporozoa and Trematoda.

While bacteria have been shown to cause disease under laboratory conditions, no evidence is at hand for bacterial diseases under *in situ* conditions. As in other host groups dealt with in this volume, the absence of information on microbial diseases appears to witness insufficient pertinent knowledge rather than host resistance to viruses, bacteria or fungi.

Experimental studies on sipunculids reveal considerable capacities of host defence. Forms such as *Phascolosoma gouldi* exhibit pronounced antibacterial activities both in the cellular and liquid components of their blood.

Among the protozoans, sporozoan agents—especially gregarines and coccidians— dominate the scene and frequently parasitize representatives of all three host phyla. Of lesser importance appear to be ciliates and, especially, flagellates. Although some data are available on protozoan agents and their interrelationships with the few sipunculids, priapulids and echiurids studied, our present knowledge is insufficient for a reasonably sound assessment of agent–host interaction and of the potential ecological role of protozoan-caused diseases.

This statement also holds for the metazoan agents—larval cestodes, molluscs and copepods. The effects of trematode metacercariae on several sipunculids has received appreciable attention. The larvae penetrate the brain of the worms leaving a path of damaged tissue behind them. Heavy metacercarial infestation can almost entirely destroy the posterior brain and deform neurosecretorial processes.

The few reports at hand on proliferative disorders and structural abnormalities in sipunculids, priapulids and echiurids are largely inconclusive and do not yet allow generalizations.

Comments on Chapter 10: Diseases of Platyhelminthes

Among the Platyhelminthes—the turbellarians, trematodes and cestodes—the latter two classes consist entirely of parasites; hence their parasitic agents represent hyperparasites. Experimentally induced hyperparasitism may provide a key for biological control and thus for limiting undesired activities of these often dangerous parasites.

In marine platyhelminths, the most frequently reported disease agents are protozoans, especially sporozoans, but also some flagellates and ciliates. The evidence for virus-caused diseases requires verification and substantiation. However, flatworms serve as vectors for viral diseases of 'higher' animals, including dogs. Under laboratory conditions, a bacterial disease—'red pest'—has been described in the acoelous turbellarian *Archaphanostoma agile*. Fungus-caused diseases have thus far become known only from limnic platyhelminths. Among the metazoan agents, other platyhelminths— especially trematodes—are of particular significance. In addition, there are a few reports concerning mesozoans, aschelminthes and copepods.

Among the sporozoan agents, members of the Microsporida have most frequently been found to be the cause of the biotic diseases of platyhelminths. Microsporidans infest particularly trematodes. In cestodes, microsporidan agents have become known only from non-marine host species. A few gregarines and coccidians have been recorded in limnic turbellarians.

Reports on proliferative disorders and structural abnormalities in platyhelminths are rare. The few data at hand refer to limnic representatives. Among non-marine forms, spontaneous tumours have been observed in planarians, and structural abnormalities—such as miracidial twinning, abnormally structured reproductive organs and unusual pigmentation—in trematodes.

Host defence may be assumed to include behavioural, mechanico-chemical and immunity mechanisms (pp. 43–55).

Comments on Chapter 11: Diseases of Nemertea

Etiological studies on nemertean diseases have remained a virgin field. No information is available on micro-organism-caused diseases, and the data on protozoan as well as metazoan symbiotes and their potential effects on nemertean hosts are sketchy at best.

Among the few facts that begin to emerge from such paucity of knowledge is the common occurrence of protozoan agents—especially sporozoans—which often inhabit the host's coelomic spaces and digestive organs, but may also be found intracellularly. The effects of these agents on their host range from interference with host motility over changes in pigmentation to parasitic castration, cellular degeneration, tissue disintegration and premature death.

In addition to protozoan agents, Mesozoa and a few Metazoa—cestodes, copepods and halacarids—have been found to parasitize Nemertea.

Thus far, only phagocytosis has been clearly demonstrated as defence mechanism available to nemertean hosts. However, cooperation of other defence mechanisms (such as encapsulation, as well as the production of antimicrobial and antibody-like substances) seems likely.

Comments on Chapter 12: Diseases of Mollusca: Gastropoda

Within the Mollusca, disease research has concentrated primarily on commercially important representatives—mostly bivalves (Volume II). Considerable information is also available on the Gastropoda. If of less or no immediate economical significance, gastropods—such as oyster drills and limpets—may seriously interfere with commercial bivalve cultivation and, hence, have been studied intensively with the primary aim of controlling their undesired activities.

Marine gastropods serve as hosts for a large variety of potential disease agents. Among these, most information is at hand on trematodes; much less on fungi, protozoans, cestodes, annelids, copepods and other molluscs, and almost nothing on protophytes, mesozoans, cnidarians, turbellarians, nematodes, isopods and pantopods. While viruses and bacteria are suspected to be capable of acting as important potential disease agents, no definitely documented cases of micro-organism-caused diseases in marine gastropods have come to our attention.

In regard to trematode agents, innumerable marine gastropods have been shown to act as first intermediate hosts for larval stages. Subsequent hosts of metacercarial stages include commercially important bivalves, crustaceans and fishes (see Volumes II, III and IV). For several trematode agents, interesting life-cycle details have been successfully worked out. Among the gastropods, littorinids—here particularly *Littorina littorea*—have been most thoroughly investigated. However, in spite of the numerous studies conducted on trematode–gastropod symbioses, the mechanisms of agent virulence and host defence are insufficiently known in most instances.

Trematode-agent effects comprise (i) structural changes, such as deformation of typical cell, tissue and organ architecture (e.g. histolysis, tissue degeneration, digestive-gland obliteration, increased shell erosion, changes in reproductive structures, abnormalities in organ and body size, gigantism); and (ii) functional changes, such as deviations in rates of growth and metabolism; in behaviour and motility; in biochemical composition and dynamics (e.g. variations in lipid composition; in total protein content of hepatopancreas, fatty-acid and amino-acid levels; glycogen depletion; variations in amounts and activities of enzymes); in reproductive processes (e.g. parasitic castration, reduction or cessation of sperm and egg production, modifications in sex ratio); reduction in overall resistance to environmental (temperature, salinity) and man-made stress (water pollutants). In all cases, extreme negative deviations may cause premature death of the host individual concerned and—where extreme situations prevail—modifications in population dynamics.

As in other symbioses, all quantitative parameters of agent virulence and host defence, as well as agent–host interactions, underlie variations as a function of environmental circumstances, including seasonal changes.

Marine gastropods serve as second intermediate hosts for trematode parasites. Typically, the cercariae emerge from their first intermediate host and then invade a new, second intermediate host. However, the cercariae may also remain in the first intermediate host and develop there into metacercariae (the same host is then, by definition, called second intermediate host); in some cases even full maturation can occur without host change (the host individual thus becoming also the final host). Such 'short cutting' in the normally more complicated host-switching procedure appears to hold advantages for the agent involved.

A few remarks must suffice here regarding potential agents on which rather limited information is at hand: Fungus infections have been observed in ova of oyster drills. Possibly, they could attain importance as biological control in oyster cultures. Several fungi also occur on the shells of living and dead gastropods. Their role as potential disease agents remains to be analyzed. The few protozoan agents known belong to the Sporozoa (gregarines and coccidians) and to the Ciliata. Several larval cestodes have been found in gastropods, e.g. in species of *Bulla*, *Patella* and *Tiedemannia*. Among the annelids, *Polydora ciliata*, which burrows in the shell of *Littorina littorea*, may possibly assume disease-causing qualities. Copepods parasitize prosobranchs, opisthobranchs and nudibranchs. Other molluscs which may cause disease in gastropods include especially small opisthobranch snails of the family Pyramidellidae. In none of the potential agents listed has detailed information been produced on agent effects or host defence.

2. DISEASES OF MARINE ANIMALS: GENERAL ASPECTS

O. KINNE

Although sporadic mention of diseases of marine animals is almost as old as are the first accounts on animal life in the seas, the history of critical research on the diseases of marine animals is rather short. Less accessible and more foreign to everyday human experience, marine animals were assumed by most ancient writers to be symbols of good health. Such an attitude is exemplified by the century-old expression: 'Gesund wie der Fisch im Wasser'. However, today we know that marine animals, including the fishes, are far from being representatives of good health. They are subject to diseases just as much as their terrestrial counterparts.

Early reports on diseases of aquatic animals include a description of a fish disease ('worms of fishes') authored by an ancient Greek physician who lived around A.D. 130 to 200 (Cheng, 1964). In 1613, Aldrovandi described a hump-headed sea perch and, in 1674, Olearius reported exostoses associated with vertebral column and spine of fishes. In his bibliography on parasites and diseases of fishes from 330 B.C. to 1923, McGregor (1963) concludes that scientific studies on fish diseases have remained largely inadequate until quite recently. This is often even more the case in regard to the diseases of other groups of aquatic animals, especially those of no immediate commercial significance.

During the last four decades, research activities directed towards the detection, description and analysis of the diseases of marine animals have increased rapidly. Sindermann (1970), for example, quotes a total of 555 references devoted to the diseases of marine fishes. Of these, only 27 appeared before 1900. The motivation for this impressive increase in disease research has rooted largely in man's interests to avoid economic losses and to disclose the life histories of agents which may interfere with human health.

Considerable additional impetus resulted from the financial support which several governments have recently channelled into aquaculture studies (Kinne, 1976b, 1977a, b). The success of aquaculture operations depends, to a large extent, on our capacity for diagnosing, counteracting or preventing the diseases of the organisms cultivated. An impressive body of knowledge has become available on the diseases of molluscs (oysters and mussels) and crustaceans (Volume II), as well as of fishes (Volume IV).

Basic research on marine animal diseases requires more attention. Even today it remains difficult to convince governments and other sponsors of reseearch that restriction to species of commercial interest is insufficient for comprehending essential ecological dynamics of life in oceans and coastal waters, for developing sound measures of environmental protection, and for understanding the principles of biotic diseases. The few species which happen to be of immediate commercial interest are 'embedded' in a multitude of interrelations with numerous other coexisting organisms. Their population dynamics, exploitability and protection can be fully assessed only in context with adequate knowledge on ecologically related organisms: predators, food organisms, competitors, associates and disease agents. The continuing, one-sided emphasis on commercially important species begins to distort the resulting picture of overall ecological dynamics and to hinder sound progress in basic ecology, so much needed for proper long-term environmental management (e.g. Kinne, in press; Kinne and Bulnheim, in press).

Of the major publications which include information on the diseases of aquatic animals we mention here Dollfus (1942), Schäperclaus (1954), Snieszko (1954a, 1970), Hopkins (1957), Dogiel and co-authors (1958, 1961, 1970), Altara (1963), Reichenbach-Klinke and Elkan (1965), Snieszko and co-authors (1965), Post (1965), Cheng (1967b, 1973; see also Cheng's 1970 book on symbiosis), Sindermann (1966, 1970), Dawe and Harshbarger (1969), Amlacher (1970, 1976), Ghittino (1970), Kabata (1970), Dailey and Brownell (1972), Halver (1972), Mawdesley-Thomas (1972a, b), Roberts and Shepherd (1974), Maramorosch and Shope (1975), Ribelin and Migaki (1975) and Pflugfelder (1977).

WHAT IS A DISEASE?

Definition and General Points

The term 'disease' denotes a demonstrable, negative deviation from the normal state (health, p. 17) of a living organism. 'Negative' implies an impairment, quantifiable in terms of a reduction in the ecological potential (e.g. survival, growth, reproduction, energy procurement, stress endurance, competition). The deviation may be functional or structural or both; it may result from a single cause or from several causes acting in concert.

The degree of a negative deviation depends on the impact of the disease-causing entity and the counteractive potential of the individual affected. In most cases, the relation between impact and counteractive potential is, in turn, subject to external influences (e.g. climate, stress) and nutrition. Both disease and health are not static concepts, but manifestations of the balance achieved between disease-causing entity and counteractive potential. A biotic disease is the expression of the status of agent–host interactions (p. 21). The ability of the agent to cause disease and the ability of the host to counteract or to resist detrimental agent effects comprise different aspects of one and the same biological principle. In terms of experimentation, the contrasting roles of agent and host can be analyzed by modifying agent impact (variable) and maintaining host resistance at a defined level (constant) and *vice versa*.

There may be a latent period between the presence (onset) of the disease-causing circumstance and the demonstrability of a disease. For example, certain substances or micro-organisms do not produce demonstrable consequences for days, weeks or even months. Can we term the condition prevailing during such a latent period a disease—unless it involves a demonstrable negative deviation from the normal state? I do not think so. Even if the causative agent can be identified, the ultimate manifestation of the disease remains a matter of predictive statistics. A disease can be expected or even predicted to occur on the basis of etiological knowledge, but its actual presence depends on demonstrable disease criteria be they ever so subtle. There are sufficient examples available which document absence of disease after the latent period, due to subnormal agent virulence or supranormal host defence, or both.

Demonstrable, negative deviation from a host's normal state requires that the agent's effects surpass a certain critical level. Critical levels of agent effects may be surpassed in various ways, for example, by (i) increase in number of a given agent per host individual; (ii) increase in a given agent's perturbative or destructive potential (virulence, p. 32); (iii) concomitant activities of several agents belonging to different taxa; (iv) decrease in host resistance due to: its physiological state (e.g. metamorphosis, reproduction, or diminution of immunity); environmental stress (e.g. light, temperature, salinity, oxygen availability, pollution); or to other additively effective disease-promoting or disease-causing conditions; (v) changes in the quantitative relations between host and agent, e.g. while an adult herring may not deviate from its normal state when parasitized by one nematode, the same nematode may kill a herring larva.

A disease is either restricted to the individual affected (non-infectious non-communicable, non-contagious disease), or transmissible from one individual to another (infectious, communicable, contagious disease). Most diseases dealt with in this treatise are transmissible. A disease may be benign or malignant, acute or chronic. The terms benign and malignant, often used to characterize the destructive potential of tumours, actually have a wider meaning. Benign diseases generally entail no complications and usually continue or end without causing critical deviations or death. In contrast malignant diseases, unless treated, tend to result in premature death. Acute diseases typically begin abruptly, develop rapidly and are soon over. In contrast, chronic diseases usually proceed more slowly, attain less pronounced intensities, but persist over longer periods of time.

In terms of epidemiology, four groups of diseases can be distinguished: (i) Enzootics, i.e. animal diseases characteristic of host populations in a certain area where they persist or reoccur, usually at low levels of overall intensity. The equivalent term in human medicine is endemics. (ii) Epizootics, i.e. temporary mass outbreaks of a communicable animal disease within a certain region. In human medicine, the equivalent term is epidemics. (iii) Panzootics, i.e. temporary mass outbreaks of a communicable animal disease which extends over wide geographical areas. In human medicine, the equivalent term is pandemics. (iv) Sporadic diseases, which manifest themselves only sporadically and in relatively few individuals; sporadic diseases are more or less untypical of the area concerned, i.e. they are ecdemic.

Many diseases are a characteristic feature of a given species, a group of species, or of closely related genera, families, or higher taxa—either within a limited area or, less frequently, over the whole area of host distribution. Certain parasites (e.g. nematodes, copepods) tend to aggregate in enzootic centres, others (e.g. trematodes) to suddenly exhibit a sharp increase in local abundance thus giving rise to epizootics.

A host may be inhabited by several different symbiotes (see also p. 21). The branching coral *Pocillopora damicornis*, for example, usually harbours a variety of animals, including several species of shrimp, crabs and the fish *Paragobiodon echinocephalus*. The coral's associates reveal different evolutionary stages of symbiosis, and close interrelationships sometimes referred to as community structure (e.g. Patton, 1974). Assemblages of different parasite populations (consisting, for example, of bacteria, fungi, protozoans and trematodes) which inhabit a given host are known as parasitocoenoses or parasite-mixes. A certain parasitocoenosis is, for instance, typical of the intestine of mammals, including those living in the marine environment. Changes in the composition or disturbances in the balance of the parasitocoenosis may affect the host in various, usually detrimental ways. The members of a given parasitocoenosis tend to affect or control each other in a manner comparable to that observed in a biocoenosis of free-living organisms.

The presence of certain parasites in the biocoenosis can interfere with the activities of parasitic competitors or even exclude these from invasion or establishment. Such interaction needs to be explored more fully. In some cases, it may hold the key for selectively excluding parasites which are particularly dangerous to a given host (see also biological control, p. 58). An example of competitive interaction of larval trematodes parasitizing the mud snail *Nassarius obsoletus* has been provided and discussed in the light of pertinent literature by De Coursey and Vernberg (1974). These authors list the following possible types of interactions between parasites competing in one and the same host individual: (i) coexistence without harmful interaction; (ii) preferential selection of different micro-habitats in the host, thus reducing the degree of competition; (iii) longitudinal or radial displacement in the tissue selected, or displacement to other tissues; (iv) unilateral cannibalism (predation) resulting in elimination or numerical reduction of the competitor.

Disease is not necessarily restricted to the host. Also the agent may 'get sick'. Since, in general, hosts are larger and more conspicuous than the agent, and since we ourselves view biotic diseases primarily from the perspective of the host, the resulting picture suffers from a tendency toward one-sidedness.

Causes of Disease

In principle, disease may have 6 different types of causes:
(i) Circumstances internal to the individual involved: innate, idiopathic or genetic diseases.
(ii) Nutritional disorders.
(iii) Negative effects due to non-living entities such as critical intensities of abiotic environmental factors (e.g. light, temperature, salinity, oxygen availability) and natural or man-made pollutants, including poisons.
(iv) Physical injuries.
(v) Coexisting organisms (agents).
(vi) A combination of the afore-mentioned conditions.

As has already been pointed out in the introduction, the present treatise is restricted to diseases caused by agents (biotic diseases), and to proliferative diseases as well as structural abnormalities. The latter often result from a variety of causes acting in concert. In the marine environment, disease-causing agents may be viruses, bacteria, fungi, protozoans, mesozoans, as well as a large variety of metazoans (p. 31).

Analysis of the causes, development and consequences (etiology) of a disease requires detailed knowledge on the biology and ecology of agent and host. For predictions regarding the potential ecological impact of epizootics, additional information must be at hand, especially on environmental and trophic dynamics. The essential analytical tools of the pathologist further include a variety of histological, biochemical and immunobiological methods.

Health

Health is a concept antonymous to disease. It denotes the normal functional and structural state of a living organism. 'Normal' implies the ability of the organism involved to accommodate itself successfully under typical ecological conditions; 'successfully' refers to adequate ecological performance, e.g. in regard to the organism's development, reproduction or competition. Both normal and successful as defined above are quantifiable (measurable) in objective terms. Ultimately, health facilitates full exploitation of an organism's ecological potential.

Healthiness is a function of innate properties, as well as of the relationships between organisms and their environment, abiotic and biotic. One and the same organism may be healthy under one set of environmental and nutritional conditions, but not under another.

The gradient between health and disease is often long and variable, and there may be wide areas of overlap. A dynamic condition resulting from a variety of compromises, health is a relative, not absolute concept. Some definitions of health, including the one offered in the preamble of the charter of the World Health Organization ('Health is a state of complete physical, mental, and social well-being and not merely the absence of disease or infirmity'), involve strongly subjective, if not utopian elements.

Disease as Ecological Principle

Disease is an important ecological principle. It can significantly modify the dynamics of organismic coexistence. Disease not only affects the relationship between agent and host. Disease of a given host, especially when of epizootic proportions, may also influence related species—such as the host's prey, predators or competitors. Disease tends to modify nutritional dynamics, reproductive potentials, distributions and abundances. In extreme cases, it can even modify essential characteristics of the local ecosystem, at least temporarily (p. 23).

Not only a biotic disease qualifies as ecological principle. Also the other basic types of diseases (p. 16)—innate, nutritional, stress-caused and injury-caused—involve ecological aspects and may appreciably affect ecological dynamics. The significance of disease as ecological principle has received insufficient attention from most biologists, whether concerned with experimentation, field work or modelling. Walford's (1958, p. 147) statement still stands:

'One of the most serious gaps in our knowledge of marine ecology is the study of diseases. To what extent do pathogenic bacteria, fungi, viruses, and other groups affect populations of plants and animals? . . . Epidemics are common occurrences in marine environments, and sometimes have devastating consequences. They may be an important cause of fluctuations, and should therefore have a prominent place in research programs.'

In terms of ecology, biotic diseases represent special cases of organismic coexistence. In principle, we can distinguish between organisms coexisting in a free-living state, characterized by predominantly multilateral interrelations and organisms coexisting in the form of symbiosis, characterized by predominantly bilateral interrelations (Fig. 2-1). All biotic diseases qualify as symbiotic interrelations, typically between two heterospecific organisms—agent (symbiote) and host.

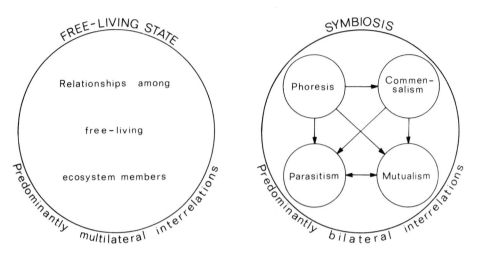

Fig. 2-1: Principal types of organismic coexistence. Symbiotic relationships typically involve close body contact of the partners concerned; they can be either facultative or obligatory. Evolutionary specialization often tends to develop from facultative to obligatory, as well as in the directions indicated by arrows. (Original.)

The term **'symbiosis'** (*syn* = together, *bios* = life) was coined in 1879 by Heinrich Anton de Bary, Professor of Botany at the German University of Strassburg. De Bary introduced the term to describe the living together of algae and fungi in the form of lichens. He defined symbiosis simply as intimate coexistence of heterospecific organisms. De Bary neither implied uni- or bilateral exploitation nor did he restrict the term 'symbiosis' to mutualism. While we use the term symbiosis in its original meaning we emphasize the intimacy ('body contact') and long standing of the predominantly bilateral relations involved, and point to the often complementary requirements of the symbiotic partners (symbiotes or symbionts). In contrast to this definition, a number of authors use the term symbiosis in the sense of mutualism (see below).

In the marine environment, both number and diversity of symbioses, including those which may lead to diseases, are extraordinarily large. The relations characteristic of a symbiosis are mostly insufficiently investigated. However, unless disproven by experimentation, we may postulate that symbiotic interrelations entail no essential elements other than those present in coexisting free-living organisms.

Terms and concepts related to the four major categories of symbiosis distinguished—phoresis, commensalism, parasitism, and mutualism (Fig. 2-1)—usually involve, in varying degrees, subjective, anthropomorphic interpretations. There is considerable need for investigating different types of organismic coexistence in detail and for defining the categories distinguished more objectively. The terms phoresis, commensalism and mutualism comprise large areas of connotation overlap. Only parasitism can presently be defined without much ambiguity (see below). Attempts to provide a more adequate terminology should, perhaps, wait until more solid information emerges on the relationships actually involved. What is needed here most is critical experimentation on interorganismic dependencies and on the flow patterns of energy and matter between the partners concerned.

For further information on pertinent symbiotic relationships consult, for example, Baer (1952), Caullery (1952), Cameron (1956), Hopkins (1957), Yonge (1957), Füller (1958), Lapage (1958), Noble and Noble (1964), Dogiel (1962), Smyth (1962), Sprent (1963), Cheng (1964, 1967a, b, 1970, 1973), Geiman (1964), Croll (1966), Dales (1966), Henry (1966, 1967), Taylor (1973), Vernberg (1974).

The term **phoresis** designates transport, shelter or other support of one type of organism (the phoront) by another (the carrier or host) without metabolic exploitation or exchange. While the phoront may enjoy the benefit of transport, shelter or substratum, no benefit is apparent for the carrier. Examples of phoresis are barnacles attached to animals such as bivalves, crustaceans, turtles or whales. High abundance of phoronts can debilitate the carrier, e.g. peritrichous ciliates on the exoskeleton of planktonic copepods. Phoresis may be facultative or, less often, obligatory.

Commensalism refers to an intimate coexistence of heterospecific organisms in which one (the commensal) obtains unilateral benefits (e.g. energy, matter, space and/or protection) from the other (the host) without causing demonstrable negative or positive effects in the latter. The latin word commensal (*com* = together, *mensa* = table) implies eating together at the same table. Numerous turbellarians, for example, live as commensals on or in a variety of marine invertebrates, such as gastropods, isopods, crabs, shrimps, echinoderms or fishes (Jennings, 1974). Commensals living on their host are called ectocommensals, those living inside their host, endocommensals. Facultative commensals can live both free and as commensals, while obligate commensals depend absolutely on their host—at least during a significant part of their life cycle.

Parasitism involves an intimate coexistence of heterospecific organisms which is characterized by the fact that one of the organisms involved (the parasite) obtains benefits (e.g. energy, matter) at the expense of the other (the host); parasitism often tends to result in demonstrable negative effects in the host. The (metabolic) dependence of the parasite may be facultative (facultative parasite) or obligate (obligate parasite).

The parasitic state can involve the agent's whole life (holoparasitism) or only part of it (meroparasitism). The parasite may live externally on the host body (ectoparasitism) or inside the host body (endoparasitism); a parasite may, in turn, be host of another parasite (hyperparasitism). Endoparasites live within cells (intracellular parasites), between cells (intercellular parasites), or in cavities, tubes, kidney, alimentary tracts, etc. of their host (extracellular parasites). All animal phyla have members which are either parasites or hosts.

Most parasites exploit host processes of energy liberation. Some even gain influence on integrative control mechanisms, involving both endocrinological and neurophysiological aspects, and thus manipulate nutritional routes as well as certain characteristics of the host environment. The effects exerted by the parasite include (i) damage due to the release of metabolic products; (ii) withdrawal of life-supporting substances, e.g. nutrients, body materials; (iii) modification or destruction of host functions, e.g. metabolic processes; (iv) deviations of host structures, including processes of morphological differentiation. Ultimately, the parasite tends to reduce the ecological potential of its host, i.e. to diminish its resistance to abiotic and biotic environmental factors, its reproductive potential, its ability to compete, and its life span.

The frequently expressed view that a parasite enjoys an effortless life in ease and comfort, abounding in food and being free of predators is, in this form, most likely incorrect. It seems that the role of a parasite is much more problematic. Many parasites must produce enormous numbers of offspring in order to compensate for the fantastic odds against life-cycle completion; in fact, in multi-host parasites only one out of billions of offspring may be able to reproduce. A parasite must continuously adjust to and counteract the host's defence mechanisms. Finally, on a long-term basis, agent activities must be dosed so delicately that critical damage leading to host annihilation—and hence to the death of the agent species itself—is avoided. In contrast to man who is about to irreversibly destroy the life-supporting properties of earth, parasites have mastered the problem of restricted, balanced long-term exploitation. Their evolutionary strategy seems to be based on the concept of limited conflict (see also p. 29).

Mutualism comprises an intimate coexistence of heterospecific organisms which results in beneficial effects for both mutualists* or partners involved. The two interacting mutualists may be, but need not be, metabolically dependent upon each other. In addition to metabolic benefits, mutualism may involve such aspects as protection or utilization, e.g. for purposes of reproduction. Mutualism may be facultative or obligatory.

Examples of metabolically dependent mutualism are the intimate partnerships between algae (zooxanthellae) and invertebrates commonly observed in shallow, tropical waters (e.g. Yonge, 1931, 1957, 1963; Taylor, 1973). The zooxanthellae release products of photosynthesis which are metabolized by their mutualist (host), for example, a cnidarian (e.g. Muscatine and Hand, 1959; Goreau and Goreau, 1960; Smith and co-authors, 1969; Taylor, 1969; Trench, 1971, 1974; Lewis and Smith, 1971; Young and co-authors, 1971; Muscatine and co-authors, 1972; Vandermeulen and Muscatine, 1974; Chalker and Taylor, 1975; Patton and co-authors, 1977). The cnidarian, in turn, provides nutrients and protection for its algal symbiotes. Such coupled use of energy and internalized recycling of essential nutrients maximizes efficient resource exploitation and minimizes the escape of utilizable energy and matter into the ambient water.

An example of metabolically independent mutualism is the association between hermit crabs and sea anemones. The latter are carried on the shells inhabited. While the crab may benefit from the deterring potential of the anemone's nematocysts, the anemone participates in the crab's meals. In addition, most of the so-called 'cleaning symbioses' (p. 43) qualify as cases of mutualism.

All four types of symbiosis distinguished—phoresis, commensalism, parasitism and mutualism—represent dynamic, not static, conditions of coexistence. They are expressions of the ecological equilibrium between the two partners concerned. The

---

*Most students of mutualism distinguish between mutualist (usually the smaller of both partners) and host. However, such differentiation seems problematic in view of the underlying phenomenon which implies mutual benefits.

equilibrium between agent and host can, at any time, shift or change, for example, due to variations in environmental (p. 24) or nutritional factors (p. 25), or due to otherwise induced changes in the partner's ecological potentials. Between the same partners, one type of symbiosis may develop into another: phoresis, for example, can turn into commensalism, or commensalism into parasitism.

In terms of survival and exploitation of life-supporting conditions, symbioses add a new dimension to the ecological limitations of a single organism. By combining the different, often reciprocal abilities and needs confined to discrete blocks of life (individuals), the intimate living together of two or more kinds of heterospecific individuals couples, complements and economizes their capabilities for making energy and material available, and provides new possibilities for space partitioning and protection.

A host harbouring several symbiotes—e.g. viruses, bacteria, protozoans, fungi, annelids and crustaceans—represents an ecological entity comparable to a small biocoenosis (p. 16). Such an organismic assemblage seems to convey essential advantages to most of the components involved. As in an ecosystem, the components change (adjust) to some extent under the impact of coexistence (Kinne, 1977d, p. 723ff.). Most of the adjustments made are not immediately reversible without losses in vitality or ecological potential. They provide directionality in the flow routes of energy and material and add new elements of system homeostasis.

Agent–Host Interactions

Although agent–host interactions remain to be thoroughly investigated and analyzed in most of the disease-causing symbioses known, we may postulate that biochemical and behavioural aspects are of particular significance. Biochemical interactions have been dealt with in a number of original papers—mostly devoted to terrestrial parasite–host combinations. Behavioural aspects, again largely restricted to non-marine animals, have received attention in Canning and Wright (1972). Behavioural adjustments can be assumed to be of considerable importance for agent and host as well as for long-term agent–host interactions. In principle, the interactions between agent and host parallel those of free-living organisms.

Life on earth is organized in the form of discrete, temporary units of specifically structured matter—individuals. At the individual level, two basic, reciprocal forces are apparent: forces which facilitate interaction and exchange between individuals, and forces which maintain discreteness and specificity (individuality) of the units concerned. Both interaction and discreteness are basic requirements of life as a whole; they are, at the same time, denominators of conflicting strategies at the individual level.

In our present context, host-related agent activities (virulence) qualify as primarily interactive forces, mechanisms of host defence as primarily discreteness-maintaining forces. We discuss agent virulence on pp. 32 to 41, host defence on pp. 41 to 56.

Both agent virulence and host defence are subject to non-genetic and genetic adaptation (e.g. Kinne, 1963, 1964a, b, 1970a, p. 435). In the course of non-genetic adaptation, an individual agent or host acquires capacities—during its individual history—which are advantageous to its own survival and reproduction. The maintenance of these capacities usually requires reinforcement lest they diminish again.

In contrast, genetic adaptation involves 'fixed', evolutionary changes in the genotype of the organism concerned. Apparently, genetic denominators of agent virulence and host defence are usually based on the function of several genes acting in concert. Only in very few cases of human diseases has host defence been demonstrated to be accomplished by a single gene.

Agent virulence and host defence are not necessarily species specific; both may be effective, to a lesser or higher degree, in groups of related organisms. Thus, a microbial agent with virulent capacities towards the European flat oyster *Ostrea edulis* may exert similar effects in American oysters *Crassostrea virginica*, or a host which has achieved resistance to a certain pathogenic bacterium may have simultaneously attained increased resistance to a related micro-organism. On the other hand, closely related races of agents or hosts may exhibit different degrees of virulence and defence.

Host specificity is a measure of the closeness or exclusiveness of an association between an agent and a given host. It implies restriction of a parasite to a certain host species. The degree of host specificity can be expressed quantitatively in terms of agent preference (quantifiable in preference experiments) or agent presence (quantifiable by examination of host samples). A more general concept of host specificity has been formulated by Noble and Noble (1964, p. 618): 'the peculiar mutual adaptation which restricts a parasite to its host species'.

Host specificity is an ecological principle comparable to food and habitat specificity of free-living organisms. While such specificity is apparent from observations in nature, its exact causes are largely unknown. They may continue to remain in the dark just as much as the causes which have led to the evolutionary development of the trunk of the elephant or the intellect of man. However, speculation seems in order about the major factors involved. Conceivably, the most important ones are (i) the essential nutritive and environmental requirements of the parasite; (ii) the defence mechanisms of the host; (iii) ecological plasticity of both parasite and host; (iv) competition among parasite candidates; and (v) time, i.e. the evolutionary span involved. Of the significant early contributions devoted to host specificity we list here Mayr (1957), who has concerned himself with evolutionary aspects, and Noble and Noble (1964), who have explored and discussed contemporary knowledge in considerable breadth and depth.

Of the conclusions conceived by Noble and Noble (1964) several are of particular importance in the present context: (i) Parasites with an indirect life cycle tend to exhibit less host specificity than those with a direct life cycle. (ii) There is less specificity in parasites with two intermediate hosts than with only one. (iii) In trematodes, specificity is more pronounced among larval stages, while the larvae of cestodes frequently tolerate a wider range of hosts than their adult counterparts. (iv) In nematodes specificity is usually greater for the intermediate host than for the definite host. (v) There seems to be less host specificity among parasites than assumed: numerous studies continue to disclose new hosts for parasites originally thought to be host specific.

In the marine environment, host specificity is particularly pronounced in trematodes (for details consult the chapters devoted to Gastropoda and Pisces). This fact may be exemplified by referring to *Meiogymnophallus minutus* (Trematoda Digenea) which utilizes *Cardium edule* as 2nd intermediate host. Near the island of Sylt (southern North Sea), 100% of the *C. edule* examined harboured metacercariae of *M. minutus*, while *C. lamarcki*—which lives side by side with *C. edule*, did not contain a single *M. minutus*

(Lauckner, personal communication). Other examples of extreme host specificity are Monogenea which parasitize marine fishes (Bychowsky, 1961; Rohde, 1977). In general, distributional ubiquitousness tends to be associated with a decrease in host specificity: Cosmopolitan hosts often harbour different agents, and cosmopolitan parasites often utilize an array of hosts.

While the marine Monogenea studied do not reveal geographic gradients in host specificity, such gradients have been documented by Rohde (1978) in marine Digenea. These exhibit increasing host specificity ranging from cold to warm seas. Rohde explains the different trends in terms of r and k strategies: Monogenea tend to follow the k strategy (great complexity of adults, few offspring) which leads to high host and site specificity; Digenea tend to follow the r strategy (simple structure of adults, many offspring) which supports infestation of a variety of hosts in a given environment. The reason for the reduction in host specificity towards cold-temperate seas is seen by Rohde in the less patchy and less restricted distribution of potential hosts in such areas.

Presumably, host specificity is based to a considerable degree on genetic factors; however, non-genetic control of host specificity may also be involved. An example of genetic control is the dependence of trematode parasites on the chemical composition of mammalian bile (Smyth and Haslewood, 1963). Examples of non-genetic control appear to be indicated in some reports on geographic or seasonal variations in host specificity. Non-genetic specificity tends to be lost again unless reinforced. Its presence and degree can be determined experimentally.

Effects at the Individual, Population and Ecosystem Levels

At the individual level, a disease can profoundly affect rates and efficiencies of metabolic processes including growth and reproduction. It may modify life-cycle dynamics as well as reduce the capacities for regulation and adaptation and, consequently, the host individual's resistance to stress, both natural and man-made (pollution). A disease can further interfere with functional and structural integration and influence morphological differentiation. Ultimately disease tends to reduce the individual's ecological potential and life span.

At the population level, a mass disease can modify population structure and diminish population size. It may influence the population's distribution, abundance and its overall reproductive capacity. Where attaining critical levels, such changes modify population dynamics and reduce the ecological potential of the population or species concerned.

At the ecosystem level, an epizootic disease of a given organism can exert concomitant influences on functionally related species such as predators, competitors or prey. In extreme cases, a disease may even change, at least temporarily, essential functions and structures of the ecosystem concerned. An example is the wasting disease of eelgrass *Zostera marina*. This disease results in rapid necrosis and disintegration of infected leaves. Especially in the years 1930 to 1932 it spread quickly, devastating *Z. marina* populations in large coastal areas (e.g. Renn, 1936a, b; Young, 1937; Tutin, 1938; Johnson and Sparrow, 1961) and changing the living conditions for other plants and for numerous animals–thus modifying essential properties of the local ecosystem.

Typically, epizootics manifest themselves in the form of oscillations, i.e. successively rising and declining abundances of diseased individuals. The wave troughs reflect temporary superiority of the agent due to cyclic growth, reproduction or augmented release of detrimental substances. Following an epizootic, the host population—after having lost most of its susceptible individuals (selection) and increased its capacity for counteracting the disease-causing agent (acquired immunity)—usually exhibits a supranormal degree of resistance. Hence, recurrence of the epizootic in the near future is unlikely. However, unless reinforced, the acquired immunity (a non-genetic adaptation to agent interference) is gradually lost again. The trend towards resistance decrease is accelerated and augmented by the disappearance of immune individuals due to emigration or death and the reappearance of susceptible individuals due to immigration or birth.

The period of time elapsing between two successive epizootics is a function of the time course of these processes, the type of disease involved and environmental circumstances affecting the agent–host relationship.

Role of Environmental Factors

Environmental factors—such as temperature and salinity—influence agent effects and host responses in numerous ways. They can affect both the degree of agent virulence (p. 32) and of host defence (p. 41), as well as the incidences of proliferative disorders and structural abnormalities.

Temperature effects on agent virulence and host defence are exemplified here by referring to (i) the vertebrate host *Triturus viridescens viridescens* and its protozoan parasite *Trypanosoma diemyctyli* (Barrow, 1958) and (ii) the invertebrate host *Homarus americanus* and its bacterial parasite *Aerococcus viridans* (Stewart and co-authors, 1969a, b). In the first example, infections are pathogenic only below 20° C; at higher temperatures, the host's metabolic rate is, apparently, high enough for successful counteraction. In the second example, the agent *A. viridans* is almost completely inactivated at low temperatures near 1° C; however, with rising temperature, its disease-causing potential increases rapidly: the median survival times of the host range from 172 days at 3° C to 2 days at 20° C.

Temperature effects on incidence and intensity of epidermal tumours (papillomas) in the European eel *Anguilla anguilla* have been reported by Peters and Peters (1977). Occurring most frequently in 15- to 35-cm long eels, the papilloma or cauliflower disease is subject to pronounced seasonal fluctuations. Both tumour abundance and tumour size attain maxima in summer and minima in winter, spring and autumn. In laboratory experiments, temperatures of 15° to 22° C induced rapid tumour growth, while temperatures of 5° to 10° C inhibited growth, or even caused tumour regression.

Differential salinity tolerances of agent and host have been found, for example, in the microsporidan parasite *Octosporea effeminans* which exerts a feminizing influence on the offspring of its host *Gammarus duebeni* (Bulnheim, 1969, 1975, 1978; see also Vol. II; for reviews on the biology of microsporidia consult Bulla and Cheng, 1976). In salinities above 25 to 30⁰/oo S, the agent's capacity to influence sex determination in host offspring becomes increasingly reduced. In 30⁰/oo, all host eggs laid are completely free of the microsporidan agent. This leads to a significant increase in the number of male offspring, provided the young developing from such eggs are raised under long-day conditions.

Seasonal variations in the abundance of disease agents and in the intensity of disease manifestation are based on environmentally controlled modifications in the dynamics of agent–host interactions. The biotic and abiotic factors involved and their effects are presumably similar, or even identical, to those controlling seasonal variations in free-living organisms. Several blood parasites exhibit seasonal as well as circadian rhythms—apparently adaptations to selection pressures exerted by characteristics of the vector (Worms, 1972).

Geographic variations in disease manifestation have been documented in numerous instances. An example is the geographic variability in tumour prevalence reported for several marine fishes by Stich and co-authors (1977). In many cases, the geographic variability revealed appears to be controlled both by genetic and environmental factors.

For the agent, the immediate environment is the host. Its chemical composition and functional as well as structural properties determine the living conditions for the agent. In many cases, this living environment responds more specifically and more directly to the agent's activities than does the abiotic and biotic environment to the activities of a free-living organism. Hence, the immediate host environment and its responsive changes must be assumed to be of paramount significance to the agent.

Pollution due to man's activities generally tends to render marine animals more vulnerable to disease. This phenomenon may be due to specific damage, or general diminution in vitality, as well as to cumulative stress. It requires detailed analysis, not least because of the rapidly increasing danger from man-made pollutants (e.g. Kinne, in press).

Role of Nutritional Factors

The role of nutritional factors in the development of biotic diseases, proliferative disorders and structural abnormalities remains to be fully investigated. Nevertheless, the information at hand on marine animals—and, more so, our pertinent knowledge on freshwater fishes, terrestrial animals and man—provides evidence that nutritional factors can significantly affect host predisposition (p. 27) and host defence (p. 41). In principle, diseases attributable to nutritional factors can be due to inadequate dietary quality, critical food shortage, or excess food uptake.

Inadequate dietary quality prevails more often under conditions of cultivation (e.g. Kinne, 1976a, b, 1977a, b) than in the field. It may significantly increase the predisposition for disease and decrease the efficiency of host defence. Inadequate dietary quality includes such phenomena as insufficient quantities or inadequate qualities of vitamins (avitominosis, e.g. Halver, 1954, 1970, 1972), minerals or amino acids, as well as insufficient protein rations. Among these, vitamin and amino-acid deficiencies seem to play the most important role in captive marine animals. Avitaminoses may not only result from insufficient amounts of vitamins taken up with the food, but also from enzymatic disorders (e.g. failure of proper vitamin processing) or gastrointestinal diseases (e.g. inadequate vitamin absorption; critical losses due to prolonged diarrhoea or vomiting).

While nutritional deficiencies tend to reduce host defence and/or agent virulence, in exceptional cases paradox responses have become known. A classical example of such a paradox response is the decrease in susceptibility to poliomyelitis virus in mice suffering from vitamin B deficiencies. Presumably, the vitamin present in the nerve cells of such mice is insufficient for supporting the virus.

For assistance in counteracting infectious agents it may be necessary to offer to the diseased animal, over extended periods of time, higher-than-normal amounts of essential substances, such as vitamins, amino acids and minerals, or to make other dietary adjustments. Noble and Noble (1964), for example, report that a decrease in carbohydrate with corresponding increase in protein intake can, in some cases, protect a host against intestinal parasites.

The nutritional requirements of marine animals have received relatively little critical attention. Only in some protozoans and in some members of commercially important groups such as molluscs, crustaceans and fishes has an appreciable amount of information accumulated (Kinne, 1977c). We may expect that adequate nutrition is a basic prerequisite for maximum host defence (p. 41). Clinical studies on man and comparative investigations on a few terrestrial mammals have shown that proteins are essential in the provision of substrates for antibody synthesis (p. 53). Similarly, vitamins and minerals play a significant role for combating microbial infections. Vitamin C, for example, tends to be an essential factor in the development of defensive inflammatory processes which usually accompany infectious diseases.

Proper nutrition is not only essential for maximizing host defence. In the agent, it must be assumed to be similarly important for its ability to counteract host defence and to establish itself on or in the host (maximization of agent virulence, p. 32).

Critical food shortage may reduce the ecological potential of the individual involved. In fact, prolonged starvation can weaken a host to an extent where its defence mechanisms become affected, thus facilitating agent establishment. In extreme cases of starvation, even organisms which are non-pathogenic under normal circumstances may attain disease-causing qualities. In contrast, shortage of food above the starvation level appears to be a rather common natural phenomenon. It stimulates competition, induces directionality into local ecological dynamics, and tends to act as evolutionary motor.

In exceptional cases, starvation can also prolong the survival span of a host. Thus, in *Homarus americanus* infected with the Gram-positive beta-haemolytic bacterium *Aerococcus viridans*, host individuals non-fed for several months contained fewer bacteria and survived much longer than their fed conspecifics (Stewart and co-authors, 1972a, b). Apparently, in this instance, a high level of nutrient supply in the host's circulatory fluid is an important prerequisite for rapid agent multiplication.

Excess food uptake appears to be unimportant as cause of disease under natural conditions. Reviewing the evidence available, Conover (1966, 1978) concludes that support for the concept of superfluous feeding in marine invertebrates is largely circumstantial. However, in cultivation and experimentation, excess food consumption can lead to phenomena similar to those observed in man, where excess eating can cause nutritional disease (obesity). In higher invertebrates and in vertebrates, obesity usually leads to high blood pressure, atherosclerosis and chronic oxygen deficiency (hypo-ventilation). These conditions tend to predispose the individual involved toward a variety of infectious diseases. Aspects of hypervitaminosis have been discussed by Halver (1954).

Host Predisposition

The predisposition of a given host for acquiring a biotic disease is a function of its innate properties (genetic adaptation), non-genetic adaptation, age, physiological state and environmental as well as nutritional circumstances.

The **innate properties (genetic adaptation)** of a host determine its resistance and its total range for counteracting potentially negative agent effects. Genetic disorders can lead to defence deficiencies and thus encourage agent entry and establishment (see also immunity deficiences, p. 44). Excessive inbreeding—a frequent consequence of long-term domestication—tends to augment the predisposition of an animal both to innate diseases (especially metabolic disorders) and to transmissible diseases. At the same time, the inbred animal's resistance to environmental and nutritional stress often decreases.

The degree of **non-genetic adaptation** (see also pp. 21 and 44) depends on the individual history of the host concerned, i.e. previous contacts and conflicts with disease agents. Non-genetic adaptation to agent activities can greatly enhance and specialize the host's counteractions and thus decrease disease predisposition.

Age influences disease predisposition in various ways. The cases studied reveal three general trends (Fig. 2-2): (i) Progressive predisposition decrease with increasing age of the host individual concerned, due to additive gain in immunity as a function of time. (ii) Progressive predisposition increase, due to increase in the chances of agent–host encounter. In several fishes, for example, the number of trematode parasites has been shown to increase with increasing age and size (e.g. Noble and Noble, 1964). (iii) Maximum predisposition in very young (newly born) and very old (senile) host individuals, due to low general resistance. As is well known, newly born and senile animals usually exhibit minimum capabilities for counteracting agent virulence and for general stress endurance.

The **physiological state** of the host depends on a number of factors—including genetically fixed properties, the presence or absence of disease agents other than the one considered, and environmental as well as nutritional conditions. Most individuals going through critical life-cycle stages—such as metamorphosis, attainment of sexual maturity, or moulting—exhibit increased degrees of disease predisposition. In mammals, numerous physiological defects—innate or acquired—are known to affect host predisposition. Reduced blood circulation, decreased local blood supply, hormonal disturbances, or disharmonization of essential body functions and structures tend to diminish host defence. In fact, whenever the efficiency of metabolic processes or the overall vitality of the host is reduced, its capacity for counteracting invasion and establishment of disease agents decreases.

Finally, capture, transport and the initial stress of captivity conditions tend to increase disease predisposition. Injuries inflicting wounds, scars or other impairments of the boundary between body surface and ambient water facilitate disease-agent entry and development (Kinne, 1977c).

The significance of **environmental** and **nutritional circumstances** for disease predisposition has been documented in numerous papers. We refer to the importance of these circumstances on pp. 24 and 25, respectively, as well as in the following chapters.

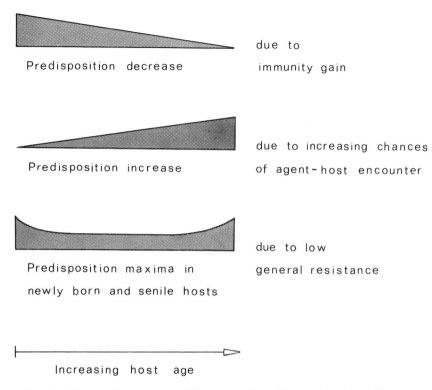

Predisposition   decrease   due to
                                             immunity gain

Predisposition   increase   due to increasing chances
                                             of agent-host encounter

Predisposition maxima in   due to low
                                             general resistance
newly born and senile hosts

Increasing   host   age

Fig. 2-2: Changes in the degree of disease predisposition as a function of host age. Schematic representation of general trends. (Original.)

Evolutionary Aspects

In terms of evolution, symbiosis is a very old phenomenon. Apparently, the first symbiotes—including the disease-causing agents among them—evolved soon after the first free-living organisms. In all probability though, symbiotes are evolutionary derivatives of free-living progenitors—with the possible exception of viruses.

In the evolution of disease-causing agents, the major driving forces for the transition from free-living to symbiotic existence seem to have been search for food and protection. Obviously nutrition and protective support can best be obtained when the agent is small and the host large; indeed, most agent–host relations are characterized by such a size gradient. Transition from free-living to symbiotic existence still occurs. Major prerequisites for such transition are spatial proximity among potential agent–host pairs, opportunism, preadaptation and genetic plasticity. In forms such as bacteria, protozoans and fungi, saprophagous nutrition facilitates the transition to parasitism. In endoparasites, capabilities for anaerobic respiration constitute an important prerequisite. Ultimately, the evolutionary success of a given symbiosis depends on the achievement of balanced interactions between the agent–host pair concerned. All long-term agent–host interrelations are based on limited-conflict strategies.

Today, marine symbioses are characterized by a wide spectrum of the agent's dependence on its host. The spectrum ranges from facultative independence, over temporary dependence to obligate dependence. Obligate host dependence prevails in all viruses, most pathogenic bacteria and fungi, as well as in many protozoan and metazoan parasites.

As all other interrelationships between coexisting organisms, agent–host inter-relations are subject to evolutionary change. A major motor for evolution, compe-tition among coexisting forms of life introduces centrifugal trends of exploitation, differentiation and specialization. While the relations between agent and host are, in essence, comparable to those among free-living organisms within a given ecosystem, in the process of evolution they tend to become more specific, more bilateral and more direct. Typically, the agent adapts so closely to its host environment that it gradually loses its ability to exist or compete over extended periods of time outside this specific 'microhabitat'. Progressive specificity is attained at the expense of versatility. The agent's adjustments to specific features of its host tend to improve the chances for contact, entry, establishment, utilization of material and energy, and for enduring or overcoming the host's defence mechanisms.

Compared to their free-living counterparts, disease agents usually augment their overall reproductive potential. This facilitates sudden, rapid enlargement of population size under favourable conditions, and increases the chances of host encounter which, under natural conditions, are often very limited. In fact, in some parasites, the odds against life-cycle completion are tremendous.

Agent–host relations can attain long-term evolutionary dimensions only if the host concomitantly evolves adequate counter measures assuring its survival at the population or species level. Indeed, we must postulate that all persisting agent–host relations entail elements of reciprocity and long-term homeostasis. Consistently very high mortalities in host populations due to a disease agent are often indicative of evolutionarily young, not yet balanced agent–host relations. They have a negative survival value for both agent and host. Being a consequence of perpetuated, sustained interorganismic action and counteraction, a disease will 'die out' where either the agent's destructive potential or the host's resistance is too high or too low. In such a case, either the agent species is unable to maintain itself (unless it finds another host) or the host species is eliminated (unless space partitioning allows part of its population to survive).

While in many cases parasitism may have evolved over phoresis or commensalism, the evolutionary avenues travelled appear to have been mostly different and multiple. Possibly, each case of parasitism or symbiosis may have had its own historical development. Convergence in terms of the state witnessed today need not imply identical or similar routes of evolution.

The common history of a given agent and its host may provide interesting cues for the analytical researcher. Careful comparative analysis of evolutionary trends in a given agent–host pair may (i) reveal insights into space–time dynamics of the symbiosis concerned; (ii) allow hypothetical extrapolations from the structural and functional organization and the phylogeny of the agent to comparable properties of its host and *vice versa*; (iii) provide indicators regarding the areas of origin, routes of dispersal and distributional ranges of agent and host. The history of agent–host developments and distributions may also be indicative of geological events, such as the origin of sea areas or the movements of continents and smaller land masses, and contribute to the understanding of biogeographic phenomena.

According to Noble and Noble (1964), the first researcher to use parasites as indicators of taxonomic relations and geographical distributions of host populations was probably Von Ihering (1891). Hence, comparative analysis of agent and host properties in different geographical areas is sometimes referred to as the 'Von Ihering method'. The evidence provided by the Von Ihering method is, of course, circumstantial and usually less reliable than direct anatomical evidence of agent and/or host structures. As Mayr (1957, p. 11) has put it:

> 'Evidence presented by parasites may be highly suggestive, but it can rarely be considered absolute proof unless corroborated by independent evidence.'

Nevertheless, the indicator capacity of agent–host relationships remains an interesting potential tool for the evolutionist. There can hardly be any doubt that long-standing agent–host relations tend to leave ineradicable marks—structural and functional—on both partners. On the other hand, agent–host parallelisms need not be restricted to taxonomically close relatives: taxonomically unrelated hosts which inhabit the same biotope and eat similar food—i.e. occupy a similar ecological niche—may share the same or similar parasites. What is needed here is a fresh, critical reassessment of the indicator value of individual agent–host relations and a refinement of pertinent analytical concepts.

The evolutionary strategies employed by parasites include changes inflicted upon their intermediate hosts which render these more available to predation by the final host. Intensified selected predation on infected individuals increases the chances of the parasite for life-cycle completion. Thus, according to Holmes and Bethel (1972), cyst-acanths of *Polymorphus paradoxus* in gammarids alter the behavioural responses of their hosts in such a way as to increase the probability of the intermediate host being consumed by the definite host. Other parasites make their intermediate hosts more conspicuous or interfere with their defensive or protective responses towards their predators. These strategies of parasites are of considerable evolutionary and ecological interest. They require detailed investigation.

Evolutionary trends of host defence (p. 41) typically reveal increasing effectiveness and specificity. In multicellular animals, the attainment of progressive complexity—ranging from sponges, cnidarians and platyhelminths to fishes, reptiles, birds and mammals—was possible only due to the concomitant elaboration of sophisticated immunity mechanisms counteracting a multitude of potentially detrimental organisms for which the host body otherwise would have provided an ideal, easily exploitable substrate.

Simple multicellular organisms such as the sponges possess 'scavenging cells' (micro-and/or macrophages) which are capable of neutralizing or removing potentially dangerous foreign substances including disease agents.

Molluscs and crustaceans contain in their circulatory fluids protein molecules capable of neutralizing or killing invading micro-organisms and of combining with, and thus inactivating, foreign materials. Primitive fishes such as the cyclostomes (hagfishes and lampreys) already exhibit chemical immune mechanisms (rejection of tissue grafts from con- and heterospecifics) as well as non-genetic adaptation of these and other immune responses, including antibody formation (p.53). While hagfishes lack thymus gland and lymph nodes, they possess a primitive spleen; their blood contains granulocytes but lacks lymphocytes. Antibody formation in hagfishes proceeds very slowly; details of this process remain to be explored. Lampreys have a small thymus gland with low numbers of lymphocytes—which are also present in spleen and bone marrow. The elasmobranch fishes studied exhibit well-developed thymus glands and possess large numbers of lymphocytes in blood and tissues; they are readily capable of producing antibodies similar to those known from higher vertebrates.

Among the fishes, antigen–antibody mechanisms attain considerable development in the teleosts. Maximum efficiency and specificity of defence mechanisms is accomplished in birds and mammals. For details on host defence, the reader is referred to p. 41 and to the following chapters.

Evolutionary aspects of host switching and of the role of intermediate hosts have been considered by numerous authors and in several reviews. While we refrain here from repetitions and hypotheses, reference is made to some interesting pertinent considerations by Odening (1974, pp. 57–76).

DISEASE AGENTS IN OCEANS AND COASTAL WATERS

The major agents known to cause biotic diseases in marine animals include viruses, bacteria, fungi, protozoans, trematodes, cestodes, nematodes, acanthocephalans and arthropods. Some agents require more than one host for the completion of their life cycle. For details consult the following chapters of this treatise.

While a few significant diseases caused by viruses, bacteria and protozoans have received appreciable attention, the ecology of the causative agents has been subject to thorough investigation in only a few cases. More knowledge is frequently available on the ecology of aquatic invertebrate parasites, especially those parasitizing fishes (e.g. Schäperclaus, 1954; Dogiel and co-authors, 1961; Hoffman, 1967; Kabata, 1970; Snieszko, 1970).

Agents such as bacteria, protozoans (particularly sporozoans) and certain metazoan parasites can transform into inactive life-cycle stages (spores, cysts). These resting stages are characterized by a reduced metabolic rate and an increased resistance to a variety of abiotic and biotic factors, including counteractive substances and the host's immunity system. Even after long periods of time (months, years) inactive agent stages may reactivate and begin or continue their role as disease agent.

Among the major agents, viruses require special attention. Of the numerous types of viruses occurring in oceans and coastal waters, a few have been shown, and several more are expected, to be capable of causing diseases in marine animals. At present, our knowledge on virus-caused diseases in marine animals is rapidly increasing. In contrast to bacterial agents, viruses are resistant to most antibiotics now available. Virus diseases of Bivalvia and of Crustacea are treated in Volume II, and of Pisces in Volume IV.

Viruses represent the most extreme case of host dependence. All are obligatory intracellular parasites. They do not possess a conventional cell structure, but only nuclear material embedded in a protein coat. Viruses are practically unable to entertain metabolic activities on their own, and can multiply only within the living cells of their host. After entering the host cell, the nuclear material of a virus parasitizes the host's metabolic processes forcing them to synthesize virus material.

Bacteria are morphologically often subdivided into several groups such as rod-shaped bacilli, spherical cocci, spiral spirochaetes, as well as branched mycobacteria and club-shaped corynebacteria. They more often cause diseases in marine animals than either viruses or fungi. There exists a very large body of information on disease-causing marine bacteria. The vast majority of bacteria are endoparasites. The nature of bacterial pathogens in fishes and the therapy of bacterial fish diseases have been discussed by Griffin (1954) and Snieszko (1954b), respectively. A partial bibliography on bacterial diseases in fishes has been prepared by Conroy (1968). For details on bacterial marine agents consult especially the chapters devoted to Mollusca, Crustacea and Pisces.

The importance of marine fungi as disease agents has received particular attention in the sections devoted to the Porifera (Chapter 5, p. 78), as well as to Mollusca, Crustacea and Pisces (Volumes II and IV). Numerous marine protozoan and metazoan parasites are dealt with, in considerable detail, throughout this treatise.

For the majority of disease agents, the spectrum of potential hosts appears to be rather limited. Numerous parasites tend to be restricted to taxonomically closely related hosts. However, we know of cases where a given agent may infect hosts which are taxonomically very remote. The fungus *Haliphtorus milfordensis*, for example, infects eggs of crustaceans and molluscs as well as the alga *Enteromorpha* sp. (Ganaros, 1957; Vishniac, 1958; Fuller and co-authors, 1964). In general, the physiological potential of disease agents for adjusting to different hosts may be larger than at present expected. The problem of host specificity has received some attention on p. 22.

For a disease-causing agent, the potential to exist on or in several hosts has considerable survival value. Host switching makes available additional, alternative sources of energy and matter. It is a phenomenon comparable to food switching, i.e. changes in food selection of free-living organisms (e.g. Kinne, 1977a, pp. 986, 995; 1977d, p. 724).

Infected host individuals may serve as 'carriers' or 'reservoirs' of a disease agent without being demonstrably affected themselves; they are simply vehicles of agent transmission. Examples are oysters which accumulate bacteria, particularly *Vibrio parahaemolyticus* and human pathogenic viruses. Marine animals acting as carriers or reservoirs for agents which can cause diseases in other animals receive attention throughout this treatise, those potentially affecting man, in Volume IV.

AGENT VIRULENCE

The term 'agent virulence' refers to the disease-producing potential of the agent. Important aspects of agent virulence are reviewed here under the headings: contact between agent and host, and agent establishment; agent reproduction; and agent distribution (Fig. 2-3). The last part of this section considers the consequences of agent virulence, i.e. the major effects exerted by disease agents on their hosts.

Contact between Agent and Host, and Agent Establishment

In the marine environment, the mechanisms facilitating contact between agent and host and subsequent agent establishment are insufficiently investigated. Both contact and establishment depend on a variety of factors involving environmental cues as well as agent and host characteristics. It is the agent which must find its host and which must exploit all chances of survival. For the host, strategies of survival or well being require agent avoidance. Where this is impossible, the host must develop appropriate strategies and mechanisms of defence (p. 41) in order to restrict or counteract critical agent effects.

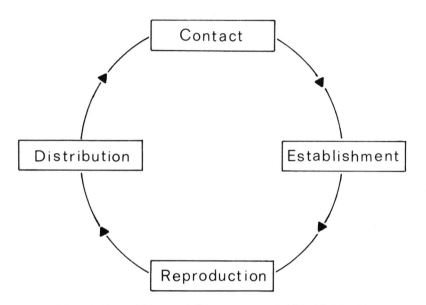

Fig. 2-3: Essential steps of disease-agent activities. (Original.)

Regarding the role of the agent, distinction is necessary between non-motile ('passive') agents and motile agents which are capable of actively moving towards the host.

Non-motile agents (non-motile agent stages) rely on host activities for contact or depend on transport, e.g. by water currents, a vector or an intermediate host. **Non-motile agents usually increase the chances of contact far above random by** associating themselves in some way or other with suitable means of translocation or with certain host characteristics—utilizing, for example, the host's feeding pattern, respiratory currents, or migratory and social behaviour. A frequently employed strategy exploits the communicable potential of host excretions, both particulate and dissolved (see also p. 38).

In motile agents, the degree of motility and orientational performance—largely based on chemoreception and its behavioural correlates—figure high in determining their strategy and potential for host localization and for achieving contact, as well as for successful attachment and establishment on or in the host. Free-swimming parasitic stages, such as trematode miracidia, seem to be guided over long or intermediate distances by host-habitat characteristics. Once near a potential host individual, the parasite appears to rely heavily on chemoreception and chemotactic behaviour. Organic substances released or leaking from the host and host-surface characteristics represent the essential cues for short-distance target orientation. Visual and auditory stimuli tend to play a less significant role. The optical and accoustical discrimination potentials are poor or lacking in most microbial agents; where present in multicellular agents, they are often less effective than in related free-living organisms. However, phototaxis and responsiveness to vibration may be important for contact and attachment, for example, in cercaria and miracidia. For details on orientational parasite behaviour consult 'Behavioural Aspects of Parasite Transmission' edited by Canning and Wright (1972) and, here, particularly the contributions by Cable, Brooker, Croll, Llewellyn and Lyons. In the present chapter, parasitic transmission is briefly referred to on p. 38.

The orientation mechanisms employed by motile agents await detailed exploration. Only in a few cases has definitive information become available (e.g. Canning and Wright, 1972). In the trematode *Cryptocotyle lingua*, cercariae are positively phototactic. In addition, vibrations caused by a passing fish induce, upon contact, immediate attachment. In contrast, for cercaria of *Renicola roscovita*, neither photo-, chemo-, rheo- or thigmotaxis, nor seismotaxis could be documented (Lauckner, personal communication). In these cercaria, contact with their second intermediate host (a bivalve) is facilitated via water propulsion and filtration of the latter, i.e. due to host activities. While it is likely that chemoreception and chemotaxis are well developed in many motile agent stages, exact evidence for such a statement remains to be provided. Host recognition seems usually restricted to short distances, e.g. centimetres or millimetres.

In principle, disease agents may be postulated to orientate in space and time by employing stimuli (cues) comparable to those utilized by their free-living counterparts (e.g. Creutzberg, 1975; Enright, 1975; Schöne, 1975; Seitz, 1975; Tesch, 1975). Among the orientation cues utilized by free-living marine organisms—e.g. light, temperature, salinity, water movement, substratum, hydrostatic pressure, dissolved gases, organic substances, gravity, sound and vibration, as well as electric and magnetic fields—only a few appear to play a major role in contact and establishment of disease agents. These include light, temperature, substratum and organic substances. As has already been said, chemoreception and chemotaxis rank highest as principal methods of close-range host finding; however, rheotaxis, thigmotaxis, skototaxis and phototaxis may also be involved. The potential significance of electric and magnetic fields requires exploration.

Random contact between agent and host which largely depends on host activities prevails in viruses as well as in non-motile resting stages (cysts, spores) of bacteria, fungi and protozoans. Similarly, in eggs of metazoan endoparasites, agent–host contact heavily relies on chance encounter. Spatial proximity and host activities—such as reproduction, crowding, feeding, migration or certain other locomotory activities—increase the chances for agent–host contact. In many cases, endoparasites are taken up with the food, e.g. in the trematode *Cryptocotyle lingua* where the eggs are swallowed by the first intermediate host, the snail *Littorina littorea*.

In the course of evolution, contact between agent and host can develop into sustained symbiotic ties only through balanced long-term adjustments of both agent and host. In the initial phase, essential prerequisites include suitable spatial and temporal interrelations (space and time coordination), availability for the agent of exploitable life-supporting conditions, and basic compatibility of the evolutionary strategies employed by agent and host.

In his review 'Marine Molluscs as Hosts for Symbioses . . . ' Cheng (1967b) distinguishes between, and discusses in some detail, four different types of agent–host contacts: accidental contact, contact dependent upon the host's feeding mechanism, contact influenced by chemotaxis, and contact influenced by other natural taxes. For details consult Cheng (pp. 19–46; see also Cheng, 1970). Since mechanisms of agent orientation are directed towards host localization and recognition, the pathologist may be well advised to consult the information available on target localization and recognition in free-living organisms; these have received detailed attention in Chapters 1, 7, 8 and 9 of Volume II of 'Marine Ecology' (Kinne, 1975a, b). In spite of several interesting recent reports, the orientation of marine disease agents has remained a virgin field. Here is fertile ground for the pathologist, behaviourist, ecologist and evolutionist. Our present knowledge on agent orientation has been documented and considered in most of the chapters of this treatise.

An agent with biological properties which would, in principle, allow contact with, and establishment on or in a given host may never reach that host because of geological, ecological, ethological or physiological barriers. For aquatic organisms, examples of geological barriers are land masses and excessive water depths; ecological barriers may result from local ecosystem dynamics, especially competitive activities; ethological barriers prevail in cases of behavioural incompatibility between agent and host, physiological barriers, in cases of biochemical incompatibility. In addition to the spatial separation implied by geological barriers, agent and host may be separated by chronological dynamics, e.g. incompatibility of life-cycle timing.

Following contact, the agent must attach or penetrate and then establish itself on or in the host. The methods employed by marine agents for attachment, penetration and establishment have received detailed attention only in very few species. Hence, generalization is difficult and highly speculative. Attachment and penetration may occur at a place different from that of the first contact and—especially in endoparasites—the place of establishment may, again, differ from that of penetration. Such site differences, as well as differences in migration routes, depend on the structural and functional characteristics of the agent–host pair involved. While ecto- and intestinal parasites often reach their target sites quickly and directly, agent migration may sometimes involve long periods of time and complicated routes. Firm establishment of microbial agents often requires preceding reproduction and increased abundance. In higher invertebrates and in vertebrates, microbial agent establishment in certain organs or tissues often occurs only after primary overall infection.

The most important routes for agent penetration and establishment on the host are through respiratory surfaces, body openings such as genital pores or ears, the outer body wall, and the digestive tract. Injuries of the host, especially its external body boundary, usually facilitate agent invasion. Agent transmission (p. 38) is often facilitated by physical contact between potential host individuals (e.g. biting, sucking, copulation), as well as by contact between the host and a substrate inhabited by the agent. The conditions provided in cultivation or experimentation tend to support agent contact, attachment, entry and establishment.

Most methods employed for agent attachment are comparable to those developed by sedentary, free-living aquatic organisms. Many agents use body protrusions, haptors or appendages for anchorage. Subsequently, they release or excrete specific substances, either cementing themselves to the host or dissolving its boundary tissues in order to facilitate penetration. However, in cases where fast moving hosts are concerned, parasitic life-cycle stages, such as miracidia, must respond very quickly. Agent attachment may be triggered by mechanical, chemical or behavioural stimuli. Agent attachment or penetration often goes hand in hand with morphological changes of the agent. Very small agents such as viruses and bacteria may not need to attach themselves, but simply get 'caught' in the host's secretions.

Agent establishment comprises movement to the proper host area and procurement of support for survival, growth, maturation or reproduction. Depending on the type of symbiosis involved, support entails such aspects as the attainment of (i) transport or shelter (phoresis, p. 19); (ii) energy, matter or protection, without negatively or positively affecting the host (commensalism, p. 19); (iii) energy, matter or protection resulting in host exploitation (parasitism, p. 19); (iv) interdependence to mutual advantage (mutualism, p. 20). In all four cases, host defence (p. 41) may interfere with agent establishment. Following penetration, e.g. through body walls, intestine, or individual cells, the agent often migrates actively to the final site. Translocation within the host may be facilitated by body-fluid circulation or by the host's muscular activities.

Successful establishment requires the ability of the agent to counteract and overcome host defence. Disease-causing organisms employ a variety of strategies for overcoming their host's immunity system. Two possibly significant hypotheses are molecular mimicry and active suppression. The molecular-mimicry hypothesis assumes that an agent can avoid recognition and hence immune responses by assuming host-like surface properties: the agent's surface characteristics mimic essential properties of the host tissue. Active suppression is assumed to be based on the production of specific substances which counteract the host's immune system (e.g. inhibitors of encapsulation or of antibody activities). Both hypotheses require verification. In view of the absence of pertinent data on marine animals further discussion is beyond the scope of this introduction.

Agent Reproduction

Typically, disease agents have large reproductive capacities. Most of them reproduce in or on their host. Viruses can reproduce only inside living cells. Bacteria and fungi usually multiply within or in direct contact with their host. In contrast, initial life-cycle stages of digenetic trematodes separate from the host inhabited during development and maturation; the reproductive cycle of these forms can proceed only if different hosts become available. Many ectoparasites reproduce in close contact with their host; however, they often move readily from one host individual to another.

The developmental stages which are the direct consequence of agent reproduction either infect new body structures of the same host or depart from the host—actively or passively. Active departure is effected by agent activities such as penetration of cell or body walls; passive departure, by host activities such as egestion, exhaling or excretion, or by certain changes in host structure, including those due to post-mortem disintegration. Departure of reproductive agent stages from the host usually initiates a phase of agent distribution (see below). The departure of reproductive agent stages from the host has been termed 'escape' by Cheng (1967b, pp. 132–133). In an attempt to classify different types of escape, Cheng introduced the terms 'active escape', 'passive escape', 'involuntary escape' and 'cellular escape'. Of these terms, the latter two seem less useful; they are difficult to define in reasonably objective terms.

The methods employed by agents for leaving their host are manifold. In most cases, the stimuli involved and the responses elicited remain to be investigated in depth. Agent reproduction including agent departure is reviewed in detail in the following chapters, in immediate context with the agent or host concerned.

Agent Distribution

The distribution of disease agents is considered here under three aspects: macrodistribution, i.e. geographic distribution, target distribution, i.e. transmission of distributional agent stages to their final target, the host, and microdistribution, i.e. topographic distribution within the body of a given host.

Macrodistribution is of basic importance to the agent's long-term ecological success. It determines to a considerable degree the availability of potential hosts, the chances of host encounter and of host switching. Studies on the macrodistributions of agent and host reveal insights into the degree of areal congruence or incongruence. Geographic aspects of agent distribution are considered throughout the chapters of this treatise.

In the aquatic environment, agent macrodistribution is effected or sustained either by passive drifting along with water currents or active locomotion (in smaller agents by gliding, undulating, pseudopodial, flagellar or ciliary movements). Over considerable distances, passive drifting is usually more important than active locomotion. Means of macrodistribution also include vectors, i.e. organisms serving as carriers or transmitters of a disease agent, and intermediate hosts, as well as man's activities such as transportation (for details on translocation of aquatic organisms by man consult Kinne, in press). In general, the agent's macrodistribution is influenced by environmental factors, biotic and abiotic, in a way comparable to that observed in free-living organisms (e.g. Kinne, 1970b, 1971, 1972).

Prerequisites for successful long-distance transport by a host or vector are parallel environmental tolerances of agent and carrier. Salmon ectoparasites, for example, must tolerate changes from limnic to marine conditions and back. In contrast, endoparasites of such potent osmoregulators as salmon are protected from excessive salinity changes; they remain in the well-controlled, little changing osmotic climate of their host's body fluids or cells. Lack of parallelism in the environmental tolerances or requirements of agent and host can sometimes lead to a reduction in agent numbers of a given host, or cause complete loss of agents during or after host migration. Thus, migratory marine birds and mammals have been shown to lose some or all of their original parasites during migration and to acquire new ones in the new locality (e.g. Delyamure, 1955). Such locality dependence of the parasitic fauna often offers interesting insights into the migratory dynamics of the host concerned. At the same time, differential agent and host tolerances constitute a basis for disease therapy (p. 58).

Target distribution comprises the transmission of distributional agent stages to their general target site on or in the host. Such transmission requires spatial proximity (contact, p. 32) between agent and host and, especially in motile agents, abilities for host recognition. We may distinguish four basic types of transmission: nutritive, respiratory, contaminative and integrated.

Nutritive transmission exploits the host's food-uptake activities and usually occurs via the mouth. Respiratory transmission utilizes the host's respiratory activities, typically exploiting respiratory water currents and the fact that respiratory surfaces are easy to penetrate. Contaminative transmission involves agent-containing body excretions of the host, such as faeces, urine, sweat or saliva, or disintegrating host tissues; in this case, transmission requires contact between the contaminated material and the new potential host individual. Integrated transmission—the most complex and sophisticated transmission mechanism—involves complete integration of the agent into the host's reproductive activities; examples are transovarial, transplacental and intra-uterine target distributions. Integrated transmission assures perpetual contact and leads to 'automatic' infection of the host's offspring. Comparable automatic offspring invasion may also occur during asexual host reproduction, e.g. via budding or fission.

The **microdistribution** of an agent within its host depends on agent preferences and requirements, means of transport or locomotion, host defence and presence or absence of competing agents. Internal transport is often facilitated by circulatory body fluids, as well as host movements or muscular activities. For details consult the following chapters.

In different geographical areas, cosmopolitan hosts may (i) harbour a given parasite in different body parts; (ii) entertain different parasites in a given microhabitat; (iii) reveal changes in taxonomic composition of their parasite fauna. The exact causes of such microdistributional changes require investigation.

Major Agent Effects

Agent effects should always be considered in the light of the reciprocity of agent–host interrelations. They arise with the agent's environmental and nutritive requirements and are limited by the host's defence mechanisms. In a given agent–host pair, balance and dynamics of interspecific coexistence are subject to differential environmental influences.

Principal agent effects include: production and release of host-life-endangering substances (toxins and related chemical compounds); competition for life-supporting substances (e.g. nutrients, vitamins, minerals); and mechanical damage. Negative effects due to utilization of host material as food have, apparently, often been overestimated. In most cases studied, only heavy infestation seems to cause critical depletion of essential nutrients. In contrast, the toxic substances released have been shown to often inflict severe damage.

Specific agent effects are, for example, deviations in physiological or morphological properties of cells, tissues and organs; detrimental influences on metabolic processes, such as respiration, growth, differentiation or reproduction; reduced resistance to infection (other diseases) and environmental stress; changes in behaviour, including orientation in time and space; interference with host movements (paralysis); disturbance of hormonal balance; and initiation of allergic reactions. Attachment or establishment of a parasite often results in mechanical pressure, tissue rupture, haemorrhage, changes in blood flow, formation of additional connective tissue, inflammation, necrosis, atrophy, and tissue liquefaction. In most cases, a variety of mechanical and chemical factors are involved, both of agent and host origin.

Depending on whether the agent affects primarily physiological processes or morphological characteristics of the host, we may distinguish functional and structural effects.

Functional agent effects comprise: (i) induction of changes in metabolic processes, endocrine balance and biochemistry of the host, resulting, for example, in modifications of rates and efficiencies of metabolism, growth, moulting and in modification of enzymatic dynamics; (ii) induction of changes in reproductive activities, including rate and mode of reproduction, 'parasitic castration', sex determination and sex reversal; (iii) induction of changes in a variety of behavioural aspects, including locomotion, social dynamics and migration.

Structural agent effects include: (i) proliferative disorders (tumours); (ii) changes in morphological differentiation, dermal structures, as well as meristic and related characteristics; (iii) changes regarding the fine architecture of organs, tissues, cells and cellular components; (iv) unusual pigmentation (colouration); (v) skeletal deformities.

Qualitatively, agent-induced modifications in the host are based on mechanical forces such as irritation, disrupture of cells or tissues, or removal of body parts, and on chemical influences, e.g. due to excretion or leakage of metabolic products (faeces, metabolites, toxins, etc.). Quantitatively, agent-induced changes depend on the outcome of the conflict between agent virulence and host defence. Both in agent and host, the capacity for adaptation, the physiological state, and environmental as well as nutritional conditions are of basic importance.

Among the different types of agents, viruses, bacteria and fungi tend to cause the most critical effects in terms of ecological dynamics regarding the host. They constitute the major source of epizootic mass mortalities and may exert tremendous influence on population dynamics within the area concerned. In contrast, most of the larger, multicellular pathogens do not often seem to cause devastating losses under natural conditions. In fact, they rarely appear to be the direct cause of death. Rather, they tend to reduce the environmental tolerance of the host involved, its reproductive potential, as well as its chances for escaping predators and for successful competition with other coexisting organisms.

As has already been pointed out, viruses are intracellular agents which can severely interfere with the host's cellular functions and structures. They may be more successful than the host's body cells in competing for vital nutrients. In fact, viruses can sometimes proliferate so intensively that they disrupt the host cell or modify essential factors of cellular and intercellular organization. Tumour-producing (oncogenic) viruses induce host cells to grow and develop beyond their normal activities. Evidence is mounting that viruses can cause cancer in invertebrates, and increasing suspicion prevails that some may also produce cancer in mammals including man.

Bacteria have been shown to cause a large variety of diseases of the skin, as well as of other vital structures including gills, kidneys, liver and reproductive organs. Well documented examples are: bacterial fin rot in fishes caused by *Vibrio* spp., and systemic infection of *Homarus americanus* by *Aerococcus viridans* (formerly *Gaffkya homari*). The effects caused by pathogenic bacteria can be grossly divided into three groups: release of life-endangering substances (either exotoxins leached or excreted from intact bacterial cells or endotoxins freed after disruption or disintegration of the bacterial cell); utilization of host substances; and induction of host-immunity (p. 44).

Fungi often attack external body surfaces of host animals, but have also been shown to infect internal organs. Mycotic infections of external body surfaces have become known especially in molluscs and crustaceans (Volume II) and in fishes (Volume IV).

The effects of disease agents belonging to different taxa are reviewed in detail in the following chapters. General, important types of effects have become known as neoplasia, hyperplasia, hypertrophy, metaplasia, gigantism, parasitic castration, sex reversal, and modifications in sex determination. These are considered below. Inflammation, a combination of defence and repair, is treated on p. 42.

Neoplasia ('new growths') result from cells which have escaped the organisms' integrating and harmonizing control. The cells grow disorderly (anarchic) and assume abnormal appearance. Neoplasms comprise benign tumours which rarely cause serious illness and malignant tumours which can produce dangerous disease conditions (cancer). Cancer cells do not remain localized but tend to invade other tissues thus forming new centres of malignant neoplasmic activities. In addition to the experimentally demonstrated (lower animals) or suspected (mammals, man) role of viruses as a cause of malignant neoplasms, cancer has been induced experimentally in vertebrates by irradiation, chemicals, chronic irritation and hormonal disorders. In microscopical sections of organs, neoplasia often reveal themselves by the presence of mitotic figures.

Neoplastic skin growths, especially papillomas, are not uncommon among fishes. Pacific flatfish from North American and Japanese coastal waters, for example, regularly manifest skin tumours (Peters and co-authors, 1978). These often develop from primary inflammatory nodules of several-month-old individuals. A bibliography on neoplasia in fishes has been presented by Mawdesley-Thomas (1969).

Hyperplasia is due to controlled, increased proliferation of normal cells. It usually results from excessive stimulation, e.g. due to chronic irritation or to hormonal factors, and leads to abnormal tissue and organ enlargement. Hyperplasia associated with parasitism often follows tissue inflammation (p. 42). Some authors have interpreted hyperplasia as a supranormal level of tissue repair. Examples of hyperplasia are (i) the callus formations often observed on the snouts of captive fishes which tend to rub against aquaria glass; (ii) the corn on a toe chronically irritated by the pressure of an ill-fitting shoe.

Hypertrophy—excessive increase in size and/or number of cells leading to supranormal development of an organ or tissue—is often caused by intracellular microbial or protozoal agents.

Metaplasia involves abnormal changes from one cell or tissue type into another without the normal intervention of embryonic tissue. An example is the formation of epithelial cells and fibroblasts in the host's lung tissue in response to fluke *(Paragonimus westermani)* invasion. The changed lung cells encapsulate the parasite.

Gigantism, i.e. enhanced growth leading to the attainment of an unusually large size of individuals or their parts, has been attributed to parasitic agents, such as trematodes (e.g. in limnic as well as marine gastropods and in sheep), nematodes (in lambs), plerocercoid larvae of the tapeworm *Spirometra mansonoides* (e.g. mice, hamsters, deer), and flagellates *Trypanosoma lewisi* (e.g. in rats). Most authors who have investigated gigantism assume some agent-produced substance to be involved—either directly or indirectly—in such unusual host growth. However, the exact causes of gigantism have remained unknown.

A common denominator of all these proliferative cellular responses to agent activities must be seen in a reduction of the inhibitory forces which, under normal circumstances, counteract the cell's tendency towards unchecked growth.

The term **'parasitic castration'** denotes the failure of a host to reproduce, due to partial or complete destruction of its gonads caused by parasitic activities. Parasitic castration has been reported from several marine invertebrates. Examples are the trematode agent *Bucephalus cuculus* which may castrate the oyster *Crassostrea virginica* and the parasitic barnacle *Sacculina carcini* which may castrate the crab *Carcinus maenas*. For details consult the chapters devoted to the diseases of molluscs and crustaceans.

Sex reversal, the change from one sex to the other in a host due to an agent—also known as feminization or masculinization—has been reported from marine molluscs and crustaceans. For examples consult the appropriate chapters.

Sex determination in host individuals may be modified by parasites. An example is the microsporidan *Octosporea effeminans* which influences the future sex in the offspring of its host, the amphipod *Gammarus duebeni* (p. 24; see also Chapter *Crustacea*).

Disease agents may live in one host without causing any demonstrable effect, but develop severe or even fatal activities in another one—either of the same or of another species. Such cases are indicative of differential capacities of the agent for causing a disease condition and/or of the host for counteraction or resistance. Some investigators have reported cases in which the intensity of the disease caused by a given agent was more pronounced in a species related to the normal host than in the typical host itself.

Commercial consequences of disease-agent effects include losses in fisheries and mariculture, and problems in public health. These points are exemplified and receive detailed attention in the various chapters of this treatise devoted to the different groups of marine animals. In commercially important animals, such as a variety of molluscs, crustaceans and fishes, diseases may significantly reduce appearance, taste, and odour. Of the disease-causing agents which often diminish the quality of sea food, sporozoans, trematodes, nematodes and copepods play a dominant role. Similarly, structural abnormalities such as tumours may significantly affect marketability. However, in general, such structural abnormalities are restricted to a limited number of host individuals.

HOST DEFENCE

Host defence refers to the potential of the host for counteracting agent virulence (p. 32); it aims at the inactivation, removal or destruction of the disease-causing forces. The evolution of efficient defence mechanisms is a basic prerequisite for the development of multicellular organisms. Where large populations of different cell types cooperate in the formation of an individual, integration, communication, recognition of 'self' and 'non-self' and concerted counteraction of potentially detrimental 'non-self' material, including disease agents, become a must.

Although the basic elements and strategies involved are comparable, the defence mechanisms investigated thus far differ in major taxonomic groupings. Thus, protozoans, invertebrates and vertebrates exhibit essential differences. Apparently, these differences are commensurate with and adjusted to differences in life span, ecological niche and organismic complexity. The long-lived, most complex forms of life—birds and mammals—have evolved defence mechanisms of maximum efficiency, specificity and complexity.

The technical terms most frequently used for describing aspects of host defence are 'immunity', 'resistance' and 'susceptibility'. While similar in connotation, these terms emphasize somewhat different perspectives: Immunity (p. 44) refers to the host's innate and/or acquired capacity for counteracting disease agents both by whole-cell (p. 47) and cell-product mechanisms (p. 50). Resistance comprises the general potential of the host to tolerate or to counteract a disease agent. Susceptibility refers to the degree of host vulnerability by a disease agent. Similar to susceptibility is the concept of 'host compatibility'. Whether a given host is compatible or incompatible with a certain agent depends, of course, on both host and agent.

The strategies and mechanisms involved in host defence—as well as in agent virulence (p. 32) and agent–host interactions (p. 21)—are based on general ecological principles which regulate the coexistence of organisms. Obviously, the pathologist can learn much from the ecologist and *vice versa*. Innate and acquired aspects of host defence, for example, can well be interpreted as special cases of genetic and non-genetic adaptation to abiotic and biotic factors.

Part of, or closely related to, host defence are repair processes such as those involved in inflammation and wound healing. In addition to these processes we consider in the following pages behavioural host defence, mechanico-chemical host defence and immunity mechanisms.

Inflammation of tissues involves both defence and repair. It is caused by local injury and/or infection and characterized by local tissue resolution, reorganization, pus formation (suppuration), tissue repair and replacement, as well as by swelling, increased sensitivity to stress and temporarily reduced efficiency of normal functions. An inflammation may be acute (highly active, intensive, rapid, short-lived) or chronic (reduced activity and intensity, often accompanied by the formation of new connective tissue, long-lived). In the few invertebrates thus far studied and in vertebrates, inflammation may have different causes, but it usually involves similar responses in the inflamed area, for example, increased permeability of blood vessels, release of blood or other circulatory fluids into the surrounding tissues, invasion of leucocytes, locally increased rates of cell division and cellular metabolism. Rapidly increasing in number, specialized cells enter the inflamed tissue and break down, inactivate, digest or remove detrimental material such as cell or tissue debris, foreign substances and invading organisms. Typically, the inflamed body part receives an increased flow of circulatory fluids containing substances counteracting the disease agents, as well as nutrients for cell repair and growth.

Wound healing in marine animals appears to involve essentially similar processes as have been described from their terrestrial counterparts. Clotting, reduction of blood flow, and wound healing have been investigated in considerable detail in *Limulus polyphemus* (Bang, 1956; Shirodkar and co-authors, 1960; Levin and Bang, 1964, 1968; see also Bang, 1970), as well as in *Sacculina carcini* (Barker and Bang, 1966) and

Crassostrea virginica (Bang, 1961; see also Levin, 1967). Clot formation (coagulation, thrombosis) involves cells or cellular products, or both. Clots of cells have been reported, for example, by Bang (1961) in *C. virginica* responding to injury due to injection. The clots formed adhered to blood-vessel walls and resolved rather slowly. Clotting tends to restrict local agent mobility, to isolate disease agents or to render them more susceptible to phagocytosis (p. 47). Wound areas are invaded by large numbers of aggregating amoebocytes that reduce or stop leakage of circulatory fluids and release substances which induce extracellular clotting. Experiments with plasma of *L. polyphemus* witness that cellular products from amoebocytes are responsible for the clotting process: cell-free plasma failed to effect coagulation.

Behavioural Host Defence

The subdivision into behavioural, mechanico-chemical and immunity mechanisms of host defence is not entirely satisfactory. The phenomena and mechanisms involved in host defence require more thorough analysis and more precise definition. We have adopted the subheadings mentioned for organizational reasons.

As has already been pointed out, behaviour is of considerable importance both for agent and host and for the development of long-term, balanced agent–host interactions. Behavioural host defence includes (i) avoidance of, or contact reduction with, the agent; (ii) removal or counteraction of attached agents by scratching, picking, shaking or locomotion of the host (some birds employ rubbing with ants, as well as sand or sunbaths); (iii) agent removal by conspecifics, e.g. in brood-carrying females attending to their eggs or young; and (iv) 'cleaning' by heterospecifics.

Brood care by conspecifics and cleaning by heterospecifics are common phenomena in the marine environment and have received attention from numerous investigators. Only heterospecific cleaning requires brief treatment in the present context, because it involves symbiotic elements. In a cleaning symbiosis, one partner 'cleans' the other, feeding on its ectoparasites, attached micro-organisms, loose tissues, or food remains adhering to its body surfaces such as mouth parts, gills, fins or appendages. Well-known examples of cleaners are the shrimp *Hippolysmata californica*, *H. grabhami*, *Periclimenes yucatanicus*, *P. pedersoni*, *Stenopus hispidus* and *S. scutellatus* and numerous species of fishes.

The animals cleaned include especially crustaceans and fishes. Apparently, at least some of these depend on their cleaners. Removal of the cleaners has been shown to result in an increased number of diseased fish and in a reduction of fish abundance (e.g. Feder, 1966; see also Limbaugh, 1961). Diving marine biologists have reported that some fishes actively search for their cleaners and even line up at 'cleaning stations' waiting for their turn to be cleaned. Individuals to be cleaned often allow the cleaner to enter their mouth, to pick their tongue, teeth or gills; they sometimes even endure minor incisions by the cleaner during its search for subcutaneous parasites. The mutual benefits obtained by both partners seem obvious: one obtains food, the other gets rid of unwanted associates or materials.

Mechanico-chemical Host Defence

Mechanical methods of host defence include, for example, the removal of agents by ciliary action, by pedicellaria activities in echinoderms or by picking in birds. A combination of mechanical and chemical mechanisms is usually involved in defence barriers such as skin, haemocoel, gut, membranes and mucous secretions.

Defence barriers consist of cells or cellular products which counteract agent invasion and establishment. In addition to specific structural arrangements, specialized cells often release antimicrobial or antiparasitic substances. The presence of antibacterial substances has been documented, for example, in mucus, saliva, genital canals and urine of a variety of marine animals; tears of birds and mammals contain the antibacterial enzyme lysozyme; sweat and other skin secretions often contain fatty and lactic acids which may counteract detrimental microbial activities (p. 50ff).

Immunity Mechanisms

The term 'immunity' refers to the capacity of a living organism for counteracting disease-causing entities such as agents or foreign substances. Immunity mechanisms are based on a variety of cellular activities which are harmonized with body-own functions and structures, but interfere with—suppress, neutralize, inactivate or eliminate—potentially detrimental foreign materials, living and non-living. Immunity is conferred upon a host by specialized cells, or cell parts, counteractive to potential disease agents and their metabolic products.

Immunity deficiencies are due either to genetic disorders or to circumstances encountered during the life of the individual concerned. Our present knowledge of immunity deficiencies is based almost exclusively on investigations conducted on a few terrestrial mammals, especially 'laboratory animals'. Under natural conditions, immunity deficiencies are likely to have a very negative selection value and to effectively eliminate the individuals concerned from successful reproduction.

General Considerations

There are two principal types of immunity: genetic immunity and non-genetic (acquired) immunity. The former depends on the genetic constitution of the host concerned, the latter on the host's individual history. We are concerned here primarily with non-genetic immunity. Prerequisites for maximizing host immunity are adequate environmental and nutritional conditions (see p. 24 and p. 25).

Non-genetic, acquired immunity is attained and reinforced due to direct contact with a specific disease-causing entity. The mechanisms involved in non-genetic immunity appear to be comparable to those operative in non-genetic adaptation to environmental factors such as temperature or salinity (Kinne, 1970a, p. 435; see also Kinne, 1963, 1964a, b). In both cases, specific adjustments are induced during the life of the individual concerned. Potentially, these affect all levels of organization (subcellular, cellular, organ, organismic) and result in a relative increase in the individual's capacity to survive, reproduce or compete. The adjustments require time to develop, as well as reinforcement for continued effectiveness; they persist beyond the circumstances which induced them.

Unless reinforced, a given non-genetic immunity is usually lost again—at least to an extent where effective protection of the host is no longer possible—during periods of time which are equivalent to only a fraction of the host's total life expectancy. However, as in non-genetic adaptation to environmental factors (Kinne, 1962), non-genetic immunity may also last—usually with somewhat decreasing effectiveness—throughout the host's life, e.g. in the case of some virus diseases of mammals, including man. Among physiologists and ecologists, such responses have become known as irreversible non-genetic adaptations.

Immunity responses are not always beneficial to the host individual. Apparently, the immune system cannot differentiate between harmful and non-harmful antigens (p.53). Responses to non-harmful antigens, as well as excessive responses to both harmful and non-harmful antigens, caused by prior (repeated) exposure to specific antigens, may lead to exaggerated responses, i.e. to allergy, often also referred to as hypersensitivity. While allergic responses are based on the principles of antigen–antibody interactions referred to on p.54, they often have negative consequences for the host individual involved.

The host body does not normally exhibit immune responses to body-own substances—a phenomenon known as self-tolerance or auto-tolerance. As does immunity, self-tolerance requires reinforcement. In the absence of reinforcement, or where self-tolerance breaks down for other reasons, immune responses may be directed against body-own cells. This can lead to 'self-allergy' or 'auto-allergy'—a phenomenon which usually produces detrimental consequences; in mammals it has been shown to damage essential body structures such as red blood cells (erythrocyte destruction, anaemia), cells of the thyroid gland, cells of the gastric mucosa, or nucleic acids.

Immunosuppression, i.e. the suppression of immune responses in the host body, becomes an important therapeutic measure where diseases due to auto-allergy prevail or where organ or tissue transplants (e.g. kidney graft in man) are necessary. The major problem of immunosuppression rests with the fact that it is still difficult or impossible to suppress a certain immune response selectively. Immunosuppression usually results in a general reduction of the host's protective immunity against potential disease agents, including viruses, bacteria, fungi, etc. According to Humphrey (1976), potential methods of selective immunosuppression include (i) long-term induction of a specific immunity tolerance; (ii) provision of excess amounts of specific antibodies before the (known) antigens can take effect (example: immunization of women against rhesus antigen is suppressed by injection of human antirhesus antibodies at the time the child is born); (iii) specific desensitization, involving careful introduction of harmless antibody which combines with the antigen in question thus preventing it from interacting with other forms of antibody. In the case of tissue transplants, immune responses are suppressed by killing lymphocytes (ionizing radiation, drugs) or by preventing the multiplication of stimulated lymphocytes (drugs interfering with nucleic-acid synthesis). However, it remains problematic to restrict such effects to lymphocytes without critically damaging other tissues.

The boundary between elements recognized as 'self' and those suppressed as 'non-self' is not absolutely fixed. Where a close mutualistic relation develops, such as between a coral and its zooxanthellae, original 'non-self' is finally accepted as 'self'. A detailed analysis of the ajustments (adaptations) involved may open up fascinating new perspectives both in medicine and ecology.

The degree of host immunity—as well as the degree of agent virulence—can be determined experimentally by infecting groups of healthy hosts with different numbers (doses) of agents under defined conditions and over defined periods of time. The dose is then determined which causes a certain response in 50% of the host individuals treated (50%-effective dose or ED_{50}). The ED_{50} is directly proportional to the degree of host immunity and inversely proportional to agent virulence.

The rate of clearance of injected immunogen from circulatory fluids has been used as criterion for assessing the efficiency of immunity responses. While circulating antibody plays a significant role in immunogen clearance, other—as yet unknown—factors appear to cooperate. In marine invertebrates, details on both whole-cell and cell-product mechanisms (see below) of immunogen clearance await exploration.

An important, sensitive criterion for assessing the immunological capacity of a given organism is the rejection or acceptance of grafts (tissue transplants) especially of allografts. In many cases, allografts—particularly orthotopic allografts—are initially accepted and heal into place like autografts. However, after several days or weeks the transplanted tissue becomes the target of immunity mechanisms and is rejected. High specificity in graft rejection appears to be largely restricted to vertebrates, but most invertebrates studied thus far are also able to distinguish between 'self' and 'non-self' tissues. The degree of graft rejection or acceptance appears to be subject to conditioning and, possibly, is a function of the tissue type involved, as well as of the physiological condition, age and genetic constitution of both donor and recipient. However, in marine invertebrates, the present status of pertinent knowledge is insufficient for drawing definite conclusions.

Ecological experience shows that natural populations often reveal differences in the degree of immunity displayed and that, within a given population, usually at least a few individuals exhibit a significantly reduced susceptibility towards an infectious agent. Such differential susceptibility is of considerable importance. It represents an expression of ecological variability and favours long-term population or species survival; at the same time it constitutes a basis for improvements in the host's evolutionary immunity strategies. The physiological causes of differences in agent susceptibility remain to be investigated.

The mechanisms involved in host immunity are often reviewed under two headings: cellular and humoural factors. However, such differentiation is problematic. Cheng (1970, p. 148), for example, defines cellular factors as 'those which involve cells, structural products of cells, or both' and humoural factors as those occurring 'in the form of the synthesis of antibodies and antibody-like molecules which, as a rule, are evenly distributed throughout the body'. Such definition is unsatisfactory because (i) all immunity mechanisms have a cellular basis, i.e. are the result of the activities of cells; (ii) structural products of cells include antibodies, i.e. substances with definable structures; (iii) none of the substances involved is evenly distributed throughout the body.

It seems somewhat more appropriate to distinguish between whole-cell mechanisms (p. 47), i.e. mechanisms involving whole cells such as phagocytes, and cell-product mechanisms (p. 50), i.e. mechanisms involving cellular products: secretions or cell fragments which are released into body fluids (humoural mechanisms*). Both whole-cell

---

*The original latin word 'humour' (or humor) means moisture or fluid. In modern medicine, humour refers to products of body cells, including hormones, released into circulating body fluids such as blood and lymph or bile. Ancient medicine distinguished 4 cardinal humours: blood, phlegm, choler (yellow bile) and melancholy (black bile). Mixtures of these humours were assumed to determine the temperaments of individuals—the predominance of one humour resulting in a sanguine, phlegmatic, choleric or melancholic temperament.

and cell-product mechanisms tend to cooperate in numerous ways; in some cases, exact distinction may be difficult or impossible. Nevertheless, such differentiation is useful for didactical reasons. While lower marine animals depend exclusively or predominantly on whole-cell mechanisms, higher vertebrates have, in addition, evolved sophisticated cell-product mechanisms; they can counteract invading agents and other foreign materials by cooperative action of both whole-cell and cell-product activities.

Whole-cell Mechanisms

Phylogenetically, whole-cell mechanisms constitute primary (original, primitive) methods of host defence. Presumably, they represent the evolutionary substrate from which the secondary, often very sophisticated cell-product mechanisms (p. 50) have evolved. Whole-cell mechanisms comprise such processes as phagocytosis, leucocytosis and encapsulation of foreign bodies. In marine animals, these processes have received attention in the reviews by Sindermann (1970), Cheng (1973), Anderson (1975), Bang (1975) and Michelson (1975).

Phagocytosis is an elementary, evolutionary old process. In unicellular animals it was, and still is, used as a means of food uptake. In multicellular animals, it often serves the additional role of excretion (uptake of waste products and transport to the outer integument, a nephridium or the intestine). A modification of these functions, 'defence phagocytosis' involves, in essence, five aspects: foreign-particle recognition, adherence, uptake (ingestion), destruction (digestion) and disposal (emigration). The specialized cells involved are collectively referred to as phagocytes or phagocytic cells.

All multicellular animals studied thus far exhibit capabilities of defence phagocytosis. This whole-cell mechanism aims at isolation and elimination of potential disease agents—e.g. bacteria, spores of fungi or protozoans, and small developmental stages of multicellular parasites. While very effective in most cases, defence phagocytosis has occasionally failed to counteract disease agents. Some agents have survived phagocytosis, and a few even reproduced inside phagocytes.

In the course of evolution, the specificity of foreign-particle recognition tends to increase. Thus, in lower invertebrates, recognition frequently reveals a rather low degree of specificity and can also occur in the absence of humoural factors. In more complex animals, recognition specificity increases and defence phagocytosis may become dependent on humoural factors (antibody and complement activities). The most significant cues for foreign-particle recognition are associated with the particle's surface characteristics.

Since the lower marine invertebrates do not possess cell-product mechanisms (p. 50), which have been evolved and increasingly sophisticated by fishes, reptiles, birds and mammals, defence phagocytosis figures very high in their ability to counteract biotic diseases.

Following the pioneer work of Metchnikoff (1884, 1893, 1905) on the function of phagocytes (amoebocytes, haemocytes) in invertebrates, the significance of phagocytosis as essential defence mechanism of invertebrates has been documented by numerous investigators, for example, by Takatsuki (1934), Stauber (1950, 1961), Tripp (1958a, b, c, 1960, 1961, 1963, 1970), Bang and Bang (1962), Bang and Lemma (1962), Feng (1962, 1967), Cheng and Rifkin (1970), Bang (1973), Hildemann and Reddy (1973) and Michelson (1975). For syntheses including information on pertinent internal defence mechanisms of marine animals consult Symposium on 'Defence Reactions in Invertebrates' (1967), Sindermann (1970), Cheng (1973) and Maramorosch and Shope (1975). Details of the mechanisms involved in phagocytosis have been explored with appreciable success under *in vitro* conditions.

The literature documenting instances of phagocytosis in protozoans, sponges, annelids, molluscs, crustaceans, echinoderms and ascidians has been reviewed by Bang (1975; see also Bang, 1961, 1967, 1970, and Anderson, 1975). Earlier detailed reports include those by Mackin (1951) who studied phagocytosis of the fungus *Labyrinthomyxa marina* (formerly *Dermocystidium marinum*) and Farley (1968) who investigated phagocytosis of the flagellate *Hexamita nelsoni* by phagocytes of the oyster *Crassostrea virginica*. According to Cheng and co-authors (1974), granulocytes of *C. virginica* and *Mercenaria mercenaria* are extremely efficient in recognizing 'self' and 'non-self' and readily phagocytize small, foreign materials. Similar results have been obtained in the gastropod *Lehmania poirieri* (Arcadi, 1968), *Littorina scabra* (Cheng and co-authors, 1969) and *Aplysia californica* (Pauley and Krassner, 1972). Gastropod amoebocytes attack allografts less readily and less intensively than xenografts (Cheng and Galloway, 1970).

Phagocytes are not only involved in phagocytosis, but play many additional roles. They are, for example, important in inflammation processes (p.42), in clotting (p. 43)—either by participating in cellular clots, or by releasing substances which act with plasma components thus producing clots of extracellular material—and in encapsulation (p.49). In molluscs they are further assumed, or have been shown, to participate in such processes as digestion, excretion, wound healing, shell repair, calcium and other ion transport, glycogen storage and transport, and initiation of encapsulation (e.g. Michelson, 1975).

The factors which control phagocytosis in marine invertebrates have largely remained unknown. In gastropod amoebocytes, particle size and haemolymph opsonins appear to play a significant role (e.g. Tripp, 1961). Apparently, organismic particles exceeding 15 μm cannot be phagocytized; they tend to induce cell aggregation and encapsulation. The mechanisms of intracellular degradation of organic particles, as well as the overall functional plasticity of phagocytes, invite further investigation. It also remains to be shown whether different types of phagocytes develop separately (multiserial) from germinal tissues or whether they have one common root (are monoserial). In any case, future studies on defence phagocytosis should pay more attention to natural pathogenic particles. While studies on 'non-natural' items such as particles of charcoal, polystyrene and thorium have revealed interesting insights, we need to know more about phagocytosis under ecologically valid conditions.

In several terrestrial animals (e.g. insects, birds, mammals), as well as in some amphibians and fishes, giant cells are formed where normal-sized phagocytes cannot deal with a large foreign particle (e.g. Pflugfelder, 1977). Origin, differentiation and exact nature of the giant cells require investigation.

Leucocytosis comprises a significant increase in number (and activity) of leucocytes. Commonly it occurs in response to disease-agent invasion as well as to heavy stress. While Farley (1968) and Cheng and co-authors (1969) have demonstrated leucocytosis to occur in various bivalves, Michelson (1975) assumes that it is a rare phenomenon in gastropods. According to Feng (1965), heart rate, leucocyte circulation and the number of circulatory haemocytes tend to increase with ambient temperature. For further details on leucocytosis in molluscs and fishes consult Sindermann (1970). Whether molluscs (or other invertebrates) can mobilize specifically activated amoebocytes is still a matter for guessing (Tripp, 1975). The following chapters contain information on the occurrence of leucocytosis in a variety of marine animals.

Where the foreign particle is too large to be engulfed by a single cell, **encapsulation** comprises an important means of isolation from the host tissues. Apparently, host cells are induced via mechanical and/or chemical stimuli to secrete substances suitable for coating and to envelop the agent by controlled cellular proliferation.

Among aquatic invertebrates, encapsulation has been studied predominantly in molluscs (Pan, 1958, 1963, 1965; Wright, 1966; Cheng and Rifkin, 1970; Meuleman, 1972; see also Michelson, 1975). An important review on encapsulation in insects, which may stimulate comparable research in marine invertebrates, has been presented by Nappi (1975). Larvae of the beetle genus *Diabrotica*, for example, respond to parasitization by the nematode *Filipjevivermis leipsandra* by forming melanotic capsules (Poinar and co-authors, 1968, quoted by Nappi, 1975): apparently due to parasite-induced autolysis, the first haemocytes contacting the nematode release their cytoplasm over the parasite's cuticle. Released cytoplasm then enters the cuticular folds and is transformed into melanin which gradually surrounds the nematode. Subsequent cell contacts lead to various degrees of necrosis and the formation of numerous membrane-bound electron-opaque inclusions (presumably intracellular stages of melanin production). After 72 h, the capsules formed reveal 4 regions: an inner noncellular melanin layer; a region of entirely necrotic haemocytes; a region consisting of extremely flattened haemocytes; and an outer layer of loosely attached cells resembling free haemocytes. The role of melanin in agent–host relationships has been considered by Lipke (1975).

In many cases, living particles tend to induce encapsulation less often and less promptly than do non-living particles. Possibly, in these cases, agent activities interfere with encapsulation: non-active or degenerating agents are often more readily encapsulated than active stages. Presumably, encapsulation is initiated by migratory amoebocytes and continued by fibroblast-like cells. Both cell types seem to originate from a common mesenchymal precursor (Sminia, 1972). Capsule formation is finally completed by myofibres, collagenous fibres and related tissue elements (Cheng and Rifkin, 1970).

Encapsulation includes nacreous depositions and pearl formation. The latter is well known from bivalves and can be induced by a variety of agents, for example, by larval helminths. According to Brooks (1969) and Cheng and Rifkin (1970), numerous particles are capable of inducing encapsulation in gastropods. The American oyster *Crassostrea virginica* responds to alimentary-tract penetration of larval tapeworms *Tylocephalum* sp. by (i) producing a concentrically arranged layer of fibres around the parasite, and (ii) local leucocyte aggregation (Cheng, 1970, p. 152). Finally, the parasite becomes immobilized by a capsule composed of cells and fibres. This encapsulation may lead to the death and eventual resorption of the parasite. Farley (1968) reports recovery of *C. virginica* from infections with the haplosporidan *Minchinia nelsoni* due to agent encapsulation, i.e. walling off in shell pustules of the previously phagocytized pathogens.

While much remains to be done before the process of encapsulation is thoroughly understood, some basic principles can now be formulated: (i) At least the initial stages of capsule formation comprise elements similar to, or based on, phagocytosis; to a large extent, cellular elements seem to be involved which are identical or comparable to those responsible for phagocytosis. Since the foreign particle concerned is too large to be phagocytized, the cells flatten and extend their surface area, thereby increasing their ability to adhere to and to cover the particle's surface. (ii) Encapsulation requires a high degree of intercellular recognition, communication and cooperation. (iii) The cellular processes and the resulting capsule structure may vary considerably, depending on the host tissue and the foreign particle (agent) concerned. Where living agents are involved, functional and structural aspects of encapsulation may be affected not only by the host but also by the agent. (iv) The activities of both host and agent usually induce modifications in normal physiological and morphological processes of the organisms concerned.

Cell-product (Humoural) Mechanisms

Cell-product mechanisms involve the release of cellular products which counteract potential disease agents and other foreign entities. Three general groups of such mechanisms may be distinguished: (i) Mechanisms involving principles which limit virus proliferation, e.g. interferon activities. In marine animals, virological research has remained a virgin field; however, in arthropods, antiviral mechanisms have received appreciable attention (see, for example, Salt, 1970; Maramorosch and Shope, 1975; Murphy and co-authors, 1975; Paschke and Summers, 1975). (ii) Mechanisms involving rather unspecific bactericidal substances which in their effects tend to mimic antibodies. (iii) Mechanisms involving specific substances, i.e. antibodies, usually produced in response to specific properties of agents or toxins.

Antibodies (p.53) are proteins which apparently can be synthesized only by vertebrates. All invertebrates investigated thus far lack mammalian-type antibodies. However, many of them possess a variety of humoural factors which often exert comparable if less specific and less powerful effects. Since invertebrates can differentiate between 'self' and 'non-self' they must have other, possibly more general, means of identifying foreign substances. Recently, Tripp (1975) has suggested the possibility that an 'all purpose' protein coats all foreign substances and thus 'tags' them for identification and further attention by amoebocytes.

In invertebrates, numerous reports on serum requirements for phagocytosis indicate the presence of a humoural recognition factor or opsonin (Anderson, 1975). Opsonizing activities are frequently associated with agglutinins, particularly haemagglutinins. Haemagglutinins (lectins) have been found in many invertebrates, including marine ones (see also below; for details consult Anderson's review).

Acquired cell-product defence mechanisms of marine invertebrates are not well investigated and much of the restricted information at hand requires reaffirmation. Details are provided in the chapters devoted to the different host taxa treated. According to Sindermann (1970, p. 270), there is some evidence for partially non-specific responses to agent contact and establishment. For example, invading trematodes render host snails more resistant to further invasion via immobilization of miracidia, and sipunculid worms produce lysis against ciliate disease agents. Antimicrobial and antitumoural substances have been found in several marine invertebrates (e.g. Skarnes and Watson, 1957; Li and co-authors, 1962, 1965; Schmeer, 1964, 1966; Schmeer and Berry, 1965; Burkholder, 1973; Maramorosch and Shope, 1975). Even sponges produce substances with antimicrobial activity (Nigrelli and co-authors, 1959; Burkholder and Ruetzler, 1969; Bergquist and Bedford, 1978). According to Bergquist and Bedford, who tested 30 species of temperate-zone sponges representative of all orders of the Demospongiae, sponge extracts inhibit the growth of marine bacteria more frequently than that of non-marine bacteria. While 46·5% of the extracts inhibit growth of Gram-negative bacteria, only 6·5% exerted comparable effects on Gram-positive bacteria. Berquist and Bedford have suggested that the antibacterial agents may play a role in enhancing the efficiency with which sponges retain their bacterial food.

In the marine invertebrates studied, cell-product mechanisms of host defence involve such substances as agglutinins, lysins and various antimicrobial factors (e.g. Bang, 1962, 1966; Sindermann, 1970; Cheng, 1973; Tripp, 1974a, b, 1975). These substances occur in body fluids, for example, of molluscs such as clams and oysters (Johnson, 1964; Tripp, 1966, 1971, 1975; Feng, 1967; Li and Fleming, 1967; Feng and Canzonier, 1970; Pauley and co-authors, 1971), of the horseshoe crab *Limulus polyphemus* (Cohen and co-authors, 1965), crustaceans (Tyler and Metz, 1945; Tyler and Scheer, 1945; Cornick and Stewart, 1966, 1968a, b; Stewart and co-authors, 1966a, 1967; Stewart and Dingle, 1968) and echinoderms (e.g. Tyler, 1946). Additional examples can be found in the following chapters. The exact role of these substances for counteracting infections cannot yet be defined precisely in most cases.

Regarding the substances involved in molluscan cell-product defence mechanisms, Tripp (1975) distinguishes antitumour and antimicrobial substances, lysozyme, and haemagglutinins. While mercenene, a substance extracted from tissues of *Mercenaria mercenaria* may exert inhibitory effects on tumourous growth, both the chemical identity and the exact functions of molluscan antitumour and antimicrobial substances remain to be investigated. Lysozyme, a mucolytic enzyme widely distributed among different kinds of organisms, comprises a class of basic, low-molecular-weight proteins capable of acting as N-acetylmuramidase and lysing certain bacteria (Chipman and Sharon, 1969). Its precise function remains to be investigated. Early documentations of lysozyme in marine invertebrates are those by Janoff and Hawrylko (1964) who studied *M. mercenaria* and *Asterias forbesi*, and by Eble and Tripp (1968) who investigated *Crassostrea virginica*. In the flatfish *Pleuronectes platessa*, Fletcher and White (1973) report lysozyme to occur in leucocytes as well as in epidermal cells.

Arimoto and Tripp (1977) found the haemolymph of *Mercenaria mercenaria* to agglutinate 4 of 30 types of bacteria tested as well as cells of a marine alga. The agglutinin involved is a (conjugated) protein with a molecular weight of ca 21,000; the presence of haemolymph was shown to enhance phagocytosis of a marine bacterium. According to Tripp (1975), the studies conducted on humoural factors in molluscs indicate that normal haemolymph may contain proteins with immunological activity, but that specific proteins for neutralizing immunogens are not synthesized. The best known invertebrate haemagglutinin is that of the horseshoe crab *Limulus polyphemus* (Cohen and co-authors, 1965; Fernandez-Moran and co-authors, 1968; Marchalonis and Edelman, 1968; Finstad and co-authors, 1972)—a uniquely configured protein (molecular weight 400,000) composed of 6 noncovalently linked subunits, arranged in a ring and with each unit consisting of 3 protein molecules (molecular weight 22,500).

In contrast to the situation prevailing in invertebrate research, there is appreciable evidence for antigen–antibody interactions in fishes and higher marine vertebrates. The chemical defence mechanisms thus far reported in these animals are quite comparable or similar to those documented in terrestrial vertebrates including mammals. For details regarding marine vertebrates consult Sindermann (1970), Cheng (1973) and the appropriate chapters of this treatise. Future studies on chemical host-defence mechanisms of marine animals, including the lower invertebrates, are likely to open up important new vistas in the field of animal diseases. Studies on forms such as sponges, cnidarians and platyhelminths may illuminate essential avenues in the evolution of agent–host relations and thus avail a new dimension for comprehending principles, strategies and ecological significance of immunity mechanisms in higher animals.

In the latter, especially the mammals, substances which are recognized as being foreign—the antigens (p. 53)—induce specialized host cells (lymphocytes) to form and release specific protein molecules—the antibodies (p. 53). Antigens and antibodies interact (p. 54), thereby neutralizing or inactivating the detrimental potential of the antigen. Most of what we know today about antigen–antibody mechanisms has been investigated in a few terrestrial mammals and man. Extrapolation of this knowledge to marine animals is not permissible without further qualification. Our review on antigen–antibody interrelations will therefore be brief and restricted to basic principles.

The cells involved in the mammal's immunity response—the lymphocytes—are derivatives of leucocytes (white blood cells). Lymphocytes are externally rather undifferentiated and featureless. In addition to the nucleus, they contain a minimum of essential cell components. The lymphocytes derive from stem cells continuously produced in the bone marrow from where they pass with the bloodstream to lymphoid tissues (e.g. thymus, spleen, lymph nodes, appendix, tonsils, Peyer's patches).

Depending on the lymphoid tissue inhabited, the lymphocytes acquire different properties. Thus, thymus-derived lymphocytes, termed T-lymphocytes, may be induced by an antigen to (i) divide into numerous large, active cells capable of reacting with the antigen; (ii) release substances which stimulate neighbouring macrophages to phagocytize and release enzymes more effectively; (iii) become inactivated. T-lymphocytes are responsible for some aspects of hypersensitivity and immunological rejection of transplanted tissues; however, they have not yet been shown to release antibodies.

Thymus-independent B-lymphocytes, i.e. those settling in lymphoid tissues without first passing through the thymus are antibody-producing cells; they release the immunoglobulins present in blood and other body fluids. There is evidence that most lymphocytes produce a specific immunoglobulin and that only the total lymphocyte population of a given host is capable of reacting with different specific antigens. Upon contact between a certain antigen and a B-lymphocyte, the latter may be induced to transform into a plasma cell which can produce immunoglobulin at very high rates (>1000 molecules sec^{-1}).

Many of the principal features of higher vertebrate immunology related to antigens and antibodies are now textbook knowledge. We summarize here only a few general aspects immediately pertinent to our topic. The summary comprises brief sections on 'Antigens', 'Antibodies' and 'Interactions between Antigens and Antibodies'; it is based on Samter and Alexander (1965), Boyd (1967), Cold Spring Harbour (1967), Burnet (1969), Humphrey and White (1970) and Humphrey (1976).

Antigens

Antigens are substances recognized as foreign by elements of the host body. They are capable of inducing antibody formation (see below) as well as interaction of antigens and antibodies (p. 54). The quality of being foreign is based on the structure of individual molecules and/or molecule composition, recognized as being different from host-body components by the responding lymphocytes. The capability of inducing antibody formation largely depends on (i) components located on antigen surfaces—the contact areas between antigen and lymphocyte—and (ii) antigen size.

Most proteins and certain carbohydrates qualify as important antigens. Hence, protein antigens such as bacterial toxins—purified and partially inactivated—are used for prophylactic immunization. In many carbohydrates, antigen effects depend to a large extent on the sugar unit at the end of the carbohydrate molecule, thus the antigenic specificity in the human blood-group substances A, B, O or H is largely a function of the terminal sugar. Glycoproteins—combinations of carbohydrates and proteins—play an important role as histocompatibility (H) antigens. H antigens have been found in all body cells of the animals investigated. They are responsible for the rejection of foreign tissue implants. H antigens vary in different individuals of the same species, except in genetically identical individuals.

In addition to being foreign to host lymphocytes, antigens must be of a certain size in order to stimulate chemical host defence. Most effective appear to be antigens with molecular weights exceeding 100,000. Antigens such as bacteria or foreign cells contain numerous, different molecules which may be antigenic. Molecules with weights below 1000 rarely trigger immunity responses, and those with molecular weights of 10,000 to 100,000 usually stimulate responses less dramatic than those observed in antigens exceeding 100,000.

Antibodies

Antibodies, also known as immunoglobulins, are cellular protein products, 'tailor-made' to counteract detrimental influences of specific antigens. Antibodies produced in response to a defined microbial agent tend to confer an increased degree of specific immunity to the host, and to suppress a subsequent reinfection by the same type of agent.

Different antibodies resemble each other in their basic structure, but vary in their properties and effects. It is assumed that an immunoglobulin molecule has a Y-shaped structure with 2 very flexible arms composed of 2 pairs of polypeptide chains. The pair of light chains (or L-chains) is smaller than that of the heavy chains (or H-chains). The 2 pairs of chains are joined by disulphide (—S—S—) linkages. Each arm carries both an antibody-combining site, as well as a region without a specific antibody function, but possessing the other properties attributed to immunoglobulins. The molecular structure assumed accounts for certain known properties of antibodies: (i) each molecule has 2 identical combining sites; (ii) treatment with a protein-digesting enzyme such as papain or pepsin separates the molecule into characteristic fragments; (iii) disruption of the disulphide linkages following mild chemical treatment liberates 2 types of polypeptide components—the light (L) and heavy (H) chains.

Immunoglobulins exhibit 2 different types of L-chains: kappa and lambda chains; however, any individual immunoglobulin molecule possesses only kappa or lambda L-chains, not both. There are 5 different types of H-chains: alpha, gamma, delta, epsilon and mu. Each type has different biological properties, but any individual immunoglobulin molecule possesses only one type of H-chain. The 5 H-chain types differ from one another in their constant parts (e.g. in terms of amino-acid sequence or carbohydrate content).

Successful combination of an immunoglobulin with an antigen requires that the configuration of the variable molecule regions of the L- and H-chains fits the shape of the specific antigen. Where such fitting is achieved, the immunoglobulin binds the antigen quite firmly, behaving as antibody (key-lock principle). Other biological effects of immunoglobulins depend on the structure of the 'constant' molecule regions (the various types of H-chains), e.g. activation of general defence mechanisms, or site selection of antibody action.

After some time of existence, all immunoglobulins are broken down and removed. At any one time, the amounts of antibodies actually present are an expression of the balance between rates of antibody formation and destruction. In man and related mammals, the life span of antibodies ranges from some 4 to 21 days.

The different classes of immunoglobulins (Ig) are termed according to the type of heavy (H) chains, i.e. alpha = IgA, gamma = IgG, delta = IgD, epsilon = IgE, or mu = IgM.

IgA antibodies are present in vertebrate secretions such as saliva, tears or nasal mucus and in blood plasma. IgA antibodies are important for local resistance to microbial agents, especially those inhabiting gut and respiratory tract. In mammals, IgA antibodies do not cross the placenta, but they are present in the first milk secreted after birth, thus providing the newly born with antibodies against microbial invasion.

IgG antibodies apparently exhibit a variety of defence functions. They are the most abundant antibodies found in human blood. Four distinct types of IgG antibodies have been detected; these await precise definition in regard to their respective biological roles.

IgD and IgE antibodies are present in small amounts. The properties of IgD remain to be investigated. IgE antibodies are cytotropic, that is, they bind firmly to the surfaces of certain cells (especially components of connective tissue); the interaction between IgE and an appropriate antigen triggers a sudden release of biologically potent substances such as histamine.

IgM antibodies (also known as macroglobulins) are larger than the other immunoglobulins. They have 10 antigen-combining sites per molecule and, therefore, can react firmly with large antigens such as bacteria or other foreign cells. IgM antibodies represent the first defence line forming in response to antigens, especially in primitive animals; they are very effective in neutralizing or killing microbial agents.

For the ecologist, such cellular immunity mechanisms within the body of multicellular animals comprise interesting models or parallels to the biochemical interactions observed among populations of free-living organisms (e.g. of protozoans).

Interactions between Antigens and Antibodies

In order that antibodies are formed and interact with antigens, the latter must be recognized by lymphocytes as being foreign. It is the recognizable difference in molecular pattern between antigen and the chemical compounds normally present in the host body concerned which triggers the interaction. In most cases, antigens differ in several or even many characteristics from body-own molecules. This fact is sometimes referred to as 'mosaic of antigenic differences' or 'antigenic mosaic'. In general, the larger the difference, the more pronounced is the response of the host's immunity mechanism. However, some antigenic characteristics may trigger a more intensive response than others. Hence, it seems that the intensity of antigen–antibody interactions is a function of the sum of both the quantity and quality of differences between antigen and body-own molecules.

Antigen–antibody interaction may also prevent or limit successful agent contact and invasion. In a virus, for example, the combination of antibodies with the active surface structures of the viral protein coat prevents the virus from penetrating and infecting host cells.

Additional aspects important to antigen–antibody interaction involve the capacities of antibodies to activate complement and to attach to macrophages. Complement refers to a property in the blood of immunized animals which inactivates or kills bacteria and other foreign cells. Comprising nine components (C_1 to C_9) in blood and tissues of mammals, complement constitutes a sequence of trigger mechanisms for supporting and modifying the basic effects of antigen–antibody interactions. While all complement components are proteins, they differ in size and properties. Similar complement systems are present in other vertebrates such as fishes, amphibians and birds. The complement system is activated by immunoglobulin G and IgM. Significantly, the action of the complement system is independent of the antigenic specificity of the antibody. The complement system activates biological defence mechanisms involved in inflammation processes (p. 42)—increased local blood flow, as well as transport or migration of macrophages and granulocytes. The second capacity of the antigen–antibody complex, i.e. attachment to macrophages, controls (typically augments) the rate at which antigens are phagocytized and digested.

Interaction and union of antigen and antibody primarily involves the appropriate determinant group of the antigen and the combining sites at the end of the flexible antibody arms. The union is firm but reversible; it does not involve chemical bonds. The forces responsible for the union of antigen and antibody include ionic bonding, van der Waals forces, and—less frequently—a shared H atom.

Major Host Effects

The effects of the host on its agent—or, in more general terms, the responses of the agent to its host environment—have received much less attention than the effects of the agent on its host (p. 38). However, since the relationship between agent and host involves reciprocal elements, many if not most of the functional and structural peculiarities of the agent must be assumed to have been influenced by the host.

In principle, host effects comprise both genetic (evolutionary) and non-genetic components. Of the stimuli involved, chemical and structural aspects appear to be of particular importance. Substances such as hormones, enzymes and antibodies have been shown or suspected to be responsible for many of the phenomena considered host effects. In marine animals, little solid information has emerged yet on this important aspect of agent–host conflicts.

In parasites, and to some extent also in other symbiotes, general trends which appear to mirror host effects or responses to the specific host environment include: (i) reductions or simplifications in locomotory and sensory mechanisms; (ii) specialization in regard to abilities related to attachment and invasion, as well as to host localization and discrimination; (iii) refinement of strategies for counteracting host defence; (iv) modifications in functions and structures related to uptake and assimilation of food; (v) enlargement of the reproductive potential; and (vi) adaptive changes in body shape. Host effects may also result in modifications of agent size, morphological differentiation, and modes of reproduction and sex determination (for examples consult Noble and Noble, 1964, and the following chapters).

Host effects on parasites further manifest themselves through the food taken up by the host. Noble and Noble (1964, pp. 554, 555) quote several cases where intestinal parasites of fishes, birds and mammals have been affected by the host's diet. For example, tapeworms of the dogfish shark lose weight when their host is starved, but such weight loss can be prevented by oral starch administration. Fishes that feed on animal plankton entertain a different parasite fauna than fishes whose diet consists of algae. When rats infested with tapeworms *Hymenolepis diminuta* received starch as sole source of carbohydrate, their tapeworms turned out to be much larger than those in rats fed only dextrose or sucrose. Additional ways in which the host environment has been shown to affect symbiotes are through changes in blood osmoregulation (pp. 24, 37) and hormone production (e.g. Noble and Noble, 1964, pp. 557–561).

DISEASE DIAGNOSIS

In most cases, biotic diseases, proliferative disorders and structural abnormalities result from several causes acting in concert. It is, therefore, often difficult to pin-point cause and effect and to make a precise diagnosis. This is especially so in instances of multiple parasitism and of additive contributions of disease agents plus environmental and nutritional factors. In addition, the physiological state and compensatory mechanisms of agent and host (regulation, adaptation), as well as interdependencies of the forces involved, often modify or mask disease manifestation. Finally, cause and manifestation of a disease may involve quite different areas of the host body concerned, thus generating problems of cause-and-effect localization.

These are not the only difficulties in disease diagnosis. Practically all disease symptoms and host characteristics involved are subject to considerable biological variability. They represent statistical means. Hence, in human medicine, normal (or standard) values are considered to lie near the centre point of a 95% range. The 2.5% above the upper limit of the 95% range and the 2.5% below the lower limit are defined as areas of abnormality or disease. Some characteristics have wide 95% ranges, others smaller ones, and a few have such narrow limits that they have become known as 'physiological constants'.

In the present treatise, disease diagnosis and disease symptoms are dealt with in context with the taxonomic host group treated. In general, four steps of disease diagnosis may be distinguished. The first step considers the diseased animal's history (its anamnesis). A case record often helps to focus the picture. The second step is a general examination, including such points as appearance and shape, posture, locomotion, behaviour, feeding pattern, amount of food intake, body colour, and smell. The third step involves the collection and analysis of samples, e.g. of urine, faeces, blood, mucus, or tissue, and the search for parasites, poisonous substances or critical deviations in host characteristics. For taxonomic identification of potential disease agents, a large variety of solid or liquid test media have been developed, as well as a number of tissue-culture methods. In transparent marine animals, careful microscopic search may reveal important clues, e.g. on the presence and activities of parasites or on structural deformities. The fourth step of disease diagnosis concentrates on measurements of a variety of metabolic performances, e.g. rates of respiration, osmoregulation and growth, as well as heart activities and stress endurance.

Where a sufficient number of diseased animals are available, a representative sample may be taken and killed for detailed examination (autopsy). Autopsy is also the final analytical tool after a diseased animal has died. It represents an important means for establishing the status of essential characteristics and, hence, for defining the cause(s) of the disease concerned. Since virological, bacteriological and haematological examinations cannot be carried out in fixed specimens, the best method of preservation for autopsy is immediate deep freezing.

Good keys for diagnosing the diseases of marine animals are rare. In most cases, symptoms and etiology remain to be studied in detail. Examples of useful keys are those presented for fishes by Reichenbach-Klinke and Elkan (1965), Reichenbach-Klinke (1975) and Amlacher (1976).

DISEASE PREVENTION

It is often easier to prevent a disease than to cure it. Hence, during the last two decades disease prevention has attracted increasing interest. The successful prevention of biotic diseases requires knowledge on the biology and ecology of both agent and host. In marine animals, successful disease prevention is thus far largely restricted to a few host groups and effectively practicable only under controlled conditions. Details regarding the prevention of the major diseases known to exist in marine animals receive attention in most of the following chapters and, especially, in Volume IV of this treatise.

In aquaculture projects, translocation of commercial animals and their disease agents creates special problems (e.g. Kinne, in press). The ecologist must insist here on protective measures which prevent organisms foreign to the area concerned escaping into the surrounding waters. Fortunately, several countries have initiated legislative measures in order to control and minimize certain communicable diseases of commercially important molluscs, crustaceans and fishes.

Biotic diseases can be prevented by (i) eliminating the agent; (ii) avoiding, reducing or interrupting contact between agent and host; (iii) reducing agent virulence (p. 32) and/or increasing host defence (p. 41). While disease prevention in natural populations of marine animals is difficult or impossible (problems of: accessibility, vastness of space, manpower, finances, and, of course, knowledge), both in research cultivation and in commercial cultivation (Kinne, 1976b, 1977a, b), disease prevention is achievable in many cases and figures high as a factor for culture success.

Under culture conditions, the first fundamental prerequisite for disease prevention is the avoidance of physical injuries and of excessive stress during capture, transport and handling. The second fundamental prerequisite is to assure that the captive organisms are offered adequate environmental and nutritional conditions. Polluted water, crowding, improper water treatment and inadequate nutrition reduce host defence, and may even turn normally non-pathogenic associated organisms into potential disease agents.

In cultures, practical measures of disease prevention include: (i) proper dimensioning of the carrying capacity of the culture system and adequate water-quality management (e.g. Kinne, 1976a, pp. 100–182); (ii) a sufficient period of quarantine for organisms newly collected in the field or obtained from sources which do not warrant the absence of disease-causing agents; (iii) disinfection or sterilization of culture medium, air, glassware and equipment (e.g. Kinne, 1976a, pp. 101–107); (iv) reduction or elimination of agent virulence through prophylactic medication; (v) increase in host resistance, e.g. via immunity induction (immunization), selective breeding (stock improvement) or via environmental management favouring the host but suppressing its agent (differential manipulation of environmental conditions); (vi) biological control, i.e. the introduction and support of organisms (predators, competitors, agents) which are counteractive to the disease-causing agent or to its reservoir or intermediate host(s). Especially in mass cultures of commercially important organisms (aquaculture), biological control may play an important role.

In all experimental studies with marine animals, quarantine should become a standard procedure, at least where organismic functions are studied with the aim of using the resulting data for assessing species-specific *in situ* performance. The length of the quarantine period must be commensurate with epidemiological and disease-historical considerations. In most cases, a period of 1 to 4 weeks should suffice. Where the presence of disease is unlikely, quarantine could parallel experiments as a control.

Agents requiring more than one host, such as digenetic trematodes, may sometimes also be controlled under natural conditions, for example, by elimination of their intermediate or final hosts; by prevention of contact between invasive stages (cercariae) and hosts; and by introduction of antagonistic (non-disease-causing) species, including hyperparasites.

DISEASE THERAPY

Therapy aims at the removal, suppression or neutralization of the disease-causing circumstance and at the restoration of the normal state (health) of the diseased organism. In infectious diseases, agent removal or agent suppression is largely based on differential reactions to treatment of agent and host. In many cases, the therapeutic treatment involves a stress (e.g. chemical or thermal) directed towards agent incapacitation. Simultaneously or alternatively, conditions are introduced in support of the host's natural defence mechanisms and of its compensatory and restorative activities, e.g. immunization; optimization of environmental and nutritive conditions; replenishment of specific substances or of energy resources exhausted due to the disease.

In marine animals, disease therapy is, in essence, restricted to special, man-controlled conditions. Here, the application of chemical remedies (drugs), the removal or incapacitation of the disease-causing agent, and the optimization of the host's environment and nutrition constitute the major therapeutic measures. Successful therapy is facilitated by early detection and exact diagnosis (p. 56).

In commercial culture projects, drug application is now being practised with appreciable success. Administered by addition to the water (topical application), by injection or per os, a variety of drugs (antibiotics, sulphonamides, nitrofurans) have produced encouraging results in combating microbial agents. However, the aquaculturist is largely limited in his choice to drugs which do not require individual application. Since topical application has often failed—because the drugs did not penetrate the host's outer integument readily enough for therapeutical success—drugs are preferred which are suitable for incorporation into the feed. Feed encapsulation offers here unique possibilities. In contrast to bacterial and fungal agents, counter measures against viral diseases are still largely restricted to prevention. In the USA, aquaculture chemotherapy is increasingly controlled through regulations issued by the Food and Drug Administration (e.g. Herman, 1970). In view of the obvious consequences for human health such control should be adopted on a world-wide basis. In fact it seems necessary to subject to formal registration all chemicals used in aquacultural disease therapy.

Presently, the Food and Drug Administration approves only of acetic acid, salt and sulphamerazine in food-fish farming. Oxytetracycline is restricted to catfish, salmon and trout cultivation. This means that the widely used chemicals acriflavine, copper sulphate, formaldehyde (formalin), furanace and potassium permanganate are excluded from legally backed-up application. Several drugs applied in aquaculture are claimed to be carcinogenic and to cause a variety of functional disorders in man. Disease control in aquaculture via vaccination holds much promise and requires more attention.

The application of antibiotics has become quite widespread. Both in research cultivation (Kinne, 1977c, see especially p. 997ff) and in commercial cultivation (Kinne and Rosenthal, 1977), antibiotics have been administered with considerable success. However, the resulting biological—and even more so the ecological—consequences of antibiotic application are insufficiently understood. Most antibiotics now in use have been developed for curing disease in man. Whether they are optimal for treating marine animals remains to be established. We need more research on antibiotic substances endemic to oceans and coastal waters.

Powerful antibiotics may seriously offset the balanced microbial dynamics normally prevailing in a multicellular living organism. They eliminate not only pathogenic bacteria but also those essential for the normal functioning of the host's body. Or they may destroy one group of micro-organisms, at the same time permitting others—now freed of their competitors—to proliferate to dangerously high levels, thus causing another disease in turn. In short, antibiotics can affect or modify in thus far still largely unpredictable ways the history, time course and final result of a disease.

Disease therapy in marine animals is a virgin field. Only in commercially important molluscs, crustaceans and fishes, as well as in some mammals, has significant information been produced. There is much need for research in this area of marine science. Our present knowledge is documented throughout this treatise in context with the animal group reviewed.

GLOSSARY

The terminology employed in marine-animal disease research derives, to a large extent, from human medicine. In essence, the glossary provided here adheres to the conventional meanings of the terms defined. However, since we visualize the biotic diseases of marine animals primarily as an ecological phenomenon, changes in perspective may result. Hence, definitions have often been modified; in several cases, new definitions or redefinitions have been provided.

Agent (syn.: pathogen): potentially pathogenic organism.

Allergy: exaggerated reaction of a living organism to certain substances or other organisms.

Anaemia: deficiency in red blood cells, haemoglobin or both; also: deficiency in total blood volume.

Anamnesis (case history): disease history and background as used for diagnosis and treatment.

Antibiotic: substance produced by an organism (e.g. bacterium, fungus), which exerts negative effects on other organisms, especially disease agents; example: penicillin.

Antibody: substance formed by the host body in response to antigen stimulation; the antibody combines with the inductive antigen thereby neutralizing its disease-causing potential.

Antigen: substance recognized as foreign by the host and capable of inducing antibody formation, as well as specific reactions with antibodies.

Aplasia: incomplete or faulty development of an organ or its parts; also: complete absence of an organ usually present in the organism concerned.

Atrophy: tissue degeneration (decrease in size or quality) due to abnormal diminution in number, size, function or structure of cells.

Autopsy (syn.: necropsy): post-mortem disease analysis; also: cause-of-death analysis.

Biopsy: removal of cells, tissues or other materials from the body for analytical purposes.

Commensalism: intimate coexistence of heterospecific organisms where one (the commensal) obtains unilateral benefits (e.g. energy, matter, protection) without causing demonstrable negative or positive effects in the latter (the host).

Endocommensals live inside their host.

Ectocommensals live on the outer body surface of their host.

Facultative commensals can live both free and as commensal.

Obligatory commensals are absolutely dependent on their host (at least during a significant part of their life cycle).

Disease: a demonstrable, negative deviation from the normal state (health) of an organism (p.14).

Biotic diseases are caused by organisms (agents) living on or in the diseased individual (host).

Endemic diseases are, at least over extended periods of time, prevalent in, or restricted to, a certain area.

Enzootic diseases—*see* Enzootics

Epizootic diseases—*see* Epizootics

Innate diseases (also known as idiopathic or genetic diseases) are caused by circumstances internal to the individual involved.

Nutritional diseases are caused by inadequate dietary quality, critical food shortage, or excess food uptake.

Sporadic diseases manifest themselves only occasionally and in relatively few individuals.

Stress diseases are due to critical intensities of environmental conditions.

Zoonotic diseases—*see* Zoonoses

Drug: a substance used in disease prevention or treatment.

Edema—*see* Oedema

Embolism: sudden blockage of a blood vessel (e.g. due to blood clot).

Endotoxin: toxic bacterial substances released, or separable, from the cell only after death (disintegration); also complex substances (protein, polysaccharide, lipid) incorporated into the surface of a bacterial cell and acting as antigen.

Enzootics: animal diseases which are characteristic in certain areas; here they persist or reoccur, usually at low levels of overall intensity.

Epibiote (*epi* = on, *bios* = life) (syn.: epibiont): an organism which lives on another one.

Epidemics: mass outbreaks of a communicable human disease at a certain time and within a certain region. Epidemics extending over wide geographical areas are called pandemics.

Epidemiology: study of incidence, distribution, abundance and control of disease; also: analysis of the interactions between disease-causing agent and its host.

Epizootics: mass outbreaks of a communicable animal disease at a certain time and within a certain region. Epizootics extending over wide geographical areas are called panzootics.

Etiology: study of cause, origin and background of a disease; also: circumstances that contribute to a disease and disease development.

Exotoxin: toxic bacterial substance released during normal cellular activities; also: secreted complex substance which acts as antigen.

Gigantism: abnormally accelerated growth of individuals or their parts leading to unusually large size.

Graft: transplanted tissue.

Allograft (syn.: homograft): tissue transplanted from one to another individual of the same species.

Autograft: tissue transplanted from its normal position to another place of one and the same individual.

Isograft: tissue transplanted from one to the other identical twin.

Xenograft (syn.: heterograft): tissue transplanted to an individual of a different species.

Granulocyte—*see* Leucocyte

Haemorrhage: copious escape of blood from blood vessel.

Health: normal functional and structural state of an organism. 'Normal' implies successful accommodation under given ecological conditions (p.17).

Host: organism serving as source of subsistence (e.g. energy, matter, space, protection) for another (symbiote, agent). Depending on its role in the life-cycle of the agent, the host is termed temporary, intermediate, intermittent, transport, alternate, final (=definitive), reservoir, facultative, or obligatory.

Hyperaemia (congestion): excess of blood (supply) in a body part, e.g. due to blood-vessel dilatation or changes in blood flow.

Hyperplasia: unusual enlargement of an organ or tissue due to controlled, increased proliferation of normal cells.

Hypertrophy: excessive development or growth of an organ or tissue, e.g. due to increase in size and/or number of cells.

Hypoplasia: arrested or incomplete development of an organ or tissue.

Immunity: capacity of an organism for counteracting disease-causing agents or substances; also: resistance to a biotic disease.

    Hyperimmunization: induction of an unusually high degree of immunity.

    Immunization: build-up of immunity.

    Immunogen: therapeutic antigen.

    Immunogenetics: study of the genetic basis of immunity.

    Immunology: study of causes and appearance of immunity.

    Immunotherapy: induction or support of immunity for therapeutic ends; also: treatment of or prophylaxis against a disease by immunological means.

    Immunotransfusion: transfer of immunized body fluids from a donor with the aim of curing an infected recipient.

Infarct: necrosis occurring in a tissue whose blood supply is blocked by a thrombus or embolus (embolism).

Infarction: process resulting in an infarct.

Infection (infestation): successful invasion of a host by an agent. While the terms 'infection' and 'infestation' are often used as synonyms, infection is preferred in this treatise where viral, bacterial and fungal agents are concerned; infestation, where protozoan or multicellular agents are involved.

    Autoinfection: self infection (reinfection) due to reproductive stages of parasites already in the host body.

    Hyperinfestation: invasion by a parasite (hyperparasite) living on another parasite; also reinfection due to reproduction of a parasite within a given host (connotation overlap with autoinfection and superinfection).

    Superinfection: invasion by an agent already represented on or in the host; also: repeated successive infection with the same type of agent (connotation overlap with hyperinfestation).

Infestation—*see* Infection

Inflammation: reaction to local injury leading to increased defence and repair activities (p. 42).

Inquilinism ('nest sharing'): a term practically identical in connotation with commensalism (sometimes also with mutualism).

Leucocyte (leukocyte): white or colourless, nucleated cell in circulating fluids (blood). Two groups are distinguished: (i) granulocytes, which are highly phagocytic and have densely granular cytoplasm as well as a complexly segmented nucleus; (ii) agranulocytes, which have nearly clear cytoplasm and a simple or kidney-shaped nucleus.

Leucocytosis (leukocytosis): increase in number and activity of leucocytes.

Medicament: substance used in medical treatment.

Medication: therapeutic treatment with medicament; provision of medical care.

Metaplasia: abnormal change of one cell (tissue) type into another, i.e. without intervention of embryonic cells.

Mutualism: intimate coexistence of heterospecific organisms resulting in beneficial effects for both partners (mutualists) involved.

Necrosis: premature death of cells or tissues, e.g. due to inadequate blood supply, poisons including those produced by micro-organisms, or extreme intensities of environmental factors.

Neoplasia (neoplasms; 'new growths'): abnormal cell growths comprising benign (harmless) and malignant (dangerous) tumours.

Oedema: abnormal accumulation of fluid in tissues.

Oncology: study of neoplasms.

Panzootics—*see* Epizootics

Parasite: organism (agent) which obtains benefits at the expense of another, heterospecific one (its host) without making compensation. The exploitation involved is based on an intimate, sustained association; it often tends to result in demonstrable negative effects in the host.

Ectoparasites live on the outer body surface of their host.

Endoparasites live inside their host.

Facultative parasites are capable of both free and parasitic life.

Holoparasites spend their whole life cycle on or in a given host.

Hyperparasites live on or in a host which is, in turn, a parasite itself.

Incidental parasites are only incidentally associated with a non-obligatory host.

Intercellular parasites live between adjacent cells.

Intracellular parasites live within cells.

Meroparasites (periodic, sporadic parasites) spend only part of their life cycle on or in a host.

Multiparasites (superparasites): these terms are applied to situations in which 2 or more species of parasites inhabit one host (e.g. a crab infected by bacteria and fungi).

Obligate parasites absolutely depend on their host, at least during a significant part of their life cycle.

Parasite-mix—*see* Parasitocoenosis

Parasitism: intimate coexistence of heterospecific organisms in which one (the parasite) obtains benefits (e.g. energy, matter) at the expense of the other (the host), ultimately often inflicting demonstrable negative effects in the latter.

Adult parasitism involves adult stages of the parasite.

Larval parasitism involves larval stages of the parasite.

Parasitocoenosis (syn.: parasite-mix): assemblage of different parasites (e.g. bacteria, fungi, protozoans and metazoans) coexisting on or in a host.

Parasitogenesis: evolutionary relationship(s) between a parasitic agent and its host.

Parasitology: study of parasites and their relations to the host.

Pathogen—*see* Agent

Pathogenesis: history (development, time course) of a disease or pathological condition.

    Pathogenic: being capable of causing a disease.

    Pathogenicity: pathogenic capacity of an organism.

Pathology: study of a disease, its causes, development and general appearance; also: study of functional and structural abnormality; analysis of a deviation from the normal organismic state.

Phagocytosis: uptake (ingestion) of particulate matter (foreign material, including small disease agents) by specialized host cells (amoebocytes, leucocytes).

Phoresis (syn.: phoresy): transport, shelter or other support of one type of organism (the phoront) by another (the carrier) without metabolic exploitation or exchange (e.g. barnacles carried along on a whale).

Phoresy—*see* Phoresis

Predisposition: a condition of increased susceptibility to a certain disease.

Premunition: resistance to infection acquired due to previous contact with a given agent (especially after acute infection by that agent has become chronic).

Remedy: substance or treatment that relieves or cures a disease condition.

Susceptibility: availability of the host to the activities of an agent; also: capacity for being affected by a disease-causing condition.

Symbiosis: intimate association (living together) of heterospecific organisms (symbiotes or symbionts).

    Symbiotic cleaning: symbiotic relation where one partner 'cleans' the other, i.e. feeds on its necrotic tissues, ectoparasites, food remains, etc.

Symptom: characteristic manifestation (sign) of a disease.

Therapy: treatment of disease.

Thrombosis: blood clot in a blood vessel (see also embolism).

Tumour: growth due to uncontrolled proliferation of abnormal cells.

    Benign tumours rarely produce serious disease.

    Malignant tumours may cause serious disease including cancer.

Vector: organism serving as passive carrier of a disease agent.

Virulence: disease-producing potential of an agent.

Zoonoses (zoonotic diseases): human diseases acquirable from or transferable to an animal. Presently, about 160 zoonoses are known. Most of the animals known to serve as reservoir hosts for zoonoses are terrestrial and domesticated.

Literature Cited (Chapter 2)

Altara, I. (1963). Symposium europeén sur les maladies des poissons et l'inspection des produits de la pêche fluviale et maritime. *Bull. Off. int. Épizoot.*, **59**, 1–152.

Amlacher, E. (1970). *Textbook of Fish Diseases* (Translated by D. A. Conroy and R. L. Herman), T. F. H. Publications, Jersey City, N. J.

Amlacher, E. (1976). *Taschenbuch der Fischkrankheiten*, G. Fischer, Stuttgart.

Anderson, R. S. (1975). Phagocytosis by invertebrate cells *in vitro*: biochemical events and other characteristics compared with vertebrate phagocytic systems. In K. Maramorosch and

R. E. Shope (Eds), *Invertebrate Immunity*. Academic Press, New York. pp. 153–180.

Arcadi, J. A. (1968). Tissue response to the injection of charcoal into the pulmonate gastropod *Lehmania poirieri*. *J. Invertebr. Pathol.*, **11**, 59–62.

Arimoto, R. and Tripp, M. R. (1977). Characterization of a bacterial agglutinin in the hemolymph of the hard clam, *Mercenaria mercenaria*. *J. Invertebr. Pathol.*, **30**, 406–413.

Baer, J. G. (1952). *Ecology of Animal Parasites*, University of Illinois Press, Urbana.

Bang, F. B. (1956). A bacterial disease of *Limulus polyphemus*. *Bull. Johns Hopkins Hosp.*, **98**, 325–351.

Bang, F. B. (1961). Reaction to injury in the oyster (*Crassostrea virginica*). *Biol. Bull. mar. biol. Lab.*, *Woods Hole*, **121**, 57–68.

Bang, F. B. (1962). Serological aspects of immunity in invertebrates. *Nature, Lond.*, **196**, 88–89.

Bang, F. B. (1966). Serologic response in a marine worm, *Sipunculus nudus*. *J. Immun.*, **96**, 960–972.

Bang, F. B. (1967). Introduction. Symposium on 'Defense Reactions in Invertebrates'. *Fedn Proc. Fedn Am. Socs exp. Biol.*, **26**, 1664–1665.

Bang, F. B. (1970). Disease mechanisms in crustacean and marine arthropods. In S. F. Snieszko (Ed.), *Symp. Diseases Fish. Shellfish. Am. Fish. Soc., Wash., Spec. Publ.*, **5**, 383–404.

Bang, F. B. (1973). Immune reactions among marine and other invertebrates. *BioScience*, **23**, 584–589.

Bang, F. B. (1975). Phagocytosis in invertebrates. In K. Maramorosch and R. E. Shope (Eds), *Invertebrate Immunity*. Academic Press, New York. pp. 137–151.

Bang, F. B. and Bang, B. G. (1962). Studies on sipunculid blood: Immunologic properties of coelomic fluid and morphology of 'urn cells'. *Cah. Biol. mar.*, **3**, 363–374.

Bang, F. B. and Lemma, A. (1962). Bacterial infection and reaction to injury in some echinoderms. *J. Insect Path.*, **4**, 401–414.

Barker, W. H., Jr. and Bang, F. B. (1966). The effect of infection by Gram-negative bacteria, and their endotoxins, on the blood-clotting mechanism of the crustacean *Sacculina carcini*, a parasite of the crab *Carcinus maenas*. *J. Invertebr. Pathol.*, **8**, 88–97.

Barrow, J. H., Jr. (1958). The biology of *Trypanosoma diemyctyli* Tobey. III. Factors influencing the cycle of *Trypanosoma diemyctyli* in the vertebrate host *Triturus v. viridescens*. *J. Protozool.*, **5**, 161–170.

Bergquist, P. R. and Bedford, J. J. (1978). The incidence of antibacterial activity in marine Demospongiae; systematic and geographic considerations. *Mar. Biol.*, **46**, 215–221.

Boyd, W. C. (1967). *Fundamentals of Immunology*, 4th ed., Interscience, London.

Brooks, W. M. (1969). Molluscan immunity to metazoan parasites. In G. J. Jackson, R. Herman and I. Singer (Eds), *Immunity to Parasitic Animals*, Vol. 1. Appelton-Century Crofts, New York. pp. 149–171.

Bulla, L. A., Jr. and Cheng, T. C. (Eds) (1976). *Comparative Pathobiology*, Vol. 1, Biology of the Microsporidia, Plenum Press, New York.

Bulnheim, H.-P. (1969). Zur Analyse geschlechtsbestimmender Faktoren bei *Gammarus duebeni* (Crustacea, Amphipoda). *Zool. Anz.*, **32** (Suppl.), 244–260 (*Verh. dt. zool. Ges., 1968*).

Bulnheim, H.-P. (1975). Intersexuality in Gammaridae and its conditions. *Pubbl. Staz. zool. Napoli*, **39** (Suppl.), 399–416.

Bulnheim, H.-P. (1978). Interaction between genetic, external and parasitic factors in sex determination of the crustacean amphipod *Gammarus duebeni*. *Helgoländer wiss. Meeresunters.*, **31**, 1–33.

Burkholder, P. R. (1973). The ecology of marine antibiotics and coral reefs. In O. A. Jones and R. Endean (Eds), *Biology and Geology of Coral Reefs*, Vol. II, Biology, 1. Academic Press, New York. pp. 117–182.

Burkholder, P. R. and Ruetzler, K. (1969). Antimicrobial activity of some marine sponges. *Nature, Lond.*, **222**, 983–984.

Burnet, F. M. (1969). *Cellular Immunology*, Cambridge University Press, London.

Bychowsky, B. E. (1961). *Monogenetic Trematodes*, American Institute of Biological Sciences, Washington.

Cameron, T. W. M. (1956). *Parasites and Parasitism*, Wiley, New York.

Canning, E. U. and Wright, C. A. (1972). *Behavioural Aspects of Parasite Transmission*, Academic Press, London.

Caullery, M. (1952). *Parasitism and Symbiosis*, Sidgwick and Jackson Ltd., London.

Chalker, B. E. and Taylor, D. L. (1975). Light enhanced calcification, and the role of oxidative phosphorylation in calcification of the coral *Acropora cervicornis*. *Proc. R. Soc.* (Ser. B), **190**, 323–331.

Cheng, T. C. (1964). *The Biology of Animal Parasites*, W. B. Saunders, Philadelphia.

Cheng, T. C. (1967a). The compatibility and incompatibility concept as related to trematodes and molluscs. *Pacif. Sci.*, **22**, 141–160.

Cheng, T. C. (1967b). Marine molluscs as hosts for symbioses with a review of known parasites of commercially important species. In F. S. Russell (Ed.), *Advances in Marine Biology*, Vol. 5. Academic Press, London. pp. 1–424.

Cheng, T. C. (1970). *Symbiosis. Organisms Living Together*, Pegasus, New York.

Cheng, T. C. (1973). *General Parasitology*, Academic Press, New York.

Cheng, T. C., Cali, A. and Foley, D. A. (1974). Cellular reactions in marine pelecypods as a factor influencing endosymbioses. In W. B. Vernberg (Ed.), *Symbiosis in the Sea*. University of South Carolina Press, Columbia.

Cheng, T. C. and Galloway, P. C. (1970). Transplantation immunity in mollusks: The histoincompatibility of *Helisoma duryi normale* with allografts and xenografts. *J. Invertebr. Pathol.*, **15**, 177–192.

Cheng, T. C. and Rifkin, E. (1970). Cellular relations in marine molluscs in response to helminth parasitism. In S. F. Snieszko (Ed.), *Symp. Diseases Fish. Shellfish. Am. Fish. Soc., Wash., Spec. Publ.*, **5**, 443–496.

Cheng, T. C., Thakur, A. S. and Rifkin, E. (1969). Phagocytosis as an internal defense mechanism in the Mollusca: with an experimental study of the role of leucocytes in the removal of ink particles in *Littorina scabra* Linn. In *Proceedings of the Symposium on Mollusca*, Part II. Marine Biological Association, India. The Bangalore Press, Bangalore, India. pp. 546–563.

Chipman, D. M. and Sharon, N. (1969). Mechanism of lysozyme action. *Science, N. Y.*, **165**, 454–465.

Cohen, E., Rowe, A. W. and Wissler, F. C. (1965). Heterogglutinins of the horseshoe crab *Limulus polyphemus*. *Life Sci.*, **4**, 2009–2016.

Cold Spring Harbour (1967). *Symposia on Quantitative Biology*, Vol. 32. Cold Spring Harbor Laboratory of Quantitative Biology, Cold Spring Harbor. L. I., New York.

Conover, R. J. (1966). Factors affecting the assimilation of organic matter by zooplankton and the question of superfluous feeding. *Limnol. Oceanogr.*, **11**, 346–354.

Conover, R. J. (1978). Transformation of organic matter. In O. Kinne (Ed.), *Marine Ecology*, Vol. IV, Dynamics. Wiley, Chichester. pp. 221–499.

Conroy, D. A. (1968). Partial bibliography on the bacterial diseases of fish. An annotated bibliography for the years 1870–1966. *F. A. O. Fish. Biol. tech. Pap.*, **FRs/T 73: 75**.

Cornick, J. W. and Stewart, J. E. (1966). Microorganisms isolated from the hemolymph of the lobster, *Homarus americanus*. *J. Fish. Res. Bd Can.*, **23**, 1451–1454.

Cornick., J. W. and Stewart, J. E. (1968a). Interaction of the pathogen *Gaffkya homari* with natural defense mechanisms of *Homarus americanus*. *J. Fish. Res. Bd Can.*, **25**, 695–709.

Cornick, J. W. and Stewart, J. E. (1968b). Pathogenicity of *Gaffkya homari* for the crab *Cancer irroratus*. *J. Fish. Res. Bd Can.*, **25**, 795–799.

Creutzberg, F. (1975). Orientation in space: Animals. Invertebrates. In O. Kinne (Ed.), *Marine Ecology*, Vol. II, Physiological Mechanisms, Part 2. Wiley, London. pp. 555–655.

Croll, N. A. (1966). *Ecology of Parasites*, Harvard University Press, Cambridge, Mass.

Dailey, M. D. and Brownell, R. L. (1972). A checklist of marine mammal parasites. In S. H. Ridgway (Ed.), *Mammals of the Sea*. C. C. Thomas, Springfield, Illinois. pp. 528–589.

Dales, R. P. (1966). Symbiosis in marine organisms. In S. M. Henry (Ed.), *Symbiosis*, Vol. I, Associations of Microorganisms, Plants, and Marine Organisms. Academic Press, New York. pp. 299–326.

Dawe, C. J. and Harshbarger, J. C. (Eds) (1969). A symposium on neoplasms and related disorders of invertebrate and lower vertebrate animals. Smithsonian Institution, Washington, D. C., June 19–21, 1968. *Natn Cancer Inst. Monogr.*, **31**.

De Bary, A. (1879). *Die Erscheinung der Symbiose*, K. J. Trubner, Strassburg.

De Coursey, P. J. and Vernberg, W. B. (1974). Double infections of larval trematodes: competitive interactions. In W. B. Vernberg (Ed.), *Symbiosis in the Sea*. University of South Carolina Press, Columbia.

Delyamure, S. L. (1955). *The Helminth Fauna of Marine Mammals in the Light of their Ecology and Phylogeny* (Russ.), Akademy of Sciences, SSSR, Moscow.

Dogiel, V. A. (1962). *General Parasitology*, Oliver & Boyd, Edinburgh.

Dogiel, V. A., Petrushevski, G. K. and Polyanski, Y. I. (Eds) (1958). *Parasitology of Fishes* (Russ.), Leningrad University Press, Leningrad.

Dogiel, V. A., Petrushevski, G. K. and Polyanski, Y. I. (Eds) (1961). *Parasitology of Fishes* (Engl. ed., transl. by Z. Kabata), Oliver & Boyd, Edinburgh.

Dogiel, V. A., Petrushevski, G. K. and Polyanski, Y. I. (Eds) (1970). *Parasitology of Fishes*, T. F. H. Publications, Neptune City, N. Y. (Translation of Russian original of 1958).

Dollfus, R. P. (1942). Études critiques sur les tétrarhynques du Muséum de Paris. *Archs Mus. natn. Hist. nat., Paris*, **19**, 1–466.

Eble, A. F. and Tripp, M. R. (1968). Enzyme histochemistry of phagosomes in oyster leucocytes. *Bull. N. J. Acad. Sci. B.*, **13**, 93.

Enright, J. T. (1975). Orientation in time: Endogenous clocks. In O. Kinne (Ed.), *Marine Ecology*, Vol. II, Physiological Mechanisms, Part 2. Wiley, London. pp. 917–944.

Farley, C. A. (1968). *Minchinia nelsoni* (Haplosporida, Haplosporidiidae) disease syndrome in the American oyster, *Crassostrea virginica*. *J. Protozool.*, **15**, 585–599.

Feder, H. M. (1966). Cleaning symbiosis in the marine environment. In S. M. Henry (Ed.), *Symbiosis*, Vol. I, Associations of Microorganisms, Plants, and Marine Organisms. Academic Press, New York. pp. 327–380.

Feng, S. Y. (1962). The response of oysters to the introduction of soluble and particulate materials and the factors modifying the response. Ph.D. Thesis, Rutgers University, New Brunswick, N. J.

Feng, S. Y. (1965). Heart rate and leucocyte circulation in *Crassostrea virginica* (Gmelin). *Biol. Bull. mar. biol. Lab., Woods Hole*, **128**, 198–210.

Feng, S. Y. (1967). Responses of molluscs to foreign bodies, with special reference to the oyster. *Fedn Proc. Fedn Am. Socs exp. Biol.*, **26**, 1685–1692.

Feng, S. Y. and Canzonier, W. J. (1970). Humoral responses in the American oyster (*Crassostrea virginica*) infected with *Bucephalus* sp. and *Minchinia nelsoni*. In S. F. Snieszko (Ed.), *Symp. Diseases Fish. Shellfish. Am. Fish. Soc., Wash., Spec. Publ.*, **5**, 497–510.

Fernandez-Moran, H., Machalonis, J. J. and Edelman, G. M. (1968). Electron microscopy of a hemagglutinin from *Limulus polyphemus*. *J. molec. Biol.*, **32**, 467–469.

Finstad, C. L., Litman, G. W., Finstad, J. and Good, R. A. (1972). The evolution of the immune response. XIII. The characterization of purified erythrocyte agglutinins from two invertebrate species. *J. Immun.*, **108**, 1704–1711.

Fletcher, T. C. and White, A. (1973). Lysozyme activity in the plaice (*Pleuronectes platessa* L.). *Experientia*, **29**, 1283–1285.

Füller, H. (1958). *Symbiose im Tierreich*, Ziemsen Verlag, Wittenberg.

Fuller, M. S., Fowles, B. E. and McLaughlin, D. J. (1964). Isolation and pure culture study of marine phycomycetes. *Mycologia*, **56**, 745–756.

Ganaros, A. E. (1957). Marine fungus infecting eggs and embryos of *Urosalpinx cinerea*. *Science, N. Y.*, **125**, 1194.

Geiman, Q. M. (1964). Comparative physiology: mutualism, symbiosis, and parasitism. *A. Rev. Physiol.*, **26**, 75–106.

Ghittino, P. (1970). *Piscicoltura e Ittiopatalogia*, Vol. 2, Ittiopatalogia, Edizione Rivista die Zootecnia, Sesto, S. G.

Goreau, T. F. and Goreau, N. I. (1960). Distribution of labeled carbon in reef-building corals with and without zooxanthellae. *Science, N. Y.*, **131**, 668–669.

Griffin, P. J. (1954). The nature of bacteria pathogenic to fish. In S. F. Snieszko (Ed.), *Symp. Diseases Fish. Shellfish Am. Fish. Soc., Wash., Spec. Publ.*, **5**, 241–253.

Halver, J. E. (1954). Fish diseases and nutrition. In S. F. Snieszko (Ed.), *Symp. Diseases Fish. Shellfish. Am. Fish. Soc., Wash., Spec. Publ.*, **5**, 254–261.

Halver, J. E. (1970). Nutrition in marine aquaculture. In W. J. McNeil (Ed.), *Marine Aquiculture*. Oregon State University Press, Corvallis. pp. 75–102.

Halver, J. E. (Ed.) (1972). *Fish Nutrition*, Academic Press, New York.

Henry, S. M. (Ed.) (1966). *Symbiosis*, Vol. I, Associations of Microorganisms, Plants, and Marine Organisms, Academic Press, New York.

Henry, S. M. (Ed.) (1967). *Symbiosis*, Vol. II, Associations of Invertebrates, Birds, Ruminants, and Other Biota, Academic Press, New York.

Herman, R. L. (1970). Prevention and control of fish diseases in hatcheries. In S. F. Snieszko (Ed.), *Symp. Diseases Fish. Shellfish. Am. Fish. Soc., Wash., Spec. Publ.*, **5**, 3–15.

Hildemann, W. H. and Reddy, A. L. (1973). Phylogeny of immune responsiveness: marine invertebrates. *Fedn Proc. Fedn Am. Socs exp. Biol.*, **32**, 2188–2194.

Hoffman, G. L. (1967). *Parasites of North American Freshwater Fishes*, University of California Press, Berkeley.

Holmes, J. C. and Bethel, W. M. (1972). Modification of intermediate host behaviour by parasites. In E. U. Canning and C. A. Wright (Eds), *Behavioural Aspects of Parasite Transmission*. Academic Press, London. pp. 123–149.

Hopkins, S. H. (1957). Interrelations of organisms. B. Parasitism. In J. W. Hedgpeth (Ed.), *Treatise in Marine Ecology and Paleoecology*, Vol. I, Ecology. pp. 413–428. (*Mem. geol. Soc. Am.*, **67**.)

Humphrey, J. H. (1976). Immunity. In *The New Encyclopaedia Britannica*. Macropaedia, Vol. 9. Encyclopaedia Britannica Inc., Chicago. pp. 247–259.

Humphrey, J. H. and White, R. G. (1970). *Immunology for Students of Medicine*, 3rd ed., Blackwell, Oxford.

Ihering, H. Von (1891). On the ancient relations between New Zealand and South America. *Trans. Proc. N. Z. Inst.*, **24**, 431–445.

Janoff, A. and Hawrylko, E. (1964). Lysosomal enzymes in invertebrate leucocytes. *J. cell. comp. Physiol.*, **63**, 267–271.

Jennings, J. B. (1974). Symbioses in the Turbellaria and their implications in studies on the evolution of parasitism. In W. B. Vernberg (Ed.), *Symbiosis in the Sea*. University of South Carolina Press, Columbia. pp. 127–160.

Johnson, H. M. (1964). Human blood group A_1 specific agglutinin of the butter clam, *Saxidomus giganteus*. *Science, N. Y.*, **146**, 548–549.

Johnson, T. W., Jr. and Sparrow, F. K., Jr. (1961). *Fungi in Oceans and Estuaries*, J. Cramer, Weinheim.

Kabata, Z. (1970). Crustacea as enemies of fishes. In S. F. Snieszko and H. R. Axelrod (Eds), *Diseases of Fishes*, Book 1. T. F. H. Publications, Jersey City, N. J. pp. 1–171.

Kinne, O. (1962). Irreversible nongenetic adaptation. *Comp. Biochem. Physiol.*, **5**, 265–282.

Kinne, O. (1963). Adaptation, a primary mechanism of evolution. In H. B. Whittington and W. D. I. Rolfe (Eds), *Physiology and Evolution of Crustacea*. Museum of Comparative Zoology (Spec. Publ.) Cambridge, Mass., USA. pp. 27–50.

Kinne, O. (1964a). Non-genetic adaptation to temperature and salinity. *Helgoländer wiss. Meeresunters.*, **9**, 433–458.

Kinne, O. (1964b). Animals in aquatic environments: crustaceans. In D. B. Dill, E. F. Adolph and C. G. Wilber (Eds), *Handbook of Physiology*. Sect. 4. Adaptation to the Environment. Am. Physiol. Soc., Washington, D. C. pp. 669–682.

Kinne, O. (1970a). Temperature: Animals. Invertebrates. In O. Kinne (Ed.), *Marine Ecology*, Vol. I, Environmental Factors, Part 1. Wiley, London. pp. 407–514.

Kinne, O. (Ed.) (1970b). *Marine Ecology*, Vol. I, Environmental Factors, Part 1. Wiley, London.

Kinne, O. (Ed.) (1971). *Marine Ecology*, Vol. I, Environmental Factors, Part 2. Wiley, London.

Kinne, O. (Ed.) (1972). *Marine Ecology*, Vol. I, Environmental Factors, Part 3. Wiley, London.

Kinne, O. (Ed.) (1975a). *Marine Ecology*, Vol. II, Physiological Mechanisms, Part 1. Wiley, London.

Kinne, O. (Ed.) (1975b). *Marine Ecology*, Vol. II, Physiological Mechanisms, Part 2. Wiley, London.

Kinne, O. (1976a). Cultivation of marine organisms: water-quality management and technology. In O. Kinne (Ed.), *Marine Ecology*, Vol. III, Cultivation, Part 1. Wiley, London. pp. 19–300.

Kinne, O. (Ed.) (1976b). *Marine Ecology*, Vol. III, Cultivation, Part 1. Wiley, London.

Kinne, O. (Ed.) (1977a). *Marine Ecology*, Vol. III, Cultivation, Part 2. Wiley, Chichester.

Kinne, O. (Ed.) (1977b). *Marine Ecology*, Vol. III, Cultivation, Part 3. Wiley, Chichester.

Kinne, O. (1977c). Cultivation of Animals. Research Cultivation. In O. Kinne (Ed.), *Marine Ecology*, Vol. III, Cultivation, Part 2. Wiley, Chichester. pp. 579–1293.

Kinne, O. (1977d). International Helgoland Symposium 'Ecosystem research': summary, conclusions and closing. *Helgoländer wiss. Meeresunters.*, **30**, 709–727.

Kinne, O. (Ed.) (in press). *Marine Ecology*, Vol. V, Ocean Management. Wiley, Chichester.

Kinne, O. and Bulnheim, H.-P. (Eds) (in press). 14th European Marine Biology Symposium 'Protection of Life in the Sea'. *Helgoländer wiss. Meeresunters.*, **33**.

Kinne, O. and Rosenthal, H. (1977). Commercial cultivation (aquaculture). In O. Kinne (Ed.), *Marine Ecology*, Vol. III, Cultivation, Part 3. Wiley, Chichester. pp. 1321–1398.

Lapage, G. (1958). *Parasitic Animals*, Heffer, Cambridge.

Levin, J. A. (1967). Blood coagulation and endotoxin in invertebrates. *Fedn Proc. Fedn Am. Socs exp. Biol.*, **26**, 1707–1712.

Levin, J. A. and Bang, F. B. (1964). A description of cellular coagulation in *Limulus*. *Bull. Johns Hopkins Hosp.*, **115**, 337–345.

Levin, J. A. and Bang, F. B. (1968). Clottable protein in *Limulus:* its localization and kinetics of its coagulation by endotoxin. *Thrombosis and Diathes. Haemorrh.*, **19**, 186–197.

Lewis, D. H. and Smith, D. C. (1971). The autotrophic nutrition of symbiotic marine coelenterates with special reference to hermatypic corals. I. Movement of photosynthetic products between the symbionts. *Proc. R. Soc.* (Ser. B), **178**, 111–129.

Li, C. P., Prescott, B., Eddy, B., Caldes, G., Green, W. R., Martino, E. C. and Young, A. M. (1965). Antiviral activity of paolins from clams. *Ann. N. Y. Acad. Sci.*, **130**, 374–382.

Li, C. P., Prescott, B., Jahnes, W. G. and Martino, E. C. (1962). Antimicrobial agents from mollusks. *Trans. N. Y. Acad. Sci.* (2), **24**, 504–509.

Li, M. F. and Fleming, C. (1967). Hemagglutinins from oyster hemolymph. *Can. J. Zool.*, **45**, 1225–1234.

Limbaugh, C. (1961). Cleaning symbiosis. *Scient. Am.*, **205**, 42–49.

Lipke, H. (1975). Melanin in host-parasite interaction. In K. Maramorosch and R. E. Shope (Eds), *Invertebrate Immunity*. Academic Press, New York. pp. 327–336.

Mackin, J. G. (1951). Histopathology of infection of *Crassostrea virginica* (Gmelin) by *Dermocystidium marinum* Mackin, Owen and Collier. *Bull. mar. Sci. Gulf Caribb.*, **1**, 72–87.

McGregor, E. A. (1963). Publications on fish parasites and diseases. 330 B.C.–A.D. 1923. *Spec. scient. Rep. U. S. Fish. Wildl. Serv.*, **474**, 1–84.

Maramorosch, K. and Shope, R. E. (Eds) (1975). *Invertebrate Immunity*, Academic Press, New York.

Marchalonis, J. J. and Edelman, G. M. (1968). Isolation and characterization of a hemagglutinin from *Limulus polyphemus*. *J. molec. Biol.*, **32**, 453–465.

Mawdesley-Thomas, L. E. (1969). Neoplasia in fish—a bibliography. *J. Fish Biol.*, **1**, 187–207.

Mawdesley-Thomas, L. E. (Ed.) (1972a). Diseases of fish. *Symp. zool. Soc. Lond.*, **30**, 1–380.

Mawdesley-Thomas, L. E. (1972b). Some tumours of fish. *Symp. zool. Soc. Lond.*, **30**, 191–283.

Mayr, E. (1957). Evolutionary aspects of host specificity among parasites of vertebrates. In *Proceedings of First Symposium on Host Specificity Among Parasites of Vertebrates*. Inst. Zool., University of Neuchâtel. pp. 5–14.

Metchnikoff, E. (1884). Über eine Sprosspelzkrankheit der Daphnien. *Virchows Arch. path. Anat. Physiol.*, **96**, 177–195.

Metchnikoff, E. (1893). *Lectures on the Comparative Pathology of Inflammation* (Transl. by F. A. and E. H. Starling), Kegan Paul, Trench, Trubner and Co., London.

Metchnikoff, E. (1905). *Immunity in Infective Diseases* (Transl. by F. G. Binnie), Cambridge University Press, London.

Meuleman, E. A. (1972). Host-parasite interrelationships between the freshwater pulmonate *Biomphalaria pfeifferi* and the trematode *Schistosoma mansoni*. *Neth. J. Zool.*, **22**, 355–427.

Michelson, E. H. (1975). Cellular defense mechanisms and tissue alterations in gastropod molluscs. In K. Maramorosch and R. E. Shope (Eds), *Invertebrate Immunity*. Academic Press, New York. pp. 181–195.

Murphy, F. A., Whitfield, S. G., Sudia, W. D. and Chamberlain, R. W. (1975). Interactions of vector with vertebrate pathogenic viruses. In K. Maramorosch and R. E. Shope (Eds), *Invertebrate Immunity*. Academic Press, New York, pp. 25–48.

Muscatine, L. and Hand, C. (1959). Direct evidence for transfer of materials from symbiotic algae to tissues of a coelenterate. *Proc. natn. Acad. Sci. U.S.A.*, **44**, 1259–1261.

Muscatine, L., Pool, R. R. and Cernichiari, E. (1972). Some factors influencing selective release of soluble organic material by zooxanthellae from reef corals. *Mar. Biol.*, **13**, 298–308.

Nappi, A. J. (1975). Parasite encapsulation in insects. In K. Maramorosch and R. E. Shope (Eds), *Invertebrate Immunity*. Academic Press, New York. pp. 293–326.

Nigrelli, R. F., Jakowska, S. and Calventi, I. (1959). Ectyonin, an antimicrobial agent from the sponge *Microciona prolifera* Verrill. *Zoologica, N. Y.*, **44**, 173–175.

Noble, E. R. and Noble, G. A. (1964). *Parasitology. The Biology of Animal Parasites*, 2nd ed., Lea and Febiger, Philadelphia.

Odening, K. (1974). *Parasitismus. Grundfragen und Grundbegriffe*, Akademie-Verlag, Berlin.

Pan, C.-T. (1958). The general histology and topographic microanatomy of *Australorbis glabratus*. *Bull. Mus. comp. Zool. Harv.*, **119**, 237–299.

Pan, C.-T. (1963). Generalized and focal tissue responses in the snail, *Australorbis glabratus*, infected with *Schistosoma mansoni*. *Ann. N. Y. Acad. Sci.*, **113**, 475–485.

Pan, C.-T. (1965). Studies on the host–parasite relationship between *Schistosoma mansoni* and the snail *Australorbis glabratus*. *Am. J. trop. Med. Hyg.*, **14**, 931–976.

Paschke, J. D. and Summers, M. D. (1975). Early events in the infection of the arthropod gut by pathogenic insect viruses. In K. Maramorosch and R. E. Shope (Eds), *Invertebrate Immunity*. Academic Press, New York. pp. 75–112.

Patton, J. S., Abraham, S. and Benson, A. A. (1977). Lipogenesis in the intact coral *Pocillopora capitata* and its isolated zooxanthellae: evidence for a light-driven carbon cycle between symbiont and host. *Mar. Biol.*, **44**, 235–247.

Patton, W. K. (1974). Community structure among the animals inhabiting the coral *Pocillopora damicornis* at Heron Island, Australia. In W. B. Vernberg (Ed.), *Symbiosis in the Sea*. University of South Carolina Press, Columbia. pp. 219–243.

Pauley, G. B., Granger, G. A. and Krassner, S. M. (1971). Characterization of a natural agglutinin present in the hemolymph of the California sea hare, *Aplysia californica*. *J. Invertebr. Pathol.*, **18**, 207–218.

Pauley, G. B. and Krassner, S. M. (1972). Cellular defense reactions to particulate materials in the California sea hare, *Aplysia californica*. *J. Invertebr. Pathol.*, **19**, 8–17.

Peters, G. and Peters, N. (1977). Temperature-dependent growth and regression of epidermal tumours in the European eel *(Anguilla anguilla* L.). *Ann. N. Y. Acad. Sci.*, **298**, 245–260.

Peters, N., Peters, G., Stich, H. F., Acton, A. B. and Bresching, G. (1978). On differences in skin tumours of Pacific and Atlantic flatfish. *J. Fish Diseases*, **1**, 3–25.

Pflugfelder, O. (1977). *Wirtstierreaktionen auf Zooparasiten*, G. Fischer, Stuttgart.

Post, G. (1965). A review of advances in the study of diseases of fish: 1954–1964. *Progve Fish Cult.*, **27**, 3–12.

Reichenbach-Klinke, H.-H. (1975). *Bestimmungsschlüssel zur Diagnose von Fischkrankheiten*, G. Fischer, Stuttgart.

Reichenbach-Klinke, H.-H. and Elkan, E. (1965). *The Principal Diseases of Lower Vertebrates*, Vol. I, Diseases of Fishes, Academic Press, London.

Renn, C. E. (1936a). The wasting disease of *Zostera marina*. I. A phytological investigation of the diseased plant. *Biol. Bull. mar. biol. Lab., Woods Hole*, **70**, 148–158.

Renn, C. E. (1936b). Persistence of the eel-grass disease and parasite on the American Atlantic coast. *Nature, Lond.*, **138**, 507–508.

Ribelin, W. E. and Migaki, G. (1975). *The Pathology of Fishes*, The University of Wisconsin Press, Wisconsin.

Roberts, R. J. and Shepherd, C. J. (1974). *Handbook of Trout and Salmon Diseases*, Fishing News (Books) Ltd., Surrey.

Rohde, K. (1977). Species diversity of monogenean gill parasites of fish on the Great Barrier Reef. *Proc. int. Symp. coral Reefs*, **3**, 585–591.

Rohde, K. (1978). Latitudinal differences in host-specificity of marine Monogenea and Digenea. *Mar. Biol.*, **47**, 125–134.

Salt, G. (1970). *The Cellular Defence Reactions of Insects*, Cambridge University Press, Cambridge. (*Cambridge Monographs in Experimental Biology*, **16**.)

Samter, M. and Alexander, H. L. (Eds) (1965). *Immunological Diseases*, Churchill Press, London.

Schäperclaus, W. (1954). *Fischkrankheiten*, Akademie-Verlag, Berlin.

Schmeer, M. R. (1964). Growth-inhibiting agents from *Mercenaria* extracts. Chemical and biological characteristics. *Science, N. Y.*, **144**, 413–414.

Schmeer, M. R. (1966). Mercenene: growth-inhibiting agent of *Mercenaria* extracts—further chemical and biological characterization. *Ann. N. Y. Acad. Sci.*, **136**, 211–218.

Schmeer, M. R. and Berry, G. (1965). Mercenene: growth-inhibitor extracted from clam *M. campechiensis*. Preliminary investigation of *in vivo* and *in vitro* activity. *Life Sci.*, **4**, 2157–2165.

Schöne, H. (1975). Orientation in space: Animals. General introduction. In O. Kinne (Ed.), *Marine Ecology*, Vol. II, Physiological Mechanisms, Part 2. Wiley, London. pp. 499–553.

Seitz, K. (1975). Orientation in space: Plants. In O. Kinne (Ed.), *Marine Ecology*, Vol. II, Physiological Mechanisms, Part 2. Wiley, London. pp. 451–916.

Shirodkar, M. V., Warwick, A. and Bang, F. B. (1960). The *in vitro* reaction of *Limulus* amebocytes to bacteria. *Biol. Bull. mar. biol. Lab., Woods Hole*, **118**, 324–337.

Sindermann, C. J. (1966). Diseases of marine fishes. In F. S. Russell (Ed.), *Advances in Marine Biology*, Vol. 4. Academic Press, London. pp. 1–89.

Sindermann, C. J. (1970). *Principal Diseases of Marine Fish and Shellfish*, Academic Press, New York.

Skarnes, R. C. and Watson, D. W. (1957). Antimicrobial factors of normal tissues and fluids. *Bact. Rev.*, **21**, 273–294.

Sminia, T. (1972). Structure and function of blood and connective tissue cells of the fresh water pulmonate *Lymnaea stagnalis* studied by electron microscopy and enzyme histochemistry. *Z. Zellforsch. mikrosk. Anat.*, **130**, 497–526.

Smith, D. C., Muscatine, L. and Lewis, D. H. (1969). Carbohydrate movement from autotrophs to heterotrophs in parasitic and mutualistic symbiosis. *Biol. Rev.*, **44**, 17–90.

Smyth, J. D. (1962). *Introduction to Animal Parasitology*, Thomas, Springfield.

Smyth, J. D. and Haslewood, G. A. D. (1963). The biochemistry of bile as a factor in determining host specificity in intestinal parasites, with particular reference to *Echinococcus granulosus*. *Ann. N. Y. Acad. Sci.*, **113**, 234–260.

Snieszko, S. F. (1954a). Symposium. Research on fish diseases: a review of progress during the past 10 years. *Trans. Am. Fish. Soc.*, **83**, 219–349.

Snieszko, S. F. (1954b). Therapy of bacterial fish diseases. In S. F. Snieszko (Ed.), *Symposium. Research on fish diseases: a review of progress during the past 10 years. Trans. Am. Fish. Soc.*, **83**, 313–330.

Snieszko, S. F. (Ed.) (1970). *A Symposium on Diseases of Fishes and Shellfishes, Am. Fish. Soc., Wash., Spec. Publ.*, **5**.

Snieszko, S. F., Nigrelli, R. F. and Wolf, K. (1965). Viral diseases of poikilothermic vertebrates. *Ann. N. Y. Acad. Sci.*, **126**, 1–680.

Sprent, J. F. A. (1963). *Parasitism*, University of Queensland Press, Australia.

Stauber, L. A. (1950). The fate of India ink injected intracardially into the oyster, *Ostrea virginica* (Gmelin). *Biol. Bull. mar. biol. Lab., Woods Hole*, **98**, 227–241.

Stauber, L. A. (1961). Immunity in invertebrates, with special reference to the oyster. *Proc. natn. Shellfish. Ass.*, **50**, 7–20.

Stewart, J. E., Arie, B., Zwicker, B. M. and Dingle, J. R. (1969a). Gaffkemia, a bacterial disease of the lobster, *Homarus americanus*: effects of the pathogen, *Gaffkya homari*, on the physiology of the host. *Can. J. Microbiol.*, **15**, 925–932.

Stewart, J. E., Cornick, J. W. and Dingle, J. R. (1967). An electronic method for counting lobster (*Homarus americanus* Milne Edwards) hemocytes and the influence of diet on hemocyte numbers and hemolymph proteins. *Can. J. Zool.*, **45**, 291–304.

Stewart, J. E., Cornick, J. W., Spears, D. I. and McLeese, D. W. (1966b). Incidence of *Gaffkya homari* in natural lobster *Homarus americanus* populations of the Atlantic region of Canada, *J. Fish. Res. Bd Can.*, **23**, 1325–1330.

Stewart, J. E., Cornick, J. W. and Zwicker, B. M. (1969b). Influence of temperature on gaffkemia, a bacterial disease of the lobster *Homarus americanus*. *J. Fish. Res. Bd. Can.*, **26**, 2503–2510.

Stewart, J. E. and Dingle, J. R. (1968). Characteristics of hemolymphs of *Cancer irroratus*, *C. borealis* and *Hyas coarctatus*. *J. Fish. Res. Bd Can.*, **25**, 607–610.

Stewart, J. E., Dingle, J. R. and Odense, P. H. (1966a). Constituents of the hemolymph of the lobster *Homarus americanus* Milne Edwards. *Can. J. Biochem.*, **44**, 1447–1459.

Stewart, J. E., Horner, G. W. and Arie, B. (1972a). Effects of temperature, food, and starvation on several physiological parameters of the lobster *Homarus americanus*. *J. Fish. Res. Bd Can.*, **29**, 439–442.

Stewart, J. E., Zwicker, B. M., Arie, B. and Horner, G. W. (1972b). Food and starvation as factors affecting the time to death of the lobster *Homarus americanus* infected with *Gaffkya homari*. *J. Fish. Res. Bd Can.*, **29**, 461–464.

Stich, H. F., Acton, A. B., Dunn, B. P., Oishi, K., Yamazaki, F., Harada, T., Peters, G. and Peters, N. (1977). Geographic variations in tumour prevalence among marine fish populations. *Int. J. Cancer*, **20**, 780–791.

Symposium on 'Defense reactions in invertebrates' (1967). *Fedn Proc. Fedn Am. Socs exp. Biol.*, **26**.

Takatsuki, S. (1934). Beiträge zur Physiologie des Austerherzens unter besonderer Berücksichtigung physiologischer Reaktionen. *Sci. Rept Tokyo Bunrika Daigaku*, **B2**, 55–62.

Taylor, D. L. (1969). The nutritional relationship of *Anemonia sulcata* (Pennant) and its dinoflagellate symbiont. *J. Cell Sci.*, **4**, 751–762.

Taylor, D. L. (1973). Algal symbionts of invertebrates. *A. Rev. Microbiol.*, **27**, 171–187.

Tesch, F.-W. (1975). Orientation in space: Animals. Fishes. In O. Kinne (Ed.), *Marine Ecology*, Vol. II, Physiological Mechanisms, Part 2. Wiley, London. pp. 657–707.

Trench, R. K. (1971). The physiology and biochemistry of zooxanthellae symbiotic with marine coelenterates. I. Assimilation of photosynthetic products of zooxanthellae by two marine coelenterates. *Proc. R. Soc.* (Ser. B), **177**, 225–235.

Trench, R. K. (1974). Nutritional potentials in *Zoanthus sociathus* (Coelenterata, Anthozoa). *Helgoländer wiss. Meeresunters.*, **26**, 174–216.

Tripp, M. R. (1958a). Studies on the defense mechanism of the oyster, *Crassostrea virginica*. Ph.D. Thesis, Rutgers University, New Brunswick, N. J.

Tripp, M. R. (1958b). Disposal by the oyster of intracardially injected red blood cells of vertebrates. *Proc. natn. Shellfish. Ass.*, **48**, 142–147.

Tripp, M. R. (1958c). Studies on the defense mechanisms of the oyster, *Crassostrea virginica*. *J. Parasit.*, **44** (Suppl.), 35–36.

Tripp, M. R. (1960). Mechanisms of removal of injected microorganisms from the American oyster, *Crassostrea virginica* (Gmelin). *Biol. Bull. mar. biol. Lab.*, *Woods Hole*, **119**, 273–282.

Tripp, M. R. (1961). The fate of foreign materials experimentally introduced into the snail *Australorbis glabratus*. *J. Parasit.*, **47**, 745–751.

Tripp, M. R. (1963). Cellular responses of mollusks. *Ann. N. Y. Acad. Sci.*, **113**, 467–474.

Tripp, M. R. (1966). Hemagglutinin in the blood of the oyster *Crassostrea virginica*. *J. Invertebr. Pathol.*, **8**, 478–484.

Tripp, M. R. (1970). Defense mechanisms of mollusks. *J. Reticuloendothel. Soc.*, **7**, 173–182.

Tripp, M. R. (1971). Immunity in invertebrates. In T. C. Cheng (Ed.), *Aspects of the Biology of Symbiosis*. University Park Press, Baltimore, Maryland. pp. 275–281.

Tripp, M. R. (1974a). Oyster hemolymph proteins. *Ann. N. Y. Acad. Sci.*, **234**, 18–22.

Tripp, M. R. (1974b). Molluscan immunity. *Ann. N. Y. Acad. Sci.*, **234**, 23–27.

Tripp, M. R. (1975). Humoral factors and molluscan immunity. In K. Maramorosch and R. E. Shope (Eds), *Invertebrate Immunity*. Academic Press, New York. pp. 201–223.

Tutin, T. G. (1938). The autecology of *Zostera marina* in relation to its wasting disease. *New Phytol.*, **37**, 50–71.

Tyler, A. (1946). Natural heteroagglutinins in the body fluids and seminal fluids of various invertebrates. *Biol. Bull. mar. biol. Lab., Woods Hole*, **90**, 213–219.

Tyler, A. and Metz, C. B. (1945). Natural heteroagglutinins in the serum of the spiny lobster, *Panulirus interruptus*. I. Taxonomic range of activity, electrophoretic and immunizing properties. *J. exp. Zool.*, **100**, 387–406.

Tyler, A. and Scheer, B. T. (1945). Natural heteroagglutinins in the serum of the spiny lobster, *Panulirus interruptus*. II. Chemical and antigenic relation to blood proteins. *Biol. Bull. mar. biol. Lab., Woods Hole*, **89**, 193–200.

Vandermeulen, J. H. and Muscatine, L. (1974). Influence of symbiotic algae on calcification in reef corals: critique and progress report. In W. B. Vernberg (Ed.), *Symbiosis in the Sea*. University of South Carolina Press, Columbia, South Carolina.

Vernberg, W. B. (Ed.) (1974). *Symbiosis in the Sea*, University of South Carolina Press, Columbia, South Carolina.

Vishniac, H. S. (1958). A new marine Phycomycete. *Mycologia*, **50**, 66–79.

Walford, L. A. (1958). *Living Resources of the Sea*, Ronald Press, New York.

Worms, M. J. (1972). Circadian and seasonal rhythms in blood parasites. In E. U. Canning and C. A. Wright (Eds), *Behavioural Aspects of Parasite Transmission*. Academic Press, London. pp. 53–67.

Wright, C. A. (1966). The pathogenesis of helminths in the Mollusca. *Helminth. Abstr.*, **35**, 207–224.

Yonge, C. M. (1931). The significance of the relationship between corals and zooxanthellae. *Nature, Lond.*, **128**, 309–311.

Yonge, C. M. (1957). Interrelations of organisms. C. Symbiosis. In J. W. Hedgpeth (Ed.), *Treatise on Marine Ecology and Paleoecology*, Vol. I, Ecology. *Mem. geol. Soc. Am.*, **67**, 429–442.

Yonge, C. M. (1963). The biology of coral reefs. In F. S. Russell (Ed.), *Advances in Marine Biology*, Vol. I. Academic Press, New York. pp. 209–260.

Young, E. L., III. (1937). Notes on the labyrinthulan parasite of the eel-grass *Zostera marina*. *Bull. Mt Desert Isl. Biol. Lab.*, **1937**, 33–35.

Young, S. Y., O'Connor, J. D. and Muscatine, L. (1971). Organic material from scleractinian coral skeletons. II. Incorporation of ^{14}C into protein, chitin and lipid. *Comp. Biochem. Physiol.*, **40B**, 945–958.

3. DISEASES OF PROTOZOA

G. LAUCKNER

Of the approximately 44,250 known species of Protozoa, about 20,200—mostly foraminiferans—are fossil. Of the remaining 24,050 recent species, some 17,300 are free-living, occupying various habitats in freshwater, marine and moist terrestrial environments. More than 6750 species are parasitic. The number of known protozoans increases steadily and rapidly (e.g. Levine, 1962).

Whereas protozoans living in freshwater habitats and parasitizing higher animals are known rather well, only a small fraction of those presumed to occur in oceans and coastal waters have, thus far, been studied in detail.

As is the case with most other phyla, the classification of the Protozoa is in continuous flux. Conservative authors—for instance Hyman (1940), Kaestner (1954-1963), Grell (1968) but also Remane and co-authors (1976)—divide the phylum Protozoa into only 5 classes. Others concede the protozoans the rank of a subkingdom Protista and establish a considerably larger number of classes. A special committee of the Society of Protozoologists (Honigberg and co-authors, 1964) has presented a detailed revised classification which, although basically adopted by most recent workers, has received some criticism and subsequent modifications (Sprague, 1966; Levine, 1970, 1971a, b; Page, 1976; and others). There can be no doubt that future studies on the ultrastructure, life cycles and physiology of a number of protozoans will necessitate shifts within and between taxonomic levels. No attempt will be made here to evaluate and discuss the various opinions (see footnote on p. 2).

Protozoans are of considerable concern as parasites of Metazoa. Some cause serious diseases, particularly among vertebrates. The flagellates and amoebae are believed to represent more ancient groups than the ciliates, with the consequence that in the former groups a considerably larger number of species have, to date, adapted to parasitism than in the latter. One group, the sporozoans, consists exclusively of endoparasites.

The Protozoa themselves may harbour viruses, bacteria, fungi, and other protozoans; and the reproductive phases of these organisms have sometimes been mistaken as those of the host. Unless autotrophic, most endobiotic forms have to be regarded as parasites in the sense that they are metabolically dependent on their hosts. In many instances, however, the protozoan host suffers no apparent detriment from the relationship, and sometimes associations between host and symbiote are constant. Even cases of mutual advantage have been observed. It is, therefore, frequently difficult to decide whether certain organisms associated with protozoans are parasites, commensals or mutualists, and for a number of associations the exact type of relationship has never been demonstrated.

Protozoan–pathogen associations represent simple biosystems, and should, therefore, be particularly suited for quantitative disease studies. Many protozoans can be cultivated under controlled experimental conditions, and for several species, adequate culture media and methods are available (Kinne, 1977). Hence, investigations on protozoan–parasite interrelationships could contribute much to our limited knowledge on physiological and biochemical mechanisms of organismic interactions, such as biological exclusion, disease and epizootiology.

Our knowledge of the biology of marine Protozoa is rather limited, and even less is known about their diseases and parasites. Consequently, some of the available information on diseases and parasites of non-marine protozoans has been included in this review. It appears reasonable to suspect that future investigations will reveal similar conditions in marine representatives of the phylum.

The literature on organisms living on and in Protozoa has been reviewed by Kirby (1941) and Ball (1969). Annotated bibliographies on pathology of invertebrates compiled by Johnson (1968) and Johnson and Chapman (1969) include more than 170 references concerning associates and diseases of Protozoa. There are a number of papers dealing with parasites and diseases of Protozoa in general, some of which include reviews of earlier literature (Mattes, 1924; Sassuchin, 1934; Kirby, 1941, 1942; Kudo, 1966; Grell, 1968).

3.1   FLAGELLATA

DISEASES CAUSED BY MICRO-ORGANISMS

Agents: Viruses

In what might be termed the pre-electron-microscopy era, small inclusions referred to as possible viruses or viral inclusions have been reported from a number of Protozoa. Since most of these structures were not found again on later occasions when they could have been examined under an electron microscope, their exact nature could not be determined. The earlier literature concerning the possible occurrence of viruses in Protozoa has been reviewed by Ball (1969).

Recently, Franca (1976) reported virus-like particles in the cytoplasm of *Gyrodinium resplendens* from Santo André lagoon (West coast of Portugal). In cell sections, clusters of particles arranged in a crystalline fashion were seen quite frequently. These particles, with a diameter of about 35 nm, presented more or less individualized circular sub-units forming a polygonal matrix of electron-dense material around a central opaque area. The aggregates occupied large areas in the cytoplasm of *G. resplendens* (Fig. 3-1). In some sections, aggregates of particles were seen with a diameter of about 20 nm and with an electron-dense periphery encircling a translucent zone with a central dense core. These clusters were surrounded by an apparently single-layered membrane (Fig. 3-2).

Cytoplasmic structures adjacent to the particle-bearing areas did not reveal any significant pathological alterations ascribable to the presence of the virus-like particles. However, in some of the more heavily affected cells, some mitochondria exhibited sparse cristae or destruction of the entire contents. In other cases, particles were seen inside modified mitochondria.

Agents: Bacteria

Bacteria, attached to the surface either by one end or in full length, occur on many flagellates, mostly on non-marine parasitic forms. Earlier workers have frequently mistaken them for pellicular differentiations, cilia or flagella (see reviews of Kirby, 1941, and Ball, 1969). Some of these associations simply represent examples of phoresis, whereas in others at least some degree of mutualistic relationship appears to exist.

The association between protozoans and bacteria that live in the cytoplasm or the nucleus is normally closer than that of the surface forms. The relationships may cover the

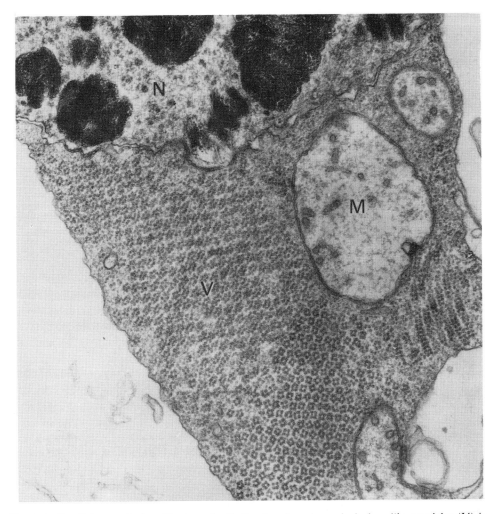

Fig. 3-1: *Gyrodinium resplendens*. Portion of cell showing densely packed virus-like particles (V) in contact with nucleus (N). Mitochondrion (M) showing small number of short cristae and fibrillar stroma. × 48,000. (After Franca, 1976; reproduced by permission of Centre National de la Recherche Scientifique.)

whole scale from mutualism to pathogenic parasitism. The latter is true particularly of the nuclear endobiotes. Bacteria are of frequent occurrence in the cytoplasm or the nucleus of flagellates. *Caryococcus hypertrophicus*, for example, causes hypertrophy of the nucleus of the flagellate *Euglena deses*, amounting to two-fifths of the body volume. The pathogen also causes destruction of the chlorophiliphorous apparatus and suppression of fission (Dangeard, 1902).

On the other hand, bacteria occurring in the cytoplasm of haemoflagellates *Blasto-crithidia culicis* and *Crithidia oncopelti* are definitely beneficial to their hosts, perhaps by supplying essential factors that are inadequate even in a rich blood medium. Elimination of the bacterial symbiotes by chloramphenicol resulted in reduced growth of the flagellates (Chang, 1975).

Agents: Fungi

The great majority of fungi attacking Protozoa belong to the Chytridiales. In some endobiotic forms, e.g. in *Sphaerita* spp. which invade the cytoplasm, as well as in *Nucleophaga* spp. which attack the nucleus, there seems to be little doubt that the relationship is one of parasite and host. Fungal infection of the nucleus appears to be invariably lethal to the protozoan host. Organisms resembling *Sphaerita* spp. or *Nucleophaga* spp. have, apparently, not yet been reported from free-living marine flagellates. With other chytrids which occur as epibiotes on Protozoa, it is a question whether the association

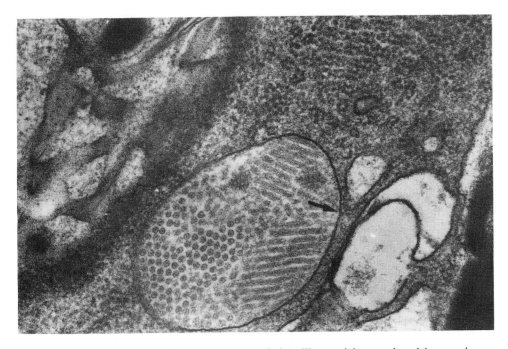

Fig. 3-2: *Gyrodinium resplendens*. Dense aggregate of virus-like particles enveloped by membrane (arrow). × 63,000. (After Franca, 1976; reproduced by permission of Centre National de la Recherche Scientifique.)

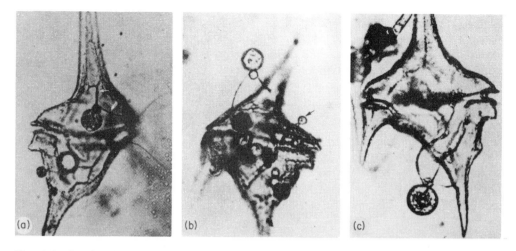

Fig. 3-3: *Ceratium hirundinella*. Individuals parasitized by chytrids *Amphicypellus elegans*. (a) Sporangium, apophysis and 2 main rhizoids (arrows) visible; (b) nearly mature individual (top) and very young stage (arrow) with its apophysis resting on host cell surface; (c) individual with 3 main rhizoids arising from apophysis. (After Ingold, 1944; reproduced by permission of British Mycological Society.)

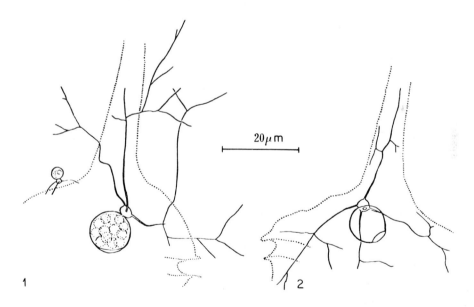

Fig. 3-4: *Amphicypellus elegans*. 1: Mature individual (centre) showing sporangium with zoospores and rhizoidal system arising from apophysis; left: very young individual. 2: Old individual in which sporangium has dehisced. Outline of host cell, *Ceratium hirundinella*, indicated by dotted lines. (After Ingold, 1944; reproduced by permission of British Mycological Society.)

should be termed one of parasite and host or of predator and prey. Sometimes these organisms are referred to as 'predaceous fungi'.

Examples of such kinds of association are *Rhizophydium* sp. attacking freshwater dino-flagellates *Glenodinium (Peridinium) cinctum* (Dangeard, 1888) and *Amphicypellus elegans* invading *Ceratium hirundinella* and *Peridinium* sp. (Ingold, 1944; Figs 3-3 and 3-4). About half the *C. hirundinella* from Windermere, England, bore the chytrid. The contents of infected cells appeared to be completely disorganized. Usually, each host cell carried several *A. elegans* and often as many as 20 occurred.

DISEASES CAUSED BY PROTOZOANS

Agents: Flagellata

An interesting case of ectoparasitism by one flagellate on another has been described by Hollande (1938). The parasite, named *Bodo perforans*, possessed a long, slender rostrum by which it was attached in a constant position near the anterior end of its host, *Chilomonas paramaecium*. The rostrum of *B. perforans* penetrated the cytoplasm only slightly but there was evidence for the passage of cellular contents from the host to the parasite. Many infested *C. paramaecium* had lost their flagella but otherwise appeared to be unaffected.

Marine euglenoids *Protoeuglena noctilucae* occurred in great numbers within the cytoplasm of *Noctiluca miliaris* from plankton samples taken off Calicut, India. Hundreds of these green flagellates which measured 5 to 6 μm in length and 4 to 4·5μm in width, were seen evenly distributed and freely moving within the host cytoplasm. During the period of observation, every *N. miliaris* collected harboured the flagellates, often in such numbers as to cause a green discolouration of the sea where patches of the dinoflagellate host occurred at the ocean surface. *P. noctilucae* was seen to reproduce within the cytoplasm of *N. miliaris* by longitudinal division. Even heavily populated hosts appeared quite healthy and active. The euglenoid, however, did not appear to be capable of existing outside the dinoflagellate (Subrahmanyan, 1954). The author believed the association to be symbiotic. Similar euglenoids, 3 to 4 μm in length, have been found to occur abundantly in *N. miliaris* from Alger, Mediterranean Sea (Cachon, 1964).

Several parasitic dinoflagellates inhabit the cytoplasm and sometimes the nucleus of other dinoflagellates. Some have either been mistaken for reproductive structures of their hosts, or their affinities have not been recognized by earlier authors. These organisms are highly modified for a parasitic mode of life and display their dinoflagellate character only during the free-living phase.

Coccidinium duboscqui invades the cytoplasm of *Peridinium balticum* from Sète, French Mediterranean cost (Fig. 3-5). When in contact with the parasite, the host nucleus degenerates and eventually disappears entirely. Individuals whose nucleus has been destroyed exhibit normal or even slightly increased motility. *P. sociale* is parasitized by another peridinean, *C. legeri*. *C. punctatum* occurs in *Ostreopsis monotis* and *C. mesnili* in *Cryptoperidinium foliaceum*; all representatives studied were collected off Sète, France (Chatton and Biecheler, 1934, 1936; Chatton, 1952).

Several parasitic dinoflagellates have been observed by Cachon (1964) in dinoflagellates from plankton samples taken off Alger, Mediterranean Sea. *Duboscquella melo* develops in the perinuclear cytoplasm of *Noctiluca miliaris*. Frequently, more than 10 trophonts occur in a single host. Affected cells exhibit marked pathological alterations. Initially, there is a retraction 'of the cytoplasmic threads which form a network within the jelly of *N. miliaris*, followed by disappearance of the tentacle and flagellum and progressive lysis of the perinuclear cytoplasm. Although *D. melo* never attacks the host nucleus directly, the latter nevertheless degenerates. Sometimes the host dies even before the parasite has completed its development.

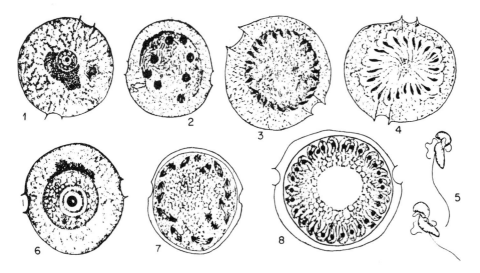

Fig. 3-5: *Coccidinium duboscqui*. 1, 2: Initial stages of parasite in *Peridinium balticum;* 3, 4: microgametogenesis; 5: dinospores; 6–8: sporulation. (After Chatton and Biecheler, 1934; reproduced by permission of Gauthier-Villars, Paris.)

Duboscquella nucleocola accomplishes its trophic development in the nucleus of *Leptodiscus medusoides*. Exceptionally, this peridinean host may harbour 2 or 3 parasites simultaneously. Size differences among individual *D. nucleocola* suggest successive infestations. In the course of the parasite's development, the host nucleus is lysed but the activity of *L. medusoides* appears unaffected. In late stages of infestation, the host's nuclear capsule is markedly distended, the enclosed *D. nucleocola* trophont attaining a diameter of up to 125 μm. Other, as yet unidentified, members of the genus *Duboscquella* have been observed in the cytoplasm or nucleus of various other gymnodinid and peridinid dinoflagellates. Surprisingly, however, the most common species in plankton samples taken off Alger, *Peridinium sociale*, *Ceratium* spp. and *Cochlodinium* spp., were never found to harbour stages of *Duboscquella* spp. (Cachon, 1964).

Dinoflagellates of the genus *Amoebophrya* have repeatedly confused zoologists and have remained a zoological enigma for decades, being either assigned to various animal groups—the orthonectid mesozoans, suctorians and other protozoan groups—or mistaken for specific body structures (mainly 'reproductive organs') of their protozoan hosts. The most amusing interpretation is doubtless that by Brooks and Kellner (1908) who believed individuals of *Amoebophrya* in *Oodinium (Gromia) appendiculariae* to represent 'embryos' of the appendicularian host, *Oikopleura tortugensis*. Resorting to imagination rather than scrutiny, they even described the presumed larval appendicularian's protochord, nervous system, mouth, digestive tract and other body structures (!). Chatton and Biecheler (1935) made a study on the life history of *Amoebophrya* and assigned the genus to the Coelomastigina, a newly established flagellate order. Grassé (1952) hesitated to group them with the dinoflagellates. It remained to Cachon (1964) to ascertain definitely the true nature of these controversial organisms.

The different species of *Amoebophrya* show a very peculiar morphological evolution. They are intracellular parasites during the first period of their life cycle, i.e. during their trophic stage, and are free-living and phagotrophic during the second period, i.e. during sporogenesis. By the end of the parasitic phase, their cellular body is completely inverted, entirely enveloping the host to which they originally had attached, and forming a large food vacuole around it, the wall of which consists of the former outer cell wall of the parasite. The external membrane of the sporont stage, in turn, corresponds to the cellular membrane which lined the mastigocoel cavity during the trophont stage (Fig. 3-6). Various aspects of the ultrastructure of *Amoebophrya* spp. have been studied by means of electron microscopy (Cachon and Cachon, 1969, 1970).

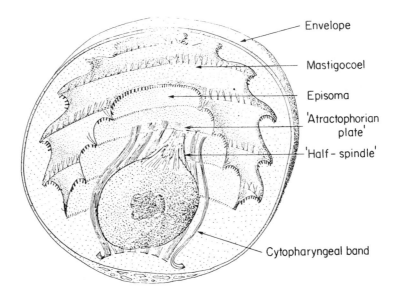

Envelope

Mastigocoel

Episoma

'Atractophorian plate'

'Half - spindle'

Cytopharyngeal band

Fig. 3-6: *Amoebophrya acanthometrae*. Sagittal section of adult trophont. (After Cachon and Cachon, 1970; reproduced by permission of Centre National de la Recherche Scientifique.)

Amoebophrya grassei lives parasitically in the cytoplasm of *Oodinium poucheti* which, in turn, is a parasite of appendicularians *Oikopleura dioica*. The parasite ramifies throughout the entire host cytoplasm, frequently pushing the nucleus against the cell wall. Multiple infestations of *O. poucheti* have been observed, sometimes comprising more than a dozen *A. grassei* within a single host cell (Cachon, 1964). In the Bay of Alger, *O. poucheti* occurred sporadically in *O. dioica*, with intermittent periods of high abundance. Abrupt decline of peridinean numbers on the appendicularians, terminating the intervals of high

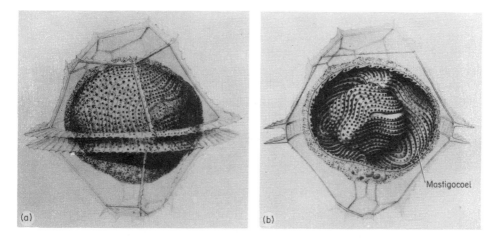

Fig. 3-7: *Godioma* sp. Individuals parasitized by *Amoebophrya ceratii*. (a) Entire view; (b) transverse
section. (After Cachon, 1964; reproduced by permission of Masson et Cie.)

abundance, invariably coincided with the appearance of the hyperparasite. It was
concluded that *A. grassei* was responsible for the rapid destruction of *O. poucheti*.

Amoebophrya ceratii, originally described as *Hyalosaccus ceratii* by Koeppen (1903),
invades the cytoplasm or the nucleus of several species of dinoflagellates. In thecate
peridineans, the parasite commences its development within the host nucleus which is

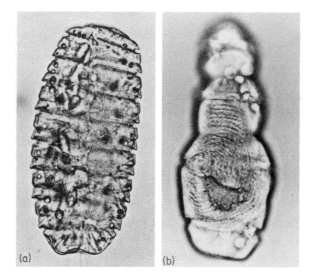

Fig. 3-8: *Polykrikos schwartzii*. (a) Healthy colony with
8 zooids showing normal shape; (b) colony
parasitized by *Amoebophrya ceratii* and exhibiting
massive body distortion. (After Drebes, 1974;
reproduced by permission of Georg Thieme
Verlag.)

lysed subsequently. Within the growing trophont, a cavity (mastigocoel) develops which is lined by a helical system of flagellated furrows. Because of its resemblance to a hypertrophied host nucleus, this stage has been termed 'parasitic giant nucleus' by the earlier authors (Fig. 3-7). The mature trophont gives rise to numerous small bilagellate dinospores. In advanced infections, the host cell wall virtually constitutes a mere 'envelope', almost entirely occupied by the parasite's body. *A ceratii* occurred in various dinoflagellates from plankton samples taken off Alger, Mediterranean Sea (Cachon, 1964). At Helgoland, German Bight, it was observed in *Polykrikos schwartzii* and *Ceratium* spp. (Drebes, 1974). Infested cells were grossly distorted and exhibited a typical 'fingerprint pattern' displayed by the parasite's helically grooved body surface (Fig. 3-8).

DISEASES CAUSED BY METAZOANS

Agents: Trematoda

A peculiar association between a peridinean and a larval trematode has been observed by Pouchet (*in*: Rebecq, 1965). At Concarneau, France, Pouchet frequently observed an unidentified 'microscopic trematode', clinging to *Noctiluca miliaris*. The parasite was also found in the stomach of sardines. According to Rebecq (1965), it was probably a metacercarian member of the Hemiuridae, who use a number of planktonic organisms—including medusae, ctenophores, chaetognaths and copepods—as intermediate hosts.

ABNORMALITIES

Can cancer occur in Protozoa? This question, apparently, was first raised by Metcalf (1928). In addition to the numerous normal nuclei, many abnormal ones were seen in *Proopalina caudata* and *Opalina obtraigona*. According to Metcalf, these nuclei closely resemble certain cancerous cells in mammals. He also observed degenerating, larger-than-normal nuclei which, again, resemble nuclei of certain neoplasms. Modern workers, however, tend to discount Metcalf's findings as examples of abnormal mitoses (Sparks, 1969).

3.2   RHIZOPODA

DISEASES CAUSED BY MICRO-ORGANISMS

Agents: Bacteria

Bacteria frequently occur on or in amoebae. A wide range of relationships appears to exist between these protozoans and their epi- and endobiotic bacterial flora—from simple phoresis through mutualism to true parasitism. A bacterium related to *Pseudomonas* has been found responsible for fatal infections in soil amoebae (Drozanski, 1956), and a Gram-negative lophotrichal rod for mortalities of free-living amoebae (Drozanski, 1963a). Drozanski (1963b) discussed the mechanism of bacterial entrance into amoebae and the effect of environmental factors. Infections with unidentified bacteria caused hypertrophy of the body, and production of multinucleate amoebae (Epstein, 1935).

Particularly bacteria occurring in the nucleus are capable of producing fatal diseases in rhizopods. Unidentified bacteria invading the marine amoeba *Paramoeba eilhardi* cause hypertrophy of the nucleus. The agent has not been observed in the cytoplasm and multiplies only in the nucleus (Fig. 3-9). Infected *P. eilhardi* stop feeding and eventually die. Upon disintegration of cytoplasm and nucleus, the bacteria are liberated. In sea water, the organisms which had been non-motile as long as they were enclosed by the host nuclear membrane, develop flagella and become active. Outside the host they may remain viable for months without multiplying. Attempts to infect experimentally amoebae other than *P. eilhardi* with this bacterium were unsuccessful (Grell, 1968, 1971).

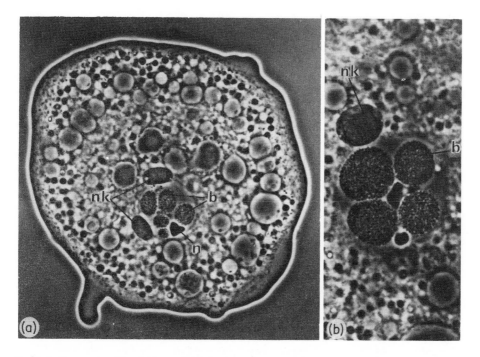

Fig. 3-9: *Paramoeba eilhardi*. Bacterial infection of macronucleus. (a) Entire view of infected individual. × 1300; (b) nuclear region showing massive concentration of bacteria. × 2600. b: Bacteria; n: nucleolus; nk: 'Nebenkörper'. (After Grell, 1968; reproduced by permission of Springer-Verlag.)

Casley-Smith and Savanat (1966) studied, by means of electron microscopy, the fate of spores, bacteria and foreign particles injected into *Amoeba proteus*. After lying free in the cytoplasm for about 2 h, the injected material was surrounded by a shell of granules which morphologically resembled ribosomes, and which were apparently transformed gradually into membranes. Bacteria and spores were digested within the membrane enclosure.

Some associations between amoebae and bacteria are of constant occurrence. So characteristic, for example, are bacteria in *Pelomyxa* spp. that Penard (1902; cited in Kirby, 1941) designated the genus as always provided with symbiotic bacteria. Leiner (1924), however, believed that when the bacteria are excessively abundant, they may become definitely injurious to the host, causing hypertrophy, structural alterations, and eventually dissolution of the nucleus. The trophic functions of affected amoebae may be disturbed and there is a decrease in stored glycogen. Upon death of *Pelomyxa palustris*, the bacteria multiply extraordinarily.

A true mutualistic relationship appears to exist between a strain of *Amoeba proteus* and its bacterial endosymbiotes. Remarkably, these endosymbiotes were originally parasitic and harmful to the hosts before they became essential cytoplasmic components of *A. proteus* over a period of several years. In amoebae treated with chloramphenicol, the average number of bacteria per cell decreased to less than 10% of that in untreated controls. No treated amoeba that lost all its endosymbiotes was viable. Comparable treatments with chloramphenicol had no adverse effect on originally symbiote-free amoebae of the same strain. Thus, death of the treated symbiote-harbouring amoebae was apparently due to the loss of their bacteria without which they could not survive (Jeon and Jeon, 1976; Jeon, 1977; Jeon and Hah, 1977).

Under certain conditions, amoebae may act as carriers of pathogenic bacteria. Jadin (1977), for example, observed incorporation into food vacuoles and subsequent digestion of enterobacteriae by axenically grown *Acanthamoeba* sp. In contrast, mycobacteria were not digested but instead multiplied within the vacuoles, sometimes entirely overwhelming the host. The pathogens also survived in cysts of *Acanthamoeba* sp. It was concluded that these amoebae may play the role of vectors of mycobacteria. Comparable mechanisms have not yet been demonstrated in marine amoebae, although they may be expected to exist.

Agents: Fungi

Several fungi, most of them nonmarine, have been reported as parasites of amoebae. A chytrid fungus, *Nucleophaga* sp., invades the nucleus of *Endolimax nana* (Brumpt and Lavier, 1935). Another chytrid, *Amoebophilus destructor*, was found in the cytoplasm of *Pelomyxa palustris*, causing epizootics and mortalities in experimental cultures (Hollande, 1945). *Sphaerita amoebae* and *S. plasmophaga* have been described from the cytoplasm and nucleus of *Amoeba sphaeronucleolus* and *A. terricola* (Mattes, 1924). The author also reviewed the earlier literature on parasites of amoebae. A chytrid of the genus *Sphaerita* has also been reported from *Endamoeba salpae* parasitic in the marine teleost *Box boops* (Léger and Duboscq, 1904). The protozoans were sometimes overwhelmed and killed by the microspheres of the fungus. Life history, structure and affinities of the genera *Nucleophaga*, *Sphaerita* and other chytrids infecting protozoans have been discussed by Chatton and Brodsky (1909) and Kirby (1941).

Branching networks of tubes and channels apparently produced by fungi have been observed to ramify through the skeletons of polythalamous foraminiferans of the genera *Operculina*, *Amphistegina*, *Heterostegina*, *Calcarina*, *Orbitolites*, *Polystomella* and *Alveolina* (Kölliker, 1860).

Galleries excavated in the calcareous tests of foraminiferans, probably caused by an organism behaving somewhat like a fungus, have also been reported by Douvillé (1930). According to Kirby (1941), this organism might be similar to or identical with *Didymella conchae*, an ascomycete reported by Bonar (1936) from shells of marine gastropods and barnacles (see section *Mollusca*). Fungal organisms are quite commonly found to invade Foraminifera and shells of marine invertebrates (Porter and Zebrowski, 1937; Zebrowski, 1937).

DISEASES CAUSED BY PROTOZOANS

Agents: Flagellata

Hertwig (1879) observed structures within the cytoplasm of Radiolaria which he believed to be integrate parts of the nucleus. Fol (1883) termed these structures 'spiral body', granting them the role of spermatophora. Their parasitic nature was first recognized by Korotneff (1891) who assigned them to the orthonectid mesozoans.

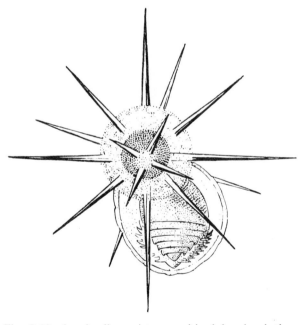

Fig. 3-10: *Acanthocolla cruciata* parasitized by *Amoebophrya acanthometrae* (in host ectoplasm). (After Borgert, 1897; reproduced by permission of Akademische Verlagsgesellschaft Geest & Portig.)

Koeppen (1894), on the other hand, believed them to be 'embryonic suctorians' and established the genus *Amoebophrya* to include 2 species, *A. acanthometrae* and *A. sticholonchae* (Figs 3-10 and 3-11). Although Borgert (1897) made further studies on the life cycles of these parasites, their affinities remained uncertain. Chatton and Biecheler (1935) noted similarities between *Amoebophrya* and *Hyalosaccus ceratii* reported from marine dinoflagellates *Ceratium tripos*, *C. fusus* and *C. horridum* by Koeppen (1903); they believed both genera to be synonymous and established a new flagellate order, the Coelomastigina, to include the genera *Amoebophrya* and *Hyalosaccus*. Finally, Cachon (1964) showed these organisms to be parasitic dinoflagellates.

Amoebophrya acanthometrae is a common parasite of Mediterranean acantharians, particularly of *Acanthometra pellucida*. The nuclei of affected hosts are entirely destroyed. Only exceptionally does a radiolarian harbour more than one parasite. On the other hand, *A. acanthometrae* has been found, on several occasions, to be hyperparasitized by another species of *Amoebophrya*: *A. ceratii* (Cachon, 1964).

Oodinium acanthometrae and *Collinella ovoides* are two further peridineans parasitic in the cytoplasm of *Acanthometra pellucida*. The trophonts of *C. ovoides*, which may attain a diameter of up to 110 μm, lie between the spicules and cause deformation of the host body (Cachon, 1964).

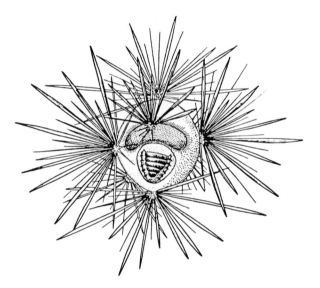

Fig. 3-11: *Sticholonche zanclea*. Individual parasitized by *Amoebophrya sticholonchae*. (After Borgert, 1897; reproduced by permission of Akademische Verlagsgesellschaft Geest & Portig.)

Peridineans of the genus *Merodinium* are known exclusively as parasites of radiolarians. *M. brandti* and *M. vernale* occur in *Collozoum inerme*, the former within and the latter outside the central capsule. *C. pelagicum* is parasitized by *M. insidiosum*; *C. fulvum*, by *M. belari*; *Myxosphaera coerulea*, by *M. mendax*; *Sphaerozoum punctatum*, by *M. dolosum*; *S. acuferum*, by *M. astatum*. All live in the cytoplasm whereas *Merodinium (Solenodinium) fallax* is an intranuclear parasite of *Thalassicolla spumida* (Chatton, 1923; Hovasse, 1923a; Hollande and Enjumet, 1953). The spores of the peridineans somewhat resemble those of their hosts (Fig. 3-12), and stages of the parasites have previously been mistaken for reproductive stages of the radiolarians (Chatton, 1920b; Hovasse and Brown, 1956).

Peridineans *Hollandella mycetoides*, *H. lobata* and *H. piriformis* have been reported from radiolarians *Spongosphaera* sp., *Plegmosphaera coronata* and *Actinosphaera* sp., respectively.

Although inhabiting the endoplasm, *H. mycetoides* and *H. lobata* cause lysis of the host nuclei. *H. piriformis*, which occurs in the ectoplasm, induces deformation of the host's central capsule (Cachon, 1964).

'Secondary nuclei', which were observed in *Aulacantha scolymantha* by Borgert (1900–1909; cited by Hollande and co-authors, 1953) and believed to represent initial stages in the formation of macro- and microspores of this radiolarian, actually represent dinocaryons of a peridinean *Syndinium borgerti*. Living on the host's cytoplasm, the parasite gradually replaces the radiolarian's cellular body whose nucleus becomes deformed, undergoes lysis and frequently disappears entirely. Fragmentation of the parasite's sporoblasts results in the formation of either macro- or microspores. Sometimes both spore types occur side by side in the central capsule of the same radiolarian. Mature spores are liberated by rupture of the host's capsule membrane (Hollande and co-authors, 1953).

Peridineans of the genus *Merodinium* are known exclusively as parasites of radiolarians. (1920a), Hovasse (1923b), Hovasse and Brown (1953) and Cachon-Enjumet (1961).

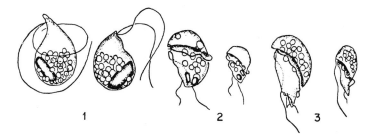

Fig. 3-12: 1: *Collozoum inerme*, isospores; 2: macro- and microspores of *Merodinium brandti*, parasite of *C. inerme;* 3: macro- and microspores of *M. mendax*, parasite of *Myxosphaera coerulea*. (After Chatton, 1923; reproduced by permission of Gauthiers-Villars, Paris.)

Hollande and Enjumet (1953) briefly mentioned and figured a flagellate, 15 μm long and 5 μm wide, which they declared to be a new species, *Bodo insidiosus*; however, they did not describe it adequately. The flagellate which, according to the authors, could not properly be termed a parasite, sometimes occurred in abundance in the ectoplasm of radiolarians of the genus *Collozoum*. The protozoan has previously been confounded with isospores of its host.

Agents: Rhizopoda

Foraminiferans *Discorbis mediterranensis* from Banyuls (French Mediterranean coast) are hosts for amoebae *Vahlkampfia discorbini* which, in their resting stage, assumed an ovoid shape of 15-μm length and 8-μm width. The foraminiferan has a normal life cycle with an alternation of schizogony and gamogony. The parasite appears to affect only the gamogonic stages of *D. mediterranensis;* it has never been found in solitary gamonts or recently established associations but paired gamonts examined after 15 h had the parasite. Infestation with *V. discorbini* may sometimes be intense, the mass of the parasite exceeding that of the host cytoplasm (Le Calvez, 1940).

Small limacine amoebae, measuring in the encysted stage 8 to 12 μm in diameter, were encountered within the test of *Spiroloculina hyalina*. Abundant in mass cultures of this foraminiferan from Panama City and in stained preparations made from these, the amoeba is distinguished by its locomotion and pseudopodial morphology, its *Endolimax*-like nucleus, and its tendency to form cysts that pass through a strongly wrinkled or deeply furrowed stage. Both trophic and encysted forms were found within the test of *S. hyalina*.

The parasite occurred most frequently either in empty host tests or in chambers from which cytoplasm was lacking altogether or had obviously been reduced in volume. The cytoplasm and nuclei remaining in such infested foraminiferans often appeared to be in a healthy condition, despite the marked reduction in cytoplasmic volume. Although the evidence was inconclusive, it was assumed that the amoeba possibly kills the foraminiferan (Arnold, 1964).

In cultures containing 2 foraminiferans, *Entosolenia marginata* (= *Oolina marginata*) and *Discorbis vilardeboanus*, the former invariably occurred on the tests of the latter. The parasite was seen to stretch its pseudopods over the ectothalamic protoplasm with which *D. vilardeboanus* covers its test, and to capture and ingest granules circulating in this portion of the host cytoplasm (Le Calvez, 1947, 1953). *E. marginata* was seen to reproduce asexually after leaving its host, forming 2 to 6 'embryos' which soon attacked other *D. vilardeboanus*. *E. marginata* is the only known parasitic foraminiferan. It is apparently host-specific since it does not attack *D. bertheloti*.

Agents: Sporozoa

Trophosphaera planorbulinae, a sporozoan parasite believed to be a coccidian, was described by Le Calvez (1938, 1939) from the cytoplasm of foraminiferans *Planorbulina mediterranensis*. A similar organism has been reported by Myers (1943). Destruction of the foraminiferans probably results from mechanical blocking of the test pores, so that the host eventually dies of starvation.

In preserved material of foraminiferans *Gypsina* spp., specimens were seen that had no cytoplasm in the chambers although the calcareous walls and the orifices between the chambers were intact. Other individuals whose chambers had not yet been emptied disclosed the presence, in the cytoplasm, of large numbers of sporozoans in various stages of development. The parasites apparently destroyed the host's cytoplasm but left the chamber walls intact, eventually escaping through the coarse mural pores of the foraminiferan's test. In some *Gypsina* populations, a very large percentage of individuals was found to carry these sporozoan infestations (Nyholm, 1962).

Examination of fixed and stained specimens of *Spiroloculina hyalina* from North and Central American coastal waters disclosed the presence of cytoplasmic inclusions (Arnold, 1964). Particularly the proloculus of adult foraminiferans may be filled with spherical bodies, 1·0 to 1·5 μm in diameter, which bear some resemblance to the spores produced by *Trophosphaera planorbulinae* in *Planorbulina mediterranensis* as described by Le Calvez (1939). Single bodies or small numbers of what appeared to be similar spore-like bodies having a deeply staining 'nucleus'—sometimes centrally, in other instances excentrically placed within an unstained cytoplasmic groundmass—not infrequently occurred within the cytoplasm of *S. hyalina*, usually within distinct vacuoles.

These structures, according to Arnold (1964), appear to be similar to sporozoan-like bodies observed in *Gypsina* sp. by Nyholm (1962) and believed by him to be the causative agent in the destruction of the foraminiferan's cytoplasm. Another clue to the coccidian nature of some of the foreign bodies in *Spiroloculina hyalina* was the observation of tests devoid of foraminiferan cytoplasm which had been replaced by ovoidal bodies, 1·25 to 2·5 μm in length and resembling stages in the development of the 'sporocytes' of *Trophosphaera planorbulinae*. Clusters of similar bodies appeared in debris of *S. hyalina* cultures.

Foreign bodies—presumably micro-organisms of uncertain taxonomic position—occur in the cytoplasm of a wide variety of other foraminiferans (Le Calvez, 1939, 1953; Thalmann, 1949; Arnold, 1964).

Two enigmatic symbiotes have been reported from marine rhizopods, one from a

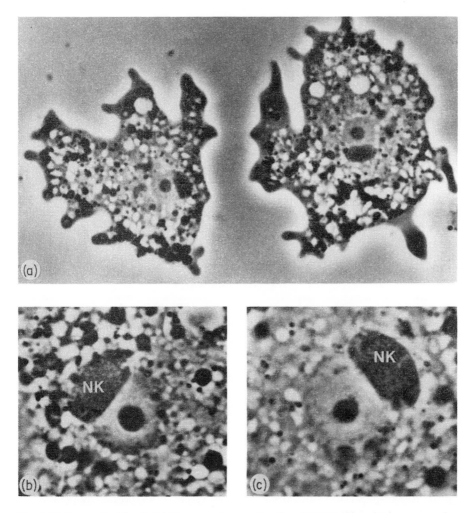

Fig. 3-13: *Paramoeba eilhardi*. (a) Two amoebae, entire view, × 1300; (b) and (c) macronucleus with 'Nebenkörper' (NK), × 3000. (After Grell, 1968; reproduced by permission of Springer-Verlag.)

radiolarian and the other from 2 amoebae. The first one, named *Caryotoma bernardi*, occurs in the endoplasm of *Thalassicolla spumida*. It lies up againt the nucleus of the radiolarian, breaking it into two parts, and engulfing one of these. The systematic position of *C. bernardi* remains unknown (Hollande, 1953; Hollande and Enjumet, 1953).

Free-living *Paramoeba eilhardi* harbour a symbiote resembling a nucleus and termed 'Nebenkörper' or 'secondary nucleus' (Fig. 3-13). Some strains of *P. eilhardi* possess only 1 or 2, but others have 4 or more of these bodies which may divide either synchronously with or independent of the host nucleus. All attempts to obtain viable amoebae without nebenkörper have thus far failed. It appears, therefore, that the symbiote has acquired the role of an 'organella' which is essential for the viability of the host. Nothing else is known about the nature of the nebenkörper (Grell, 1961, 1968). It should, however, be termed 'mutualistic' rather than 'parasitic' (Grell, personal communication).

An endosymbiote of the same kind has been observed in *Paramoeba perniciosa*, a parasitic amoeba causing 'gray crab disease' in decapods *Callinectes sapidus* along the North American Atlantic coast (Sprague and Beckett, 1966, 1968; Sprague and co-authors, 1969). Studies of its nebenkörper by means of electron microscopy (Perkins and Castagna, 1971) ascertained its nature as a discrete organism but revealed nothing else about the interrelationship.

DISEASES CAUSED BY METAZOANS

Agents: Nematoda

An undetermined, minute nematode attacking the foraminiferans *Rotalia turbinata* and *Iridia lucida* was briefly mentioned by Le Calvez (1953). The nematode enters the protozoans through the stomostyl and curls up in the cytoplasm where its eggs are deposited. Infested hosts degenerate slowly.

3.3   SPOROZOA

The sporozoans represent a heterogenous group of Protozoa whose representatives are exclusively parasitic. Hence, reports on parasites of sporozoans actually describe instances of hyperparasitism. Most of the cases described concern gregarines.

DISEASES CAUSED BY MICRO-ORGANISMS

Agents: Bacteria

In the cytoplasm of trophozoites of gregarines *Cystobia* sp., parasitic in sea-cucumbers *Holothuria tubulosa*, Changeux (1961) observed what he believed to be bacteria. Tiny motile micro-organisms have also been reported from *Cystobia stichopi* occurring in holothurians *Stichopus tremulus*, about 1% of the endospores of the gregarine being infected. Such spores were always somewhat larger than normal ones and slightly deformed (Lützen, 1968).

Bacteria were also found by Hesse (1909) in the cytoplasm of monocystid gregarines parasitic in the seminal vesicles of several species of oligochaetes. Each gregarine species appeared to have its own peculiar bacteria, varying in shape from ovoid to filamentous. Bacterial infections were uncommon among the gregarines studied; however, when present, they involved most individuals of a population and frequently led to the destruction of affected hosts.

Agents: Fungi

Several papers report invasion of non-marine gregarines by chytrid fungi, some resembling *Sphaerita* spp. For a detailed review and discussion consult Ball (1969). Records of fungal diseases in sporozoans from marine hosts have not come to the reviewer's attention.

DISEASES CAUSED BY PROTOZOANS

Agents: Sporozoa

Marine gregarines are frequently parasitized by microsporidans. *Nosema frenzelinae* occurs in *Cephaloidophora conformis*, which is parasitic in marine crabs *Pachygrapsus marmoratus* in France (Léger and Duboscq, 1909a, b). Infestations are most frequent in older associated pairs of *C. conformis* but also occur in the gregarine's cysts. Sporulation of the microsporidan is synchronized with sexual reproduction of the host. Infested gamonts associate, encyst and initially behave like healthy ones but eventually gamete formation is inhibited. The authors interpreted this as parasitic castration of the protozoan host. Spores of *N. frenzelinae* are extremely small, measuring only 2·8 µm in length. The microsporidan was fairly common in crab-infesting *C. conformis* from Cavalière (French Mediterranean coast). When present in a crab it destroyed all the gregarines of that host.

Another microsporidan, *Perezia lankesteriae*, a hyperparasite of gregarines *Lankesteria ascidiae* from ascidians *Ciona intestinalis* has also been described by Léger and Duboscq (1909c). A further *Nosema* species, *N. vivieri*, was found hyperparasitic in an unidentified monocystid gregarine living in the coelom of a likewise unspecified marine nemertean from Wimereux (French coast of the English Channel). The spores of this species were ovoidal, measuring 3·5 × 1·2 µm (Vinckier and co-authors, 1970).

Dogiel (1906) assigned to the Coccidia a parasite, named *Hyalosphaera gregarinicola*, of gregarines *Cystobia chiridotae* parasitizing holothurians. Caullery and Mesnil (1919) considered this classification doubtful but were certain that the organism is not a member of the Metchnikovellidae.

The family Metchnikovellidae is abundantly represented in the marine environment; most of the records are from gregarines parasitizing polychaetes (Fig. 3-14). Caullery and Mesnil (1897) first described metchnikovellids from a gregarine, probably *Gregarina spionis* inhabiting the gut of *Spio filicornis (S. martinensis)* collected near Vauville (French coast of the English Channel); they could not, at that time, assign these organisms to any known group. A subsequent series of intense studies (Caullery and Mesnil, 1905, 1914, 1919; Dogiel, 1922) attempted to trace the taxonomic position of the Metchnikovellidae. The authors discussed their affinities with various protistan groups including higher fungi and haplosporidans, but finally concluded that the taxonomic status of these organisms remains uncertain. Later, Caullery (1953)—with all reservations—assigned the metchnikovellids to the Haplosporida but maintained that they could also be included in the Fungi.

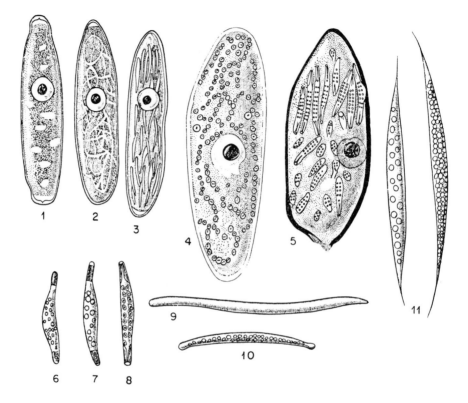

Fig. 3-14: Metchnikovellidae. 1-8: *Metchnikovella spionis* from *Polyrhabdina spionis*, a gregarine parasitic in polychaetes *Spio martinensis;* vegetative stages (1, 2) and sporulation (3); living individuals; 4, 5: sections through fixed and stained specimens, vegetative stage (4) and sporulation (5); 6, 7: living cysts; 8: fixed and stained cyst. 9: *Metchnikovella (Amphiamblys) capitella*; living cyst from unidentified gregarine in *Capitella capitata*. 10: *M. (Amphiamblys) capitellidis*; living cyst from unidentified gregarine in *Capitellides giardi*. 11: *M. (Amphiacantha) longa*; living cysts from *Ophioidina elongata*, a gregarine parasite of *Lumbrineris tingens*. (After Caullery, 1953; reproduced by permission of Masson et Cie.)

On the basis of extensive life-cycle studies of *Amphiacantha ovalis* and *A. attenuata* hyperparasitic in *Lecudina* sp. from Californian polychaetes *Lumbrineris latreilli* and *L. zonata* (Figs 3-15 and 3-16), Stubblefield (1955) arrived at the conclusion that the Metchnikovellidae have to be assigned to the Haplosporida. Vivier (1965), however, studying the ultrastructure of the spore of *Metchnikovella hovassei* hyperparasitic in gregarines *Lecudina pellucida* from *Perinereis cultrifera* in French waters, showed these protozoans to belong to the Microsporida.

The information available on Metchnikovellidae and their respective hosts has been reviewed and presented in tabular form by Caullery and Mesnil (1914, 1919) and

Stubblefield (1955). Thus far, 21 species—members of the genera *Metchnikovella*, *Amphiamblys*, *Amphiacantha* and *Caulleryetta*—have been reported from gregarines in marine polychaetes. *M. hessei* occurs in *Monocystis mitis*, a gregarine parasite in terrestrial oligochaetes *Fridericia polychaeta* (Hesse, 1909).

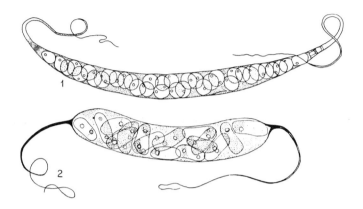

Fig. 3-15: Metchnikovellidae. Gametocysts of 2 species of *Amphiacantha*, parasitic in gregarines *Lecudina* sp. from *Lumbrineris latreilli*. 1: *A. attenuata*; 2: *A. ovalis*. (After Stubblefield, 1955; reproduced by permission of Journal of Parasitology.)

Metchnikovella berliozi (Fig. 3-17) is the first representative of its group reported from gregarines living in a non-annelid host. Arvy (1952) described it as a hyperparasite of *Lecudina franciana* occurring in the intestine of sipunculids *Phascolion strombi* from Dinard (French coast of the English Channel). While infested gregarines are found quite frequently in annelids, the sipunculid hyperparasite appeared to be of rare occurrence, the gregarine population in only 8 of 300 *P. strombi* being invaded by *M. berliozi*. Mackinnon and Ray (1931), who often observed metchnikovellids in gregarines from polychaetes *Malacoceros (Scolelepis) fuliginosa* and *Polydora flava* from Plymouth (England), emphasized that they never encountered similar organisms in gregarines *Hentschelia thalassemae* and *Lecythion thalassemae* recorded from the alimentary tract of *Phascolion strombi* in the same area.

Little information is available regarding the effects that metchnikovellids exert on their gregarine hosts. According to Caullery and Mesnil (1897, 1914, 1919) injury is but slight, particularly in the host's vegetative stages. What effect there is appears to be mainly mechanical. Heavily infested gamonts, however, are believed to be incapable of completing their sexual development.

Metchnikovella spionis and *M. caulleryi*, infesting *Polyrhabdina spionis* and *P. polydora*, in the polychaetes *Malacoceros fuliginosa* and *Polydora flava*, respectively, apparently cause degeneration of the host nucleus (Mackinnon and Ray, 1931). Ganapati and Aiyar (1937) observed a metchnikovellid (according to Stubblefield, 1955, possibly a species of *Amphiacantha*) in *Lecudina brasili* from *Lumbrineris* sp. They stated that during heavy infestations the entire host cytoplasm may be packed with cysts, the body of the gregarine becomes misshapen and the nucleus seemingly degenerates. Parasitized indi-

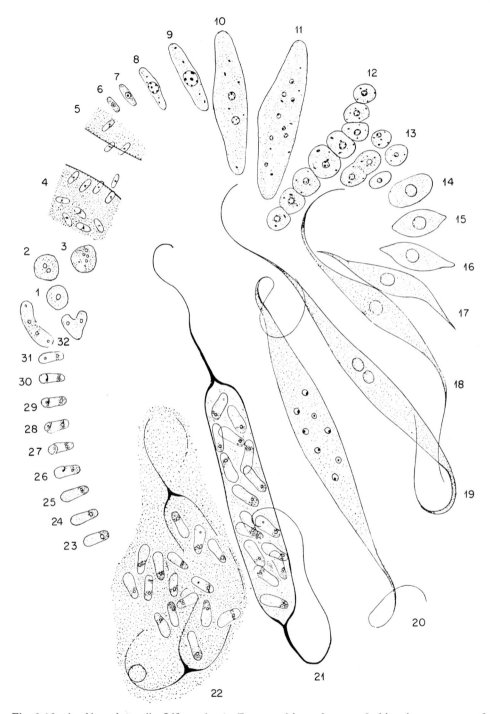

Fig. 3-16: *Amphiacantha ovalis*. Life cycle. 1: Zygote with synkaryon; 2: binucleate sporont; 3: tetranucleate sporont; 4, 5: sporozoites in host cytoplasm, and probable method of transfer from host to host; 6-11: growth stages developing from sporozoites; 12, 13: conclusion of

viduals of *L. brasili* were not observed to associate. Stubblefield (1955), studying *Amphiacantha ovalis* and *A. attenuata* hyperparasitic in *Lecudina* sp. from the polychaete *Lumbrineris* sp., believed that impoverishment of the gregarine cytoplasm, as a direct result of overcrowding, appears to be the only specific evidence of the destructive action of these microsporidans.

A number of further hyperparasites of gregarines, most of them with microsporidan affinities, have been briefly mentioned by Caullery and Mesnil (1919).

Microsporida have also been noted as hyperparasites of Myxosporida. Kudo (1924, 1944) reported *Nosema marionis* in *Ceratomyxa (Leptotheca) coris* from the gall bladder of Mediterranean teleosts *Coris julis*. *N. notabilis* was found to invade *Sphaerospora polymorpha*, parasitizing the fishes *Opsanus tau* and *O. beta*. The hosts' generative nuclei were found to be hypertrophied and degenerate, and no spore formation took place.

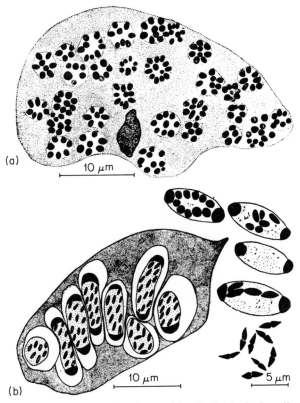

Fig. 3-17: *Lecudina franciana*. (a) Individual heavily parasitized by *Metchnikovella berliozi*; transverse section through cysts containing parasites. (b) Longitudinal section through cysts. (After Arvy, 1952; reproduced by permission of Laboratoire maritime de Dinard.)

schizogony to produce trophozoites; 14-21: gametocyst development; 22: disintegration of gametocyst within cytoplasm of host, *Lecudina* sp.; 23-31: maturation of gametocytes; 32: cytoplasmic fusion of isogametes to produce prozygote. (After Stubblefield, 1955; reproduced by permission of American Society of Parasitologists.)

3.4   CILIATA

DISEASES CAUSED BY MICRO-ORGANISMS

Agents: Viruses

Apparently, no true virus diseases of ciliates have been described. Several species are, however, known as carriers and vectors of virus diseases of higher animals, including man. Kovacs and co-authors (1966) reported on experimental propagation of mammalian EMC virus in the ciliate genus *Tetrahymena*, and Kovacs and Bucz (1967) isolated complete picornaviruses from species of *Tetrahymena* experimentally infected with picornaviral particles or their infectious RNA. In a third paper, Kovacs and co-authors (1967) reported on changes in population density, viability and multiplication of human encephalomyocarditis virus from experimentally infected *Tetrahymena*.

Experiments of this kind have been extended considerably during the past years, and it has been shown that a variety of animal and human viruses are capable of not only persisting but also of multiplying in free-living ciliates, flagellates and amoebae.

Serial laboratory experiments employing picorna-, adeno- and myxoviruses, as well as a number of protozoans, demonstrated that in 104 out of 130 such combinations between protozoans and viruses no interaction occurred among both partners. In the remaining 26 associations, either inactivation or multiplication and persistence of the viruses were observed. Depending on the nature of the association, one particular protozoan species may be indifferent to one or several types of viruses whereas other viruses can multiply or be inactivated (Teras and co-authors, 1977).

Ciliate cultures exposed to suspensions of picornaviruses and having incorporated the pathogens, remained infectious for 10 to 14 days. In the course of the following 30 passages no essential changes were observed in the infectivity of either ciliate cultures or suspensions prepared from them although, beginning with the second passage, the protozoans were cultivated without the addition of picornaviruses. It was suspected that associations of this kind between protozoans and viruses may occur in nature, and that free-living protozoans may, under certain circumstances, become potential sources of virus infections (Kesa and Teras, 1977).

Marine hymenostomes *Miamiensis avidus*, experimentally infected with IPN virus in trout-cell tissue cultures, were able to transmit the virus to sea horses. Although it has not been demonstrated that *M. avidus* serves as an IPN carrier in nature, its role as a potential virus vector should be taken into consideration. The protozoan lives as a facultative parasite in skin tumours of sea horses (Moewus, 1963; Moewus-Kobb, 1965a, b).

Agents: Bacteria

A great number of bacteria are associated ectobiotically or endobiotically with ciliates. The interrelationships in many of these associations have not yet been studied closely enough to reveal their proper nature but at least part of them are obviously mutualistic. The older literature discussing ciliate–bacteria associations has been reviewed by Kirby (1941) and Ball (1969).

More recently, Fenchel and co-authors (1977) studied, by means of electron microscopy, the relationship between marine estuarine anaerobic ciliates and their bacterial ecto- and endosymbiotes. It was speculated that the bacteria may utilize the metabolic end products of the Protozoa for growth and energy yielding processes.

Epibiotic bacteria, adhering longitudinally to the pellicle of their hosts, have also been described from ciliates of the genus *Cyclidium* inhabiting the gut of Atlantic and Pacific sea urchins—a different type from each species (Powers, 1933, 1936; Fig. 3-18). Kahl (1933) maintained that adherent bacteria are advantageous symbiotes, contributing somehow to the nutrition of their ciliate hosts. Even though this is mere speculation, there appear, on the other hand, to arise no detrimental effects upon the host from this association.

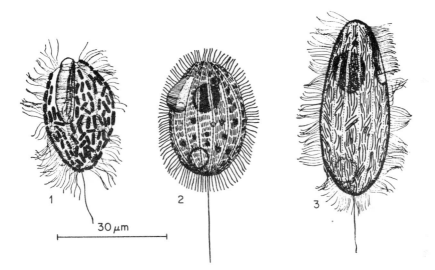

30 μm

Fig. 3-18: *Cyclidium* spp. Characteristic bacteria adhering to pellicle. 1: *C. rhabdotectum*; 2: *C. ozakii*; 3: *C. stercoris*. (After Powers, 1936; reproduced by permission of Carnegie Institution, Washington.)

The relationship between ciliates and bacteria living in the cytoplasm or in the nucleus is closer than that of surface forms since these endobiotes must derive all nutriment from, and discharge their metabolic wastes into, the body of the host. Associations of this kind cover the entire range of interorganismic relationships—from mutualism to true parasitism, i.e. pathogenicity.

Flexuous rods, 8 to 20 μm long, were seen in the cytoplasm of all individuals of peritrichs *Ellobiophrya donacis* from marine bivalves *Donax vittatus* but did not occur in the mantle cavity of the ciliates' host (Chatton and Lwoff, 1929). The bacteria were not corroded and frequently showed division. The authors concluded that these micro-organisms are specific symbiotes.

Bacteria from the macronucleus of the non-marine peritrich *Vorticella* sp. *(similis?)* have been described by Kirby (1942). Infection caused hypertrophy, particularly in the region of highest pathogen concentrations (Fig. 3-19). Von Stein (1859) mistook similar fine straight rods in hypertrophied macronuclei of *Paramecium caudatum* for reproductive elements of the ciliate.

Bacterial endosymbiotes, as well as bacteria-like 'particles' and associated viral structures have been most thoroughly studied in members of the non-marine genus *Paramecium* (Sonneborn, 1959; Soldo, 1963, 1974; van Wagtendonk, 1969; Soldo and Merlin, 1972; Stevenson, 1972; and others). These will not here be considered further.

An interesting case of immunity of a ciliate to bacterial infection has been reported by Roux and co-authors (1964). When grown with *Escherichia coli, Tetrahymena pyriformis* developed into a strain resistant to a toxic factor produced by the bacteria. Moreover, a specific agglutination by *Tetrahymena* sp. of various species of *Salmonella* occurs. For instance, a strain grown with *S. paratyphi* B will agglutinate this strain, but not *S. paratyphi* A.

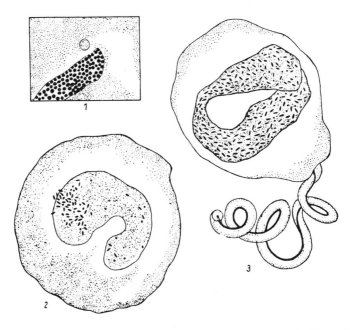

Fig. 3-19: *Vorticella* sp. *(similis?)*. Bacterial infection of macronucleus. 1: Normal macronucleus with deep-staining chromatin granules. 2: Macronucleus with bacteria, showing hypertrophy mainly in region of greatest pathogen numbers; few bacteria occur in host cytoplasm. 3: Macronucleus with heavy bacterial infection. (After Kirby, 1942; reproduced by permission of Journal of Parasitology.)

Ninety-five percent of the zooids of *Zoothamnium pelagicum*, a planktonic colonial marine peritrich, displayed brownish pigmentation. This discolouration was most obvious in structurally modified macrozooids. Electron-microscopic examination revealed that the pigment accumulation was caused by the presence of bacteria which occurred in the macronucleus but never in the micronucleus. Two types of micro-organisms—'B1' measuring 0.4×1 μm and 'B2', 0.45×1.5 μm—could be distinguished. 'B1' always maintained direct contact with the host nucleoplasm and frequently with the nucleolar region; this type was frequently seen dividing. In contrast, Type 'B2' was never observed to divide. Its position within the macronucleus was variable, generally in the centre, but also in contact with the nuclear membrane which was then deformed, suggesting passage of the bacterium across the membrane into the cytoplasm. Transitional stages between 'B1' and 'B2' were also observed and it was assumed that bacteria of the first type gradually transform into Type 'B2' and pass from the macronucleus into the cytoplasm of infected macrozooids where they degenerate, leaving behind a distinct pigment granule (Laval, 1970).

Rod-shaped structures appear in the loricae of degenerating peritrichs *Lagenophrys lunatus* which live on the carapace of brackish-water palaemonid shrimps (Debaisieux, 1958). The structure of these bodies leads one to speculate that they might be bacteria.

Agents: Fungi

A fungus assigned to the Saprolegniales infected more than 50% of a population of the marine suctorian *Acineta tuberosa* from Roscoff (France). Developing within the cytoplasm, the agent destroys the cell and forms isolated spheres in the empty lorica. Subsequently, these spheres give rise to long tubes, coiled up in the lorica or projecting to the exterior. One of the tubes terminated in a large, spherical sporangium (Sand, 1899).

DISEASES CAUSED BY PROTOZOANS

Agents: Flagellata

The flagellate *Leptomonas karyophilus* parasitizes *Paramecium trichium*. There is a certain balance in the host-parasite system as long as division rates of the ciliate are high. Under conditions of semi-starvation, the host's macronucleus becomes so overrun with dividing flagellates that they eventually fill the entire nucleus and kill the ciliate (Gillies and Hanson, 1963). Cultures of the peritrich *Stentor coeruleus*, fed on colourless euglenoids of the genus *Astasia*, were destroyed by the 'food' organism. Instead of being digested, the flagellates moved about in the food vacuoles for several hours without being destroyed. When liberated from the food vacuoles by the experimentor, they exhibited normal behaviour and no signs of damage. In heavily infested *S. coeruleus*, the cytoplasm was totally overrun with flagellates which obviously had escaped from the surrounding food vacuoles. Infested stentors remained in a semi-contracted state, while the cytoplasm exhibited progressive vacuolization, which finally resulted in degeneration and death of the host. In some instances, intact flagellates abandoned hosts undergoing lysis. Schönfeld (1959) suggests that the parasite might be responsible for the dissolution of the vacuole membrane. He was able to demonstrate a direct toxic effect of the flagellate's metabolic products on the ciliate. Addition of filtered *Astasia* culture medium caused degeneration and death of *S. coeruleus*.

Marine ciliates are hosts for a variety of parasitic peridineans. *Amoebophrya rosei* has been reported from foettingeriids which, in turn, parasitize Mediterranean siphonophores *Abylopsis tetragona*. *A. tintinni* occurs in Mediterranean tintinnids *Xystonella lohmanni* (Cachon, 1964).

Several peridineans of the genus *Duboscquella* have been described, mainly from marine tintinnids. Early authors mistook these endoparasitic dinoflagellates for stages in the hosts' life cycle. Thus, Haeckel (1873; cited by Cachon, 1964) believed them to be 'embryos', and Laackmann (1906) took them for sporocysts with micro- and macrospores. Finally, Lohmann (1908) and Entz (1909) recognized their peridinean nature by the morphology of their spores; Duboscq and Collin (1910) made the first life-cycle studies.

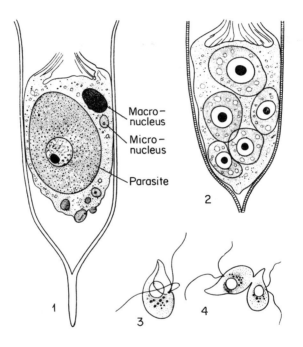

Fig. 3-20: *Favella ehrenbergii*. 1: Individual parasitized by *Duboscquella tintinnicola*; 2: individual harbouring 5 parasites; 3: *D. tintinnicola*, gamete; 4: copulation of 2 gametes differing slightly in size. (After Chatton, 1952; reproduced by permission of Masson et Cie.)

Duboscquella tintinnicola and *D. anisospora* (Figs 3-20 and 3-21) parasitize tintinnids of the genera *Codonella*, *Tintinnopsis*, *Favella* (*Cyttarocylis*), *Tintinnus* and *Rhabdonella* (Chatton, 1920b, 1952). Hofker (1931) found *D. tintinnicola* in *Favella ehrenbergii* and *F. helgolandica*. In waters off Alger (Mediterranean Sea), *F. ehrenbergii* frequently harbours *D. aspida* and *D. cnemata*. In some plankton samples virtually no uninfested individuals are found. *D. aspida* also parasitizes tintinnids *Coxliella lacinosa*, *Codonella campanula* and *Tintinnus fraknoii* in the Mediterranean (Cachon, 1964).

Infestation of tintinnids by *Duboscquella aspida* appears to occur passively, in that spores of the parasite are ingested and phagocytized like normal food organisms. Growth within the host is fast; trophonts reach the adult stage within 3 to 4 days. Towards the end of its development, the parasite becomes phagotrophic, devouring most of the host's cytoplasm. Eventually, it becomes extracytoplasmic but completes its sporulation within the tintinnid's lorica. Multiple infestations may be seen in individual hosts, size differences among the parasites reflecting successive infestations (Fig. 3-20). Normally, *Duboscquella aspida* infestations are fatal for the tintinnids, and loricae may be seen in the plankton which only harbour the parasite. Mature spores escape from the empty lorica, sometimes completing their last divisions in the open water.

Duboscq and Collin (1910), who observed *Duboscquella tintinnicola* to occur abundantly in *Favella ehrenbergii* from Sète (French Mediterranean coast), stated that the parasite's

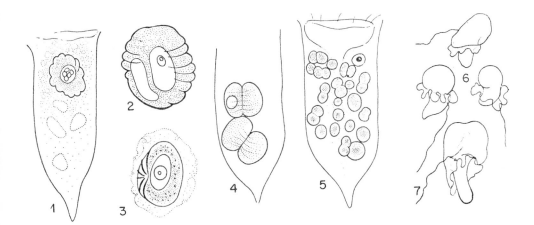

Fig. 3-21: *Favella ehrenbergii*. 1: Individual parasitized by *Duboscquella anisospora*; 2, 3: parasite excised from host showing cuticular striations; 4: bipartition of parasite; 5: gamete differentiation; 6: microgametes; 7: macrogamete. (After Chatton, 1952; reproduced by permission of Masson et Cie.)

subspherical body grew to a large size (about 100 μm) without apparent inconvenience to the host. Cachon (1964), on the other hand, reported that rapid population declines of *F. ehrenbergii* in previously flourishing populations observed off Alger coincided with maximum infestation incidences of *D. aspida*. The disappearance of *F. ehrenbergii* from the plankton was, therefore, attributed to *Duboscquella* attacks.

If *Favella ehrenbergii* happens to survive a *Duboscquella aspida* infestation, it rejects the parasite, which may then be found degenerated and clinging to the peduncle of the host. Sometimes, tintinnids may rid themselves of an infestation. Expelled trophonts usually succumb but if they have developed to almost maturity (although still being osmotrophic), they may complete their development outside the host (Cachon, 1964).

Holotrichs of the genus *Prorodon* and oligotrichs of the genera *Strombidium* and *Strombilidium* from inshore waters off Alger (Mediterranean Sea) harbour another *Duboscquella* species, *D. caryophaga* which, although living in the cytoplasm, attacks the macronucleus from the outside. From infested ciliates, the macronucleus disappears almost entirely (Cachon, 1964).

Parasitic peridineans of the genus *Duboscquodinium*, which is similar to but distinct from *Duboscquella*, have been described from tintinnids. Thus, *Duboscquodinium collini* parasitizes *Tintinnus fraknoii*, and *Codonella campanula* is host for *D. kofoidi* (Chatton, 1952; Fig. 3-22).

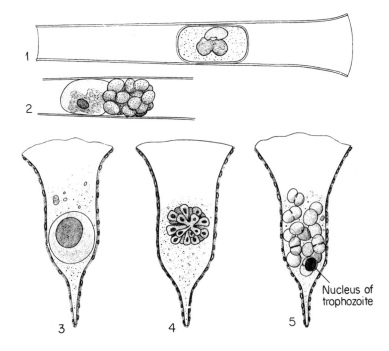

Fig. 3-22: 1, 2: *Tintinnus fraknoi*; individuals parasitized by *Duboscquodinium collini*; nuclear division (1) resulting in gymnospore formation (2); left: degenerating trophozoite. 3-5: *Codonella campanula*; individuals parasitized by *Duboscquodium kofoid*; 3: trophozoite within host body; 4: gametocyte formation; 5: gymnospores in process of differentiation. (After Chatton, 1952; reproduced by permission of Masson et Cie.)

A parasite of vague dinoflagellate affinities has been seen in *Tintinnopsis nucula* by Campbell (1926). Named *Karyoclastis tintinni*, the organism is primarily an intranuclear parasite but it also has a cytoplasmic phase. In the host's macronucleus the parasite occurs in the form of numerous small bodies. During multiplication, the nuclear membrane undergoes partial disintegration and the parasites emerge, forming a cloud-like mass in the host's cytoplasm. According to Kirby (1941), the dinoflagellate affinities of this organism are doubted by most authorities. However, Cachon (1964) noticed some resemblances of certain developmental stages of *K. tintinni* to corresponding stages in the life cycle of *Duboscquella aspida*, and Hofker (1931) referred to similarities between *K. tintinni* and small round bodies, which appeared to be the end-product of a fragmentation phenomenon, in the lorica of *Tintinnopsis fimbriata*.

Enigmatic parasites recorded from marine ciliates include *Sporomonas infusorium* (Fig. 3-23), encountered in *Folliculina elegans*, *Vortucella* sp. and once in *Lacrymaria lagenula* in French waters by Chatton and Lwoff (1924). Potts (cited by Kirby, 1941) found *S. infusorium* in *Folliculina ampulla* near Woods Hole (Massachusetts, USA). In its early stage, the parasite occurs as reniform bodies, 5 to 6 μm long, constantly rotating due to the action of a laterally inserted flagellum which disappears when the organism has attained a size of 10 to 12 μm. Growth terminates at a body length of about 70 μm, when the parasite is expelled and undergoes multiplication outside the host. Repeated nuclear and cytoplasmic divisions without growth (palintomy) result in a great number of small, virgulate bodies provided with a single lateral flagellum. Chatton and Lwoff (1924) considered *S. infusorium* a flagellate but discussed its resemblance to chytrid fungi. Although provisionally grouping this parasite with zoo-flagellates of uncertain systematic position, Grassé (1952) suggests it should possibly be included in the Chytridiales.

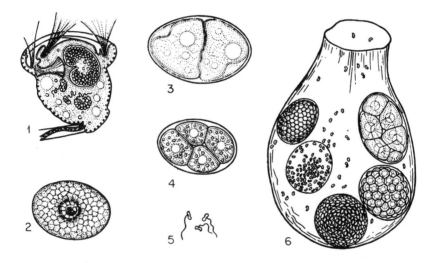

Fig. 3-23: *Sporomonas infusorium*. 1: *Vorticella* sp. containing 4 *S. infusorium* of which 3 are very young and flagellated; 2: large *S. infusorium* liberated from host; 3, 4: first and second division; 5: free flagellated spores; 6: posterior body end of *Folliculina elegans* containing *S. infusorium* in various stages of development. (After Chatton and Lwoff, from Grassé, 1952; reproduced by permission of Masson et Cie.)

Gregarella fabrearum (Fig. 3-24) is another enigmatic organism reported from halophilic ciliates *Fabrea salina* by Chatton and Brachon (1936) and Chatton and Villeneuve (1937), who considered it to represent a much regressed flagellate. Individuals of *G. fabrearum* occur either within the host's food vacuoles or adhere to the outside of its body, mostly near the cytopyge. The organisms are capable of slowly changing their shape; they contain large refractile inclusions, and are devoid of flagella or other permanent differentiations. *G. fabrearum* can survive for some time independent of their host; after a while, they assume a spherical shape but remain unencysted.

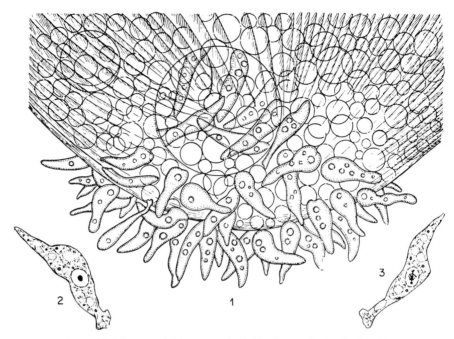

Fig. 3-24: *Gregarella fabrearum.* 1: Numerous individuals attached to body of *Fabrea salina;*
2, 3: fixed and stained specimens; ×1500. (After Chatton and Villeneuve, 1937;
reproduced by permission of Centre National de la Recherche Scientifique.)

Agents: Rhizopoda

Parasitization of ciliates by rhizopods appears to be extremely rare. Chatton (1910)
described the very small species *Amoeba mucicola* as an endoparasite of peritrichs
Trichodina labrorum which, in turn, live on the gills of labrid fishes. Wetzel (1926) reported
on heliozoans *Raphidocystis infestans* which normally prey upon small flagellates but can,
under certain conditions, attack various species of freshwater ciliates and become
temporary parasites.

Agents: Sporozoa

Sporozoan infestations seem to be rare in ciliates. Krüger (1956) described
microsporidan spores which he observed in freshwater peritrichs *Campanella umbellaria*;
these had been considered to be 'nematocysts' by previous investigators. Krüger
proposed the name *Glugea campanellae* for this inadequately described species, known
only in the spore stage.

Cytoplasmic parasites of *Lagenophrys lunatus*, a peritrich living on the carapace of
brackish-water palaemonid shrimps, appear in the form of chains, spheres, morulae or
plasmodia. The organism, which has not been identified, seems to be pathogenic to its
host (Debaisieux, 1958). Whether it can be assigned to the sporozoans remains to be
investigated.

About 70% of astomatids *Spirobütschliella chattoni*, parasitizing serpulid polychaetes *Pomatoceros triqueter* at Banyuls (French Mediterranean coast), were found to be hyperparasitized by microsporidans *Gurleya nova*. The smallest stages found, about 2 µm in diameter, were amoeboid and occurred either within the cytoplasm or in the macronucleus of *S. chattoni* where they were seen to divide abundantly. Larger stages, apparently sporoblasts, produced bi- and tetranucleated forms which developed into spores. Infested hosts seemingly divided as frequently as healthy individuals. If, however, the macronucleus was invaded, signs of nuclear degeneration became apparent (Hovasse, 1950).

Agents: Ciliata

Parasitic ciliates belong to various orders. Those attacking marine ciliates are mostly holotrichs of the orders Thigmotrichida and Apostomatida, as well as a variety of Suctoria.

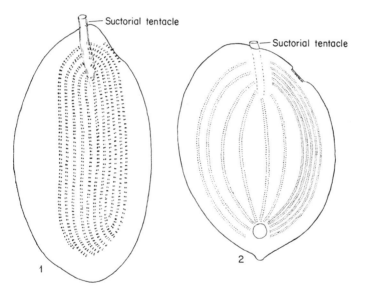

Fig. 3-25: 1: *Hypocoma parasitica* from *Zoothamnium* spp.; 2: *Heterocoma hyperparasitica* from *Trichophrya salparum*. (After Chatton and Lwoff, 1939; reproduced by permission of Gauthiers-Villars, Paris.)

While members of the Hypocomidae—like most other thigmotrichs—usually occur on molluscs, the genus *Hypocoma* is engaged in a parasitic relationship with other Protozoa. *Hypocoma parasitica* (Fig. 3-25, 1) is known from Mediterranean colonial peritrichs of the genus *Zoothamnium* (Gruber, 1884). Plate (1888) recognized a second species, *H.* (*'Acinetoides'*) *zoothamni*. The generic name chosen by Plate (1888) indicates that, at that time, the hypocomids were believed to be acinetid suctorians (Collin, 1907). However, there can be no doubt that they belong to the Hypocomidae (Chatton and Lwoff, 1923).

Hypocoma acinetarum attacks *Ephelota gemmipara*, *Acineta papillifera*, as well as several other free-living suctorians (Collin, 1907). *Heterocoma hyperparasitica* (Fig. 3-25, 2) has been reported from *Trichophrya salparum* parasitizing a species of *Salpa* (Chatton and Lwoff, 1939). As has been emphasized by Ball (1969), these associations represent an interesting relationship since suctorians usually parasitize ciliates, rather than ciliates parasitizing suctorians. The parasites firmly attach to the host, chiefly at the base of the stalk, pierce the pellicle by means of their anterior suctorial tentacle, and suck out the cytoplasm. The presence of *H. acinetarum* on *E. gemmipara* may lead to a fragmentation of the nucleus and to degeneration of the entire cytoplasmic mass.

Individual *Ephelota gemmipara* may have numerous *Hypocoma acinetarum* attached to their outside. In other cases, hypocomids occur within the host cell, eating away the cytoplasm from the interior. These 'endoparasites' probably originate from an individual that had succeeded in penetrating, in some unknown fashion, through the pellicle of *E. gemmipara* (Grell, 1967).

Members of the apostomatid genus *Phtorophrya* are characteristically hyperparasitic or live phoretic on the phoronts of other apostomes (Chatton and Lwoff, 1935). *Phtorophrya fallax* occurs on *Gymnodinioides inkystans* on shore crabs *Carcinus maenas*, and *P. insidiosa* on the phoronts of *G. corophii* on amphipods (Chatton and co-authors, 1930). It is interesting to note that both host and parasite—or parasite and hyper-parasite—are members of the same family, the Foettingeriidae.

Suctorians may be associated with ciliates as ecto- and endoparasites; other associations have been reported which merely represent cases of phoresis or, taking into account the relative sizes of the partners involved, assume the relationship of predator and prey, rather than that of parasite and host.

Ectoparasitic suctorians *Pottsia infusoriorum* have been found mainly on spirotrichs *Folliculina ampulla* and—rarely—*F. elegans*, but they occurred also on the peritrichs *Cothurnia socialis* and *C. ingenita*. In the aquarium of Monaco, up to 75% of the *F. ampulla* were infested with as many as 22 suctorians. The parasites occurred on the body surface of the folliculinid, within the lorica, their 4 tentacles deeply penetrating into the host's cytoplasm. Embryos, developing endogenously by budding, swim actively when released from the parent individual, and attach to the same folliculinid by means of terminal sucking tubes (Chatton and Lwoff, 1927). When the number of *P. infusoriorum* is large, the host may undergo degeneration and eventually die. The suctorians can survive for some time among the remains but gradually perish within the lorica.

A suctorian, similar to or identical with *Pottsia infusoriorum*, parasitizes folliculinids *Platyfolliculina paguri* which live attached to hermit crabs *Pagurus pubescens* from Frenchman's Bay (Maine, USA), as well as *Parafolliculina amphora* and *Metafolliculina andrewsi* from Chesapeake Bay (Maryland, USA). Fatal infestations by these suctorians were believed to account for the many empty *Platyfolliculina paguri* loricae seen on *Pagurus pubescens* (Andrews and Reinhard, 1943).

Of particular interest are associations involving suctorians which are parasitized by other suctorians. Several such cases, a few marine, have been reported.

Suctorians of the genus *Pseudogemma* occur, attached by a short, stout peduncle, on the body of suctorians of the genus *Acineta*. *P. fraiponti* lives on *A. dirisa*, *P. pachystyla* on *A. tuberosa* and *P. keppeni* on *A. papillifera* (Collin, 1909, 1912). They reproduce by internal budding. Since tentacles are absent in the epiphoront, and since the fixation organella is deeply embedded in the host cytoplasm, Collin (1912) has suggested that the *Pseudogemma* peduncle may have an absorptive function. Some stages in the development of *P. keppeni*—sometimes external and sometimes almost entirely internal in position—remind one of similar stages occurring in the life cycle of *Tachyblaston ephelotensis*. Collin (1912) assumes that they might furnish a natural transition from *Pseudogemma* to *Endosphaera* (see below).

Complex situations, illustrating the diversity of protozoan–protozoan interrelationships, arise from associations which involve more than 2 partners. One such example is that described by Fauré-Fremiet (1943) from a non-marine association. A peritrich, *Glossatella piscicola*, living attached to the fins of a stickleback, carried another peritrich, *Epistylis lwoffi*, as epiphoront. The latter was attached to the fish epibiote by means of a rigid 'ring'. Also attached to *G. piscicola* was the suctorian *Erastophrya chattoni* (Fig. 3-26). It is possible that, in such associations, the suctorian feeds, at least occasionally or to a limited extent, on its living substrate.

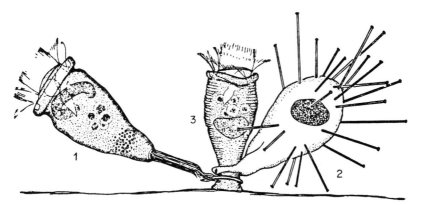

Fig. 3-26: Vorticellid *Epistylis lwoffi* (1) and suctorian *Erastophrya chattoni* (2), attached to vorticellid *Glossatella piscicola* (3). (After Fauré-Fremiet, 1943; reproduced by permission of Société Zoologique de France.)

Tachyblaston ephelotensis, as described by Martin (1909), has a curious, aberrant life cycle, involving both an external phoretic existence on suctorians *Ephelota gemmipara* with multiplication and an endoparasitic phase, also with multiplication. Discussing Martin's (1909) findings, Kirby (1941, p. 1085) stated that

'It seems not impossible that reinvestigation will show that two organisms have been confused in this cycle, since it is so unlike the life histories of other Suctoria'.

Restudying the species, Grell (1950), ascertained that the life cycle of *Tachyblaston ephelotensis* is characterized by an alternation of 2 asexually reproducing generations (Figs 3-27 to 3-30). The early free-swimming—so-called dactylozoite—stage, devoid of cilia and equipped with a single finger-like tentacle, becomes attached to the pellicle of *Ephelota gemmipara*. The suctorial organella penetrates the pellicle and the young parasite sucks out host cytoplasm. As it grows to a considerable size, a deep pellicular invagination forms in the host body which accommodates the entire body of *T. ephelotensis*, leaving only a narrow connection to the exterior. This 'obscured ectoparasitic' stage has been interpreted as endoparasitic (Martin, 1909). Ciliated 'swarmers' (called 'spores' by Martin) form by consecutive external budding and leave the parent individual. They are, however, not able to invade a new host directly but become attached after a brief period of free existence, to an *E. gemmipara* peduncle. There they develop a stalked, club-shaped capsule within which about 16 dactylozoites are formed consecutively from the mother cell by continuous budding.

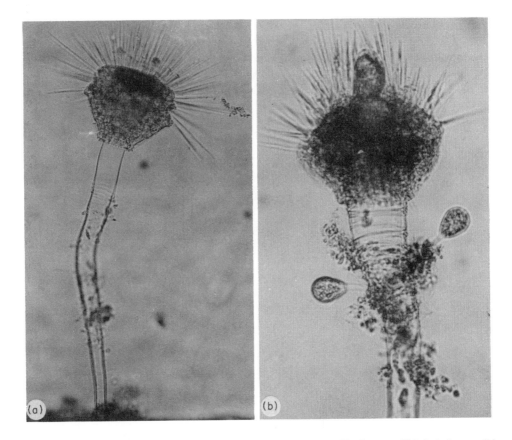

Fig. 3-27: *Ephelota gemmipara*. (a) Individual attached to stolon of hydrozoan *Tubularia larynx*; (b) individual parasitized by suctorian *Tachyblaston ephelotensis*. One swarmer on top and 2 young *Dactylophrya* stages on stalk. (After Grell, 1968; reproduced by permission of Springer-Verlag.)

No food is taken up at this stage and no further growth occurs. The epiphoretic stage of *Tachyblaston ephelotensis* has already been described by Collin (1909) who believed it to be a separate species of suctorian and named it *Dactylophrya roscovita*. Before the budding process is terminated, the distal portion of the lorica-like capsule dissolves and the dactylozoites are released, singly or in groups, to the exterior. Frequently, numerous empty *Dactylophrya* capsules may be seen attached to the stalks of infested *Ephelota gemmipara*. Transport of dactylozoites, which are not capable of individual locomotion, and infestation of new hosts probably occur passively. *T. ephelotensis* is strictly host-specific, infesting only *E. gemmipara* (Grell, 1949, 1950, 1967, 1969).

Suctorians of the genera *Sphaerophrya* and *Endosphaera* live as internal parasites of other Ciliophora and have a wide variety of hosts, mostly in fresh water. Of these endobiotes, *Endosphaera* has more thoroughly adapted to a parasitic way of life. It does not occur free-living, except for a brief motile phase serving the parasite's dissemination. *Endosphaera* has been reported from a variety of freshwater vorticellids of the genera *Vorticella*, *Zoothamnium*, *Epistylis*, *Carchesium*, *Trichodina* and *Opisthonecta*. All these forms were

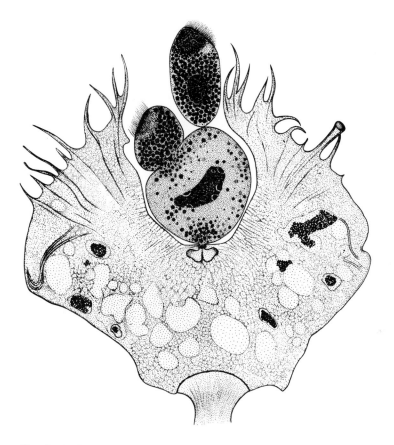

Fig. 3-28: *Ephelota gemmipara*. Individual parasitized by *Tachyblaston ephelotensis*. Note suctorial tentacle of parasite (with bud and fully developed embryo or 'swarmer') embedded in host's cytoplasm. × 580. (After Grell, 1950; reproduced by permission of Springer-Verlag.)

assigned to 1 species, *E. engelmanni* (Lynch and Noble, 1931). Other species have been described from suctorians.

Endosphaera engelmanni is also known from marine peritrichs *Trichodina spheroidesi* and *T. halli* infesting puffer fishes *Sphaeroides maculatus* (Padnos and Nigrelli, 1947). The parasite enters the host by penetrating its pellicle to which it remains attached by a short **stalk through which passes** a canal terminating in a birth pore (Fig. 3-31). The young form of *E. engelmanni*, as well as the free-living swarmer and the bud within the parent

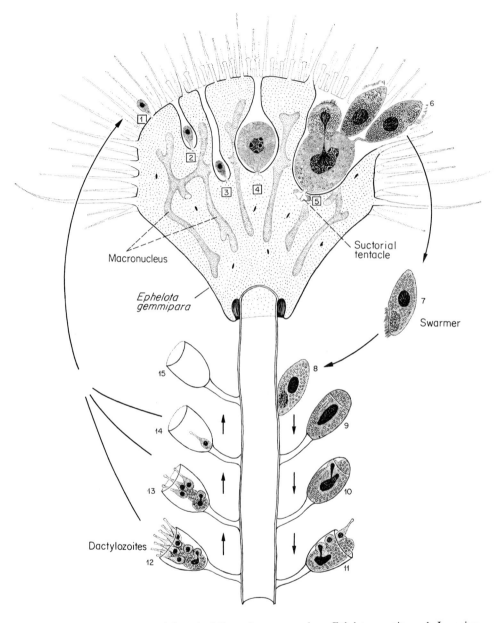

Fig. 3-29: *Tachyblaston ephelotensis*. Life-cycle stages on host *Ephelota gemmipara*. 1: Invasive stage (dactylozoite) attaching to and piercing host pellicle; 2-4: growing dactylozoites inducing deep invaginations in host pellicle; 5: fully grown individual forming several external buds; 6: swarmer detaching from parent individual; 7: free-swimming swarmer; 8: swarmer attaching to substrate (here: peduncle of host); 9: swarmer developing into stalked *Dactylophrya* stage; 10-11: dissolution of anterior capsule portion and formation of dactylozoites; 12-14: *Dactylophrya* stage liberating fully developed dactylozoites; 15: empty residual capsule. (After Grell, 1950; reproduced by permission of Springer-Verlag.)

cell, measure from 9 to 16 μm in diameter. During reproduction by endogenous budding, the cell diameter increases to twice its original size.

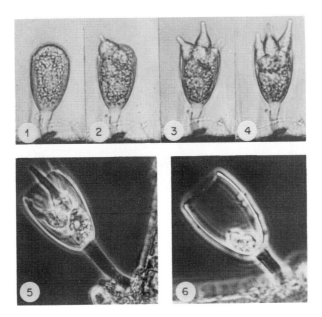

Fig. 3-30: *Tachyblaston ephelotensis. Dactylophrya* stages
attached to peduncle of host *Ephelota gemmipara.* 1: Young
individual with closed, stalked capsule; 2-4: dissolution
of anterior capsule portion and formation of
dactylozoites; × 460. 5: *Dactylophrya* showing capsule
aperture and a few remaining dactylozoites; 6: empty
residual capsule; × 500. (After Grell, 1968; reproduced
by permission of Springer-Verlag.)

Endosphaera engelmanni occurred in about 20% of the *Trichodina spheroidesi* and in 2% of
the *T. halli* examined. Up to 3 parasites were seen in a single host. The parasite apparently interferes with the normal development of the ciliate by exerting pressure on its
cytoplasm and macronucleus. In many of the single infestations and in all of the double
and triple infestations, the host macronucleus is displaced and distorted (Fig. 3-32). The
normal trophic macronucleus of *Trichodina* is horseshoe shaped. An extreme case of
malfunctioning was noted in parasitized *Trichodina* undergoing binary fission. Under
such conditions, the macronucleus was forced into the upper third of the cell and
therefore was prevented from participating in the fission process, resulting in its failure
to pull apart (Fig. 3-32, 3).

In addition to mechanical distortion, internal changes occur in the macronucleus of
infested *Trichodina*. In the normal macronucleus, chromatin granules are homogenously
distributed throughout the matrix, whereas in parasitized individuals the nucleus
contains large chromatin clumps within vacuolated areas. These changes become

apparent when the parasite occupies about half of the volume of the peritrich. This is indicative of macronuclear disintegration, ending in death of the host.

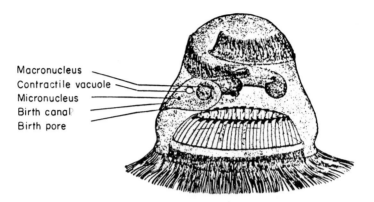

Macronucleus
Contractile vacuole
Micronucleus
Birth canal
Birth pore

Fig. 3-31: *Trichodina spheroidesi* parasitized by *Endosphaera engelmanni*. (After Padnos and Nigrelli, 1947; reproduced by permission of New York Zoological Society.)

ABNORMALITIES

Considerable morphological abnormalities have been observed in *Paramecium caudatum*. They include giant individuals, nuclear aberrations, distortion of the contractile vacuole, and other phenomena. Some clones produced offspring, while others failed to survive (Bovee, 1960).

Monstrous *Tetrahymena pyriformis* have been obtained after exposure of normal cells to numerous heat shocks, to flattening on agar or gelatin plates, or to viscous solutions of methyl cellulose. It was shown that in some cases the abnormalities are inherited and that this results in clones where the cells are different from each other and reveal various abnormalities with respect to cortical pattern, swimming and feeding behaviour, and generation time. Growth without subsequent division was found to be important for the production of the abnormal individuals (Hjelm, 1977).

Mottram (1940) noted similarities between tumour formation and certain changes observed in *Paramecium* sp. exposed to benzo[α] pyrene. In only a few of the exposed animals did long-term exposure to the carcinogen result in accelerated growth rates. Once a change had occurred, it persisted for many generations after the hydrocarbon had been removed. Abnormal individuals produced abnormal offspring, and the resulting cells showed wide morphological variation. Tittler (1948), on the other hand, found no observable effect of carcinogens on the growth of *Tetrahymena geleii*. He believes that the results of Mottram and other workers were due to improper cultivation methods.

No reports on structural abnormalities in marine ciliates have come to the reviewer's attention.

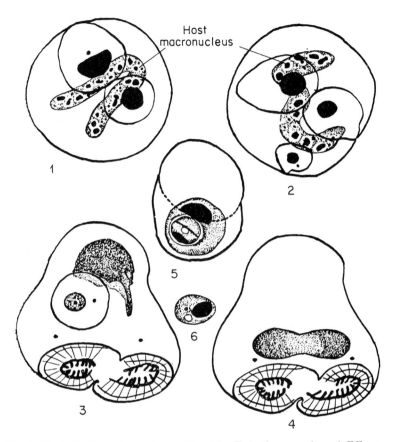

Fig. 3-32: *Trichodina spheroidesi* parasitized by *Endosphaera engelmanni*. Effects of parasite on host. 1, 2: Host macronucleus distorted and vacuolated; 3: host macronucleus displaced in dividing cell; 4: normal position of macronucleus during division; 5: parent cell showing completely formed bud; 6: free-living swarmer. × 680. (After Padnos and Nigrelli, 1947; reproduced by permission of New York Zoological Society.)

3.5   ANNEX TO DISEASES OF PROTOZOA: PROTOPHYTA

Although not members of the Protozoa, some Protophyta hosts are discussed here briefly for the following reasons: (i) Protozoa and Protophyta are often closely related; in some forms proper distinction is not possible—the temporary predominance of animal- or plant-like features of one and the same organism may depend on environmental or nutritional circumstances; (ii) organisms similar or even closely related to disease-causing associates of marine Protophyta also occur in marine invertebrates and may be expected to inhabit marine Protozoa; (iii) possibly enigmatic structures reported from the cytoplasm or nuclei of some Protozoa actually represent stages in the life cycles of such organisms; (iv) Protophyta may act as vectors or carriers of agents causing diseases in marine invertebrates, vertebrates or even man.

DISEASES CAUSED BY MICRO-ORGANISMS

Agents: Viruses

Roughly 30% of the cells of a marine *Platymonas* sp. (Chlorophyta, Prasinophyceae) from Santa Catalina Island (California, USA) observed in thin section with the electron microscope revealed signs of intranuclear virus-like particles. These are hexagonal in cross section, measure between 51 and 57·5 μm in diameter, and have a single electron-dense core surrounded by a lighter matrix all enclosed by a shell. Some particles have 3 or 4 electron-dense areas within a gray matrix surrounded by an outer layer and still others show no electron-dense material in the core but a uniform matrix enclosed by a shell.

The particles have been seen only in the nucleus. In some cells, the nucleoplasm retains a close-to-normal granular density with patches of closely packed hexagonal particles scattered throughout. In others, the nucleoplasm has lost much of its density and granularity, becoming very loosely fibrillar in nature. Nuclei in this condition contain virus-like particles individually dispersed throughout the nucleoplasm and not aggregated in crystalline arrays. Although the inner membrane of the nuclear envelope persists in all conditions thus far observed, the perinuclear space becomes quite enlarged in some cases, and in a few *Platymonas* individuals the outer nuclear envelope membrane no longer exists, or only fragments remain. Frequently, apparent cytoplasmic inclusions are observed in this enlarged perinuclear space.

In some cells, the cytoplasm appears to degenerate leaving a large nucleus, some chloroplast material and a few mitochondria, all enclosed by the persistent theca. This apparent cytoplasmic degeneration is evident in all cells with an enlarged perinuclear space. On the other hand, many cells with severe nuclear alterations exhibit no signs of cytoplasmic degeneration or enlarged perinuclear space. When viewed with the light microscope, some cells show partial loss of their pigmentation and, less frequently, clear areas devoid of internal structures. These areas are probably effects of the virus infection.

There was no evidence for the mechanism of infection or release of the virus-like particles from affected *Platymonas* sp. It was assumed, however, that infected nuclei prevent normal cell operation leading to gradual cytoplasmic degeneration and resulting in whole-cell lysis, thereby releasing the particles to the surrounding medium (Pearson and Norris, 1974).

This is the first decisive evidence provided for intranuclear virus-like particles in marine algae. The particles observed in *Platymonas* sp. are similar to a herpes-type virus infecting American oysters *Crassostrea virginica* (Farley and co-authors, 1972). As emphasized by Pearson and Norris (1974), the occurrence of virus-like particles in *Platymonas* sp. and of similar agents in oysters provide a basis for speculation that such marine algae may act as vectors for diseases of marine animals. Experimental studies on the transmission and mode of infection of these viruses are needed to prove this hypothesis. As is well known, human hepatitis viruses are retained by marine pelecypods, and infection occurs when raw or insufficiently cooked shellfish are eaten (Schäfer and Witt, 1973). Since these animals are suspension feeders living on planktonic algae, it seems worthwhile to investigate the possible role of the latter organisms as carriers of hepatitis virus.

Other virus diseases in algae, both prokaryotic and eukaryotic, marine and freshwater, have been reviewed and summarized by Brown (1972). Schnepf and co-authors (1970, 1971) described an interesting association involving a freshwater alga, a fungus-like parasite and a virus. Polyhedral virus-like particles, about 200 nm in diameter, were seen in the thalli of *Aphelidium* sp. *(chlorococcarum?)*, a protistan parasite of possible protomyxidan affinities (Schnepf, 1974), as well as in the cytoplasm of its host, the unicellular green alga *Scenedesmus armatus*. It was assumed that *Aphelidium* sp. acts as a vector for the virus disease of *S. armatus*.

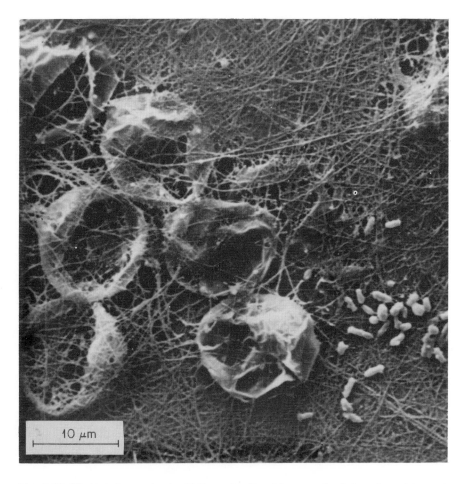

Fig. 3-33: *Thalassiosira partheneia*. Collapsed cells with network of threads and bacteria adhering to threads. (SEM photograph courtesy Dr. M. Elbrächter.)

Agents: Bacteria

No reports on bacterial diseases of marine Protophyta have come to the reviewer's attention. However, such diseases are known to affect non-marine algae (see, for example, Schnepf and co-authors, 1974), and must be expected to occur in oceans and coastal waters. On the other hand, the antibiotic activity of many—if not most—phytoplankters (e.g. Sieburth, 1959) may account for the apparent scantiness of reports on bacterial diseases in marine Protophyta. One known case of a probably ecologically significant association between a marine diatom and bacteria is considered below.

Thalassiosira partheneia occurs abundantly in the north-west African upwelling area. It produces colonies measuring up to 5 cm in length, and consisting of from several hundred to some 25,000 cells, each 7 to 15 μm in diameter. Some 8 to 128 individual cells are interconnected by a thick central thread to form long, straight chains. In addition, groups of chains adhering alongside each other by means of the cells' twisted marginal threads form tube-like aggregates up to 2 cm in diameter.

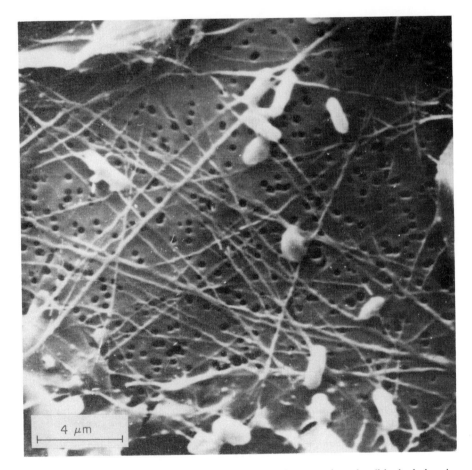

Fig. 3-34: *Thalassiosira partheneia*. Bacteria adhering to threads (black holes in background: membrane filter pores). (SEM photograph courtesy Dr. M. Elbrächter.)

As revealed by epifluorescent techniques and scanning electron microscopy, bacteria are present on the surface as well as on the threads of living *Thalassiosira partheneia* cells (Figs 3-33 and 3-34). On one colony of about 1000 cells, approximately 20,000 bacteria were counted. The significance of these microbial epibiotes is not clear. Perhaps they use the diatom's threads merely for attachment. Elbrächter and Boje (1978), however, hypothesize that these—possibly chitinoclastic—bacteria are responsible for the disintegration of larger *T. partheneia* aggregates into shorter chains or even single cells, thus making the otherwise undevourable colonies available to zooplankters. The central, as well as the marginal, threads of *T. partheneia* probably consist of chitan, as do those of *T. fluviatilis* (McLachlan and co-authors, 1965). Since chitan is similar to chitin, chitinoclastic bacteria may also be capable of utilizing chitan as growth substrate.

As has been demonstrated by means of radioactive tracer techniques, large intact *Thalassiosira partheneia* colonies are not utilized as food by marine zooplankters, such as copepods and euphausiids. However, short chains and single cells represent a good diet which is readily accepted by filter feeders, as well as ciliates such as tintinnids. Since it is generally assumed that a considerable proportion of the marine nanoplankton is transferred to larger omnivores via tintinnids, bacterial breakdown of *T. partheneia* colonies may be of ecological significance (Elbrächter, personal communication).

Agents: Fungi

Lagenisma coscinodisci, a phycomycete of the order Lagenidiales, is a common endobiotic parasite of marine centric diatoms belonging to the genera *Coscinodiscus* and *Palmeria* (Fig. 3-35). Zoospores of the fungus enter the algal cells by means of an infecting tube which penetrates the cell through the gap between epi- and hypotheca. Developing thalli, which may grow to a length of 550 μm within 3 days, are irregularly branched and non-septate. Upon completion of their development, during which they use up the entire host-cell contents by means of osmotrophy, they transform into a single large zoosporangium. The zoospores, which are released to the exterior through a discharge tube, pass through 2 different cyst stages. The primary zoospores are kidney-shaped and laterally biflagellated. They form a primary cyst with a spiny wall within which isomorphic secondary zoospores develop. The latter produce a smooth-walled secondary cyst. Upon germination, the secondary cyst infects a new diatom cell. Sexual reproduction of *L. coscinodisci* is induced in ageing host cells.

Lagenisma coscinodisci was first described from North Sea diatoms *Coscinodiscus granii*, *C. concinnus* and *C. pavillardii* by Drebes (1966, 1968) and was subsequently observed by Gotelli (1971) to infect Pacific *C. concinnus*, *C. wailesii* and *C. centralis*. Grahame (1976) reported *L. coscinodisci* from *Palmeria hardmaniana* in Kingston (Jamaica).

Aspects of the development and mode of infection of *Lagenisma coscinodisci* have been explored by Drebes (1966, 1968), Gotelli (1971), Grahame (1976) and Schnepf and Drebes (1977), and its ultrastructure by Schnepf and co-authors (1978a, b); Chakravarty (1969) studied aspects of cultivation, and Chakravarty (1974) its ecology.

Lagenisma coscinodisci is capable of producing disease effects of epiphytotic proportions in diatom populations. The mass occurrence of this fungus appears to be associated with blooms of the host diatoms. While during the onset of a 1969 *Coscinodiscus* bloom in Sequim Bay (Washington, USA) no infected cells were seen, one week later diseased diatoms occurred. The fungus appeared to be extremely virulent and was believed to have affected the size or duration of the bloom. Shortly after the detection of infected cells, the number of *Coscinodiscus* rapidly declined to pre-bloom levels (Gotelli, 1971). Infection of *Palmeria hardmaniana* from Kingston Harbor (Jamaica) with *L. coscinodisci* only occurred during 2 or 3 blooms of that species. Cell concentrations reached 1400 to 1700 cells l^{-1} at the peak of the blooms (normal concentration: less than 50 cells l^{-1}). The fungus spread rapidly through the diatom population, and 76 to 92% of the cells became parasitized. In both instances, the *P. hardmaniana* populations were severely reduced, sometimes up to a point where they disappeared from the sampling area (Grahame, 1976).

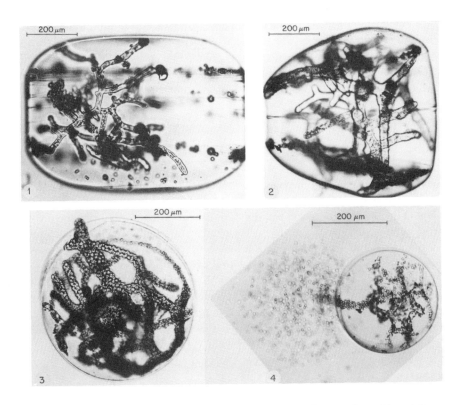

Fig. 3-35. *Lagenisma coscinodisci*. Mycelium in cell of *Coscinodiscus concinnus* (1) and *C. granii* (2); 3: mycelium with numerous zoospores; 4: release of zoospores through discharge tube. (After Drebes, 1974; reproduced by permission of Georg Thieme Verlag.)

The development of the fungus appears to be favoured by high water temperatures (Chakravarty, 1974; Grahame, 1976). In *Coscinodiscus granii* from Helgoland (southern North Sea) the temperature range in which infection occurred under experimental conditions is 10° to 20° C, but the rate of infection—as well as the number of zoospores released from zoosporangia—was higher at and above 15° C. The diatoms are comparatively more tolerant to salinity changes; they can multiply even at 20°/oo S. The tolerance range of the fungus is much more limited. No infections occurred at salinities below 25°/oo S (Chakravarty, 1974).

According to Gotelli (1971), *Lagenisma coscinodisci* is probably identical with fungi tentatively identified as *Lagenidium* sp. from *Coscinodiscus centralis* in Pacific northwest waters by Parsons (1962) and Johnson (1966). Taylor (1976) reported the occurrence of a fungus, provisionally identified as *Lagenidium* sp., in *C. oculus-iridis* from New Zealand waters.

In the order Saprolegniales, the genus *Ectrogella* (Fig. 3-36) is almost exclusively confined to diatoms as hosts. The vegetative development of these fungi is similar to that described for *Lagenisma coscinodisci*. Details are available in Sparrow (1960).

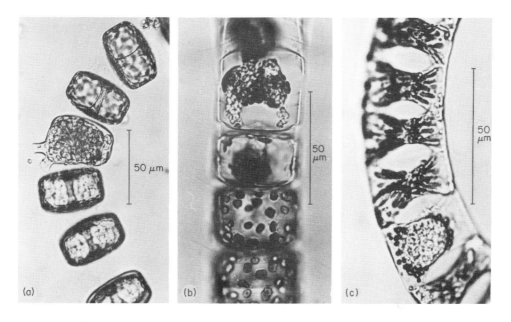

Fig. 3-36: *Ectrogella* spp. (a) One cell in chain of *Podosira glacialis* invaded by fungus; saclike thallus filled with zoospores; two discharge tubes open up to exterior. (b) Mature zoosporangium with zoospores in *Schroederella schroederi* cell. (c) *Ectrogella* sp. in *Eucampia zoodiacus*. (After Drebes, 1974; reproduced by permission of Georg Thieme Verlag.)

Among the Chytridiales, several species provisionally assigned to the genus *Rhizophydium* have been observed as parasites of marine centric diatoms *Bacteriastrum hyalinum* and *Chaetoceros densus* from the North Sea (Fig. 3-37; Drebes, 1974). Other members of the genus have been reported from freshwater phytoplankters (Paterson, 1958).

Some pathogenic fungi exhibit a broad host range. Although species parasitic in marine Protophyta have hitherto not been recorded from Protozoa or Invertebrata, such an extension of the host spectrum cannot entirely be ruled out. Thus, *Haliphtorus milfordensis*, a phycomycete originally observed by Ganaros (1957) on the eggs of gastropods *Urosalpinx cinerea*, is also capable of invading crustacean ova (Vishniac, 1958; Fisher and co-authors, 1975). It has furthermore been reported from *Enteromorpha* sp., a benthic green alga (Fuller and co-authors, 1964).

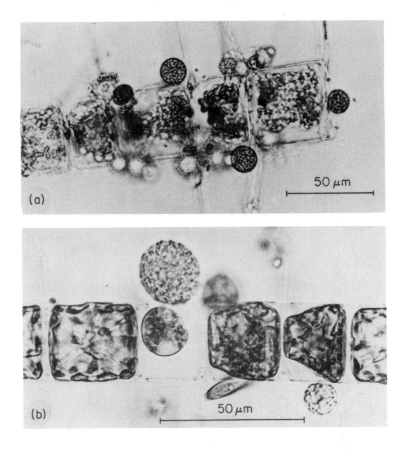

Fig. 3-37: Chytridiales (*Rhizophydium* sp.) infecting centric diatoms. (a) Heavily infected chain of *Chaetoceros densus*; (b) *Bacteriastrum hyalinum*. (After Drebes, 1974; reproduced by permission of Georg Thieme Verlag.)

DISEASES CAUSED BY PROTOZOANS

Of the protozoans associated with, or causing diseases in, marine Protophyta, only a few will be discussed here in passing—in particular representatives of groups which have counterparts affecting marine Protozoa, Invertebrata or Vertebrata.

Agents: Flagellata

Several dinoflagellates are common parasites of marine protozoans, invertebrates and vertebrates, and some attack marine Protophyta.

Chytriodinids *Myxodinium pipiens* occur ectoparasitically on *Halosphaera viridis* and *H. minor*, two abundant Mediterranean unicellular prasinophycean green algae. In summer 1967, often all *Halosphaera* spp. in the plankton from the French Mediterranean coast were found to be infested. The invasive stage of the peridinean, grossly spherical in

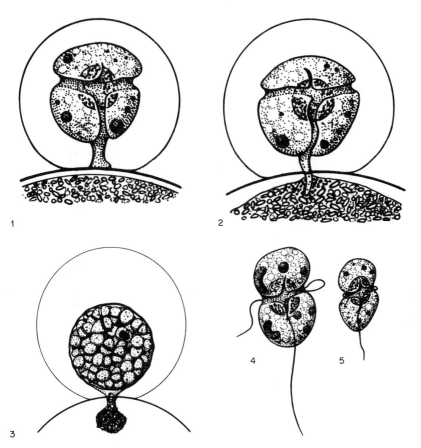

Fig. 3-38: *Myxodinium pipiens*. 1: Young invasive stage attaching externally to
Halosphaera sp. cyst; 2: trophont extending suctorial tentacle into host cytoplasm; 3: sporocyst formation; 4: free-swimming 'sporocyst'; 5: spore
(microspore). (After Cachon and co-authors, 1969; reproduced by permission
of Blackwell, Oxford.)

shape and 10 to 15 μm in diameter, attaches to the external membrane of the host cyst.
The parasite then emits a short, stout tentacle which—upon contact with the host
membrane—broadens to form a holdfast, and subsequently penetrates the external and
internal membranes of the host (Fig. 3-38, 1 and 2). By means of this suctorial tentacle
M. pipiens sucks out the cytoplasmic content of the host cyst which gradually diminishes
in size. Infested *Halosphaera* cysts are easily distinguishable from healthy ones by their
distinct opacity.

Uninucleate *Myxodinium pipiens* rarely exceed 30 μm in diameter. During growth, the
parasite becomes surrounded by a mucopolysaccharide capsule, 8 to 10 μm in thickness.
Exhaustion of the food source, i.e. complete absorption of the host cytoplasm, initiates
spore formation. The resulting mass of 'sporocysts' attains a diameter of up to
approximately 130 μm, its surrounding capsule reaching or even slightly surpassing the
size of the host cyst (230 μm) (Fig. 3-38, 3). The 'sporocysts' which measure about 12 to
15 × 25 to 27 μm (Fig. 3-38, 4) are liberated upon rupture of the enclosing capsule.
Free-swimming 'sporocysts' develop into macrospores, measuring 12 × 25 to 27 μm, or

divide several times to form microspores of 8×16 μm (Fig. 3-38, 5). Whether sporogenesis in *M. pipiens* actually represents a gametogenesis resulting in anisogamy remains to be studied. Gamete copulation has not yet been seen, but the invasive stage of the parasite requires a maturation period of approximately 10 days in order to become infective for *Halosphaera* spp. (Cachon and co-authors, 1969).

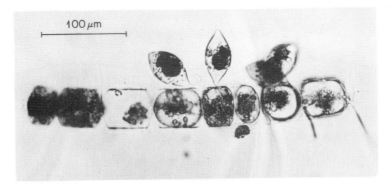

Fig. 3-39: *Amphidinium sphenoides* (?) attached to *Chaetoceros eibenii*. Dark contents of parasite cells consist of host cytoplasm and chromatophores. (After Drebes, 1974; reproduced by permission of Georg Thieme Verlag.)

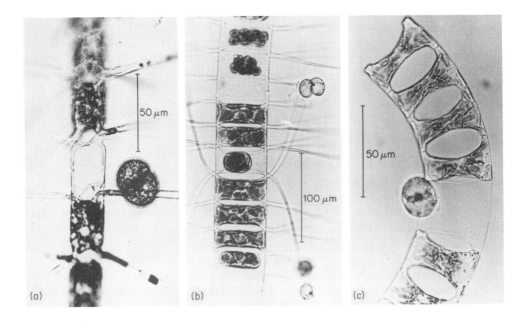

Fig. 3-40: Dinoflagellates parasitizing diatoms. (a) *Paulsenella chaetoceratis* attached to bristle of *Chaetoceros borealis*. Note emptied host cell and accumulation of host material inside parasite. (b) *P. chaetoceratis* (?) attached to *C. decipiens*. Note partially or entirely emptied host cells. (c) *Paulsenella* sp. on *Eucampia zoodiacus*. (After Drebes, 1974; reproduced by permission of Georg Thieme Verlag.)

Dinoflagellates living ectoparasitically on North Sea plankton diatoms include *Paulsenella chaetoceratis* attaching to the bristles of *Chaetoceros borealis* and *C. decipiens*, as well as *Amphidinium sphenoides* attaching to the cell walls of *C. eibenii* (Figs 3-39 and 3-40; Drebes, 1974). Colonial diatoms *Thalassiosira partheneia* from the northwest African

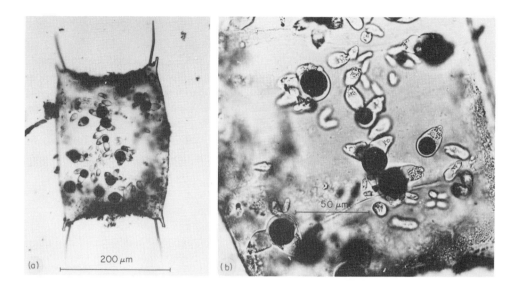

Fig. 3-41: *Biddulphia sinensis*. (a) Individual parasitized by *Pronoctiluca* sp. cf. *phaeocysticola*; (b) enlarged portion of host cell harbouring flagellates. Note characteristic dark spheres consisting of partially digested host chromatophores. (Photograph courtesy Dr. M. Elbrächter.)

upwelling area are attacked by *Amphidinium phaeocysticola*, *Gymnodinium heterostriatum* and *Glenodinium* sp. (Elbrächter and Boje, 1978).

Coscinodiscus concinnus and other centric diatoms from North Sea plankton are frequently parasitized by *Pronoctiluca* sp., a colourless flagellate which feeds phagotrophically on the host's cell content (Drebes, 1974). *Pronoctiluca* sp. is probably not a dinoflagellate but a cryptomonad (Elbrächter, personal communication). *P. phaeocysticola* has been found as endoparasite of *Phaeocystis pouchetii* and occurs ectoparasitically on *Thalassiosira partheneia*. A very similar form, *Pronoctiluca* sp. cf. *phaeocysticola* parasitizes *Biddulphia sinensis*. Dark spherules within the organism's cytoplasm consist of host chromatophores which are ingested, aggregated into dense masses, and then expelled. Their uniform reddish-black colour, which differs from that of the original host chromatophores, indicates that they are partially digested by the parasite (Fig. 3-41; Elbrächter, personal communication).

Palisporomonas apodinium, a colourless flagellate, pyriform in shape and up to 27 μm in length, is an ectoparasite of the Mediterranean diatoms *Actinocyclus subtilis*, *Striatella* sp. and *Licmophora* sp. Upon attachment by means of a suctorial tentacle, the parasite feeds on the host's cytoplasm. After a period of rapid growth, the flagellate divides once, forming a so-called trophocyte and a gonocyte. Only the trophocyte remains in contact with the host, whereas the gonocyte gives rise to numerous generations of sporocytes. These, in turn, undergo several mitoses to produce 16 to 32 zoospores. The development of the latter has not been followed but it is assumed that they represent the invasive stage (de Saedeleer, 1947). The taxonomic position of *P. apodinium* remains uncertain; it is probably a chrysomonad.

Agents: Rhizopoda

Diatoms *Biddulphia sinensis* from the North Sea are frequently parasitized by *Amoeba biddulphiae* (Fig. 3-42). Young individuals occur free in the plankton. As soon as an amoeba has penetrated a diatom's frustule, the host cytoplasm undergoes plasmolysis, eventually forming a densely pigmented mass in the centre of the cell. Amoebae feeding on the diatom's cell contents grow rapidly and divide repeatedly so that, after 2 to 3 days, 18 to 32 parasites are present in a single frustule. When the entire cell contents are used up, the amoebae abandon the disintegrating empty frustule and invade new hosts.

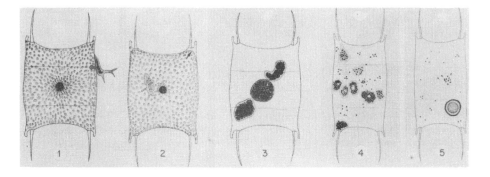

Fig. 3-42: *Biddulphia sinensis*. 1: *Amoeba biddulphiae* penetrating host frustule. 2: *A. biddulphiae* within cytosplasm of *B. sinensis*; note beginning parasite-induced plasmolysis (arrow). 3: Same individual after 32·5 h; host cytoplasm contracted into round mass in centre of cell; amoeba divided into 2 individuals feeding on ball of cytoplasm; note accumulation of host chromatophores within body of parasites. 4: *B. sinensis* 3 days p. i.; eight amoebae present; large portion of host chromatophores already digested; starving amoeba becoming progressively hyaline. 5: Empty *B. sinensis* frustule with encysted *A. biddulphiae*. (After Zuelzer, 1927; reproduced by permission of VEB Gustav Fischer Verlag.)

Amoeba biddulphiae infestations are invariably fatal to *Biddulphia sinensis*. The agent appears to be host specific; no other plankton algae from the same haul harboured the amoeba. *A. biddulphiae* seems to be nutritionally dependent on its host. Under laboratory conditions, individuals kept without *B. sinensis* succumbed. In the North Sea, *A. biddulphiae* incidences displayed a distinct seasonality with peak infestations involving 16 to 20% of the population by the end of September (Zuelzer, 1927).

Unidentified proteomyxidan amoeboflagellates, possibly close to the genus *Pseudospora*, are not uncommon in *Halosphaera* cysts from the western English Channel and the Bay of Biscay. *H. viridis* is more frequently infested than either *H. minor* or *H. russellii*. The parasite has a non-motile phase of up to $30 \times 16 \, \mu$m and an ovoid-to-pyriform motile phase, 15 to 18 × 5 to 8 μm, with 2 very unequal flagella—one attaining body length, the other 3 times body length. Both phases are amoeboid. The parasite usually completely devours the contents of the *Halosphaera* cyst, filling it with motile cells by rapid multiplication. The colourless parasites with the ingested green host plastids and carotenoid granules look very much like motile *Halosphaera* stages and have been mistaken for these by early workers (Parke and Den Hartog-Adams, 1965).

Literature Cited (Chapter 3)

Andrews, E. A. and Reinhard, E. G. (1943). A folliculinid associated with a hermit crab. *J. Wash. Acad. Sci.*, **33**, 216–223.

Arnold, Z. M. (1964). Biological observations on the foraminifer *Spiroloculina hyalina* Schulze. *Univ. Calif. Publs Zool.*, **72**, 1–93.

Arvy, L. (1952). Sur deux parasites de *Phascolion strombi* Montagu. *Bull. Lab. marit. Dinard*, **36**, 7–13.

Ball, G. H. (1969). Organisms living on and in Protozoa. In T.-T. Chen (Ed.), *Research in Protozoology*, Vol. 3. Pergamon Press, New York. pp. 566–718.

Bonar, L. (1936). An unusual ascomycete in the shell of marine animals. *Univ. Calif. Publs Bot.*, **19**, 187–193.

Borgert, A. (1897). Beiträge zur Kenntnis der in *Sticholonche zanclea* und Acanthometridenarten vorkommenden Parasiten (Spiralkörper Fol, *Amoebophrya* Köppen). *Z. wiss. Zool.*, **63**, 141–186.

Bovee, E. C. (1960). Morphological anomalies in a population of large *Paramecium caudatum*. *J. Protozool.*, **7** (Suppl.), 16.

Brooks, W. K. and Kellner, C. (1908). On *Oikopleura tortugensis*, a new appendicularian from the Tortugas, Florida, with notes on its embryology. *Pap. Tortugas Lab.*, **1**, 89–94.

Brown, R. M. (1972). Algal viruses. *Adv. Virus Res.*, **17**, 243–274.

Brumpt, E. and Lavier, G. (1935). Sur une *Nucleophaga* parasite d'*Endolimax nana*. *Annls Parasit. hum. comp.*, **13**, 439–444.

Cachon, J. (1964). Contribution à l'étude des péridiniens parasites. Cytologie. Cycles évolutifs. *Annls Sci. nat.* (Zool., Ser. 12), **6**, 1–158.

Cachon, J. and Cachon, M. (1969). Ultrastructures des Amoebophryidae (péridiniens Duboscquodinida). I. Manifestations des rapports entre l'hôte et le parasite. *Protistologica*, **5**, 535–547.

Cachon, J. and Cachon M. (1970). Ultrastructure des Amoebophryidae (péridiniens Duboscquodinida). II. Systèmes atractophoriens et microtubulaires; leur intervention dans la mitose.) *Protistologica*, **6**, 57–70.

Cachon, J., Cachon, M. and Bouquaheux, F. (1969). *Myxodinium pipiens* gen. nov., sp. nov., péridinien parasite d'*Halosphaera*. *Phycologia*, **8**, 157–164.

Cachon-Enjumet, M. (1961). Contribution à l'étude des radiolaires phaeodariés. *Archs. Zool. exp. gén.*, **100**, 151–237.

Campbell, A. S. (1926). The cytology of *Tintinnopsis nucula* (Fol) Laachmann, with an account of its neuromotor apparatus, division, and a new intranuclear parasite. *Univ. Calif. Publ. Zool.*, **29**, 179–236.

Casley-Smith, J. R. and Savanat, T. (1966). The formation of membranes around micro-organisms and particles injected into amoebae: Support for the "reticulosome" concept. *Aust. J. exp. Biol. med. Sci.*, **44**, 111–122.

Caullery, M. (1953). Classe des haplosporidies. In P. P. Grassé (Ed.), *Traité de Zoologie*, Vol.I, Part 2. Masson, Paris. pp. 922–934.

Caullery, M. and Mesnil, F. (1897). Sur un type nouveau (*Metchnikovella* n.g.) d'organismes parasites des grégarines. *C. r. hebd. Séanc. Acad. Sci., Paris*, **125**, 787–790.

Caullery, M. and Mesnil, F. (1905). Sur quelques nouvelles haplosporidies d'annélides. *C. r. Séanc. Soc. Biol.*, **58**, 580–583.

Caullery, M. and Mesnil, F. (1914). Sur les Metchnikovellidae et autres protistes parasites des grégarines d'annélides. *C. r. Séanc. Soc. Biol.*, **77**, 527–532.

Caullery, M. and Mesnil, F. (1919). Metchnikovellidae et autres protistes parasites des grégarines d'annélides. *Annls Inst. Pasteur, Paris*, **33**, 209–240.

Chakravarty, D. K. (1969). Zum Kulturverhalten des marinen parasitischen Pilzes *Lagenisma coscinodisci*. *Veröff. Inst. Meeresforsch. Bremerh.*, **11**, 309–312.

Chakravarty, D. K. (1974). On the ecology of the infection of the marine diatom *Coscinodiscus granii* by *Lagenisma coscinodisci* in the Weser estuary. *Veröff. Inst. Meeresforsch. Bremerh.*, **5** (Suppl.), 115–122.

Chang, K.-P. (1975). Reduced growth of *Blastocrithidia culicis* and *Crithidia oncopelti* freed of intracellular symbiotes by chloramphenicol. *J. Protozool.*, **22**, 271–276.

Changeux, J.-P. (1961). Contribution à l'étude des animaux associés aux holothurides. *Actual. scient. ind.*, **1961**, 1284.

Chatton, É. (1910). Protozoaires parasites des branchies des labres: *Amoeba mucicola* Chatton, *Trichodina labrorum* n.sp. Appendice: parasites des trichodines. *Archs Zool. exp. gén.* (Ser. 5), **5**, 239–266.

Chatton, É. (1920a). Les péridiniens parasites. *Archs Zool. exp. gén.*, **59**, 1–475.

Chatton, É. (1920b). Existence chez les radiolaires de péridiniens parasites considérés comme formes de reproduction de leurs hôtes. *C. r. hebd. Séanc. Acad. Sci., Paris*, **170**, 413.

Chatton, É. (1923). Les péridiniens parasites des radiolaires. *C. r. hebd. Séanc. Acad. Sci., Paris*, **177**, 1246–1249.

Chatton, É. (1952). Classe des dinoflagelles ou péridiniens. In P.-P. Grassé (Ed.), *Traité de Zoologie*, Vol. I. pp. 309–406.

Chatton, É. and Biecheler, B. (1934). Les Coccidinidae, dinoflagellés coccidiomorphes parasites de dinoflagellés, et le phylum des Phytodinozoa. *C. r. hebd. Séanc. Acad. Sci., Paris*, **199**, 252–255.

Chatton, É. and Biecheler, B. (1935). Les *Amoebophrya* et le *Hyalosaccus;* leur cycle evolutif. L'ordre nouveau des Coelomastigina dans les flagellés. *C. r. hebd. Séanc. Acad. Sci., Paris*, **200**, 505–507.

Chatton, É. and Biecheler, B. (1936). Documents nouveaux relatifs aux coccidinides (dinoflagellés parasites). La sexualité du *Coccidinium mesnili* n.sp. *C. r. hebd. Séanc. Acad. Sci., Paris*, **203**, 573–576.

Chatton, É. and Brachon. S. (1936). Sur un protiste parasite du cilié *Fabrea salina* Henneguy: *Gregarella fabrearum* n. gen., n. sp., et son évolution. *C. r. hebd. Séanc. Acad. Sci., Paris*, **203**, 525–527.

Chatton, É. and Brodsky, A. (1909). Le parasitisme d'une chytridinée du genre *Sphaerita* Dangeard chez *Amoeba limax* Dujard. Étude comparative. *Arch. Protistenk.*, **17**, 1–18.

Chatton, É. and Lwoff, A. (1923). Sur l'évolution des infusoires des lamellibranches. Relations des hypocomidés avec les ancistridés. Le genre *Hypocomides* n.g. *C.r. hebd. Séanc. Acad. Sci., Paris*, **177**, 787–790.

Chatton, É. and Lwoff, A. (1924). Sur un flagellé hypertrophique et palintomique parasite des infusoires marins: *Sporomonas infusorium* (n.g., n.sp.). *C. r. Séanc. Soc. Biol.*, **91**, 186–190.

Chatton, É. and Lwoff, A. (1927). *Pottsia infusoriorum* n.g., n.sp., acinétien parasite des folliculines et des cothurnies. *Bull. Inst. océanogr. Monaco*, **489**, 1–12.

Chatton, É. and Lwoff, A. (1929). Contribution à l'étude de l'adaptation. *Ellobiophrya donacis* Ch. et Lw. péritriche vivant sur les branchies de l'acéphale *Donax vittatus* da Costa. *Biol. Bull. mar. biol. Lab., Woods Hole*, **63**, 321–349.

Chatton, É. and Lwoff, A. (1935). Les ciliés apostomes. Morphologie, cytologie, éthologie, évolution, systématique. I. Aperçu historique et général; étude monographique des genres et des espèces. *Archs Zool. exp. gén.*, **77**, 1–453.

Chatton, É. and Lwoff, A. (1939). Sur la systématique de la tribu des thigmotriches rhynchoidés. Les deux familles des Hypocomidae Bütschli et des Ancistrocomidae n.fam. Les deux genres nouveaux, *Heterocoma* et *Parhypocoma*. *C. r. hebd. Séanc. Acad. Sci., Paris*, **209**, 429–431.

Chatton, É., Lwoff, A. and Lwoff, M. (1930). Les *Phtorophrya* n.g., ciliés Foettingeriidae hyperparasites des *Gymnodinioides*, Foettingeriidae parasites des crustacés. *C. r. hebd. Séanc. Acad. Sci., Paris*, **180**, 1080–1082.

Chatton, É. and Villeneuve, S. (1937). *Gregarella fabrearum* Chatton et Brachon protiste parasite du cilié *Fabrea salina* Henneguy. La notion de dépolarisation chez les flagellés et la conception des apomastigines. *Archs Zool. exp. gén.*, **78**, 216–237.

Collin, B. (1907). Note préliminaire sur quelques acinétiens. I. *Ephelota gemmipara* (Hertwig); II. *Hypocoma acinetarum* n. sp. *Archs Zool. exp. gén.* (Ser. 4), **7**, 93–103.
Collin, B. (1909). Diagnoses préliminaires d'acinétiens nouveau ou mal connus. *C. r. hebd. Séanc. Acad. Sci., Paris*, **149**, 1094–1095.
Collin, B. (1912). Étude monographique sur les acinétiens. II. Morphologie, physiologie, systématique. *Archs Zool. exp. gén.*, **51**, 1–457.
Dangeard, P. A. (1888). Les péridiniens et leurs parasites. *J. Bot., Paris*, **2**, 126–132.
Dangeard, P. A. (1902). Sur la caryophysème des eugléniens. *C. r. hebd. Séanc. Acad. Sci., Paris*, **134**, 1365–1366.
Debaisieux, P. (1958). *Lagenophrys lunatus* Ima. (Ciliate peritriche). *Cellule*, **59**, 361–383.
Dogiel, V. A. (1906). Beiträge zur Kenntnis der Peridineen. *Mitt. zool. Stn Neapel*, **18**, 1–45.
Dogiel, V. A. (1922). Sur un nouveau genre de Metchnikovellidae. *Annls Inst. Pasteur, Paris*, **36**, 574-577.
Douvillé, N. (1930). Parasitisme ou commensalisme chez les foraminifères. Les canaux chez les Nummulitides. *Bull. Soc. geol. Fr., Livre jubilaire 1830–1930*, **1**, 257–262.
Drebes, G. (1966). Ein parasitischer Phycomycet (Lagenidiales) in *Coscinodiscus. Helgoländer wiss. Meeresunters.*, **13**, 426–435.
Drebes, G. (1968). *Lagenisma coscinodisci* gen. nov. sp. nov., ein Vertreter der Lagenidiales in der marinen Diatomee *Coscinodiscus. Veröff. Inst. Meeresforsch. Bremerh.*, **3**, 67–70.
Drebes, G. (1974). *Marines Phytoplankton*, Georg Thieme Verlag, Stuttgart.
Drożański, W. (1956). Fatal bacterial infection in soil amoebae. *Acta microbiol. pol.*, **5**, 315–317.
Drożański, W. (1963a). Studies of intracellular parasites of free-living amoebae. *Acta microbiol. pol.*, **12**, 3–8.
Drożański, W. (1963b). Observations on intracellular infection of amoebae by bacteria. *Acta microbiol. pol.*, **12**, 9–23.
Duboscq, O. and Collin, B. (1910). Sur la reproduction sexuée d'un protiste parasite des tintinnides. *C. r. hebd. Séanc. Acad. Sci., Paris*, **151**, 340–341.
Elbrächter, M. and Boje, R. (1978). On the ecological significance of *Thalassiosira partheneia* in the Northwest African upwelling area. In R. Boje and M. Tomzschak (Eds), *Upwelling Systems*. Springer-Verlag, Berlin. pp. 24–31.
Entz, G. (1909). Studien über Organisation und Biologie der Tintinniden. *Arch. Protistenk.*, **15**, 93–226.
Epstein, E. W. (1935). Bacterial infection in an amoeba. *Jl R. microsc. Soc.*, **55**, 86–94.
Farley, C. A., Banfield, W. G., Kasnic, G. and Foster, W. S. (1972). Oyster herpes-type virus. *Science, N.Y.*, **178**, 759–760.
Fauré-Fremiet, E. (1943). Commensalisme et adaptation chez une vorticellide: *Epistylis lwoffi*, n.sp. *Bull. Soc. zool. Fr.*, **68**, 154–157.
Fenchel, T., Perry, T. and Thane, A. (1977). Anaerobiosis and symbiosis with bacteria in free-living ciliates. *J. Protozool.*, **24**, 154–163.
Fisher, W. S., Nilson, E. H. and Shleser, R. A. (1975). Effect of the fungus *Haliphthoros milfordensis* on the juvenile stages of the American lobster *Homarus americanus*. *J. Invertebr. Pathol.*, **26**, 41–45.
Fol, H. (1883). Sur le *Sticholonche zanclea* et un nouvel ordre de rhizopodes. *Mém. Inst. nat. Genève*, **15**.
Franca, S. (1976). On the presence of virus-like particles in the dinoflagellate *Gyrodinium resplendens* (Hulburt). *Protistologica*, **12**, 425–430.
Fuller, M. S., Fowles, B. E. and McLaughlin, D. J. (1964). Isolation and pure culture study of marine phycomycetes. *Mycologia*, **56**, 745–756.
Ganapati, P. N. and Aiyar, R. G. (1937). Life-history of a dicystid gregarine, *Lecudina brasili* n.sp. parasitic in the gut of *Lumbriconereis* sp. *Arch. Protistenk.*, **89**, 113–132.
Ganaros, A. E. (1957). Marine fungus infecting eggs and embryos of *Urosalpinx cinerea. Science, N.Y.*, **125**, 1194.
Gillies, C. and Hanson, E. D. (1963). A new species of *Leptomonas* parasitizing the macronucleus of *Paramecium trichium. J. Protozool.*, **10**, 467–473.
Gotelli, D. (1971). *Lagenisma coscinodisci*, a parasite of the marine diatom *Coscinodiscus* occurring in the Puget Sound, Washington. *Mycologia*, **63**, 171–174.

Grahame, E. S. (1976). The occurrence of *Lagenisma coscinodisci* in *Palmeria hardmaniana* from Kingston Harbour, Jamaica. *Br. phycol. J.*, **11**, 57–61.

Grassé, P.-P. (1952). Zooflagellés de position systématique incertaine. In P.-P. Grassé (Ed.), *Traité de Zoologie*, Vol. I, Part 1. Masson, Paris. pp. 1005–1022.

Grell, K.-G. (1949): Der Parasitismus bei den Suktorien. *Forsch. Fortschr.*, **25**, 214–215.

Grell, K.-G. (1950). Der Generationswechsel des parasitischen Suktors *Tachyblaston ephelotensis* Martin. *Z. ParasitKde*, **14**, 499–534.

Grell, K.-G. (1961). Über den "Nebenkörper" von *Paramoeba eilhardi* Schaudinn. *Arch. Protistenk.*, **105**, 303–312.

Grell, K.-G. (1967). Parasiten und Räuber von *Ephelota gemmipara* (Suctoria). Begleitveröffentlichung zum wissenschaftlichen Film C907/1965. *Publ. wiss. Film*, **2A**, 117–126.

Grell, K.-G. (1968). *Protozoologie*, 2nd ed., Springer, Berlin.

Grell, K.-G. (1969). Fortpflanzung der Suktorien. Begleitveröffentlichung zum wissenschaftlichen Film C 913/1966. *Publ. wiss. Film.* **2A**, 653–668.

Grell, K.-G. (1971). *Paramoeba eilhardi* (Amoebina). Parasitische Bakterien im Zellkern. *Encyclop. Cinematogr.*, **E 1174/1967.**

Gruber, A. (1884). Die Protozoen des Hafens von Genua. *Nova Acta K. Leop. Carol.*, **46**, 475–539.

Hertwig, R. (1879). *Der Organismus der Radiolarien*, Fischer, Jena.

Hesse, E. (1909). Contribution à l'étude des monocystidées des oligochètes. *Archs Zool. exp. gén.* (Ser. 5), **3**, 27–301.

Hjelm, K. K. (1977). Monstrous *Tetrahymena* with intraclonal variation in structure produced by hereditary modification of normal cells, *J. Protozool.*, **24**, 420–425.

Hofker, J. (1931). Studien über Tintinnoidea. *Arch. Protistenk.*, **75**, 315–402.

Hollande, A. (1938). *Bodo perforans* n.sp. flagellé nouveau parasite externe du *Chilomonas paramaecium* Ehrenb. *Archs Zool. exp. gén.*, **79**, 75–81.

Hollande, A. (1945). Biologie et reproduction des rhizopodes des genres *Pelomyxa* et *Amoeba* et cycle évolutif de l'*Amoebophilus destructor* nov. gen., nov. sp., chytridinée parasite de *Pelomyxa palustris* Greeff. *Bull. biol. Fr. Belg.*, **79**, 31–66.

Hollande, A. (1953). Compléments à l'étude cytologique des radiolaires. In P.-P. Grassé (Ed.), *Traité de Zoologie*, Vol. I, Part 2. Masson, Paris. pp. 1089–1100.

Hollande, A. and Enjumet, M. (1953). Contribution à l'étude biologique des sphaerocollides (radiolaires collodaires et radiolaires polycyttaires) et de leurs parasites. Partie I: Thalassicollidae, Physematidae, Thalassophysidae. *Annls Sci. nat.* (Zoologie, Ser. 11), **15**, 99–183.

Hollande, A., Enjumet, M. and Manciet, J. (1953). Les péridiniens parasites des phaeodariés et le problème de la sporogénèse chez ces radiolaires. *C. r. hebd. Séanc. Acad. Sci., Paris*, **336**, 1607–1609.

Honigberg, B. M., Balamuth, W., Bovee, E. C., Corliss, J. O., Gojdics, M., Hall, R. P., Kudo, R. R., Levine, N. D., Loeblich, A. R., Weiser, J. and Wenrich, D. H. (1964). A revised classification of the phylum Protozoa. *J. Protozool.*, **11**, 7–20.

Hovasse, R. (1923a). Sur les péridiniens parasites des radiolaires coloniaux. *Bull. Soc. zool. Fr.*, **48**, 337–338.

Hovasse, R. (1923b). Les péridiniens intracellulaires. Zooxanthelles et *Syndinium* chez les radiolaires coloniaux. Remarques sur la reproduction des radiolaires. *Bull. Soc. zool. Fr.*, **48**, 247–254.

Hovasse, R. (1950). *Spirobütschliella chattoni*, nov.gen., nov.sp., cilié apostome, parasite en Méditerranée du serpulien *Pomatoceros triqueter* L., et parasité par la microsporidie *Gurleya nova*, sp.nov. *Bull. Inst. océanogr., Monaco*, **962**, 1–10.

Hovasse, R. and Brown, E. M. (1953). Contribution à la connaissance des radiolaires et de leurs parasites syndiniens. *Annls Sci. nat.* (Ser. 11), **15**, 405–438.

Hovasse, R. and Brown, E. M. (1956). La reproduction des radiolaires et de leurs parasites péridiniens. *Proc. int. Congr. Zool.*, **1953**, **14**, 448–449.

Hyman, L. H. (1940). *The Invertebrates*, Vol. I, Protozoa through Ctenophora, McGraw-Hill, New York.

Ingold, C. T. (1944). Studies on British chytrids. II. A new chytrid on *Ceratium* and *Peridinium*. *Trans. Br. mycol. Soc.*, **27**, 93–96.

Jadin, J. B. (1977). Résistance et multiplication des mycobactéries dans les vacuoles des amibes *"Limax"*. (Abstract.) In *Proceedings of the 5th International Congress of Protozoology*, No. 239.

Jeon, K. W. (1977). Further evidence for the host cell's dependence on newly acquired cytoplasmic components in amoebae. (Abstract.) In *Proceedings of the 5th International Congress of Protozoology*, No. 445.

Jeon, K. W. and Hah, J. C. (1977). Effect of chloramphenicol on bacterial endosymbiotes in a strain of *Amoeba proteus*. *J. Protozool.*, **24**, 289–293.

Jeon, K. W. and Jeon, M. S. (1976). Endosymbiosis in amoebae: Recently established endosymbionts have become required cytoplasmic components. *J. cell. comp. Physiol.*, **89**, 337–344.

Johnson, P. T. (1968). *An Annotated Bibliography of Pathology in Invertebrates other than Insects*, Burgess, Minneapolis.

Johnson, P. T. and Chapman, F. A. (1969). *An Annotated Bibliography of Pathology in Invertebrates other than Insects*. (Suppl.) Misc. Publ., Center for Pathobiology, University of California, Irvine, **1**, 1–76.

Johnson, T. W. (1966). A *Lagenidium* in the marine diatom *Coscinodiscus centralis*. *Mycologia*, **58**, 131–135.

Kaestner, A. (1954-1963). *Lehrbuch der Speziellen Zoologie*, Fischer, Jena.

Kahl, A. (1933). Ciliata libera et ectocommensalia. In G. Grimpe and E. Wagler (Eds), *Die Tierwelt der Nord- und Ostsee*. Lief. 23, II, C3. Akad. Verlagsgesellschaft, Leipzig. pp. 29–146

Kesa, L. and Teras, J. (1977). Pathogenicity of free-living Protozoa in interaction with viruses in vitro. (Abstract.) In *Proceedings of the 5th International Congress of Protozoology*, No. 126.

Kinne, O. (1977). Cultivation of animals. Research cultivation. In O. Kinne (Ed.), *Marine Ecology*, Vol. III, Cultivation, Part 2. Wiley, Chichester. pp. 579–1293.

Kirby, H. (1941). Organisms living on and in Protozoa. In S. N. Calkins and F. M. Summers (Eds), *Protozoa in Biological Research*. Columbia Univ. Press, New York. pp. 1009–1113.

Kirby, H. (1942). A parasite of the macronucleus of *Vorticella*. *J. Parasit.*, **28**, 311–314.

Kölliker, A. (1860). Über das ausgebreitete Vorkommen von pflanzlichen Parasiten in den Hartgebilden niederer Thiere. *Z. wiss. Zool.*, **10**, 215–232.

Koeppen, N. (1894). *Amoebophrya sticholonchae* n.gen. et sp. *Zool. Anz.*, **17**, 417-424.

Koeppen, N. (1903). *Hyalosaccus ceratii* nov.gen., nov.sp., parasit dinoflagellat. *Zapiski Kiev. obshch.*, **16**, 89–135.

Korotneff, A. (1891). Zoologische Paradoxen. *Z. wiss. Zool.*, **51**, 613–628.

Kovács, E. and Bucz, B. (1967). Propagation of mammalian viruses in Protista. II. Isolation of complete virus from yeast and *Tetrahymena* experimentally infected with Picorna viral particles or their infectious RNA. *Life Sci.*, **6**, 347–358.

Kovács, E., Bucz, B. and Kolompár, G. (1966). Propagation of mammalian viruses in Protista. I. Visualization of fluorochrome labelled EMC virus in yeast and *Tetrahymena*. *Life Sci.*, **5**, 2117–2126.

Kovács, E., Kolompár, F. and Bucz, B. (1967). Propagation of mammalian viruses in Protista. III. Change in population densities, viability and multiplication of yeasts and *Tetrahymena* experimentally infected with encephalomyocarditis virus. *Life Sci.*, **6**, 2359–2372.

Krüger, F. (1956). Über die Microsporidien-Infektion von *Campanella umbellaria* (Ciliata Peritricha). *Zool. Anz.*, **156**, 125–129.

Kudo, R. R. (1924). A biologic and taxonomic study of the Microsporidia. *Illinois biol. Monogr.*, **9**, 1–268.

Kudo, R. R. (1944). Morphology and development of *Nosema notabilis* Kudo, parasitic in *Sphaerospora polymorpha* Davis, a parasite of *Opsanus tau* and *O. beta*. *Illinois biol. Monogr.*, **20**, 7–57.

Kudo, R. R. (1966). *Protozoology*, Thomas, Springfield.

Laackmann, H. (1906). Ungeschlechtliche und geschlechtliche Fortpflanzung der Tintinniden. *Zool. Anz.*, **30**, 440–443.

Laval, M. (1970). Présence de bactéries intranucléaires chez *Zoothamnium pelagicum* (cilié péritriche). Leur rôle dans la formation des pigments intracytoplasmiques des zoides. *VII. Congr. int. Microsc. électronique, Grenoble*, No. 403.

Le Calvez, J. (1938). Recherches sur les foraminifères. *Archs Zool. exp. gén.*, **80**, 163–333.

Le Calvez, J. (1939) *Trophosphaera planorbulinae* n.gen., n.sp., protiste parasite du foraminifère *Planorbulina mediterranensis* d'Orb. *Archs Zool. exp. gén.*, **80**, 425–443.

Le Calvez, J. (1940). Une amibe, *Vahlkampfia discorbini*, n.sp. parasite du foraminifère *Discorbis mediterranensis* (D'Orbigny). *Archs Zool. exp. gén.*, **81**, 123–129.

Le Calvez, J. (1947). *Entosolenia marginata*, foraminifère apogamique ectoparasite d'un autre foraminifère *Discorbis vilardeboanus*. *C. r. hebd. Séanc. Acad. Sci., Paris*, **224**, 1448–1450.

Le Calvez, J. (1953). Ordre des foraminifères. In P.-P. Grassé (Ed.), *Traité de Zoologie*, Vol. I, Part 2. Masson, Paris. pp. 149–265.

Léger, L. and Duboscq, O. (1904). Notes sur les infusoires endoparasites. *Archs Zool. exp. gén.* (Ser. 4), **2**, 343–356.

Léger, L. and Duboscq, O. (1909a). Sur une microsporidie parasite d'une grégarine. *C. r. hebd. Séanc. Acad. Sci., Paris*, **148**, 733–734.

Léger, L. and Duboscq, O. (1909b). Études sur la sexualité chez les grégarines. *Arch. Protistenk.*, **17**, 19–134.

Léger, L. and Duboscq, O. (1909c). *Perezia lankesteriae* n.g.n.sp., microsporidie parasite de *Lankesteria ascidiae* Ray Lank. *Archs Zool. exp. gén.* (Ser. 5), **1**, 1–5.

Leiner, M. (1924). Das Glycogen in *Pelomyxa palustris* Greeff, mit Beiträgen zur Kenntnis des Tieres. *Arch. Protistenk.*, **47**, 253–307.

Levine, N. D. (1962). Protozoology today. *J. Protozool.*, **9**, 1–6.

Levine, N. D. (1970). Taxonomy of the Sporozoa. *J. Parasit.*, **56**, 208–209.

Levine, N. D. (1971a). Taxonomy of the Archigregarinorida and Selenidiidae (Protozoa, Apicomplexa). *J. Protozool.*, **18**, 707–717.

Levine, N. D. (1971b). Taxonomy of the piroplasms. *Trans. Am. microsc. Soc.*, **90**, 2–33.

Lohmann, H. (1908). Untersuchungen zur Feststellung des vollständigen Gehaltes des Meeres an Plankton. *Wiss. Meeresunters. (Kiel)*, **10**, 129–370.

Lützen, J. (1968). Biology and structure of *Cystobia stichopi*, n.sp., (Eugregarina, family Urosporidae), a parasite of the holothurian *Stichopus tremulus* (Gunnerus). *Norw. J. Zool.*, **16**, 14–19.

Lynch, J. E. and Noble, A. E. (1931). Notes on the genus *Endosphaera* Engelmann and on its occasional host *Opisthonecta henneguyi* Fauré-Fremiet. *Univ. Calif. Publs Zool.*, **36**, 97–114.

Mackinnon, D. L. and Ray, H. N. (1931). Observations on dicystid gregarines from marine worms. *Q. Jl microsc. Sci.* (Ser. 2), **74**, 439–466.

McLachlan, J., McInnes, A. G. and Falk, M. (1965). Studies on the chitan (chitin: poly-N-acetylglucosamine) fibres of the diatom *Thalassiosira fluviatilis* Hustedt. *Can. J. Bot.*, **43**, 707–713.

Martin, C. H. (1909). Some observations on Acinetaria. I. The 'Tinctinkörper' of Acinetaria and the conjugation of *Acineta papillifera*. II. The life-cycle of *Tachyblaston ephelotensis* (gen. et spec. nov.), with a possible identification of *Acinetopsis rara* Robin. *Q. Jl microsc. Sci. (N. S.)*, **53**, 351–389.

Mattes, O. (1924). Über Chytridineen im Plasma und Kern von *Amoeba sphaeronucleolus* und *Amoeba terricola*. *Arch. Protistenk.*, **47**, 413–430.

Metcalf, M. M. (1928). Cancer (?) in certain Protozoa. *Am. J. trop. Med.*, **8**, 545–557.

Moewus, L. (1963). Studies on a marine parasitic ciliate as a potential virus vector. In C. Oppenheimer (Ed.), *Symposium on Marine Microbiology*. Thomas, Springfield, Ill. pp. 366–379.

Moewus-Kobb, L. (1965a). Studies with IPN virus in marine hosts. *Ann. N.Y. Acad. Sci.*, **126**, 328–342.

Moewus-Kobb, L. (1965b). Experimental parasitization of fishes with *Miamiensis avidus* (Thompson and Moewus 1964), a holotrichous marine ciliate. In *Progress in Protozoology*. Abstracts of papers from 2nd int. Conf. Protozool., Lond., 1965. pp. 252–253.

Mottram, J. C. (1940). 3,4-benzpyrene, *Paramecium* and the production of tumours. *Nature, Lond.*, **145**, 184–185.

Myers, E. H. (1943). Life activities of Foraminifera in relation to marine ecology. *Proc. Am. phil. Soc.*, **86**, 439–458.

Nyholm, K. G. (1962). A study of the foraminifer *Gypsina*. *Zool. Bidr. Upps.*, **33**, 201–206.

Padnos, M. and Nigrelli, R. F. (1947). *Endosphaera engelmanni* endoparasitic in *Trichodina spheroidesi* infecting the puffer, *Sphaeroides maculatus*. *Zoologica, N.Y.*, **32**, 169–172.

Page, F. C. (1976). A revised classification of the Gymnamoebia. *Zool. J. Linn. Soc.*, **58**, 61–77.

Parke, M. and Den Hartog-Adams, J. (1965). Three species of *Halosphaera. J. mar. biol. Ass. U.K.*, **45**, 537–557.

Parsons, T. R. (1962). Infection of a marine diatom by *Lagenidium* sp. *Can. J. Bot.*, **40**, 523.

Paterson, R. A. (1958). Parasitic and saprophytic phycomycetes which invade planktonic organisms. I. New taxa and records of chytridiaceous fungi. *Mycologia*, **50**, 85–96.

Pearson, B. R. and Norris, R. E. (1974). Intranuclear virus-like particles in the marine alga *Platymonas* sp. (Chlorophyta, Prasinophyceae). *Phycologia*, **13**, 5–9.

Perkins, F. O. and Castagna, M. (1971). Ultrastructure of the Nebenkörper or 'secondary nucleus' of the parasitic amoeba *Paramoeba perniciosa* (Amoebida, Paramoebidae). *J. Invertebr. Pathol.*, **17**, 186–193.

Plate, L. (1888). The genus *Acinetoides*, g.n., an intermediate form between the ciliated Infusoria and the Acinetae. *Ann. Mag. nat. Hist.* (Ser. 6), **2**, 201–208.

Porter, C. L. and Zebrowski, G. (1937). Lime-loving molds from Australian sands. *Mycologia*, **29**, 252–257.

Powers, P. B. A. (1933). Studies on the ciliates from sea urchins. I. *Biol. Bull. mar. biol. Lab., Woods Hole*, **65**, 106–121.

Powers, P. B. A. (1936). Studies on the ciliates of sea-urchins: A general survey of the infestations occurring in Tortugas echinoids. *Pap. Tortugas Lab.*, **29**, 293–326.

Rebecq, J. (1965). Considérations sur la place des trématodes dans le zooplancton marin. *Annls Fac. Sci. Marseille*, **38**, 61–84.

Remane, A., Storch, V. and Welsch, U. (1976). *Systematische Zoologie*, Gustav Fischer Verlag, Stuttgart.

Roux, J., Serre, A. and Bassouls, C. (1964). Mise en évidence d'un phénomène d'immunité cellulaire chez un protozaire: *Tetrahymena pyriformis. C. r. Séanc. Soc. Biol.*, **158**, 613–615

Saedeleer, H. de (1946). *Palisporomonas apodinium* n.g., n.sp., flagellé parasite épibiotique de diatomées marines. *Annls Soc. r. zool. Belg.*, **77**, 90–162.

Sand, R. (1899). Étude monographique sur le groupe des infusoires tentaculifères. *Ann. Soc. belg. Micr.*, **25**, 7–205.

Sassuchin, D. N. (1934). Hyperparasitism in Protozoa. *Q. Rev. Biol.*, **9**, 215–224.

Schäfer, E. and Witt, E. (1973). Austern und Muscheln als Virus-Vektoren. *Umweltmedizin*, **1973**, 21–23.

Schnepf, E. (1974). Die Feinstruktur der *Scenedesmus*-Parasiten *Chytridium* und *Aphelidium. Veröff. Inst. Meeresforsch. Bremerh.*, **5** (Suppl.), 65–81.

Schnepf, E., Deichgräber, G. and Drebes, G. (1978a). Development and ultrastructure of the marine parasitic oomycete, *Lagenisma coscinodisci* Drebes (Lagenidiales). The infection. *Arch. Mikrobiol.*, **116**, 133–139.

Schnepf, E., Deichgräber, G. and Drebes, G. (1978b). Development and ultrastructure of the marine parasitic oomycete, *Lagenisma coscinodisci* Drebes (Lagenidiales). Thallus, zoosporangium, mitosis, and meiosis. *Arch. Mikrobiol.*, **116**, 141–150.

Schnepf, E. and Drebes, G. (1977). Über die Entwicklung des marinen parasitischen Phycomyceten *Lagenisma coscinodisci* (Lagenidiales). *Helgoländer wiss. Meeresunters.*, **29**, 291–301.

Schnepf, E., Hegewald, E. and Soeder, C.-J. (1971). Elektronenmikroskopische Beobachtungen an Parasiten aus *Scenedesmus*-Massenkulturen. 2. Über Entwicklung und Parasit-Wirt-Kontakt von *Aphelidium* und virusartige Partikel im Cytoplasma infizierter *Scenedesmus*-Zellen. *Arch. Mikrobiol.*, **75**, 209–229.

Schnepf, E., Hegewald, E. and Soeder, C.-J. (1974). Elektronenmikroskopische Beobachtungen an Parasiten aus *Scenedesmus*-Massenkulturen. *Arch. Mikrobiol.*, **98**, 133–145.

Schnepf, E., Soeder, C.-J. and Hegewald, E. (1970). Polyhedral viruslike particles lysing the aquatic phycomycete *Aphelidium* sp., a parasite of the green alga *Scenedesmus armatus. Virology*, **42**, 482–487.

Schönfeld, C. (1959). Über das parasitische Verhalten einer *Astasia*-Art in *Stentor coeruleus. Arch. Protistenk.*, **104**, 261–264.

Sieburth, J. McN. (1959). Antibacterial activity of Antarctic marine phytoplankton. *Limnol. Oceanogr.*, **4**, 419–424.

Soldo, A. T. (1963). Axenic culture of *Paramecium*. Some observations on the growth, behavior and nutritional requirements of a particle-bearing strain of *Paramecium aurelia* 299 λ. *Ann. N.Y. Acad. Sci.*, **108**, 380–388.

Soldo, A. T. (1974). Intracellular particles in *Paramecium*. In W. J. van Wagtendonk (Ed.), *Paramecium, A Current Survey*. Elsevier, Amsterdam. pp. 377–442.

Soldo, A. T. and Merlin, E. J. (1972). The cultivation of symbiote-free marine ciliates in axenic medium. *J. Protozool.*, **19**, 519–524.

Sonneborn, T. M. (1959). Kappa and related particles in *Paramecium*. *Adv. Virus Res.*, **6**, 229–356.

Sparks, A. K. (1969). Review of tumors and tumor-like conditions in Protozoa, Coelenterata, Platyhelminthes, Annelida, Sipunculida, and Arthropoda, excluding insects. *Natn. Cancer Inst. Monogr.*, **31**, 671–682.

Sparrow, F. K. (1960). *Aquatic Phycomycetes*, University of Michigan Press, Ann Arbor.

Sprague, V. (1966). Suggested changes in "A revised classification of the phylum Protozoa", with particular reference to the position of the haplosporidans. *Syst. Zool.*, **15**, 345–349.

Sprague, V. and Beckett, R. L. (1966). A disease of blue crabs *(Callinectes sapidus)* in Maryland and Virginia. *J. Invertebr. Pathol.*, **8**, 287–289.

Sprague, V. and Beckett, R. L. (1968). The nature of the etiological agent of 'Gray Crab' disease. *J. Invertebr. Pathol.*, **11**, 503.

Sprague, V., Beckett, R. L. and Sawyer, T. K. (1969). A new species of *Paramoeba* (Amoebida, Paramoebidae) parasitic in the crab *Callinectes sapidus*. *J. Invertebr. Pathol.*, **14**, 167–174.

Stein, F. v. (1859). *Der Organismus der Infusionsthiere*, I, Abtheilung, Allgemeiner Theil und Naturgeschichte der hypotrichen Infusionsthiere, Engelmann, Leipzig.

Stevenson, I. (1972). Bacterial endosymbiosis in *Paramecium aurelia*: Bacteriophage-like inclusions in a kappa symbiont. *J. gen. Microbiol.*, **71**, 69–76.

Stubblefield, J. W. (1955). The morphology and life history of *Amphiacantha ovalis* and *A. attenuata*, two new haplosporidian parasites of gregarines. *J. Parasit.*, **41**, 443–459.

Subrahmanyan, R. (1954). A new member of the Euglenineae, *Proteoeuglena noctilucae* gen. et sp. nov., occurring in *Noctiluca miliaris* Surivay, causing green discoloration of the sea off Calicut. *Proc. Indian Acad. Sci.* (Sect. B), **39**, 118–127.

Taylor, F. J. (1976). A fungal parasite in the marine diatom *Coscinodiscus oculus-iridis*. *Botanica mar.*, **19**, 61–62.

Teras, J., Kesa, L., Kallas, E. and Jogiste, A. (1977). On the relationship between some free-living and parasitic Protozoa and the RNA and DNA viruses. (Abstract.) In *Proceedings of the 5th International Congress of Protozoology*, N.Y. No. 446.

Thalmann, H. E. (1949). Mitteilungen über Foraminifera. VII. *Eclogae geol., Helvetiae*, **41**, 366–372.

Tittler, I. A. (1948). An investigation of the effects of carcinogens on *Tetrahymena geleii*. *J. exp. Zool.*, **108**, 309–325.

Vinckier, D., Devauchelle, G. and Prensier, G. (1970). *Nosema vivieri* n.sp. (Microsporida, Nosematidae) hyperparasite d'une grégarine vivant dans le coelome d'une némerte. *C. r. hebd. Séanc. Acad. Sci., Paris* (Ser. D), **270**, 821–823.

Vishniac, H. S. (1958). A new marine Phycomycete. *Mycologia*, **50**, 66–79.

Vivier, E. (1965). Étude, au microscope électronique, de la spore de *Metchnikovella hovassei* n.sp.; appartenance des Metchnikovellidae aux microsporidies. *C. r. hebd. Séanc. Acad. Sci., Paris*, **260**, 6982–6984.

Wagtendonk, W. J. van (1969). Neoplastic equivalents of Protozoa. *Natn. Cancer Inst. Monogr.*, **31**, 751–768.

Wetzel, A. (1926). Zur Morphologie und Biologie von *Raphidocystis infestans* n.sp., einem temporär auf Ciliaten parasitierenden Heliozoon. *Arch. Protistenk.*, **53**, 135–182.

Zebrowski, G. (1937). New genera of Cladochystriaceae. *Ann. Mo. bot. Gdn*, **23**, 553–564.

Zuelzer, M. (1927). Über *Amoeba biddulphiae* n.sp., eine in der marinen Diatomee *Biddulphia sinensis* Grev. parasitierende Amöbe. *Arch. Protistenk.*, **57**, 247–289.

4. DISEASES OF MESOZOA

G. Lauckner

The phylum Mesozoa contains only some 50 species of structurally simple organisms. It remains open to debate whether their structural characteristics must be considered to be primitive or whether they are the result of parasitic degeneration.

Stunkard (1954) provides evidence that the simplicity of mesozoans is secondary and the result of parasitic adaptation. He suggests that they be included as a class in the phylum Platyhelminthes. On the other hand, the parasitic status of the mesozoan order Dicyemida has been questioned: Lapan (1975) hypothesizes that dicyemids engage in a symbiotic, rather than a parasitic, relationship with their cephalopod hosts. For a more detailed discussion on this subject consult the section *Cephalopoda*.

Mesozoans are, without exception, parasites of marine invertebrates. Although this group has been studied in detail by many authors—most of whom were quite familiar with parasitology—reports on parasites or diseases of Mesozoa have not come to the reviewer's attention.

A great variety of structural abnormalities of dicyemids have been reported by Gersch (1938a, b, 1941a, b), Nouvel (1938, 1948), McConnaughey (1951) and McConnaughey and Kritzler (1952). Nouvel (1948) described and figured nematogens of *Dicyemennea lameerei* with two axial cells and increased numbers of peripheral cells, as well as double monsters of *Dicyema moschatum* nematogens, and other abnormalities in stages of *D. misakiense*, *D. typus* and *D. schulzianum*. Abnormal *Dicyemennea granularis*, *D. californica* and *D. abelis* (Fig. 4-1) have been observed by McConnaughey (1951). A curious vermiform larva was found in *Dicyema aegira* from *Octopus vulgaris* in Florida (USA). It was fully developed and with the characteristic number of somatic cells, but the calotte had become divided longitudinally during early development. This resulted in two half calottes, separated by several trunk cells and pointing in opposite directions, giving the appearance of a two-headed embryo (Fig. 4-2, 1). In the same species, a giant infusoriform larva, approximately double the usual size, was seen (Fig. 4-2, 2 and 3; McConnaughey and Kritzler, 1952).

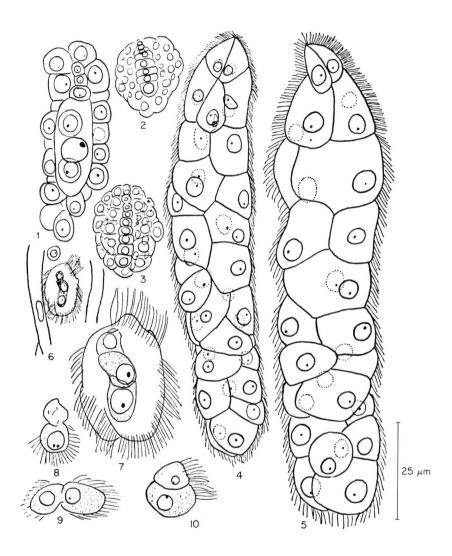

Fig. 4-1: Abnormalities in Dicyemida. 1: *Dicyemennea granularis* larva with 3 abortive axial cells anterior to definite axial cell; 2, 3: unusual *D. granularis* larvae with supranormal cell numbers; 4, 5: fully formed *D. californica* larvae without axial cell and with abnormal calotte in 5; 6: unusual body in axial cell of mature *D. abelis* nematogen; 7: enlarged view of body in 6; 8-10: other unusual cells scattered in axial cell of same nematogen, apparently derived from disaggregation of a fully formed larva prior to its escape from nematogen axial cell. (After McConnaughey, 1951; reproduced by permission of University of California Press.)

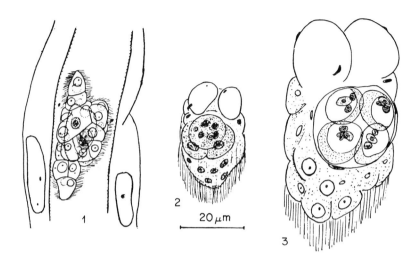

Fig. 4-2: *Dicyema aegira*. 1: Abnormal vermiform larva with divided calotte, the 2 half-calottes pointing in opposite directions; 2: frontal optical section through normal infusoriform larva; 3: abnormal giant infusoriform larva approximately double the usual size. (After McConnaughey and Kritzler, 1952; reproduced by permission of American Society of Parasitologists.)

Literature Cited (Chapter 4)

Gersch, M. (1938a). Untersuchungen über die Fortpflanzung der Dicyemiden. *Zool. Anz.*, **11** (Suppl.), 64–71.

Gersch, M. (1938b). Der Entwicklungszyklus der Dicyemiden. *Z. wiss. Zool.*, **151**, 515–605.

Gersch, M. (1941a). Weitere Untersuchungen über die Dicyemiden (Die Zerfallsformen). *Z. wiss. Zool.* (Abt. A), **154**, 409–441.

Gersch, M. (1941b). Die Entartungen der Brut bei Degeneration und beim Abklingen der Entwicklungsphase bestimmter tierischer Parasiten (Dicyemiden). *Z. Altersforsch.*, **3**, 147–155.

Lapan, E. A. (1975). Studies on the chemistry of the octopus renal system and an observation on the symbiotic relationship of the dicyemid Mesozoa. *Comp. Biochem. Physiol.*, **52**(A), 651–657.

McConnaughey, B. H. (1951). The life cycle of the dicyemid Mesozoa. *Univ. Calif. Publ. Zool.*, **55**, 295–336.

McConnaughey, B. H. and Kritzler, H. (1952). Mesozoan parasites of *Octopus vulgaris* Lam. from Florida. *J. Parasit.*, **38**, 59–64.

Nouvel, H. (1938). Sur une anomalie observée chez un dicyémide du genre *Dicyema*. *Bull. Inst. océanogr. Monaco*, **747**, 1–3.

Nouvel, H. (1948). Les dicyémides. 2e partie: Infusoriforme, tératologie, spécificité du parasitisme, affinités. *Archs Biol.*, **59**, 147–223.

Stunkard, H. W. (1954). The life-history and systematic relations of the Mesozoa. *Q. Rev. Biol.*, **29**, 230–244.

5. DISEASES OF PORIFERA

G. LAUCKNER

The phylum Porifera comprises 3 classes—the Calcarea or Calcispongia, the Demospongia, and the Hexactinellida or Hyalospongia. Some 1400 genera (about 5000 species) of sponges have been described. All except one subfamily, the Spongillinae, are marine. Only 2 genera of Demospongia produce skeletons that have market value.

Only a few parasites and diseases have been reported from calcareous sponges and from hexactinellid glass sponges. All three classes are, therefore, treated together.

Although cultivated sponges, as well as natural populations, have been subject to sometimes devastating microbial diseases in various parts of the world, very little is known about the etiology of these maladies. Fungi and bacteria appear to be involved in most of the mortalities. So far, viruses have, apparently, not been reported from marine sponges.

DISEASES CAUSED BY MICRO-ORGANISMS

Agents: Bacteria

Allemand-Martin (1906) reports moribund *Hippospongia equina* from the Mediterranean coast of Tunisia, which were presumably suffering from bacterial invasion. The dermal cortex of dying specimens was covered with white, greyish or greenish liquid. When placed in clean, running sea water, some of the diseased sponges recovered. Bacteria isolated from affected *H. equina* in the field resembled those found in moribund individuals maintained in aquaria. It appeared that the disease was favoured by insufficient water exchange in the spongocoel and predominated at shallower depths (Allemand-Martin, 1914).

Boliek (1935) describes mortalities in cultivated sponge larvae caused by bacterial contamination. In some cultures of *Lissodendoryx carolinensis* a number of attached larvae were partially destroyed. The basal region of the sponges was most commonly affected, although the invasion may extend over most of the surface, resulting in destruction of the epidermis and exposure of the sponge mass.

The parenchyma of calcareous sponges frequently harbours great numbers of possibly pathogenic micro-organisms. Thus, polymorphic bacilli, less than 1 μm in length, were seen in *Leucosolenia falcata*. *L. clathra* harboured rod-shaped bacteria, 3 to 4·5μm long. Spirochaetes, believed to be a species of *Treponema* and named *T. brevis*, occurred in *Clathrina coriacea* (Duboscq and Tuzet, 1936b).

Dosse (1940) reports great numbers of undetermined bacteria from diseased Caribbean *Hippospongia communis* var. *meandriformis*, as well as from healthy Mediterranean *Spongia officinalis* and *Cacospongia cavernosa*. He suspects these

micro-organisms, primarily associated with lesions, to be responsible for the
destruction observed. Based on the mere examination of microscopical sections, his
findings are, however, inconclusive since healthy sponges also harbour a rich microflora.
Colwell and Liston (1962) examined the natural bacterial flora of the crumb-of-bread
sponge *Halichondria panicea*. They detected pseudomonads, flavobacteria, micrococci,
bacilli and others. No *Vibrio, Achromobacter, Corynebacterium* or enterobacteria were found.

In contrast, Madri and co-authors (1967) report corynebacteria and enterobacteria,
notably *Escherichia coli*, in addition to pseudomonads and flavobacteria as members of
the indigenous microflora of the redbeard sponge *Microciona prolifera* from the Great
South Bay area of New York (USA). All bacteria found were in a viable state within the
sponge at the time of catch, but were eventually digested.

Microciona prolifera proved effective in concentrating and eliminating large quantities of
bacteria, notably *E. coli*, from sea water. The filtering capacity of the sponge was found
to depend on the initial concentration of bacteria present in the surroundings, and it was
shown that the more bacteria present, the more efficiently the sponge utilizes them. It
was suggested that red-beard sponges could be used to combat microbial pollution in
estuaries resulting from faecal contamination (Claus and co-authors, 1967; Madri and
co-authors, 1967).

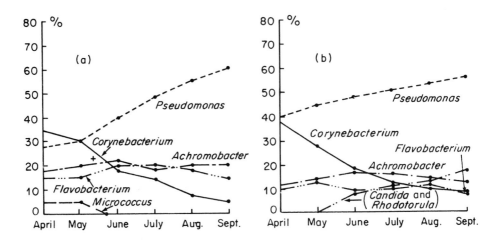

Fig. 5-1: *Microciona prolifera*. Seasonal variations in percentage of dominant genera of
micro-organisms in sponge filtrate (a) and sea water (b). (After Madri and co-authors, 1971;
reproduced by permission of Walter de Gruyter & Co., Berlin.)

In a subsequent paper, Madri and co-authors (1971) studied the seasonal variation of
bacterial concentrations in sea water and in *Microciona prolifera* from Long Island
(New York, USA). Organisms isolated from the sponge and the surrounding sea
water consisted of the following genera: *Pseudomonas, Achromobacter, Flavobacterium,
Corynebacterium, Micrococcus, Vibrio* and *Aeromonas*, as well as of unidentified non-
fermentative Gram-negative rods. Quantitative differences occurred from month to
month (Fig. 5-1). In April and May, the predominating groups were the coryneforms
and pseudomonads, present in almost equal numbers. In late May the coryneform level

dropped, with a corresponding increase in the number of pseudomonads. *Flavobacterium* and *Achromobacter* levels remained relatively constant. In general, the bacterial flora in sponge filtrates is qualitatively similar to that in the surrounding sea water.

Interestingly, however, no yeasts or other fungi were isolated in any of the sponge samples cultured whereas various *Candida* and *Rhodotorula* spp. were found in the surrounding sea water (Fig. 5-1, b). In a series of papers (consult Claus and co-authors, 1967, for references), it has been shown that lower fungi such as *Candida albicans* not only survive in sea water but retain their viability and infectivity to mice almost indefinitely. Hence, estuarine waters containing waste effluents could be a reservoir for the dissemination of these potentially harmful organisms.

Claus and co-authors (1967) demonstrated experimentally that *Microciona prolifera* is able to ingest and utilize *Candida albicans* and *Cryptococcus neoformans* as food in the same fashion as *Escherichia coli* in the experiments conducted by Madri and co-authors (1967). *In vitro* studies have shown what seemed to be chitinolytic activity in sponge tissues which effectively lysed the fungal cells.

In the light of these findings, it is difficult to interpret the earlier authors' statements regarding the pathogenicity of bacteria for sponges. In fact, sponges possess very active internal defense mechanisms (Duboscq and Tuzet, 1936b; Cheng and co-authors, 1967, 1968a, b, c; Connes, 1967).

Tethya lyncurium, for instance, is capable of isolating and casting off portions of its cortex which have been invaded by pathogenic bacteria. Motions of the spicules play a predominant role in eliminating the affected areas (Connes, 1967).

In addition to cellular defense mechanisms which result in mechanical elimination of foreign material, sponges possess biochemical means capable of inactivating pathogenic micro-organisms. Thus, Jakowska and Nigrelli (1960) isolated antimicrobial substances from several species of marine sponges, namely *Halichondria panicea*, *Cliona celata*, *Haliclona viridis* and others. An antimicrobially very active substance, ectyonin, had previously been extracted from the North Atlantic redbeard sponge *Microciona prolifera* (Nigrelli and co-authors, 1959). The materials obtained from all the sponges were active against the Gram-negative *Escherichia coli*, and some also inhibited other micro-organisms. The active substances were produced only by living sponge tissue.

Not all marine Porifera elaborate antimicrobially active substances, and in those which have been found to synthesize such compounds activities may vary considerably. Of 31 Mediterranean sponges, only 18 showed biological activity against one or more of the test organisms. The marine bacterium B-746 exhibited the greatest susceptibility to growth inhibitors of these sponges, and *Candida albicans* showed the least. Some of the poriferans tested, for example *Verongia aerophoba*, *Crambe crambe* and *Aplysilla sulfurea*, apparently contain substances capable of inhibiting both Gram-positive and negative bacteria. Non-antibiotic sponges were: *Ircinia oros*, *I. (Sarcotragus) spinulosa*, *Gellius fibulatus*, *Hymedesmia versicolor*, *Suberites domuncula*, *Cliona viridis*, *Tethya aurantium*, *Erylus discoporus*, *Pachastrella monolifera*, *Chondrilla nucula*, *Leuconia solida*, *Leucosolenia complicata* and *Clathrina blanca* (Burkholder and Ruetzler, 1969).

In the experiments conducted by Madri and co-authors (1971; see above), every bacterial species isolated was susceptible to all tested quantities of *Microciona prolifera* fluid in marine agar, whereas growth on control plates was luxuriant in all cases. Pre-inoculated semi-solid marine agar plates into which small portions of sponge had been placed did not show any zones of inhibition for any of the organisms originally isolated. Hence, it appears that the antibiotic is a non-diffusable constituent of the sponges' tissues.

Madri and co-authors (1971) further note that *Microciona prolifera* maintains its overall bacterial flora to a relatively constant level. Gross changes in the number of one large group, the coryneforms, closely correspond with a complementary shift in the pseudomonads (Fig. 5-1). One may assume that the constancy of the total colony counts of the sponge liquid obtained in the experiments is due to the antibiotic properties of *M. prolifera*.

Beside the usual microflora which, more or less, reflects the bacterial spectrum of the surrounding sea water, very intimate associations exist between Porifera and bacteria. Thus, photosynthetic bacteria, as well as a species of *Thiocystis*, have been isolated from *Halichondria panicea* (Eimhjellen, 1967). The abundant occurrence of certain bacteria in sponges has long been noticed (for review consult Dosse, 1940) but its biological implications have become apparent only from recent electron microscopical studies (Lévi and Lévi, 1965; Bertrand and Vacelet, 1971).

As revealed by electron microscopy, bacteria present in the intercellular spaces of *Verongia cavernicola* constitute as much as 38% of the total living matter of the sponge, which is approximately the volume of the intercellular substance (41%) and almost twice the volume of the sponge cells proper (21%). The proportion was found to be remarkably constant in all individuals of *V. cavernicola* examined, and regardless of the fixation procedure. Sponges fixed *in situ*, i.e. under water, by application of

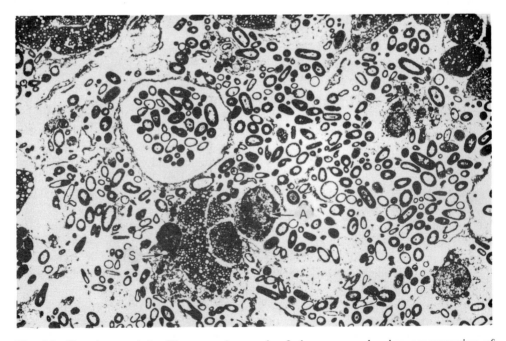

Fig. 5-2: *Verongia cavernicola*. Electron micrograph of choanosome showing concentration of extracellular symbiotic bacteria. A = archaeocyte; P = 'pocket cell'; S = spherule cell. × 4500. (After Sarà and Vacelet, 1973; reproduced by permission of Masson et Cie.)

glutaraldehyde, gave exactly the same results as those fixed in the laboratory (Fig. 5-2; Bertrand and Vacelet, 1971).

The ectosome of *Verongia cavernicola* contained maximum bacterial concentrations as well as highest concentrations of spherule cells. In contrast, bacteria were lacking almost entirely in the outermost layers of *V. aerophoba* where symbiotic cyanophyceans were numerous. Vacelet (1971) attributes these conditions to the presence, in these parts, of antimicrobial substances elaborated by the cyanophyceans.

The bacteria observed in the intercellular spaces of *Verongia cavernicola* obviously represent characteristic (symbiotic) associates of the sponge. In dying and disintegrating individuals their number decreased and the typical microflora was gradually replaced by other, rod-shaped bacteria not normally present in healthy sponges.

In healthy *Verongia cavernicola*, bacteria of the kind normally seen extracellularly were sometimes seen to occur intracellularly; these were obviously in a process of being phagocytized, indicating that the sponge may feed on its bacterial endosymbiotes. Others were seen to be engulfed by so-called 'pocket cells' (Fig. 5-2). These bacteria were not digested but instead continued to multiply within the 'pockets' whose function remained uncertain.

By means of electron microscopy, 8 principal types of bacteria could be distinguished, mainly with respect to the morphology of their cell wall. Cultivation yielded 260 isolates which could be grouped into 16 types. Fourteen of these were species of *Aeromonas* and *Pseudomonas* which exhibited a low degree of specialization and could easily be cultured. They showed, however, several characteristics that distinguished them from bacteria present in the surroundings of the sponges.

Bacteria similar to those isolated from *Verongia cavernicola* have also been observed in Mediterranean and Indian Ocean sponges of the genera *Spongia*, *Hippospongia*, *Cacospongia* and *Ircinia*, as well as in other unrelated species of Demospongia. Transfer of the symbiotic micro-organisms appears to occur directly from the parent sponges to their brood. Thus, larvae of *Ircinia variabilis* still enclosed in the maternal tissues were already found to be infested (Bertrand and Vacelet, 1971).

The interrelationships between sponges and their indigenous bacterial flora are not yet readily understood, but are beyond doubt mutualistic. The micro-organisms live, at least in part, on the sponge's metabolic waste products and the sponge, in turn, lives on the microbial protein by phagocytizing excessive symbiotes, thereby maintaining its bacterial population at a constant level. As long as they remain within the intercellular space, the bacteria are not affected since digestion in sponges is strictly intracellular.

The ecological potential of the association is certainly greater than that of the sponge alone because the micro-organisms are capable of utilizing the dissolved organic substances abundantly present in the surrounding water (Schmidt, 1970). Lévi and Lévi (1965) have pointed out that such large quantities of bacteria intimately associated with sponges could significantly influence the results of biochemical analyses conducted on whole sponge homogenates. Since not all sponges thus far examined possess a rich indigenous bacterial flora and, on the other hand, not all sponges yield antibiotically active substances, one might speculate whether there could exist a correlation between bacterial flora and biological activity in sponges.

In addition to the normal extracellular bacterial population, intranuclear symbiotes occurred in some of the cells of *Verongia aerophoba* and *V. cavernicola*. These consisted of long bacteria-like filaments, 150 to 350 mμ in diameter, situated between the nucleoplasm and the nuclear membranes and very dissimilar to the normal symbiotic bacteria. Two types of infected cells could be distinguished. Most of them occurred in the superficial layers of the ectosome and next to the central exhalant canal. Isolation and cultivation of the bacteria-like filaments met with difficulties since they could not readily be isolated from host cells, due to the superfluous presence of normal symbiotic bacteria.

Bacteriocytes were usually of rare occurrence in *Verongia cavernicola* but their number seemingly increased during the period of maturation, i.e. in April and May. They also seemed to be more numerous in sponges kept in aquaria for several days. In a single case, attack of the symbiotes by an apparent bacteriophage was seen. No intranuclear micro-organisms were found in other horny sponges of the genera *Spongia*, *Cacospongia* and *Ircinia*. The origin, fate and significance of the 'bacteriocytes' and their microbial contents could not be traced. The conditions observed in *V. cavernicola* were, however, believed to be pathological, although the overall vitality of the sponges did not appear to be affected (Vacelet, 1970).

Agents: Fungi

A fungus-like organism in tissues of the sponge genus *Ircinia* has been reported by Carter (1878) and described as a minute, short nematoid filament with a bulb at each end. Named *Spongiophaga communis*, this pathogen destroys the entire sponge body, leaving only a crust of spongin fibres. Carter's early description has been supplemented by Polejaeff (1884), who illustrates the bursting of the 'heads' of the filaments and the escape of small corpuscles in a fungus-invaded *Cacospongia* from the Indian Ocean. Polejaeff also includes further comments regarding the nature of the filaments. However, since it was not possible to cultivate the organism, it could not definitely be assigned to any particular group of fungi. Further accounts of this sponge disease have been given by Smith (1941) and Osorio Tafall and Cardenas (1945).

A peculiar malady, possibly of fungal etiology, occurred among commercial sponges on fishing grounds between Knight Key and Cape Sable (Florida, USA) in 1895. The sponges appeared normal until brought to the surface, when the whole inside dropped out, leaving nothing but a mere 'shell' (Brice, 1896).

Mass mortalities of Porifera, occurring along the Atlantic coast of North America and in the Mediterranean Sea, have been ascribed to fungus invasion. In 1938 and 1939, a sponge disease, occurring in the Bahamas and British Honduras, assumed epizootic proportions (Galtsoff and co-authors, 1939; Smith, 1939, 1941, 1947, 1954; Galtsoff, 1942; Osorio Tafall and Cardenas, 1945). Mortalities were first observed in Bahamian waters. Shortly afterwards, a similar phenomenon was reported on the north coast of Cuba and, during March, 1939, the sponge grounds of the Florida Keys (USA) were also severely depleted. Similar outbreaks of lesser degree occurred later in the Tarpon Springs area, between Cedar Keys and Carabelle. In June, 1939, the sponge fisheries of British Honduras suffered heavy losses (Smith, 1941). The sheepswool sponge *Hippospongia lachne*, as well as the velvet *H. gossypina*, yellow *Spongia barbara*, hardhead *S. dura* and grass *S. graminea* sponges were involved in the mortalities.

The epizootics observed were associated with high salinities during June, 1939. Least damage was encountered, however, in areas with maximum salinities. No other physical conditions were found which could conceivably account for such heavy mortality.

Microscopical examination of sponge sections disclosed the presence of fungal filaments, associated with mortalities in the Bahamas (Galtsoff and co-authors, 1939). These filaments, between 0·001 and 0·002 mm in diameter, were observed in the narrow zone between the living and dead 'tissues' of diseased sponges; they were found neither in the living tissue, nor in healthy sponges. The filaments were colourless, and did not reveal any definite structure, although granular inclusions were sometimes present. First signs of damage were only observed when a sponge was cut open, and a patch of rotten, evil-smelling tissue was disclosed, imbedded in the sponge body. During the peak of the epizootic, affected specimens rotted completely within a week of the initial appearance of a diseased patch (Fig. 5-3).

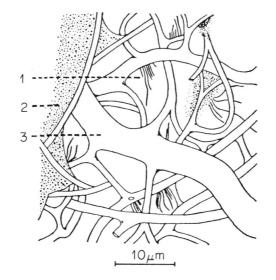

Fig. 5-3: *Hippospongia gossypina*. Portion of diseased individual. 1: Filamentous disease organism; 2: unaffected sponge tissue; 3: spongin fibre. (After Smith, 1941; reproduced by permission of Duke University Press.)

Although most sponges affected were killed, many recovered before the rot had spread very far. In these cases, the rotten area became separated off as a pocket of dead tissue by a skin or callous, similar in structure to the lining of the main oscula. This callous was frequently observed whenever local damage occurred to a sponge, and is, by no means, diagnostic of fungus disease. The decay of the sponge was confined almost entirely to the soft parts and, in most cases, the spongin fibres were not appreciably affected. For this reason, many of the dead sponges were still marketable.

Closer examination of the diseased sponges revealed no unusual parasites visible to the naked eye. The typical commensals, polychaete worms, ophiuroids and crustaceans were present in the canal systems, and began to desert the sponge as the disease advanced. Bacteria and Cyanophyceae occurred in the later stages of decay. They were present in decaying sponges at all times, irrespective of the cause of death, and were not confined to victims of the mortality cause considered here (Smith, 1941).

Incidence and spread of the epizootic suggested that it was contagious, and transmitted by water currents. The pathogen involved might have been *Spongiophaga communis*(Smith, 1954). It has been suggested that this organism is always present, becoming sufficiently virulent to kill the sponges only under abnormal stress conditions (Smith, 1941). According to de Laubenfels (1952), the 1939 to 1940 epizootics reduced the Gulf of Mexico stock of commercial sponges to approximately 5% of its previous number. Yellow sponges *Spongia barbara*, for instance, were collected at only 1 out of 22 stations where they had been abundant before. Over wide areas, the disease had wiped out the entire commercial sponge population. From 1944 to 1954, American sponges practically vanished from the market (de Laubenfels and Storr, 1958). Survivors of the epizootics showed large, healed-over lesions; the commercial stocks recovered but slowly (Galtsoff, 1942; Dawson and Smith, 1953). Velvet and wire sponges, however, never resumed commercial importance again; for all practical purposes, they had disappeared (Storr, 1957).

According to Arndt (1937), sponge diseases of epizootic proportions, but of unknown etiology, have previously been reported from Florida (1895 and 1900) and from the Mediterranean Sea (Sfax: 1911 to 1912; Egypt: 1920; Tunisia: 1920–1927). While the majority of the outbreaks were confined to shallow waters, the Tunisian epizootic also involved sponges from greater depths. In infected specimens, the skeleton became brittle like touchwood, while the soft parts remained virtually unaffected. The disease appeared to be etiologically different from the one occurring in shallow-water sponges. Thus, Dosse (1940), who published a detailed histological study of healthy, diseased and decaying sponges (from Gulf of Mexico mortalities and from healthy Mediterranean specimens), found virtually the same pathological conditions in the soft parts previously described by Galtsoff and co-authors (1939), while the skeletal fibres remained unaffected.

Provided that fungi are the causative agents responsible for the reported sponge epizootics, it is evident that the mechanisms leading to the destruction of *Candida albicans* and *Cryptococcus neoformans*, as reported by Claus and co-authors (1967) and Kunen and co-authors (1971; see section *Bacteria*), are not active against these sponge-pathogenic fungi.

Fungi affecting sponge skeletons have been described by Kölliker (1860), Porter and Zebrowski (1937) and Zebrowski (1937).

DISEASES CAUSED BY PROTOZOANS

Agents: Flagellata

Syncrypta spongiarum is a common parasite of *Grantia compressa* and *Sycon ciliatum*, inhabiting the choanocytes or the lumen of the radial channels of the sponges. Cysts of a euglenoid flagellate were seen in choanocytes of *Sycon elegans* (Tuzet, 1973a).

Agents: Rhizopoda

An amoeba, about 80 μm in length, 40 μm in width and similar to *Amoeba cristalligera*, has been observed in *Sycon coronatum* (Orton, 1913, 1914; Tuzet, 1973a). Dendy (1913) erroneously interpreted these organisms as metamorphosed sponge choanocytes, and Bidder (1920), who saw the same or similar amoebae in *Clathrina coriacea* believed them to be sponge spermatozoids. *Topsentella fallax*, a minute amoeboid organism of uncertain affinities, occurs in the parenchyma of *Sycon raphanus*. It is very variable in size and shape (Fig. 5-4). Large vermiform stages may attain a length of 5 to 15 μm; pyriform or ovoid stages are about 2 μm in diameter (Duboscq and Tuzet, 1936a). Tuzet (1973a) provisionally grouped *T. fallax* with the chytrid fungi.

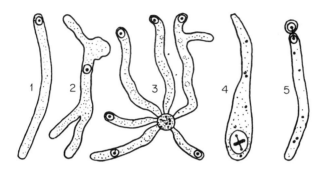

Fig. 5-4: *Topsentella fallax*. Various aspects of individuals from parenchyma of *Sycon raphanus*. 1: Normal straight individual; 2: bifurcated form; 3: gregarious specimens; 4: stage in nuclear division; 5: budding (?). (After Duboscq and Tuzet, 1936a; reproduced by permission of Centre National de la Recherche Scientifique.)

Agents: Sporozoa

According to Tuzet (1973a), eggs of *Leucandra nivea* have been found to be parasitized by an unidentified microsporidan.

Agents: Ciliata

Wenzel (1961a) studied the ciliate fauna of several species of Mediterranean poriferans. Representatives of 33 ciliate species were obtained from 12 to 26 freshly collected sponges. *Suberites domuncula*, *Mycale* sp., *Dysidea avara* and *Spongia officinalis* were found to be devoid of protozoans. No explanation was offered for this observation. Upon collection, most of the sponges that carried ciliates were but lightly populated. Protozoan numbers increased, however, after 24 h of storage in aquaria. It was concluded that the density of the ciliate fauna was largely dependent on bacterial numbers present. None of the ciliates seemed to be an obligate sponge associate, with the possible exception of *Ophryodendron multiramosum*, a suctorian that possibly feeds on the contents of sponge cells (Wenzel, 1961a, b).

Agents: Protophyta

The occurrence of algae within sponge tissues has long been known. Carter (1878) observed Cyanophyceae in sponges and believed them to be parasitic, but Feldmann (1933) found the relationship to be mutualistic. *Phormidium spongeliae*, *Aphanocapsa feldmanni* and *A. raspaigellae* are commonly engaged in a mutualistic relationship with Mediterranean demosponges. The association between sponges and blue-green algae is of particular interest since it is the only known case of mutualism between Metazoa and Cyanophyceae. Ultrastructural aspects of this association have been studied—among others—by Sarà (1971).

The literature on associations between sponges and other protophytes—mainly dinoflagellates (zooxanthellae)—has been discussed by Arndt (1928) and reviewed by Sarà and Vacelet (1973).

DISEASES CAUSED BY METAZOANS

A great variety of invertebrates, primarily ophiuroids, crustaceans and polychaetes are closely associated with marine sponges, but also cnidarians, nematodes, alpheids, crabs, shrimps, stomatopods, clams, echinoids and fishes, as well as represenatatives of numerous other invertebrate groups, have been reported as sponge inquilines or lodgers in various parts of the world (Carter, 1878; Santucci, 1922; de Laubenfels, 1947; Bakus, 1966; Fishelson, 1966; Pansini, 1970; Băcescu, 1971; Al Nimeh and Vitiello, 1976; further authors are cited below).

The number of associates populating individual sponges may reach very high levels. Thus, Pearse (1935) recorded 6282, 13,504 and 17,128 inhabitants, representing 21 species, from 3 large loggerhead sponges *Speciospongia vespara* (with volumes of 50,000 cm^3, 50,000 cm^3 and 185,000 cm^3, respectively) from Dry Tortugas (Florida, USA). These numbers correspond to 0·13, 0·27 and 0·09 animals per cm^3 of sponge volume. Much lower figures were obtained, however, from *S. vespara* and other sponges at Bimini, Bahamas (Pearse, 1950). De Laubenfels (1947), on the other hand, reported at least 3 inhabitants per cm^3 in *Hymeniacidon heliophila* and 5 individuals per cm^3 in *Lissodendoryx isodictyalis* from Beaufort (North Carolina, USA). Băcescu (1971) found 21,000 *Syllis spongicola* in a grapefruit-sized sponge from the Gulf of Mexico. Large sponges with good-sized internal canals may serve as veritable 'living hotels' (Pearse, 1935).

The trophic relationships between sponges and their associates are little understood. According to Sarà and Vacelet (1973), they may cover all transitions from superficial inquilinism to true parasitism. Even in loose associations, in which the inhabitants merely seek shelter but are otherwise metabolically independent of the 'host', high population densities of lodgers can cause at least some degree of irritation and evoke responses which may be termed 'diseased conditions'.

Tissue reactions to the presence of parasites and commensals have been studied in several marine sponges (Gravier, 1922; Tuzet and Paris, 1964; Connes, 1967; Connes and co-authors, 1971).

The number of individuals, as well as the number of species populating sponges may vary with host species, sponge volume, niche structure, water depth and other macro- and microecological factors. Thus, *Speciospongia vespara* from deeper waters off Dry Tortugas had three times as many associates as sponges of the same species from shallower depths (Pearse, 1935). Pansini (1970) recorded seasonal variations in the population density of dwellers from 3 species of Mediterranean sponges, with a minimum in winter.

Some associates apparently exhibit some degree of preference for certain sponge species. Long (1968), for example, recorded the spionid *Polydora socialis* from within the sponge *Suberites lata*, as well as several species of amphipods, sabellids, nereids and nematodes from *Microciona prolifera*. The crumb-of-bread sponge *Halichondria panicea* harboured the richest associate fauna, comprising 52 species from 9 phyla. Most common were the amphipods *Corophium acherusicum* and various caprellids. The inhabitants of various Caribbean sponges have been described by Pearse (1935, 1950). None of these associations has been claimed to be truly parasitic, although close scrutiny might possibly reveal such relationships in some cases.

Agents: Cnidaria

Several species of cnidarians—members of different classes—are known to be associated with marine sponges. Some of these associations are merely superficial and may represent cases of simple phoresis; others are more intimate, with the cnidarian penetrating the sponge body.

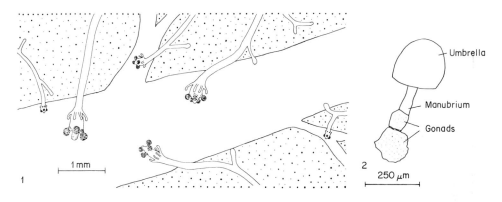

Fig. 5-5: *Dipurena spongicola*. 1: Stolons and hydranths in host sponge *Halichondria panicea*; 2: young medusa. (After Anger, 1972; reproduced by permission of Institut für Meereskunde, Kiel.)

Scyphozoans of the genus *Stephanoscyphus* are closely associated with various sponges. The stolons which are surrounded by chitinous tubes, ramify throughout the sponge parenchyma, only the polyps rising above the host cortex. The free-swimming medusal stage of *Stephanoscyphus* sp. is known under the name *Nausithoë punctata*. *S. mirabilis* has been reported from *Spirastrella* spp. collected during the Siboga Expedition (Vosmaer, 1911), as well as from a number of other sponges (Carter, 1878). In the Mediterranean, *Stephanoscyphus* sp. has been found in *Crambe crambe*, *Antho involvens*, *Dysidea avara* and *Cacospongia scalaris*, as well as in several other Keratosa (Riedl, 1966). Sponges inhabited by *S. mirabilis* frequently exhibit club-shaped distortions (Vosmaer, 1911).

Hydrozoans *Dipurena halterata* develop in *Chalina montagui*, with their stolons embedded in the sponge parenchyma and the adult polyps protruding from the host's body surface (Rees, 1939). *Suberites carnosus typicus* from the French Mediterranean coast frequently harbours this hydrozoan (Connes and co-authors, 1971). *D. strangulata* shows similar stages in *Microciona prolifera* (Calder, 1970), whereas *D. simulans* develops in the oscula of *Adocia simulans* (Bouillon, 1971).

In contrast, *Dipurena spongicola* completes its entire polyp stage within the parenchyma and water passages of *Halichondria panicea* from the western Baltic Sea. The delicate and irregularly branched stolons of this species, 100 to 180 μm in diameter and up to 1 cm or more in length, ramify throughout the sponge parenchyma. Stolon tips that come into contact with the water passages transform into hydranths which measure 400 to 800 μm in length and 120 to 350 μm in width (Fig. 5-5, 1). On one occasion, a young medusa of *D. spongicola* was found within a host sponge. Its dome-shaped umbrella, 220 μm in diameter and 220 μm in height, bore a tube-like manubrium, 350 μm in length and supporting the gonads at its distal end (Fig. 5-5, 2). Crumb-of-bread sponges occupied by *D. spongicola* showed no signs of detriment. The hydrozoan apparently feeds on matter brought in by the sponge's filter current, as well as on cyclopoids, harpacticoids, ostracods, ciliates, turbellarians and nematodes inhabiting the water passages of *H. panicea* (Anger, 1972).

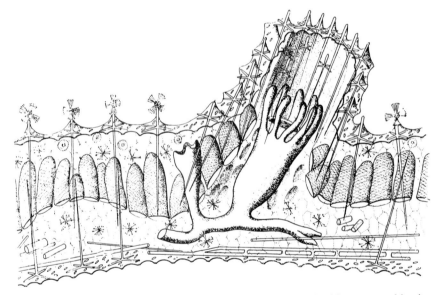

Fig. 5-6: *Walteria flemmingi.* Section showing individual parasitized by a gymnoblastic hydrozoan. (After Tuzet, 1973b; reproduced by permission of Masson et Cie.)

Three other known members of the genus *Dipurena*, *D. reesi*, *D. ophiogaster*, and *D. bicircella*, have not yet been reported as inhabitants of marine sponges (Vannucci, 1956; Kramp, 1959; Rees, 1977). An undetermined gymnoblastic hydrozoan, morphologically different but in behaviour similar to *D. spongicola*, occurs in *Walteria flemmingi* and *W. leuckarti*. It is this endobiote with its stolonial ramifications that determines the special shape of these hexactinellid sponges (Fig. 5-6).

Zoantharians of the genus *Palythoa* frequently attach to the outer surface of Demospongia and Hexactinellida. *Thoracactis topsenti*, an actinian, occurs on hexactinellids *Sarostegia oculata* (Tuzet, 1973b). There are several other records of associations between cnidarians and Porifera (Carter, 1878; Arndt and Pax, 1936).

Agents: Rotifera

Rotifers have been reported as true parasites of freshwater sponges, feeding on their epidermal tissues (Bērziņš, 1950). No such associates have, thus far, been described from marine Porifera.

Agents: Mollusca

Bivalve molluscs are frequently found embedded in the cortex of marine sponges. *Stelletta grubii* from the northern Gulf of Mexico, for example, were found to harbour *Ostrea permollis*. Adults live crowded on the sponge surface or embedded in the choanosome with the shell margins protruding (Figs 5-7 and 5-8). Most *S. grubii* collected

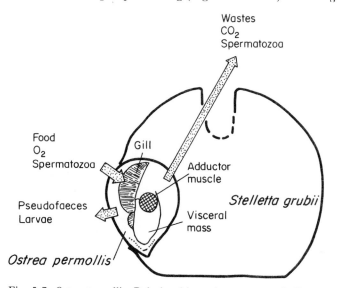

Fig. 5-7: *Ostrea permollis*. Relationship to host sponge, *Stelletta grubii*. (After Forbes, 1966; modified; reproduced by permission of Rosenstiel School of Marine and Atmospheric Science, University of Miami.)

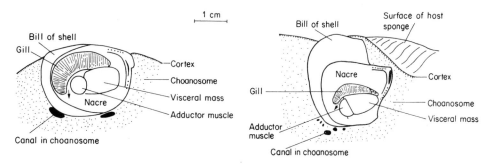

Fig. 5-8: *Ostrea permollis* within *Stelletta grubii*. Sagittal sections, right valves *in situ*. Arrows: inferred path of excurrent stream. (After Forbes, 1966; modified; reproduced by permission of Rosenstiel School of Marine and Atmospheric Science, University of Miami.)

contained from a few to several hundred *O. permollis*. The bivalves did not occur outside sponges and were found in a sponge other than *S. grubii* only once, thus exhibiting a marked degree of host-specificity. On the other hand, *O. permollis* did not appear to depend on *S. grubii* for nutrition (Forbes, 1964, 1966).

Agents: Annelida

Polychaete annelids—mostly syllids, nereids and cirratulids—occur as lodgers or commensals in the water passages of a great variety of demosponges. Records of polychaetes are included in virtually all published lists of sponge inhabitants. Some species populate marine Porifera in vast numbers. Polychaetes have also been recorded in hexactinellid sponges. *Hermadion fauveli*, for example, lives in *Sarostegia oculata* (Tuzet, 1973b).

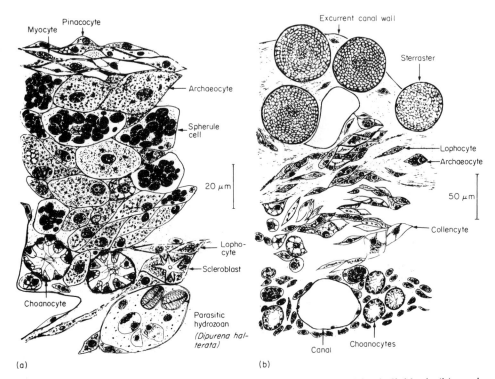

Fig. 5-9: *Geodia cydonium*. (a) Section through osculum wall of healthy individual; (b) section through osculum wall of individual harbouring *Eunice siciliensis*. (After Connes and co-authors, 1971; reproduced by permission of Le Naturaliste canadien.)

Usually, annelids are regarded as harmless inquilines that do not affect their hosts in any way. However, Connes and co-authors (1971) demonstrated that polychaetes in the water passages may induce considerable irritation leading to structural alterations in the host sponge. Thus, *Geodia cydonium* reacts to the presence of *Eunice siciliensis* by a massive proliferation of microscleres and increased fibrogenesis (Fig. 5-9). The wall of a normal exhalant canal is practically devoid of sterrasters and oxyasters. In sponges harbouring annelids, great numbers of sterrasters, 70 to 80 μm in diameter, accumulate in the region occupied by the worms. Simultaneously, the number of oxyasters increases. Microscleres are formed in abundance within the pinacocyte layer, and numerous archaeocytes and lophocytes participate in fibrogenesis.

Excurrent canals occupied by *Eunice siciliensis* lose their normal function of water transport. Contractile cells (myocytes) and spherule cells diminish in number. The former play a major role in the regulation of the water circulation whereas the latter have an excretory function. The formation of sterrasters and oxyasters occurs in response to the mechanical irritation provoked by the annelid and may contribute to seclude the parasite from contact with the sponge body.

Agents: Copepoda

Numerous siphonostome cyclopoid copepods—mostly but slightly transformed or almost untransformed representatives of the families Asterocheridae, Acontiophoridae, Artotrogidae, Myzopontiidae, Dyspontiidae and Entomolepidae—are associated with marine sponges (Leigh-Sharpe, 1935; Stock and Kleeton, 1964; Stock, 1965; Hamond, 1968; Yeatman, 1970). Schirl (1973) assembled a list of known sponge–siphonostome associations.

Siphonostomes and other representatives of the Copepoda sometimes populate the outer surfaces and water passages of sponges in considerable numbers. Although their trophic relationships with their host sponges have rarely been studied in depth, these crustaceans are generally listed as harmless commensals or lodgers. Host-specificity, observed in a great number of these associations, however, points towards a more intimate relationship rather than mere commensalism or phoresis. It must be borne in mind that among the Copepoda associated with other animals can be found the entire scale of symbiotic relationships, with gradual transitions ranging from commensalism to true parasitism. Among the spongicolous siphonostomes, at least some species are histophagic.

Cryptopontius gracilis was collected from *Halichondria bowerbanki*, *Craniella gravida*, *Microciona prolifera* and *Haliclona permollis* from Chesapeake Bay (Virginia, USA). Sponge cells were seen in the digestive tracts of several individuals indicating that *C. gracilis* is definitely histophagic on species of poriferans on which they were found. The red-pigmented cells of *Microciona prolifera* were especially easy to locate in the copepods' gut. *Asterocheres jeanyeatmanae* is another siphonostome histophagic on its host sponges, *H. bowerbanki* and *M. prolifera* (Yeatman, 1970).

Hemicyclops perinsignis, a new poecilostome copepod, from the sponge *Agelas* sp. from Madagascar, has been described by Humes (1973). Poecilostomes *Pseudoclausia longiseta* were reported by Bocquet and Stock (1963) from the Mediterranean. Although the sponge hosts were not identified, the authors stated that they belong to different species. Thus, *P. longiseta* does not appear to exhibit any marked degree of host-specificity. Both papers are merely taxonomic; neither of the authors reports on pathological effects (Fig. 5-10).

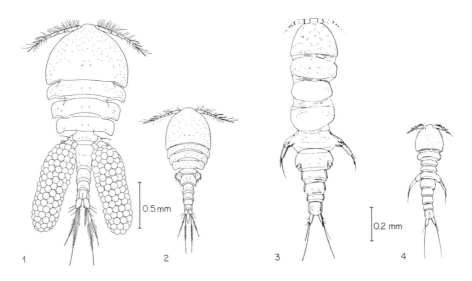

Fig. 5-10: Copepods from marine sponges. Female (1) and male (2) *Hemicyclops perinsignis* from *Agelas* sp.; female (3) and male (4) *Pseudoclausia longiseta* from undetermined Mediterranean sponge. (1 and 2 after Humes, 1973; reproduced by permission of Biological Society of Washington; 3 and 4 after Bocquet and Stock, 1963; reproduced by permission of Koninklijke Nederlandse Akademie van Wetenschappen.)

The sponginticolid *Clionophilus vermicularis* (Fig. 5-11), a copepod about 1 mm in length and almost completely vermiform, inhabits the canal system of the boring sponge *Cliona celata* (Silén, 1963). Its adaptations to this specialized niche are extensive. Pereiopods are entirely lacking, mouth parts are greatly reduced, and the furca has almost vanished. The body shape of living *C. vermicularis* may vary considerably due to the elastic nature of the cuticle and the contractability of its body. *C. vermicularis* possesses a suctorial pharynx; this strongly suggests that it is a true parasite.The copepod was first described by Silén (1963) from Gullmar Fjord (Sweden), and was later recorded from Strangford Lough (Northern Ireland) by Gotto (1965). About 75% of the *C. celata* from Gullmar Fjord harboured *C. vermicularis*. The adult parasites were always found in the large canals of the sponge, in contrast to eggs and embryos, which were invariably situated in the sponge tissue itself, though near the canals.

Clionophilus vermicularis does not appear to thrive outside the sponge. Copepods removed from the host and suspended in sea water were dead within 2 to 5 h. The parasite's mode of feeding could not be determined with confidence. It was assumed, however, that the maxillipeds, which perform incessant scratching movements, tear small portions from the canal wall, which are immediately ingested by means of the suctorial pharynx (Silén, 1963).

Another copepod, similar to *Clionophilus vermicularis* in being vermiform in shape and lacking appendages, has superficially been described from *Cliona celata* (French coast of the English Channel), as well as from *Mycale macilenta* and *Stylopus coriaceus* (French Mediterranean coast) under the name *Sponginticola uncifera* (Topsent, 1928). Stock and Kleeton (1964) confirmed that both copepods are identical. Hence, the generic name *Clionophilus* has to be suppressed as a synonym.

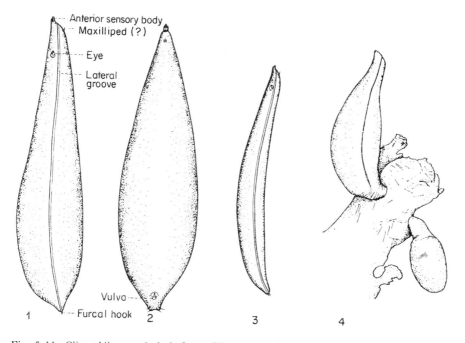

Fig. 5-11: *Clionophilus vermicularis* from *Cliona celata*. Mature female in lateral (1) and ventral (2) view, and male in lateral view (3); × 100. 4: Two individuals adhering with their furcal hooks to a piece of sponge body; × 60. (After Silén, 1963; reproduced by permission of E. J. Brill, Leiden.)

Stock and Kleeton (1964) established the new family Spongiocnizontidae to include a single, unique species collected from the tissues of *Hemimycale columella* at Port-Vendres (French Mediterranean coast). Named *Spongiocnizon petiti*, this copepod is entirely vermiform, devoid of segmentation and exhibits an almost complete reduction of body appendages. Females measure about 2·5 mm, males about 1·75 mm in length. Nothing is reported on the relationship between *S. petiti* and its host but it appears likely that the copepod feeds on sponge tissue.

Tuzet and Paris (1964) studied the response of *Suberites domuncula* to *Sponginticola uncifera*. There was an intense accumulation of host cells in the region surrounding the copepods, resulting in the formation of a capsule-like structure. The histological changes were virtually identical to those exhibited by *Sycon raphanus* in response to the presence of foreign bodies (Duboscq and Tuzet, 1936b).

As has been pointed out, little is known about the interrelationships between sponges and their copepod associates. A few cases of apparent host-specificity have been reported: Siphonostomes *Asterocheres simplex* showed a preference for *Clathrina clathrus* and *C. lacunosa*; *Myzopontius pungens* for *C. contorta*; and *A. mucronipes* for *Oscarella lobularis*. *A. corneliae* was most abundant on *C. primordialis*, but the same host species also harboured *M. pungens* (Schirl, 1973).

With the exception of the siphonostome cyclopoids *Cryptopontius gracilis* and *Asterocheres jeanyeatmanae* (Yeatman, 1970) and the lamippid *Clionophilus vermicularis* (Silén, 1963), feeding habits have, apparently, not yet been studied in spongicolous copepods. It must be borne in mind that the mouth parts of siphonostomes are well suited for the piercing of cell walls and sucking of cell contents. Several siphonostomes are known as true parasites of members of other invertebrate phyla.

Agents: Amphipoda

Suberites carnosus typicus from Sète, French Mediterranean coast, occasionally harbour lysianassid amphipods *Perrierella audouiniana*. The crustaceans lie, curled up, in ovoid depressions, about 3×1 mm in dimension and deeply embedded in the sponge tissue. The cavities possess a connection with the sponge's water passages, thus supplying the inhabitant with a constant flow of nutrient-rich water. The cavity walls are formed by a discontinuous layer of pinacocytes which appears to be altered structurally by the presence of the amphipod. Immediately below this superficial pinacocyte layer, 4 to 5 layers of lophocytes and collencytes form a conspicuous envelope surrounding the cavities (Connes and co-authors, 1971).

A similar reaction has been observed in *Tethya lyncurium* in response to *Leucothoë spinicarpa*. These amphipods settle in gall-like structures, about 13 mm in diameter, on the outer surface of the sponge. The inner wall of cavities occupied by *L. spinicarpa* is lined by a kind of 'cuticle', 2·5 to 3 μm in thickness and apparently originating from flattened cells that had lost their contours. No pinacocytes occur in the vicinity of the cavity. The sponge does not attempt to eliminate the intruder but instead mobilizes a repair mechanism. Local tissue disintegration occurs, accompanied by a dedifferentiation of cells. Choanocytes are absent but there is a marked increase in amoebocyte concentration around the cavity. The amphipod becomes isolated by a successive reinforcement of the reactive tissue (Connes, 1967).

Tritaeta gibbosa was frequently found in depressions in the cortex of Mediterranean sponges, particularly in *Ircinia* spp. and *Suberites* spp. (Fage, 1928; Riedl, 1966). Such depressions may, upon superficial inspection and in the absence of their inhabitants, sometimes be taken for oscula (Carter, 1878; Vosmaer, 1911). Host reactions against *T. gibbosa*, studied in *Suberites domuncula*, are essentially the same as those evoked by other spongicolous amphipods (Tuzet and Paris, 1964).

Agents: Cirripedia

Structural modifications of the sponge body comparable to those produced by amphipods may also be caused by cirripeds. The latter sometimes become overgrown by sponge tissue, forming wart-like excrescences with a hole in the summit for the projection of the cirri (Carter, 1878; Vosmaer, 1911; Gravier, 1922).

Most of the individuals of *Ircinia fasciculata* collected off Sète harboured cirripeds *Balanus perforatus* which were found to provoke a moderate tissue reaction (Fig. 5-12). In response to the attachment of the basal plate, a tissue resembling normal ectosoma in some respects is formed between the sponge's choanosome and the balanid. The sponge tissue in immediate contact with the crustacean forms a delicate layer, 1 to 2 μm in thickness and devoid of cellular elements. The most conspicuous host response is represented by the abundance of spongin filaments within the underlying tissue, which

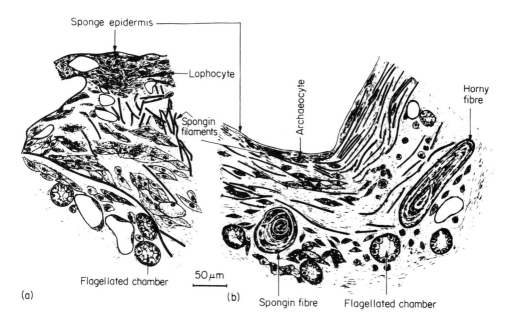

Fig. 5-12: *Ircinia fasciculata*. (a) Transverse section through ectosome of healthy individual; (b) longitudinal section through ectosome in contact with *Balanus perforatus*. (After Connes and co-authors, 1971; reproduced by permission of Le Naturaliste canadien.)

form a fibrous barrier against the intruder. The latter, however, is not eliminated or suffocated (Connes and co-authors, 1971).

In contrast, the reaction of *Cacospongia scalaris* to invasion by the cirriped *Acasta spongites* is much more pronounced (Fig. 5-13). When this crustacean settles within the lumen of an osculum, the perioscular stratum becomes reinforced by numerous spongin fibres and increases in thickness from 70 to 80 μm in normal oscula to about 100 to 250 μm. In addition, a delicate spongin layer, about 2 to 3 μm in thickness, begins to form immediately beneath the superficial pellicle lining the inner walls of the osculum. Some time after the intrusion of the cirriped, the sponge overgrows the invader by formation of new cortex and choanosome material. Although the crustacean eventually dies from suffocation, the occupied osculum does not resume its function. Instead, new excurrent canals and oscula open in the vicinity of the obstructed one (Gravier, 1922; Connes and co-authors, 1971).

Hammer (1906) observed that individuals of *Ircinia variabilis* populated by cirripeds (probably *Acasta spongites*) do not become sexually mature. However, the existence of 'parasitic castration' in sponges remains very doubtful. *A. spongites* has been reported from a variety of Mediterranean sponges (Gravier, 1922; von Kolosváry, 1940; Tuzet and Paris, 1964; Riedl, 1966).

Agents: Mysidacea

Numerous mysidaceans are commensal with sponges, particularly in tropical and subtropical waters. Some—like species of *Heteromysis* and *Heteromysoides* living in the

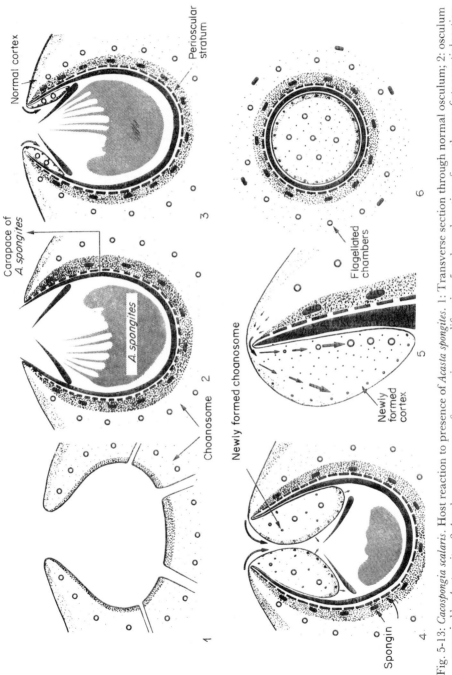

Fig. 5-13: *Cacospongia scalaris*. Host reaction to presence of *Acasta spongites*. 1: Transverse section through normal osculum; 2: osculum occupied by *A. spongites*; 3, 4: subsequent stages of sponge tissue proliferation; 5: enlarged portion of growth zone; 6: tangential section through osculum after suffocation of inhabitant. (After Connes and co-authors, 1971; reproduced by permission of Le Naturaliste canadien.)

water passages of Gulf of Mexico sponges—exhibit varying degrees of adaptation to their special mode of life and display host-specificity (Băcescu, 1968, 1971).

Agents: Decapoda

Decapod crustaceans constitute an important portion of sponge inquilines (Carter, 1878; Hunt, 1925; Arndt, 1933; Pearse, 1935, 1950; Schmitt, 1935; Forbes, 1966; Castro, 1971; Sarà and Vacelet, 1973; Bruce, 1976; consult these papers for further references). Arndt (1933) reviewed the older literature on biological relationships between crustaceans and sponges.

Shrimps *Synalpheus laevimanus* and *Typton spongicola* have been found associated with Mediterranean demosponges (Riedl, 1966). Females and males of *Spongicola venusta* live in pairs enclosed in hexactinellids, mostly members of the genus *Euplectella* (Ijima, 1901). An unidentified palaemonid shrimp occupies the subdermal cavities of *E. marshalli* and *Semperella schulzei* (Tuzet, 1973b).

'Crustaceans' occurring in the water passages of *Grantia ciliata* and *G. compressa* were seen to devour sponge gastrulae, as well as portions of the mother sponge itself (Carter, 1878). Analyses of the stomach contents of decapods *Typton spongicola*, which occur in several sponge species, also revealed remains of sponge tissue (Hunt, 1925). It appears probable that comparable analyses of the stomach and gut contents of other crustaceans from sponges will reveal these 'commensals' to be true parasites (Arndt, 1933).

Agents: Arachnida and Pantopoda

A list of mites, both freshwater and marine, and of their respective sponge hosts was published by Arndt and Viets (1939). While, in most cases, the relationship of the freshwater sponge–mite associations is truly parasitic, such parasitism is less pronounced in comparable marine associations. Pathological conditions, caused by Acari, have, so far, not been reported from marine sponges. Various representatives of the Pantopoda live in association with marine sponges but the nature of these associations is not clear (Arndt and Viets, 1939).

Agents: Pisces

Various fishes live as inquilines in the water passages of marine sponges. Radcliffe (1917) reported gobies *Evermannichthys (Garmannia) spongicola* from unidentified poriferans collected off North Carolina (USA). Böhlke and Robins (1969) gave a detailed account of the genus *Evermannichthys* whose 4 known species all inhabit western Atlantic sponges. Blennies *Starksia ocellata* live in *Ircinia*-type sponges off South Carolina. The blennies are also common among corals and sea-urchins at Tortugas (Gulf of Mexico) and hence are not in any way dependent on the sponge (Dawson, 1960). *Blennius tentacularis* and *Gobius* sp. have been reported as inquilines from Mediterranean *Geodia cydonium* (Santucci, 1922). Gudger (1950) and Fishelson (1966) listed further teleosts associated with Porifera. The sponges do not appear to suffer any negative effects from their piscean lodgers.

TUMOURS AND ABNORMALITIES

No information is available concerning tumours or related neoplastic growth in the Porifera. According to Sparks (1969), it is uncertain whether sponges do indeed lack such growth or whether investigators have failed to seek, recognize or report neoplastic abnormalities in the sponges.

Small 'granulomata' developed in the parenchyma of *Sycon raphanus* in response to intruded foreign material which was surrounded by archaeocytes and broken down by the sponge (Duboscq and Tuzet, 1936b; Fig. 5-14). Structural abnormalities, probably due to injury, occur in glass sponges of the family Euplectellidae (Ijima, 1901).

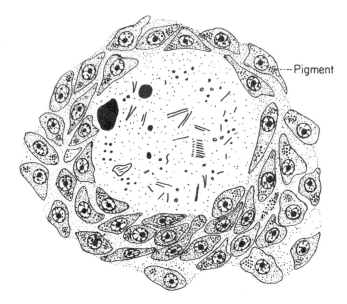

Fig. 5-14: *Sycon raphanus*. Small 'granuloma' developing in response to and enclosing intruded foreign body. (After Duboscq and Tuzet, 1936b; reproduced by permission of Patrimoine de l'Institut Royal des Sciences Naturelles de Belgique.)

Skeletal abnormalities in *Hippospongia communis* from the Gulf of Mexico have been observed by Dosse (1940). While the secondary fibres are round and smooth in healthy sponges, a single aberrant specimen was found with 'collars' surrounding the fibres, which appeared 'inflated' in the affected areas. Abnormal spicules in the freshwater sponge *Ephydatia fluviatilis* have been reported by Wierzejki (1912) and Tuzet and Connes (1962). Boliek (1935) described abnormal larvae of cultivated *Lissodendoryx carolinensis*.

Literature Cited (Chapter 5)

Allemand-Martin, A. (1906). Étude de physiologie appliquée sur la spongiculture sur le côtes de Tunisie. Thèse, Univ. Lyon.

Allemand-Martin, A. (1914). Contribution à l'étude de la culture des éponges. *C. r. Ass. Advmt Sci. Tunis*, **1914**, 375–377.

Al Nimeh, M. and Vitiello, P. (1976). Premières observations sur le peuplement nématologique associé aux éponges de la 'biocoenose précoralligène'. *C. r. hebd. Séanc. Acad. Sci., Paris*, **283**, 1775–1778.

Anger, K. (1972). *Dipurena spongicola* sp. n. (Hydrozoa, Corynidae), ein in Schwämmen lebender Hydroidpolyp aus dem Kattegat und der nördlichen Kieler Bucht. *Kieler Meeresforsch.*, **28**, 80–83.

Arndt, W. (1928). Lebensdauer, Altern und Tod der Schwämme. *Sitz. ber. Naturforsch. Ges.*, **1928**, 23-44.

Arndt, W. (1933). Die biologischen Beziehungen zwischen Schwämmen und Krebsen. *Mitt. zool. Mus. Berl.*, **19**, 221–305.

Arndt, W. (1937). Schwämme. In F. Pax and W. Arndt (Eds), *Die Rohstoffe des Tierreiches*. Bornträger, Berlin.

Arndt, W. and Pax, F. (1936). Das Zusammenleben von Krustenanemonen und Schwämmen im Mittelmeer. *Thalassia*, **2**, 1–34.

Arndt, W. and Viets, K. (1939). Die biologischen (parasitologischen) Beziehungen zwischen Arachnoideen und Spongien. *Z. ParasitKde*, **10**, 67–93.

Băcescu, M. (1968). Heteromysini nouveaux des eaux cubaines: trois espèces nouvelles de *Heteromysis* et *Heteromysoides spongicola* n.g., n.sp. *Rev. Roumaine Biol., Zool.*, **13**, 221–237.

Băcescu, M. (1971). Les spongiaires; un des plus intéressants biotopes benthiques marins. *Rapp. Comm. int. mer Médit.*, **20**, 239–241.

Bakus, G. J. (1966). Marine poeciloscleridan sponges of the San Juan Archipelago, Washington. *J. Zool.*, **149**, 415–531.

Bertrand, J. C. and Vacelet, J. (1971). L'association entre éponges cornées et bactéries. *C. r. hebd. Séanc. Acad. Sci., Paris*, **273**, 638–641.

Bērziņš, B. (1950). Observations on rotifers on sponges. *Trans. Am. microsc. Soc.*, **69**, 189–193.

Bidder, G.-P. (1920). The fragrance of calcinean sponges and spermatozoa of *Guancha* and *Sycon*. *Proc. Linn. Soc., Lond.*, **34**, 299–304.

Bocquet, C. and Stock, J. H. (1963). Copépodes parasites d'invertébrés des côtes de France. XVI. Description de *Pseudoclausia longiseta* n.sp. (Copépode cyclopoide, famille des Clausiidae). *Proc. K. ned. Akad. Wet.* (Ser. C), **66**, 139–152.

Böhlke, J. E. and Robins, R. H. (1969). Western Atlantic sponge-dwelling gobies of the genus *Evermannichthys*: their taxonomy, habits and relationships. *Proc. Acad. nat. Sci. Philadelphia*, **121**, 1–24.

Boliek, M. I. (1935). Syncytial structures in sponge larvae and lymph plasmodia of sea urchins. *J. Elisha Mitchell Sci. Soc.*, **51**, 252–288.

Bouillon, J. (1971). Sur quelques hydroides de Roscoff. *Cah. Biol. mar.*, **12**, 323–364.

Brice, J. J. (1896). The fish and fisheries of the coastal waters of Florida. *U.S. Bur. Fisheries, Rept. Comm. Fish.*, **22**, 263–342.

Bruce, A. J. (1976). *Discias mvitae* sp. nov., a new sponge associate from Kenya (Decapoda Natantia, Disciadidae). *Crustaceana*, **31**, 119–130.

Burkholder, P. R. and Ruetzler, K. (1969). Antimicrobial activity of some marine sponges. *Nature, Lond.*, **222**, 983–984.

Calder, D. R. (1970). Hydroid and young medusa stages of *Dipurena strangulata* (Hydrozoa, Corynidae). *Biol. Bull. mar. biol. Lab., Woods Hole*, **138**, 109–114.

Carter, H. J. (1878). Parasites of the Spongida. *Ann. Mag. nat. Hist.* (Ser. 5), **2**, 157–172.

Castro, P. (1971). The natantian shrimps (Crustacea, Decapoda) associated with invertebrates in Hawaii. *Pacif. Sci.*, **25**, 395–403.

Cheng, T. C., Rifkin, E. and Yee, H. W. F. (1967). The role of certain parenchymal cells of *Terpios zeteki* (Porifera: Demospongiae) in phagocytosis and elimination of foreign particles. *Am. Zool.*, **7**, 771–772.

Cheng, T. C., Rifkin, E. and Yee, H. W. F. (1968a). Studies on the internal defense mechanisms of sponges. II. Phagocytosis and elimination of India ink and carmine particles by certain parenchymal cells of *Terpios zeteki*. *J. Invertebr. Pathol.*, **11**, 302–309.

Cheng, T. C., Yee, H. W. F. and Rifkin, E. (1968b). Studies on the internal defense mechanisms of sponges. I. The cell types occurring in the mesoglea of *Terpios zeteki* (de Laubenfels)(Porifera: Demospongiae). *Pacif. Sci.*, **22**, 395–401.

Cheng, T. C., Yee, H. W. F., Rifkin, E. and Kramer, M. D. (1968c). Studies on the internal defense mechanisms of sponges. III. Cellular reactions in *Terpios zeteki* to implanted heterologous biological materials. *J. Invertebr. Pathol.*, **12**, 29–35.

Claus, G., Madri, P. and Kunen, S. (1967). Removal of microbial pollutants from waste effluents by the redbeard sponge. *Nature, Lond.*, **216**, 712–714.

Colwell, R. R. and Liston, J. (1962). The natural bacterial flora of certain marine invertebrates. *J. Insect Pathol.*, **4**, 23–33.

Connes, R. (1967). Réactions de défense de l'éponge *Tethya lyncurium* Lamarck, vis-à-vis des micro-organismes et de l'amphipode *Leucothoë spinicarpa* Abildg. *Vie Milieu* (Ser. A), **18**, 281–289.

Connes, R., Paris, J. and Sube, J. (1971). Réactions tissulaires de quelques démosponges vis-à-vis de leurs commensaux et parasites. *Naturaliste can.*, **98**, 928–935.

Dawson, C. E. (1960). *Starksia ocellata* (Steindachner), a new sponge inquiline from South Carolina. *Copeia*, **1960**, 75.

Dawson, C. E. and Smith, F. G. W. (1953). The Gulf of Mexico sponge investigation. *Tech. Ser. Fla St. Bd Conserv.*, **1**, 1–27.

Dendy, A. (1913). Amoebocytes in calcareous sponges. *Nature, Lond.*, **92**, 339.

Dosse, G. (1940). Bakterien- und Pilzbefunde sowie pathologische und Fäulnisvorgänge in Meeres- und Süsswasserschwämmen. Untersuchungen im Zusammenhang mit dem gegenwärtigen Sterben der Badeschwämme in Westindien. *Z. ParasitKde*, **11**, 331–356.

Duboscq, O. and Tuzet, O. (1936a). *Topsentella fallax* n.g., n.sp. parasite du mésenchyme de *Sycon raphanus* O. S. *Archs Zool. exp. gén.*, **78**, 137–144.

Duboscq, O. and Tuzet, O. (1936b). Les amoebocytes et les cellules germinales des éponges calcaires. *Mém. Mus. r. Hist. nat. Belg.* (Ser. 2), **3**, 209–226.

Eimhjellen, K. E. (1967). Photosynthetic bacteria and carotenoids from a sea sponge *Halichondria panicea*. *Acta chem. scand.*, **21**, 2280–2287.

Fage, L. (1928). Remarques sur le comportement du *Tritaeta gibbosa* (Bate), crustacé amphipode, commensal des éponges. *Bull. Soc. zool. Fr.*, **53**, 285–291.

Feldmann, J. (1933). Sur quelques cyanophycées vivant dans le tissu des éponges de Banyuls. *Archs Zool. exp. gén.*, **75**, 381–404.

Fishelson, L. (1966). *Spirastrella inconstans* Dendy (Porifera) as an ecological niche in the littoral zone of the Dahlak Archipelago (Eritrea). *Sea Fish. Res. Sta. Haifa*, **41**, 17–25.

Forbes, M. L. (1964). Distribution of the commensal oyster, *Ostrea permollis*, and its host sponge. *Bull. mar. Sci. Gulf Caribb.*, **14**, 453–464.

Forbes, M. L. (1966). Life cycle of *Ostrea permollis* and its relationship to the host sponge, *Stelletta grubii*. *Bull. mar. Sci. Gulf Caribb.*, **16**, 273–301.

Galtsoff, P. S. (1942). Wasting disease causing mortality of sponges in the West Indies and Gulf of Mexico. In *Proceedings of the 8th American Scientific Congress*, **3**, 411–421.

Galtsoff, P. S., Brown, H. H., Smith, C. L. and Smith, F. G. W. (1939). Sponge mortality in the Bahamas. *Nature, Lond.*, **143**, 807–808.

Gotto, R. V. (1965). *Clionophilus vermicularis*: a sponge-dwelling copepod new to the British Isles. *Ir. Nat. J.*, **15**, 20.

Gravier, C. J. (1922). Sur les relations du crustacé et de l'éponge chez les cirripèdes spongicoles. *C. r. hebd. Séanc. Acad. Sci., Paris*, **174**, 830–832.

Gudger, E. W. (1950). Fishes that live as inquilines (lodgers) in sponges. *Zoologica, N.Y.*, **35**, 121–126.

Hammer, E. (1906). Zur Kenntnis von *Hircinia variabilis*. *Sber. Ges. naturf. Freunde Berl.*, **6**, 149–155.

Hammond, R. (1968). Some marine copepods (Misophrioida, Cyclopoida, and Notodelphyoida) from Norfolk, Great Britain. *Crustaceana*, **1968** (Suppl. 1), 37–60.

Humes, A. G. (1973). *Hemicyclops perinsignis*, a new cyclopoid copepod from a sponge in Madagascar. *Proc. biol. Soc. Wash.*, **86**, 315–328.

Hunt, O. D. (1925). The food of the bottom fauna of the Plymouth fishing grounds. *J. mar. biol. Ass. U.K.*, **13**, 560–598.

Ijima, I. (1901). Studies on Hexactinellida. Contribution I. Euplectellidae. *J. Coll. Sci. imp. Univ. Tokyo*, **15**, 1–299.

Jakowska, S. and Nigrelli, R. F. (1960). Antimicrobial substances from sponges. *Ann. N.Y. Acad. Sci.*, **90**, 913–916.

Kölliker, A. (1860). Über das ausgebreitete Vorkommen von pflanzlichen Parasiten in den Hartgebilden niederer Thiere. *Z. wiss. Zool.*, **10**, 215–232.

Kolosváry, G. von (1940). Biologische Angaben zu den Ansiedlungsverhältnissen der Acasten in *Hircinia*. *Zool. Anz.*, **129**, 219–222.

Kramp, P. L. (1959). The hydromedusae of the Atlantic Ocean and adjacent waters. *Dana Rep., Carlsberg Found.*, **46**, 1–283.

Kunen, S., Claus, G., Madri, P. and Peyser, L. (1971). The ingestion and digestion of yeast-like fungi by the sponge, *Microciona prolifera*. *Hydrobiologia*, **38**, 565–576.

Laubenfels, M. W. de (1947). Ecology of the sponges of a brackish water environment, at Beaufort, N.C. *Ecol. Monogr.*, **17**, 31–46.

Laubenfels, M. W. de (1952). Sponges from the Gulf of Mexico. *Bull. mar. Sci. Gulf Caribb.*, **2**, 511–557.

Laubenfels, M. W. de and Storr, J. F. (1958). The taxonomy of American commercial sponges. *Bull. mar. Sci. Gulf Caribb.*, **8**, 99–117.

Leigh-Sharpe, W. H. (1935). A list of British invertebrates with their characteristic parasitic and commensal Copepoda. *J. mar. biol. Ass. U.K.*, **20**, 47–48.

Lévi, C. and Lévi, P. (1965). Populations bactériennes dans les éponges. *J. Microsc.*, **4**, 60.

Long, E. R. (1968). The associates of four species of marine sponges of Oregon and Washington. *Pacif. Sci.*, **22**, 347–351.

Madri, P. P., Claus, G., Kunen, S. M. and Moss, E. E. (1967). Preliminary studies on the *Escherichia coli* uptake of the redbeard sponge (*Microciona prolifera* Verrill). *Life Sci.*, **6**, 889–894.

Madri, P. P., Hermel, M. and Claus, G. (1971). The microbial flora of the sponge *Microciona prolifera* Verrill and its ecological implications. *Botanica marina*, **14**, 1–5.

Nigrelli, R. F., Jakowska, S. and Calventi, J. (1959). Ectyonin, an antimicrobial agent from the sponge, *Microciona prolifera* Verrill. *Zoologica, N.Y.*, **44**, 173–176.

Orton, J. H. (1913). On the habitat of a marine amoeba. *Nature, Lond.*, **92**, 371.

Orton, J. H. (1914). Some habitats of marine amoeba. *Nature, Lond.*, **92**, 606.

Osorio Tafall, B. F. and Cardenas, F. M. (1945). Sobre las esponjas comerciales de Quintana Roo y una enfermedad que las destruye. *Ciencia, Mex.*, **6**, 25–31.

Pansini, M. (1970). Inquilinismo in *Spongia officinalis*, *Ircinia fasciculata* e *Petrosia ficiformis* della Riviera Ligure di Levante. *Boll. Musei Ist. biol. Univ. Genova*, **38**, 5–17.

Pearse, A. S. (1935). Inhabitants of certain sponges at Dry Tortugas. *Pap. Tortugas Lab.*, **28**, 117–122.

Pearse, A. S. (1950). Notes on the inhabitants of certain sponges at Bimini. *Ecology*, **31**, 149–151.

Poléjaeff, N. (1884). Report on the Keratosa collected by H.M.S. 'Challenger' during the years 1873–1876. *Challenger Reps. Zool.*, **11**, 1–88.

Porter, C. L. and Zebrowski, G. (1937). Lime-loving molds from Australian sands. *Mycologia*, **29**, 252–257.

Radcliffe, L. (1917). Description of a new goby, *Garmannia spongicola*, from North Carolina. *Proc. U.S. natn. Mus.*, **52**, 423–425.

Rees, J. T. (1977). Polyp and medusa of *Dipurena bicircella* n.sp. (Hydrozoa: Corynidae) from Northern California. *Mar. Biol.*, **39**, 197–202.

Rees, W. J. (1939). The hydroid of the medusa *Dipurena halterata* (Forbes). *J. mar. biol. Ass. U.K.*, **23**, 343–346.

Riedl, R. (1966). *Biologie der Meereshöhlen*, Parey, Hamburg.

Santucci, R. (1922). La *Geodia cydonium* come centro di associazione biologica. *R. Comitato Talassogr. Ital.*, **103**, 5–19.

Sarà, M. (1971). Ultrastructural aspects of the symbiosis between two species of the genus *Aphanocapsa* (Cyanophyceae) and *Ircinia variabilis* (Demospongiae). *Mar. Biol.*, **11**, 214–221.

Sarà, M. and Vacelet, J. (1973). Écologie des Démosponges. In P.-P. Grassé (Ed.), *Traité de Zoologie*. Masson, Paris. pp. 462–576.

Schirl, K. (1973). Cyclopoida Siphonostomata (Crustacea) von Banyuls (Frankreich, Pyrénées orientales) mit besonderer Berücksichtigung des Gast-Wirtverhältnisses. *Bijdr. Dierk.*, **43**, 64–92.

Schmidt, I. (1970). Phagocytose et pinocytose chez les Spongillidae. Étude *in vivo* de l'ingestion de bactéries et de protéines marquées à l'aide d'un colorant fluorescent en lumière ultra-violette. *Z. vergl. Physiol.*, **66**, 398–420.

Schmitt, W. (1935). *Coralliocaris pearsei* Schmitt new species. Appendix (to Pearse, 1935). *Pap. Tortugas Lab.*, **28**, 123–124.

Silén, L. (1963). *Clionophilus vermicularis* n.gen., n.sp., a copepod infecting the burrowing sponge, *Cliona. Zool. Bidr. Upps.*, **35**, 269–288.

Smith, F. G. W. (1939). Sponge mortality at British Honduras. *Nature, Lond.*, **144**, 785.

Smith, F. G. W. (1941). Sponge disease in British Honduras, and its transmission by water currents. *Ecology*, **22**, 415–421.

Smith, F. G. W. (1947). Preliminary report on the Tarpon Springs sponge industry. *Sponge Inst. Trade Rep.*, **46**.

Smith, F. G. W. (1954). Biology of the commercial sponges. *Fishery Bull. Fish Wildl. Serv. U.S.*, **55**, 263–266.

Sparks, A. K. (1969). Review of tumors and tumor-like conditions in Protozoa, Coelenterata, Platyhelminthes, Annelida, Sipunculida, and Arthropoda, excluding insects. *Natn. Cancer Inst. Monogr.*, **31**, 671–682.

Stock, J. H. (1960). Sur quelques copépodes associés aux invertébrés des côtes du Roussillon. *Crustaceana*, **1**, 218–257.

Stock, J. H. (1965). Copépodes associés aux invertébrés des côtes du Roussillon. V. Cyclopoides siphonostomes spongicoles rares et nouveaux. *Vie Milieu*, **16**, 295–324.

Stock, J. H. and Kleeton, G. (1964). Copépodes associés aux invertébrés des côtes du Roussillon. IV. Description de *Spongiocnizon petiti* gen. nov., sp. nov., copépode spongicole remarquable. *Vie Milieu*, **17** (Suppl.), 325–336.

Storr, J. F. (1957). The sponge industry of Florida. *Educ. Ser. Fla St. Bd Conserv.*, **9**, 28.

Topsent, E. (1928). Note sur *Sponginticola uncifera*, n.g., n.sp., crustacé parasite d'éponges marines. *Bull. Soc. zool. Fr.*, **53**.

Tuzet, O. (1973a). Éponges calcaires. In P.-P. Grassé (Ed.), *Traité de Zoologie*, Vol. III. Masson, Paris. pp. 27–132.

Tuzet, O. (1973b). Hexactinellides ou hyalosponges. In P.-P. Grassé (Ed), *Traité de Zoologie*, Vol. III. Masson, Paris. pp. 633–690.

Tuzet, O. and Connes, R. (1962). Spicules anormaux d'une variété écologique d'*Ephydatia fluviatilis* L. *Vie Milieu*, **13**, 467–470.

Tuzet, O. and Paris, J. (1964). Réactions tissulaires de l'éponge *Suberites domuncula* (Olivi) Nardo, vis-à-vis de ses commensaux et parasites. *Vie Milieu*, **17** (Suppl.), 147–155.

Vacelet, J. (1970). Description de cellules à bactéries intranucléaires chez des éponges *Verongia*. *J. Microsc.*, **9**, 333–346.

Vacelet, J. (1971). Étude en microscopie électronique de l'association entre une cyanophycée chroococcale et une éponge du genre *Verongia*. *J. Microsc.*, **12**, 363–380.

Vannucci, M. (1956). Biological notes and description of a new species of *Dipurena* (Hydrozoa, Corynidae). *Proc. zool. Soc. Lond.*, **127**, 479–487.

Vosmaer, G. C. J. (1911). The genus *Spirastrella. Siboga Exped.*, **64**, 1–69.

Wenzel, F. (1961a). Ciliaten aus marinen Schwämmen. *Pubbl. Staz. zool. Napoli*, **32**, 272–277.

Wenzel, F. (1961b). Notizen über *Ophryodendron multiramosum* n.sp. und seine Konjugation. *Arch. Protistenk.*, **105**, 269–272.

Wierzejki, A. (1912). Über Abnormitäten bei Spongiliden. *Zool. Anz.*, **39**, 290–295.

Yeatman, H. C. (1970). Copepods from Chesapeake Bay sponges including *Asterocheres jeanyeatmanae* n.sp. *Trans. Am. microsc. Soc.*, **89**, 27–38.

Zebrowski, G. (1937). New genera of Cladochystriaceae. *Ann. Mo. bot. Gdn*, **23**, 553–564.

6. DISEASES OF CNIDARIA

G. LAUCKNER

The phylum Cnidaria comprises 4 recent classes—the Scyphozoa (about 250 species), the Cubozoa (some 15 species), the Hydrozoa (more than 2700 species) and the Anthozoa (approximately 6000 species). All except a few hydrozoans are marine. The systematics of the cnidarian classes have been subject to much scientific controversy. According to recent investigations (Werner, 1973), the Scyphozoa constitute the most primitive group, whereas the Hydrozoa—previously believed to represent the most simple type of cnidarian organization—contain species with the greatest diversity of morphological structures and complexity of life histories (Uchida, 1963). The Cubozoa, previously grouped with the Scyphozoa, are now regarded as a separate class positioned intermediate between Scyphozoa and Hydrozoa (Werner, 1976).

A number of Cnidaria can now be cultivated successfully over several generations (Kinne, 1977). This fact makes numerous disease phenomena available for critical analysis and facilitates long-term studies on agent–host dynamics.

DISEASES CAUSED BY MICRO-ORGANISMS

Agents: Viruses and Bacteria

No viral or bacterial diseases are known to occur among marine cnidarians. However, with a considerable degree of probability, such diseases should be expected to exist, even though a number of cnidarians are capable of secreting antimicrobial substances. Burkholder and Burkholder (1958), for example, showed that extracts from several corals and seawhips *Antillogorgia turgida* inhibited numerous marine bacteria. Extracts from fresh and dried seawhips were equally active. The substances appeared to be produced by the outer grey-purple cortex, not by the brown core of the horny corals. Extracts from stony corals exhibited lesser activity.

Inhibited micro-organisms included *Clostridium feseri*, *Micrococcus aureus*, *Bacillus subtilis*, *Escherichia coli* and various marine bacteria. Strains of penicillin-resistant *Micrococcus* were equally susceptible to inhibition by extracts from *Antillogorgia turgida*. Unsusceptible organisms included *Lactobacillus casei*, *Candida albicans*, *Kloeckera brevis*, *Cryptococcus neoformans* and *Saccharomyces cerevisiae*. In contrast to the results with gorgonian corals, little or no antimicrobial activity could be detected in the species of stony corals that were tested. Examples of inactive species were *Acropora palmata*, *Porites porites*, *Montastrea* sp. and hydrozoans *Millepora alcicornis*.

Evidence for the presence of antibody-like substances has been reported for the sea anemone *Anthopleura elegantissima* by Phillips and Yardley (1960). Phillips (1963) claims that there are immune mechanisms in cnidarians, which are not essentially different from those existing in vertebrates.

Agents: Fungi

Higher marine fungi were found as degraders of dead chitinous exoskeletons of undetermined Hydrozoa from deep waters of the Atlantic Ocean. Fruiting bodies and hyphae of ascomycetes *Abyssomyces hydrozoicus* (Figs 6-1 to 6-3) occurred on hydrozoans at a depth of 631 to 641 m near the South Orkney Islands. Sterile mycelia, some of them resembling *Dictyonema zoophytarum*, were collected on hydrozoans off the North Carolina coast at depths between 46 and 73 m (Kohlmeyer, 1972). Whether these or other fungi attack the exoskeletons of living Hydrozoa is unknown.

Fungi can penetrate the calcareous skeletons of stony corals. Thus, *Porites clavaria* was found to harbour moderately branched mycelia carrying numerous sporangia. Similar fungi were frequently seen to ramify in the skeletons of *Astraea annularis*, *Maeandrina* sp., *Fungia* sp., *Corallium rubrum*, *Madrepora muricata*, *Tubipora musica* and other stony corals, as well as in the coral-like hydrozoan *Millepora alcicornis* (Kölliker, 1860).

DISEASES CAUSED BY PROTOZOANS: SCYPHOZOA

Only a few protozoans are known to be associated with Scyphozoa. The reports either concern enigmatic—possibly host-specific—structures or commensals rather than parasites. Thus far, protozoans have not been definitely shown to produce disease in scyphozoans. 'Sporozoans', reported by Vallentin (1888) as occurring in white, spherical masses of 0·3 to 1·25 mm diameter on the exumbrella and subumbrella of *Lucernaria auricula* and *L. cyathiformis*, are more likely to represent masses of nematocysts enclosed by nematoblasts (Weill, 1935). Weill also mentioned apostome ciliates on *Rhizostoma* sp. and unidentified amoebae on *Haliclystus octoradiatus* as 'occasional commensals'.

DISEASES CAUSED BY PROTOZOANS: HYDROZOA

From hydrozoans, parasitic Protozoa have frequently been reported. Some are capable of exerting control over abundance and distribution of their host populations. Our pertinent knowledge stems, however, almost exclusively from freshwater species of the genus *Hydra* (some of which have previously been named *Pelmatohydra* or *Chlorohydra*). Some interrelationships between protozoans and freshwater hydrozoans will be discussed briefly since comparable investigations on marine associations of this kind are lacking.

Agents: Flagellata

Trypanophis grobbeni, a bodonid flagellate, parasitizes in the somatocyst of *Nanomia bijuga (Halistemma tergestinum)*, *Monophyes gracilis* and other siphonophores from the Mediterranean Sea (Poche, 1903; Keysselitz, 1904; Floyd, 1916). The organism, which measures 50 to 83 μm in length and 9 to 11·3 μm in width, has been regarded as an

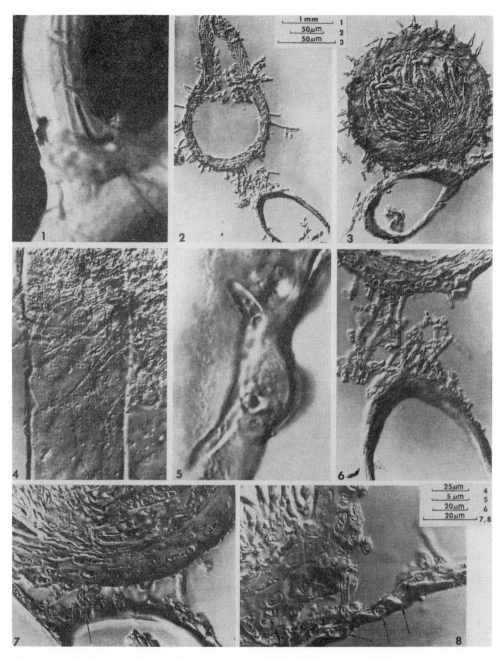

Fig. 6-1: 1–8: Fungi affecting Hydrozoa. *Abyssomyces hydrozoicus* on hydrozoan exoskeleton. 1: Dark ascocarps on hydrorhiza attached to white stony coral; 2 and 3: ascocarps in longitudinal section (above) attached to hydrozoan exoskeleton in cross section; 4: hyphae near ascocarp on surface of hydrorhiza; 5: section through exoskeleton with hyphae growing within wall; 6: wall of ascocarp (above) attached with hypae to hydrorhiza (in cross section, below); 7 and 8: hyphae near ascocarp, on and in wall (arrows) of hydrozoan exoskeleton. Interference contrast. (After Kohlmeyer, 1972; reproduced by permission of Springer-Verlag.)

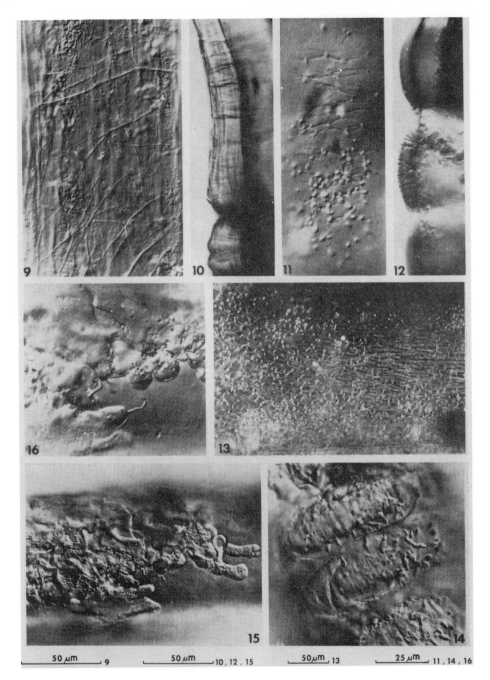

Fig. 6-2: 9–16: Fungi affecting Hydrozoa. Four different types of biodeterioration caused by fungi (and possibly bacteria) in hydrozoan exoskeletons. 9, 10: First type, delicate filaments in surface view (9) and in optical cross section through wall (10); 11-13: second type, network of hyphae in surface view (11, 13) and in optical section through wall (12); 14: third type, corrosion within walls of hydrozoan annuli; 15, 16: fourth type, wide channels within exoskeleton (15), thin filament connected to large cavity (16); 13 in phase contrast, others in interference contrast. (After Kohlmeyer, 1972; reproduced by permission of Springer-Verlag.)

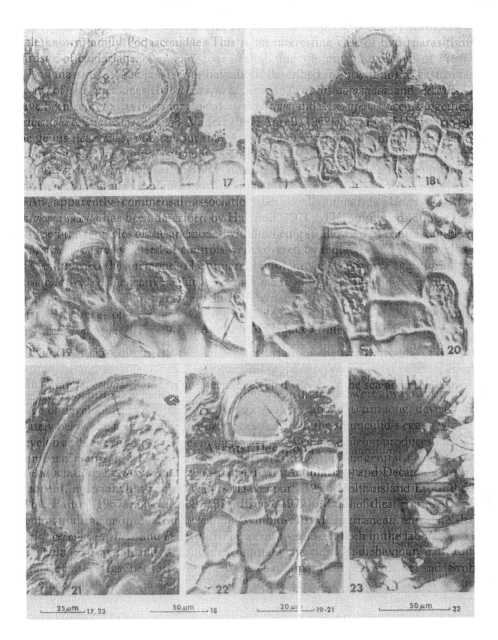

Fig. 6-3: 17–23: Fungi affecting Hydrozoa. Sterile mycelium on *Sargassum* sp. and hydrozoan exoskeleton. 17, 18 and 22: Dark hyphal mat, covering alga and partly surrounding hydrorhiza, hypha (arrow) enclosed by hydrozoan wall in 22. 19. Section through *Sargassum* sp., brown hyphal cells above, hyaline nutritional filaments penetrating (arrows). 20: Thin nutritional hyphae within algal walls (arrow), brown surface hypha left. 21: Section through hydrorhiza on algal host with hyaline hyphae penetrating wall (arrows). 23: Hyphal mat in surface view. 17 and 23 in brightfield, others in interference contrast. (After Kohlmeyer, 1972; reproduced by permission of Springer-Verlag.)

'intestinal worm' by earlier authors (see Poche, 1911). In addition to the flagellated form, Duboscq and Rose (1927, 1933) observed a gregarine-like parasite, as well as what they believed to be a transitional stage between flagellate and 'gregarine'. The flagellates always occurred in the liquid contents of the gastrovascular cavity whereas the 'gregarines' were found either attached to the outer wall of the somatocyst or free in the host's mesogloea. The transitional amoeboid form was believed to penetrate the somatocyst wall and give rise to the 'gregarine' stage outside the gastrovascular cavity.

Rose (1939a, b, 1947) attempted to follow the transformation of the flagellated into the 'gregarine' form and gave some dubious interpretations of amoeboid and mycelial structures which he linked with the life cycle of *Trypanophis grobbeni*. Cachon and co-authors (1972), who restudied the parasite by means of electron microscopy, confirmed the flagellate nature of *T. grobbeni* which they frequently encountered in the somatocysts of siphonophores of the genera *Chelophyes*, *Diphyes*, *Muggia* and *Lensia*. Transitional stages were not found, and the 'gregarines' which were most numerous in *C. appendiculata* but rare in other siphonophores, were identified as a second species of protozoan parasite, probably the stage of a sporozoan.

A second species of *Trypanophis*, *T. major*, has been reported as a parasite of siphonophores *Abylopsis pentagona* (Duboscq and Rose, 1926, 1933).

In addition to *Trypanophis grobbeni*, Mediterranean siphonophores *Diphyes elongata*, *Monophyes gracilis* and *Nanomia bijuga* harboured, in their gastrovascular cavities, parasitic peridineans named *Oxyrrhis parasitica* by Poche (1903). Chatton (1920) included these forms in the genus *Gymnodinium* as *G. parasiticum*.

Velella velella from the French Mediterranean coast were found to be infested, in great numbers, by a parasitic peridinean named *Endodinium chattonii* (Hovasse, 1922, 1923). The spherical non-motile cells of the parasite, 7 to 12 μm in diameter, occurred intracellularly in the endothelium lining the siphonophore's gastrozooids and gonozooids. Sometimes 2 parasites were seen in a single host cell. Infestation caused considerable hypertrophy of the nucleus and cytoplasm, and cessation of cell division. Host buds were seen to be destroyed, and the possibility of parasitic castration was discussed. Hovasse (1923) also noted similarities of *E. chattonii* with *Blastodinium* spp. parasitizing in the intestinal tracts of various marine copepods (Chatton, 1906).

Later, Hovasse (1924) identified the presumed parasite as a mutualistic symbiote and changed its name to *Zooxanthella chattonii*. On the basis of ultrastructural studies, Taylor (1971) concluded that the *Velella velella* symbiote belongs to the genus *Amphidinium* and renamed it *A. chattonii*—a view rejected by Sournia and co-authors (1975), who maintain that the ultrastructure of *Endodinium chattonii* differs from that of members of the genus *Amphidinium*. Symbioses between siphonophores and zooxanthellae have been discussed by Kuskop (1921).

Another peridinean, *Protoodinium chattoni*, is an external parasite of hydromedusae *Lizzia blondina* and occasionally of *Sarsia* sp., *Obelia dichotoma*, *Podocoryne carnea* and *P. minima* in the Black and Mediterranean Seas. It occurs on the manubrium, umbrella, velum and exceptionally on the exumbrella, attached by means of a peduncle provided with rhizoid-like processes anchoring the parasite in the host's epithelial cells. While most parasitic dinoflagellates are osmotrophic, *P. chattoni* is phagotrophic, ingesting host cytoplasm by means of its attachment organella which functions as a suctorial tentacle (Fig. 6-4). Although a true ectoparasite which completes its entire life cycle on hydromedusae, *P. chattoni* has retained all the morphological characters typical of free-living dinoflagellates, i.e. a theca with typical tabulation, girdle, sulcus and two well-developed flagella (Hovasse, 1935; Cachon and Cachon, 1971). A related species, *P. hovassei*, parasitizes siphonophores (Cachon, 1964).

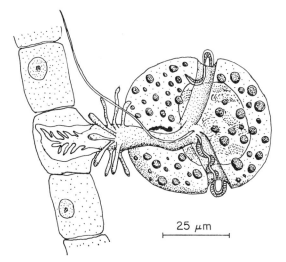

Fig. 6-4: *Protoodinium chattoni*. Individual with its funnel-shaped suctorial tentacle inserted into ectodermal cell of host *Podocoryne minima* medusa. (After Cachon and Cachon, 1971; reproduced by permission of VEB Gustav Fischer Verlag.)

Abylopsis tetragona, Forskålia contorta, Chelophyes sp. and other siphonophores from the French and Algerian coasts of the Mediterranean Sea were found to harbour a curious protistan parasite. Unable to assign it to any known group of organisms, Rose and Cachon (1951, 1952a, b) named it *Diplomorpha paradoxa*. Eventually, life-cycle studies conducted by Cachon (1953) revealed its peridinean nature. Trophozoites of *D. paradoxa*, 25 to 130 μm long, occur—attached to the host's ectoderm by means of a rhizoid-like holdfast—in the bell of the siphonophores (Fig. 6-5, 1). When fed experimentally to gastrozooids of *Abylopsis tetragona*, the parasite extrudes numerous filamentous processes into which the cytoplasm expands (Fig. 6-5, 2). Upon discharge of the organism into the ambient sea water, the mass of cytoplasm withdraws into the centre of the cell and becomes enclosed by a rapidly forming double membrane (Fig. 6-5, 3). Disintegration of the original cell wall and its filamentous processes is followed by a series of palintomic divisions (divisions without subsequent growth; Fig 6-6, 1), resulting in the formation of several hundred small spherical cells. The last generation of these cells gives rise to flagellated and actively swimming zoospores measuring about 20 μm in diameter (Fig. 6-6, 3). At each division, the cells abandon their old envelopes to form new ones. Under experimental conditions, the cells remain attached to their old envelopes which degenerate into chains of wrinkled stalks (Fig. 6-6, 2).

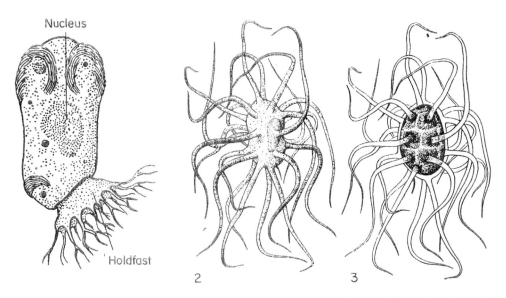

Fig. 6-5: *Diplomorpha paradoxa*. 1: Trophozoite (× 350); 2: stage developing in siphonophore's gastric cavity (× 130); 3: free-living stage (× 130). Note concentration of cytoplasm in centre of cell. (After Cachon, 1953; reproduced by permission of Société zoologique de France.)

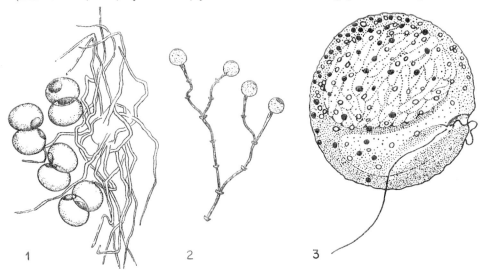

Fig. 6-6: *Diplomorpha paradoxa*. 1, 2: Palintomy (× 150); 3: zoospore (× 2500). (After Cachon, 1953; reproduced by permission of Société zoologique de France.)

The further fate of the *Diplomorpha paradoxa* spores remains unknown. Cachon (1953) believed that they represent a stage in the life cycle of a species of *Actinodinium*, a parasite of pelagic crustaceans. However, Sournia and co-authors (1975) listed *D. paradoxa* under the name *Cachonella paradoxa*.

Refringent bodies resembling oil droplets in the cavities of gastrozooids of siphonophores *Abylopsis tetragona*, *Chelophyes* sp. and *Sulculeolaria* sp. from the Mediterranean Sea turned out to be dinococcid peridineans of the genus *Stylodinium*, named *S. gastrophilum*. The ovoid cells, which measured up to 100 μm in length and 50 μm in width, were attached to the siphonophores' gastric epithelium by means of a delicate, flexible stalk, 2 to 3 μm in diameter and 10 to 15 μm long, and terminating in a funnel-shaped holdfast (Fig. 6-7). *S. gastrophilum* feeds on the contents of the

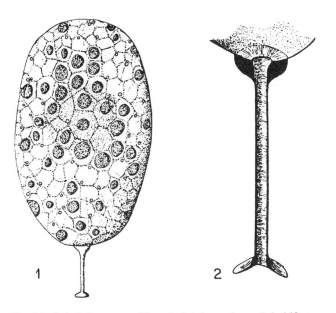

Fig. 6-7: *Stylodinium gastrophilum*. 1: Adult trophont; 2: holdfast (After Cachon and co-authors, 1965; reproduced by permission of Institut océanographique de Monaco.)

siphonophores' epithelial cells, its tubular attachment organella functioning as a suctorial tentacle. Sporogenesis is initiated by the detachment of the peridinean from its host, i.e. by interruption of the food supply. Free spores, measuring 12 to 15 μm in length and 7 μm in width, remain active in sea water for one or two days but eventually encyst and lose their flagella. Spores fed to *Abylopsis tetragona* did not develop. Hence, the further life-cycle stages of the parasite remain unknown. Other members of the genus *Stylodinium* are known only from fresh water and are non-parasitic (Cachon and co-authors, 1965).

Agents: Rhizopoda

Reports on associations between hydrozoans and amoebae appear to be confined to fresh water. *Hydramoeba hydroxena* (originally described as *Amoeba hydroxena* by Entz, 1912), in infection experiments conducted by Reynolds and Looper (1928), killed 65 out of 66 infested *Hydra oligactis* and *H. viridis* within 3 to 30 days. Bryden (1952) reports the appearance of large numbers of hydramoebae in a population of *H. oligactis*. Within a short time, the entire host population was wiped out, apparently due to the detrimental effects of the parasite. In several *Hydra* species, a relationship between temperature and pathogenicity of *Hydramoeba hydroxena* was established (Stiven, 1962, 1964a), the response of the host–parasite system being more pronounced at low temperatures and low initial infestation. The parasites appear to break down the intracellular matrix, and gradually consume the host's cells. The size of the hydra decreases until, eventually, disintegration occurs. *Hydra pseudoligactis* and *H. oligactis* were the most susceptible, while *H. viridissima* exhibited a marked resistance, and *H. littoralis* appeared to be almost immune. Temperature increase caused early cessation of feeding in infested *H. viridissima*, as well as decrease in the budding period and survival time (Stiven, 1964b). Normal *H. viridissima* were more resistant under stress than albino ones, and lived longer when infested with *Hydramoeba hydroxena* and exposed to light. Survival rates were, however, identical with those of individuals kept in darkness (Stiven, 1965). The pathogenicity of *H. hydroxena* on *H. oligactis* depends on hydrogen-ion concentrations: pH values between 5·2 and 5·6, and between 8·6 and 9·6 are inhibitory (Threlkeld and Reynolds, 1929). Transmission of *H. hydroxena* occurs not, as previously assumed, by cysts, but by amoeboid trophozoites (Beers, 1963). Rice (1960) described *H. hydroxena* as a parasite of the freshwater medusa *Craspedacusta sowerbii*. Adult medusae were destroyed in 6 days, while polyps and other developmental stages were not attacked by the parasite.

Agents: Sporozoa

Microsporidan infestations of *Hydra littoralis* have been described by Spangenberg and Claybrook (1961). The causative agent, a species of *Pleistophora*, was transmitted through the egg. It was not found to be fatal to the host, although infested individuals appeared slightly smaller and paler than parasite-free specimens. On the other hand, *in vitro* cultures of *Hydra* cells infested with *Pleistophora* sp. were destroyed by the microsporidan (Li and co-authors, 1963).

During the examination of sections of *Boreohydra simplex* from Swedish waters, Nyholm (1963) observed that the entoderm of 9 of 800 specimens was greatly modified, due to intracellular infestation by stages of an unidentified sporozoan parasite, probably a coccidian. Young trophozoites with a single nucleus were seen to become multinucleate and differentiate into meroblasts which then developed into merozoites. Sexual stages also occurred abundantly in *B. simplex*. The morphology of the parasite suggested affinities with the coccidian families Aggregatidae or Caryotrophidae.

Agents: Ciliata

The interrelationships between ciliates and hydrozoans are not quite clear. *Kerona pediculus*, for instance, was believed to be a harmless commensal (Hyman, 1940). Schulze (1913), on the other hand, showed it to be a parasite causing hypertrophy of the tentacles of *Hydra oligactis*, when present in large numbers. In choice experiments, *K. pediculus* exhibited a preference for *Hydra fusca* and *H. vulgaris*, rather than for *H. viridis* (Uhlemeyer, 1922).

Coleman (1966) attempted to determine the factors regulating the distribution and abundance of *K. pediculus* on *Hydra* spp. Hypotrich abundance varied inversely with their population density per hydra over a wide range, the density increasing abnormally when the hosts were infested with *Hydramoeba hydroxena* or with small histiophagic ciliates and flagellates. Only amoebic infestation led to increases in the absolute number of hypotrichs. The study confirmed that *K. pediculus* depends on hydra for some food requirements, but apparently does not damage the host. Ciliate populations could not be sustained on starved hydras, indicating that the availability of undetermined food substances from the host seems to limit the numbers of *Kerona* per *Hydra*. Coleman regards the relationship as commensalistic, not mutualistic.

Other ciliates described from freshwater hydrozoans include *Trichodina pediculus* (Fulton, 1923) and *Costia necatrix* (Deckart and Löfflath, 1954). In both cases, hydrozoans appear to act as reservoir hosts. *T. pediculus* also occurs on the branchial appendages of amphibians, and *C. necatrix* produces skin disturbances in fishes.

Trophonts of *Spirophrya subparasitica*, an apostome ciliate of the family Foettingeriidae, occur in the gastric cavity of hydropolyps *Cladonema radiatum* at Banyuls-sur-Mer (France). The phoront attaches to harpacticoid copepods *Idya furcata* (Chatton and Lwoff, 1924, 1935). The life cycle of these curious ciliates involves an alternation of hosts (Fig. 6-8). The cnidarian harbours the trophont stage. This is expelled together with undigestible food remains. Outside the cnidarian, the trophonts encyst to form the so-called tomont stage. The tomont differentiates into numerous tomites by palintomy (division without growth). The tomites encyst on the exoskeletons of various crustaceans, mostly copepods, to become phoronts. Hatching of the phoronts and considerable subsequent growth occurs when the crustacean host is ingested by a cnidarian. Since the foettingeriids live on the copepods' body fluids, which are liberated during their digestion by the cnidarian, these protozoans should more correctly be termed commensals.

Foettingeriids have also been observed to invade the statocyst of Mediterranean siphonophores *Galeolaria quadrivalvis*. Upon experimental liberation from the host, the trophonts encyst in sea water. The life cycle of the unnamed parasite remains unknown but it is assumed that the phoront stage occurs on pelagic copepods which carry the invasive stage to other siphonophores (Rose, 1933). Unspecified foettingeriid ciliates have been reported from siphonophores *Abylopsis tetragona* (Rose, 1937; cited in Cachon, 1964).

DISEASES CAUSED BY PROTOZOANS: ANTHOZOA

Judging from the literature, associations between anthozoans and protozoans appear to be either of rare occurrence, or have—more likely—consistently been overlooked. At least apostomatid ciliates of the family Foettingeriidae should be expected to occur in a greater number of Anthozoa than hitherto reported.

Agents: Sporozoa

Danielsen (1890) reported on the occurrence of spores of a dubious 'gregarine' in ovocytes of *Epizoanthus glacialis*. Weill (1935), however, stated that the structures observed by this author could either have been an immature cnidarian ovum, an immature nematocyst or an accidentally introduced diatom.

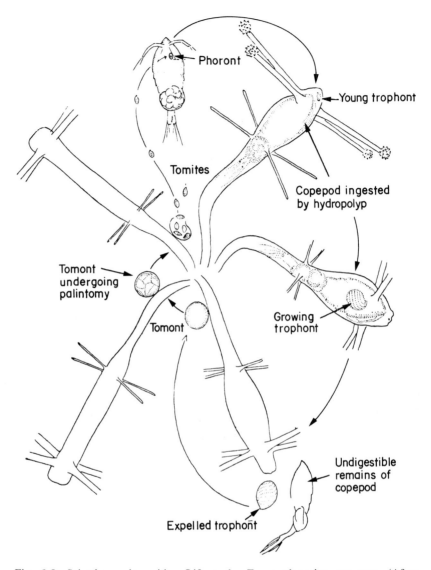

Fig. 6-8: *Spirophrya subparasitica*. Life cycle. For explanation see text. (After Chatton and Lwoff, 1935; modified; reproduced by permission of Centre National de la Recherche Scientifique.)

Agents: Ciliata

Trophonts of *Gymnodinioides* sp., a foettingeriid, have been described from the gastrovascular cavity of sea anemones *Sagartia parasitica* found attached to snail shells inhabited by hermit crabs *Eupagurus prideauxi* at Roscoff (France). *Foettingeria actiniarum* parasitizes various European actinians, namely *Actinia equina*, *Anemonia sulcata*, *Tealia crassicornis*, *Heliactis bellis*, *Sagartia parasitica*, *S. troglodytes*, *Adamsia palliata*, *Bunodes gemmaceus* and *Metridium dianthus* collected along the coasts of France. Infestation of the cnidarian hosts occurs congenitally and *F. actiniarum* has been seen in even the smallest actinian buds. *Metridium marginatum*, *Sagartia leucolena* and *Astrangia danae* from Woods Hole (Massachusetts, USA) were never found to harbour foettingeriids (de Morgan, 1925; Chatton and Lwoff, 1935).

Another species of *Foettingeria*, specifically distinct from the European form, occurs commonly in the coelenteron of *Anthopleura xanthogrammica* in southern California (Ball and Moebius, 1955). Trophonts range from 55 × 32 μm to 250 × 200 μm in size, averaging 123 × 91 μm. Development in general followed that described for *F. actiniarum* by Chatton and Lwoff (1935).

Weill (1935) discussed further reports of protozoans parasitic or commensal in or on Cnidaria.

DISEASES CAUSED BY METAZOANS: SCYPHOZOA

A great number of metazoan associates and parasites, including enigmatic and imperfectly described forms, have been reported from various representatives of all classes of the Cnidaria (Dollfus, 1923c, 1926, 1963; Thiel, M. E., 1970, 1976).

There are numerous associations between scyphomedusae and invertebrates belonging to various phyla. Some of the pertinent observations date back into the 18th century; many have not been documented in detail; others—studied more closely—revealed no evidence for parasitism. Only a few of the scyphomedusa–invertebrate associations reported which are known or assumed to be parasitic in nature will be considered here. Thiel, M. E. (1970, 1976) reviewed the literature on associations between Scyphozoa and other metazoan organisms.

Agents: Cnidaria

Scyphomedusae may be parasitized by other cnidarians. Larval actinians of the genus *Peachia* have been reported from *Cyanea capillata* in Australian and European waters (Blackburn, 1948, Künne, 1948). Badham (1917) observed larval *Peachia hilli* within the gastrovascular system of *Catostylus mosaicus* in Australian waters. The larvae, which fed on digested gastrovascular contents of their host, increased in size from about 3 to 40 mm and then bored holes in the subumbrellar wall through which they escaped from the host. In the same area, adult *P. hilli* existed in the free-living state.

Philomedusa vogtii, reported as an actinian parasitizing scyphomedusae *Chrysaora hysoscella* by Müller (1860), is probably identical with *Halcampa medusophila*, described by Graeffe (1884) from various hydromedusae. According to McMurrich (1913), both forms undoubtedly belong to the genus *Bicidium*.

Agents: Trematoda

In addition to several species of hydromedusae, Stunkard (1967, 1968, 1969) reported the scyphomedusa *Dactylometra quinquecirrha* as host for metacercariae of *Neopechona pyriforme*. In spite of numerous trials, Stunkard (1969) could not obtain experimental infestation in the scyphozoan *Aurelia aurita*. The cercariae made no attempt to penetrate, whereas they attacked *D. quinquecirrha*, as well as hydromedusae *Gonionemus vertens*, in vast numbers (Fig. 6-18). The metacercariae penetrate the host's mesogloea but do not encyst. The scyphomedusa *Pelagia noctiluca* was also susceptible. The adult stage of *N. pyriforme* occurs in the pyloric caeca and intestine of rudderfish *Palinurichthys perciformis* and scup *Stenotomus chrysops* (Linton, 1900; Stunkard, 1967, 1968, 1969).

Another unencysted trematode metacercaria reported from scyphozoans is *Lepocreadium setiferoides*. Of the scyphomedusae common in the Woods Hole (Massachusetts, USA) area, *Dactylometra quinquecirrha* was the only species invaded. Ctenophores *Mnemiopsis leidyi*, which harboured metacercariae of *Neopechona pyriforme* (likewise a member of the family Lepocreadiidae), were not attacked. Ophthalmotrichocercous cercariae of *L. setiferoides* (Fig. 12-29; see also sections *Mollusca* and *Annelida* of this review) emerge from snails *Nassarius obsoletus*. Definite hosts are various fish species, particularly flatfishes. In addition to *D. quinquecirrha*, several turbellarians and annelids serve as second intermediate hosts for *L. setiferoides* (Miller and Northup, 1926; Martin, 1938; Stunkard, 1972).

Ophthalmotrichocercous—probably lepocreadiid—cercariae, named *Cercaria tuticorina*, were found attached along the marginal lappets of *Ephyra* larvae of *Aurelia* sp. from Tuticorin (South India). Out of a large number of *Ephyra* larvae, only 3 contained these cercariae, some of which had shed their tails and migrated to the host's central cavity where they developed into the metacercarial stage (Thapar, 1964). Without supporting evidence, the author linked this metacercaria with adult *Lepocreadioides indicum*, an intestinal parasite of the marine teleost *Platycephalus insidiator*.

Dollfus (1960, 1963) and Rebecq (1965) listed a number of inadequately described larval trematodes from *Pelagia noctiluca*, *Rhizostoma cuvieri*, *Cotylorhiza tuberculata* and other Mediterranean scyphomedusae.

Some temperate-water fishes, particularly members of the *Carangidae*, live in association with scyphozoans, gaining shelter from these cnidarians, and feeding on their gonads and tissues (Fig. 6-14). It seems likely, therefore, that the adult stages of the trematodes parasitizing the medusae can be found by examining the intestinal tracts of these fish associates.

Agents: Cestoda

Rhizostomes *Stomolophus meleagris* and *Lichnorhiza* sp. from waters off Santos, Brazil, have been found to harbour larval tetrarhynchidean cestodes embedded in the mesogloea. There appeared to be some larval growth and development in the scyphozoan intermediate host—from a small cylindrical form into a larger, rounded one. The latter was considered a tailless cysticercoid. Believed to belong to the genus *Dibothriorhynchus* they were named *D. dinoi*. The further life-cycle stages remain unknown (Vannucci Mendes, 1944).

Rhizostomes *Acromitus rabanchatu* from Lake Chilka (India) served as intermediate or paratenic hosts for tetraphyllidean plerocercoids of unknown specific identity (Fig. 6-9). Measuring 2 to 2·5 mm in length and 0·34 mm in diameter, the larvae were cylindrical in shape and embedded in cavities of host jelly, but not encysted, although there was a slight condensation of cells around them. Internally, the larvae consisted of a stroma framework enclosing a few large cells. These cells were at first granular but, later on, calcareous corpuscles developed within them, gradually filling the entire lumen and eventually being liberated (Southwell, 1921).

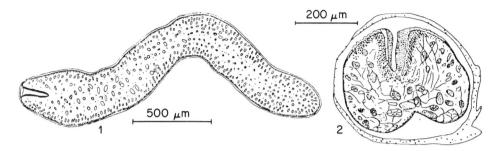

Fig. 6-9: Tetraphyllidea. Unidentified plerocercoid from *Acromitus rabanchatu*. 1: Entire larva, optical section; 2: anterior region, oblique section. (After Southwell, 1921; reproduced by permission of Zoological Survey of India.)

A tetraphyllidean plerocercoid—very similar to if not identical with that reported by Southwell (1921)—has been described by Moestafa and McConnaughey (1966) from another rhizostome, *Catostylus ouwensi*, collected off Irian (New Guinea). All 5 *C. ouwensi* specimens examined were heavily invaded by these worms which measured 'about 3 mm long when mature' and were situated in the jelly just beneath the subumbrellar musculature, along the bell margins, in the subgenital porticus and in the upper parts of the oral lappets. 'Mature' individuals were commonly found with their anterior end projecting slightly through a small pore in the jelly through which the channel in which they were situated opened to the exterior.

Even though the authors made a detailed study on the morphology of the parasite—interpreting structures as 'mouth', 'eye', 'gland cells', etc. (Fig. 6-10)—they were unable to assign the organism to any known group:

'. . . . . this parasite does not fit well the morphological pattern of any group with which we are familiar. Several zoologists, both here and abroad, have been consulted but none have come forth with a definite answer as to the identity or affinities of this parasite' (p. 6).

This is a good example of the difficulties and problems parasitologists are sometimes confronted with in identifying 'foreign structures' even at the metazoan level. Although apparently unaware of Southwell's (1921) doubtlessly correct interpretation and unfamiliar with the morphology of larval Tetraphyllidea, Moestafa and McConnaughey (1966) established the genus *Ouwensia* to include *O. catostyli*, the 'enigmatic' parasite from *Catostylus ouwensi*, as type species. Until the adult of this larval cestode is determined, the generic as well as the specific name must be considered provisional.

Another tetraphyllidean-like plerocercoid was recovered from the mesogloea of an oral lappet of 1 of 6 deep-water coronate medusae, *Periphylla periphylla*, in the Gulf of Mexico. Other oceanic coronate medusae, including *Atolla wyvillei*, *A. vanhoffeni*, *Periphyllopsis braueri* and *Nausithoë punctata*, were not infested (Phillips and Levin, 1973).

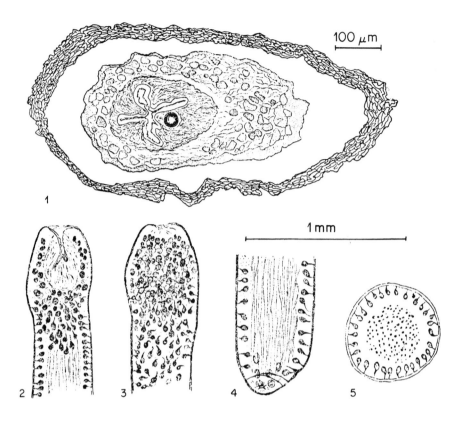

Fig. 6-10: *Ouwensia catostyli*. 1: Transverse section through anterior body end showing cruciform 'mouth', 'eye' and gland cells. Worm *in situ* within channel in jelly of host, *Catostylus ouwensi*; 2: median longitudinal section through anterior body end of *O. catostyli*; 3: optical section through anterior end; 4: posterior end; 5: diagrammatic transverse section through trunk. (After Moestafa and McConnaughey, 1966; reproduced by permission of Lembaga Biologi Nasional LIPI.)

Cabbagehead rhizostomes *Stomolophus meleagris* from coastal waters of Texas, Louisiana and Mississippi (USA) turned out to be commonly infested with an unidentified larval cestode measuring up to 4·5 mm in length. All of more than 500 medusae with a bell diameter greater than 30 mm carried the parasite. The worms had an inverted scolex which was often everted and used in grasping host tissues when the parasites tunnelled through the jelly. Vacant burrows were seen from which the worms had apparently been lost by burrowing completely through to the exterior. These empty tunnels appeared in many cases to contain large bacterial populations. In *S. meleagris* with a large plerocercoid burden there were tangled masses of worms in mesogloeal pockets, 3 to 5 mm in diameter, in the vicinity of the bell margin. Each clump contained as many as 10 worms (Phillips and Levin, 1973).

The larvae could be maintained in the laboratory, surviving up to 3 weeks in host tissue at 4° to 16° C; they could also be maintained in sea water at the same temperatures and in salinities ranging from 10⁰/₀₀ to 37⁰/₀₀. Above 20° C, they became markedly active. When mechanically removed from host tissue, the worms actively invade any suitable gelatinous substrate including sea-water agar. Burrowing is rapid at 16° C, a 4-mm larva penetrates 6 mm into a block of medusal tissue within 10 min. This plerocercoid was apparently limited to Rhizostomae. Species other than *Stomolophus meleagris*, however, were not found to be infested. Even though these larval cestodes are excellent material for tetraphyllidean life-cycle studies, no such work has as yet been undertaken.

The further fate of all plerocercoids reported from scyphozoans remains unknown. Similar larvae are, however, found encysted in the gastric and intestinal walls of deep-sea fishes of the family Macrouridae (Phillips and Levin, 1973). The latter authors assume that for larval cestodes from *Stomolophus meleagris* teleost fishes of the genera *Caranx, Peprilus, Poronotus* and *Chloroscombrus*, which commonly associate with *S. meleagris*, may well serve as paratenic or definite hosts. A large variety of teleosts utilize *S. meleagris* as a food source. Additional early reports on the occurrence of larval cestodes in planktonic Cnidaria, including Scyphozoa, have been cited and commented upon by Dollfus (1931).

Agents: Copepoda

Only a few harpacticoid and cyclopoid copepods have been described as 'semiparasitic' associates of scyphomedusae. Harpacticoids *Nitocra medusae* inhabit small pits in the exumbrellar surface of *Aurelia aurita* from Portsmouth, New Hampshire (USA). Approximately 1030 individuals of both sexes were recovered from a single small host, about 7·5 cm in diameter. When undisturbed, the copepods remained in their flask-shaped pits in the exumbrella, the largest pit being about 1 to 1·5 mm deep and 1 mm in diameter. There were more than 30 depressions on this medusa, each with 10 to 30 or more copepods. Since the copepods, massed together in their pits, were opaque or slightly cream-coloured, the medusa appeared to the unaided eye as though there were sand grains in the jelly. Whether or not the copepods excavate the pits has not been determined. When examined under intense illumination or when disturbed with a needle, the copepods became active, crawling in and out of the pits and over the exumbrellar surface, clinging tenaciously to bits of debris and jelly fragments (Humes, 1953).

Lichomolgoids *Paramacrochiron sewelli* and *P. rhizostomae* have been reported from the medusae *Lichnorhiza malayensis* and *Rhizostoma* sp., respectively, in southeastern Indian waters (Reddiah, 1968). *Pseudomacrochiron stocki* occurred on *Dactylometra quinquecirrha* from the same area (Reddiah, 1969).

Sewellochiron fidens was discovered in Puerto Rico (USA), where it associated with the medusa *Cassiopea xamachana* (Humes, 1969c). From Japanese waters, Humes (1970) described *Paramacrochiron japonicum* as an associate of *Thysanostoma thysanura*. No details are available on the nature of these associations; some of them have been termed 'semiparasitic'.

Agents: Amphipoda

The cosmopolitan hyperiid *Hyperia galba* associates with various scyphomedusae. It has been reported from *Aurelia aurita, Cyanea capillata, Chrysaora hysoscella, Pelagia noctiluca* and *Rhizostoma pulmo* var. *octopus* in the North and Baltic Seas and the English Channel (Franc, 1951; Buchholz, 1953; Haahtela and Lassig, 1967; Goormaghtigh and Parmentier, 1973) as well as in the Mediterranean Sea (Laval, 1972). It was also associated with *A. aurita* and *C. capillata* at the North American Atlantic coast (Holmes, 1905; Bowman and co-authors, 1963), as well as with *Desmonema gaudichaudi* in the Antarctic Ocean (White and Bone, 1972). There are further records from various parts of the world ocean with the exception of lower latitudes.

The relation between *Hyperia galba* and scyphomedusae has been described as commensal (Hollowday, 1946), semi-parasitic (Stephensen, 1923) and parasitic (Dahl, 1959a, b; Agrawal, 1963, 1967; Metz, 1967; White and Bone, 1972). Orton (1922) suggested that *H. galba* is an opportunistic, faculative, food parasite of *Aurelia aurita*. However, little if any evidence for the various viewpoints was presented in the earlier papers.

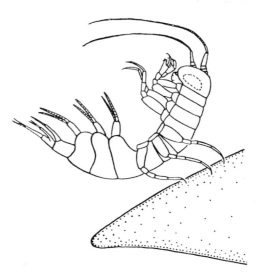

Fig. 6-11: *Hyperia galba*. Adult male in resting posture on edge of *Cyanea capillata* bell. (After Bowman and co-authors, 1963; not copyrighted.)

During the examination of sections and smear preparations of the digestive tracts of 25 *Hyperia galba* collected from the bell of *Cyanea capillata* in Norwegian waters, Dahl (1959a, b) was struck by the presence of numerous empty nematocysts in virtually all formed food remains encountered in the amphipods' gut. Their dimensions agreed well with those from the host and were quite different from nematocysts of all other medusae collected in the same area. On his slides, Dahl furthermore observed pieces of host tissue that had passed the mandibles and were in the process of being swallowed. He concluded that *H. galba* is a true ectoparasite of *C. capillata* and other scypho- and hydromedusae.

Observing living *Hyperia galba* to hold on and move in an inverted position (Fig. 6-11) while attached to the exumbrellar surface of individuals of *Cyanea capillata* from North American waters, Bowman and co-authors (1963) questioned Dahl's (1959a, b) findings. They stressed that the mouth parts face away from the substrate and that if *H. galba* is parasitic it would probably feed on tentacles or oral lappets rather than the bell of the medusa. The amphipod, however, occurs most frequently not on the exumbrellar surface but in the subgenital pouches (Hollowday, 1946; Agrawal, 1963; Laval, 1965; Metz, 1967; White and Bone, 1972), and has previously been seen devouring *Aurelia aurita* tissues, and feeding in the gastric pouches of this scyphozoan (Romanes, 1877; Lambert, 1936).

Substantiating Dahl's (1959a, b) original opinion regarding the parasitic nature of the *Hyperia galba*–scyphozoan association, White and Bone (1972) found adult and adolescent stages of the amphipod on the subumbrella around the manubrium of *Desmonema gaudichaudi*, which fed on the epidermal tissues. Newly released instars without eye pigment and functional swimming appendages, as well as instars up to 6 mm long, were found in the terminal ramifications of the gastrovascular system of the host. It was assumed that the ovigerous females deposit their brood in the manubrium from where they are conveyed to the peripheral portions of the gastrovascular system by the host's normal ingestive or locomotory activities. According to White and Bone, the assumption of an endoparasitic development of *H. galba* is in accordance with observations by Brusca (1967b) and other investigators which indicate that individuals up to the 6 mm stage are absent from the plankton. Furthermore, Laval (1965) demonstrated that, after experimental release from the brood pouch, young instars of hyperiids are incapable of independent existence. Lack of young stages in the plankton also supports White and Bone's idea that dispersal to new hosts does not take place until adolescent and adult stages are attained.

Invasion by *Hyperia galba* may cause considerable damage or even death of the scyphozoan host. Metz (1967) found large numbers of adult amphipods in the subgenital cavities or the gonads proper of *Aurelia aurita* from Isefjord (Denmark). In many cases, the host's reproductive organs were half or almost completely eaten away. The author believed that in this particular area *H. galba* is entirely dependent on *A. aurita,* exerting definite control over the host population. Once the host population is destroyed, the parasite also vanishes from the fjord (Fig. 6-12).

Hyperia galba infestations can locally reach epizootic proportions. Thus, the entire Isefjord population of mature *Aurelia aurita* acquired the parasite within a few weeks after its arrival from the neighbouring Kattegat, with which the Isefjord is connected by a narrow sound. Infested *Cyanea capillata,* drifted in from Kattegat by the wind, served as source of initial infestation for the Isefjord scyphozoans (Metz, 1967). *C. capillata* collected in the fjord were likewise almost invariably and heavily parasitized by this amphipod. In one case, a medusa, 20 cm in diameter, harboured a total of 327 *H. galba* of different sizes (Rasmussen, 1973). In massive infestations, the medusal gonads were entirely destroyed.

Temperature has a marked influence on the parasite–host system: lower water temperatures favour infestation by *Hyperia galba*. As a result, *Aurelia aurita* disappears from the Isefjord much earlier in cool (August to September) than in warm summers (October to November). Periods between attainment of a 90% infestation incidence and the total breakdown of the *A. aurita* population are brief, indicating great impact of the parasite on its host (Fig. 6-12). During periods of heavy infestation, *H. galba* is sometimes found free-swimming—apparently in search of a new host (Metz, 1967). Brusca (1967a, b) recorded free-swimming *H. galba* in 31 plankton samples collected at depths of 85 to 1100 m off southern California (USA). There was an obvious diurnal vertical migration with concentrations above the 500-m level at night. While individuals

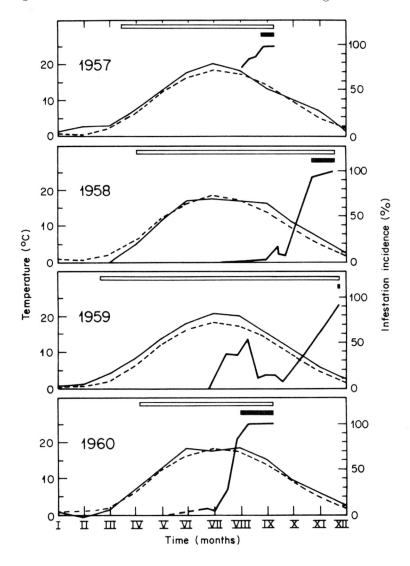

Fig. 6-12. *Aurelia aurita.* Infestation by *Hyperia galba* in Isefjord, Denmark. Open horizontal bars: period during which medusae occur in fjord; solid bars: interval between 90% infestation incidence and disappearance of medusae; heavy line: infestation incidence; light line: mean monthly water temperatures; broken line: monthly mean water temperatures for period 1895–1930. (After Metz, 1967; reproduced by permission of Dansk Naturhistorisk Forening.)

associated with medusae are usually translucent, free-living *H. galba* are reddish-brown in colour, probably due to an extension of their chromatophores (Rasmussen, 1973).

Diurnal vertical migrations displayed by *Hyperia galba* in the western Baltic Sea have been studied *in situ* by means of saturation diving (Schriever, 1975). The amphipods migrated from the surface to the bottom (15-m depth) about 0·5 h after sunset and returned to the surface 0· 5 h before sunrise. Males reached both the bottom and the surface earlier than females. Of 592 *H. galba*, collected from *Aurelia aurita* trapped near the Underwater Laboratory 'Helgoland', 62·5% were adult ovigerous females, 19·8% adult males and 17·7% juveniles.

As has been demonstrated by Metz (1967), *Hyperia galba* vanishes from the Isefjord as soon as the *Aurelia aurita* and *Cyanea capillata* population has been extinguished. The author theorized about the hibernation and possible replenishment of the Isefjord stock of the parasite. According to Buchholz (1953), overwintering *H. galba* have been found in hydromedusae *Melicertum octocostatum*, *Halitholus cirratus* and *Sarsia tubulosa*, as well as in the ctenophore *Beroë cucumis*. *H. galba* thereby changes its host in the sequence of occurrences of the particular hydromedusae. The amphipod shows, however, a definite preference for the greater scyphomedusae, and changes over to *A. aurita* and *C. capillata*, as soon as these have attained a diameter of about 2 cm during April to May (Rasmussen, 1973). Thiel, H. (1970) confirmed, by underwater *in situ* observations, that *H. galba* is capable of overwintering on the dense pads of *A. aurita* scyphistomae populating hard substrates in shallow water. The amphipods were seen to lie on their dorsal sides among the polyps, attaching to them by means of their posterior pereiopods and devouring their tentacles from the tips down to the bases. Hence, *H. galba* can shift, in the absence of suitable medusal hosts, from its normal pelagic life to a benthic one.

Scyphomedusae, particularly *Aurelia aurita* and *Cyanea capillata*, have become a threat to the fishery, especially in the Baltic Sea, where, in recent years, trawls sometimes contain nothing but jellyfish. The utilization of *H. galba* in the biological control of *Aurelia* merits investigation.

Another hyperiid, *Hyperoche medusarum*, has been found associated with *Aurelia aurita*, *Cyanea capillata* and other scyphomedusae from the European and American Atlantic coasts (Sars, 1895; Stephensen, 1923; Bowman and co-authors, 1963). It has also been reported from North Pacific and North Atlantic hydromedusae but appears to occur most frequently associated with comb-jellies (see Chapter 7).

Associations between gammarid and caprellid amphipods and scyphomedusae have been listed and discussed by Vader (1972). There is little evidence of parasitism in most of these.

Agents: Isopoda

An association between deep-sea scyphomedusae *Deepstaria enigmatica* and a giant isopod, *Anuropus* sp., has been documented on photographs taken by the submersible 'Deepstar' (Barham and Pickwell, 1969). The photos show an 8-cm isopod clinging to the subumbrellar surface of the medusa at the time of capture. The authors suggested that the isopod feeds on host tissues, incapacitates medusa movement and creates a 'floating protective environment'. They did not, however, demonstrate the presence of *D. enigmatica* nematocysts in the stomach contents of *Anuropus* sp. associated with the medusa. Phillips (1973) rejected Barham and Pickwell's interpretation and emphasized that—as has been shown by Phillips and co-authors (1969)—medusae can serve as hosts for a wide variety of crustaceans and other metazoans without incapacitation.

Examination of the *Deepstaria enigmatica* specimen on which the above-mentioned isopod was found by Russell (1967) revealed that at the time of its capture various parts were missing, i.e. the stomach portion of the umbrella, the epithelial lining, and large parts of the coronal muscle. Russell suggested that the specimen was moribund, although he noted what appeared to be viable cellular elements.

The damage observed in the *Deepstaria enigmatica* specimen could well have been caused by the attached *Anuropus* sp. but direct evidence is lacking. Barham and Pickwell (1969) were unable to detect nematocysts in the yellow, waxy-like mass taken from the gut of their *Anuropus* sp. Menzies and Dow (1958), on the other hand, found nematocysts in the alimentary tract of 1 of the 5 specimens of *A. bathypelagicus* studied by them. Hence, these anuropids feed at least occasionally on cnidarians.

According to Barham and Pickwell (1969), several anatomical features of the genus *Anuropus* are striking. The distal portions of the second to seventh pairs of thoracic appendages are curved inward and armed with sharp dactyls that appear to be admirably suited for clinging to objects. The pointed, laterally extended epimeral plates may also be an adaptation for lodging fast to the host medusa.

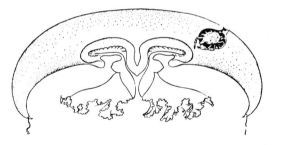

Fig. 6-13: *Aurelia aurita*. Cross section through medusa showing typical mesogloeal excavation occupied by *Libinia dubia*. (After Jachowski, 1963; not copyrighted.)

Agents: Decapoda

Spider crabs *Libinia dubia* have been found on the subumbrellar surface, as well as in pits in the exumbrella of *Aurelia aurita* from Chesapeake Bay (Fig. 6-13). The pits had apparently been excavated by the crabs. Eleven juvenile *L. dubia* were collected from 10 medusae. Their carapace lengths ranged from 10 to 25 mm, with an average of 15 mm. By comparison, the carapace length of a large adult female crab is over 100 mm.

The medusae were apparently in good condition, except for the holes that the crabs had cut in them. Several *Libinia dubia* appeared to be feeding upon a living medusa when later observed in the laboratory. The crabs pulled tissue fragments from the exumbrella with their chelipeds and transferred them to their mouth parts (Jachowski, 1963). Even though *L. dubia* invaded *Cyanea capillata* and *Dactylometra quinquecirrha* in Mississippi Sound, it did not produce pits in these scyphomedusae (Phillips and co-authors, 1969). *L. dubia* has also been reported from other scyphomedusae (Corrington, 1927; Gutsell, 1928; Thiel, 1976).

Young blue crabs *Callinectes sapidus* may be found clinging to the umbrellas of *Dactylometra quinquecirrha* but have never been observed to feed upon them (Jachowski, 1963). On the other hand, adult *Carcinus maenas* were very frequently seen to feed upon tissues of *Aurelia aurita* in the Baltic Sea (Lauckner, unpublished underwater observation).

Phyllosoma larvae of the scyllarid lobster *Ibacus* sp. were observed firmly attached to the exumbrellar surface of *Pelagia panopyra* in Sydney Harbour. The larvae clung tenaciously to the host's bell and were difficult to remove without injuring them. Phyllosomes removed from their sites of attachment and placed among the tentacles remained unharmed and rapidly climbed back to the upper surface of the bell (Thomas, 1963).

Ibacus sp. phyllosoma larvae collected from the subumbrellar surface of *Catostylus mosaicus* in New South Wales waters contained the same purple pigment as the host. Apparently, the crustaceans fed on the body tissues of the medusa (Thomas, 1963). Shojima (1963) observed phyllosoma larvae of *I. ciliatus* attached to *Aurelia aurita* and *Dactylometra pacifica* in Japanese waters. The bodies of these medusae were sometimes damaged; some lacked their mouth tentacles. Although no direct observations on the feeding of the larval crustaceans were made, it appeared probable that the damage to the hosts' bodies was caused by them.

In this context, it is interesting to note that Sims and Brown (1968) reported faecal masses from a giant, 6·9-cm scyllarid phyllosoma taken north of Bermuda, which consisted entirely of undigested nematocysts. This clearly indicates that phyllosoma larvae may, at least occasionally, feed on cnidarian tissues.

Hayashi and Miyake (1968) reported on the association of caridean shrimps *Chlorotocella gracilis*, *Latreutes anoplonyx* and *L. mucronatus* with rhizostomes *Mastigias papua* in Japanese waters. Although no detailed observations regarding the interrelationship were made, it was—probably rightly so—termed commensalistic. For further references on associations between shrimps and scyphozoans consult Hayashi and Miyake (1968).

Mysids are among the less well-known associates of Cnidaria. *Idiomysis tsurnamali* has been found associated with Red Sea rhizostomes *Cassiopea andromeda*, as well as with sea anemones *Megalactis hemprichti* (Băcescu, 1973).

A number of other invertebrates—including representatives of the Turbellaria, Nematoda, Cirripedia, Schizopoda, Stomatopoda, Decapoda, Pycnogonida, Arachnida, Echinodermata and Cephalopoda—have been found to be associated with Scyphozoa, either occasionally or permanently. The literature concerning these associations has been reviewed by Thiel (1976).

Agents: Pisces

A great number of small—mostly juvenile—teleostean fishes are known to associate with semaeostome and rhizostome scyphozoans. A considerable body of information witnessing such associations has accumulated in the past decades; numerous publications date back to the 19th century. The pertinent literature has been extensively reviewed by Mansueti (1963) and Thiel, M. E. (1970).

Evidently, the majority of the Semaeostomae is associated with fishes of the family Gadidae whereas most Rhizostomae are accompanied by Carangidae (Fig. 6-14). This may, at least in part, be due to differences in the geographical distribution of both medusae and fishes. According to Thiel, M. E. (1970), there appears to exist a fundamental difference between these two groups of associations. Evidence suggests that the relationship between rhizostomes and fishes is primarily a mutualistic one, frequently assuming the nature of cleaning symbioses, whereas the semaeostome–fish associations are truly parasitic.

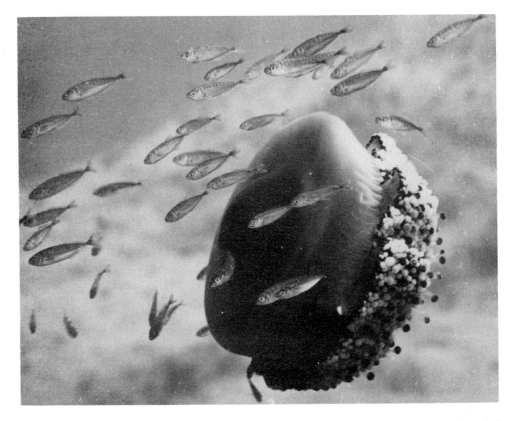

Fig. 6-14: *Cotylorhiza tuberculata* accompanied by numerous *Trachurus trachurus*. Isle of Capri (Gulf of Naples, Italy), 5 m depth. (Original.)

The latter hypothesis has been substantiated by various observations and experiments, although results and interpretations of such experiments have sometimes been controversial. For a detailed discussion see Mansueti (1963) and Thiel, M. E. (1970). Only a few examples will be discussed here.

Young North Sea whiting *Merlangius merlangus* frequently congregate below the bell and among the tentacles of *Cyanea capillata* without being harmed. A dozen or more of these small fish may accompany a single large medusa. Scheuring (1915) demonstrated experimentally that whiting feed on *C. capillata* tissues, particularly on the gonads, when kept under aquarium conditions. The fishes even refused copepods and amphipods *Hyperia galba*. The author concluded that young *M. merlangus* depend on *C. capillata* as main food, and hence, that the relationship is a parasitic one.

However Dahl (1961), using the same species in a series of aquarium studies, obtained quite opposite results. His *Merlangius merlangus* fed on planktonic organisms, mainly copepods, and took *Hyperia galba* when offered. Associated *Cyanea capillata*, on the other hand, were not attacked although *M. merlangus* took minced jellyfish. The alimentary tracts of young whiting caught in the sea together with *C. capillata* contained zooplankton, mostly copepods, but no remnants of scyphozoan tissue were found.

Merlangius merlangus appeared to have acquired a certain degree of immunity from the nematocysts of *Cyanea capillata*. Histological examination of whiting exposed to tentacles of the medusa revealed only a few and scattered nematocysts attached to the skin. To *Gobius flavescens* a similar experience was fatal. Great numbers of nematocysts were encountered in the skin, indicating the discharge of entire nematocyst batteries (Dahl, 1961). Rees (1966), however, reported that also *M. merlangus* were stung to death when the host medusa, *C. capillata*, was disturbed. The latter observation has been confirmed by several underwater experiments conducted in Norwegian waters (Lauckner, unpublished).

In support of Scheuring's (1915) findings, Mansueti (1963) noted remains of host tissue and gonads in the stomachs of young harvestfish *Peprilus alepidotus* associated with *Dactylometra quinquecirrha* in Chesapeake Bay (USA). *P. alepidotus* was not immune to the jellyfish toxin. Jachowski (1963) observed young harvestfish in Chesapeake Bay feeding on *Aurelia aurita*.

Butterfish *Peprilus triacanthus* from the North American Atlantic coast have been observed to associate with *Cyanea capillata* (Haedrich, 1967). Gulf butterfish *Poronotus burti* from Mississippi Sound (USA) fed on *C. capillata* and were immune to the toxin of this medusa. In contrast, all other fishes in that area living in association with scyphomedusae possessed no immunity to jellyfish toxins (Phillips and co-authors, 1969). Protective mechanisms giving the illusion of immunity are probably identical to those reported for anemone fishes by Schlichter (1975).

These divergent results cannot yet be explained adequately. According to Mansueti (1963), fish–jellyfish symbioses are temporary phenomena resulting from a series of extrinsic factors; the fishes act as active opportunists while the scyphomedusae are essentially passive hosts. Associations may be initially commensal, become ectoparasitic as the fish feed upon the host and finally, as its ecological requirements change, may develop into a non-symbiotic predatory relationship.

DISEASES CAUSED BY METAZOANS: CUBOZOA

No definite cases of metazoan-caused diseases in cubozoans have come to the reviewer's attention. Unidentified larval trematodes have been observed in the mesogloea of *Carybdea marsupialis* off Agadir, Northwest Africa (H. Thiel, personal communication to Thiel, 1976). Spider crabs *Libinia dubia* have been reported from the outside and from within the umbrella of *Chiropsalmus quadrumanus* in Mississippi Sound (Phillips and co-authors, 1969).

DISEASES CAUSED BY METAZOANS: HYDROZOA

Agents: Cnidaria

Phialidium hemisphaericum from the Isle of Man (England) were found to be infested by larval anthozoans *Peachia hastata*. The larvae were seen not only to take food from the hosts' stomachs but also to devour parts of their gonads (Werner, 1959). Künne (1948) had previously reported this parasitic actinian from *Eutonina indicans* in the North Sea (Fig. 6-15). A large percentage of these small leptomedusae were found to be infested. The adult of *P. hastata* has been described by Gosse (1855).

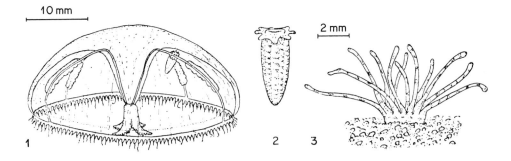

Fig. 6–15: 1: *Eutonina indicans*. Larval *Peachia hastata* attached to radial channel of medusa; 2, 3: *P. hastata*, larva (2) and adult (3) burrowed in sediment. (After Künne, 1948; reproduced by permission of Senckenbergische Naturforschende Gesellschaft.)

In *Peachia quinquecapitata* infesting *Phialidium gregarium* along the North American Pacific coast, the entire life cycle was elucidated experimentally. A free-swimming planula larva, when ingested by a suitable medusa, begins to grow and differentiate in the gastrovascular cavity of the host. Planulae which are not ingested fail to develop. The larvae remain endoparasitic for an average of 11 days at 12° to 15° C and probably feed on material in the gastrovascular cavity. After 11 days the larvae become ectoparasitic and feed on the gonads of the medusae. A larval anemone, 2 mm in length, is able to eat all 4 gonads off a host in 2 days. It will then generally proceed to eat the manubrium, stomach and tentacles and, in some cases, the mesogloea of the bell itself. If given the opportunity under laboratory conditions, larval *P. quinquecapitata* may transfer from one host to another. Complete transfer from initial contact to release of the old host medusa may take from 10 s to more than 1 h. During transfer, *P. quinquecapitata* is able to hold two actively swimming medusae in spite of very small contact areas. Given transfer opportunity, the anemones ate an average of 14·6 *Phialidium gregarium* gonads during their development, involving about three transfers. After an average of 31 days of ectoparasitism the anemones measure about 4·2 mm in length and 2·3 mm in diameter, acquire adult characteristics and drop off the host to become free-living (Spaulding, 1972). Once off the host, the anemones burrow quickly into the sediment in the manner described for *P. hastata* by Ansell and Trueman (1968).

Between 5·0 and 62·5% of the *Phialidium gregarium*, collected at different times of the year near Friday Harbor (Washington, U.S.A.), were found to harbour larval *Peachia quinquecapitata*. *Phialidium hemisphaericum, Aequorea aequorea, Halistaura cellularia* and *Mitrocomella polydiademata* from the same area were also infested. Dip-net collections of *P. gregarium* indicated that female medusae were more heavily parasitized than males. Although *Peachia quinquecapitata* showed no preference for either host sex in transfer, parasites which ate a larger proportion of female gonads became free-living more quickly. Those restricted to male medusae took an average of 41·2 days for the ectoparasitic phase, ate about 15·2 gonads, and were approximately 4·6 mm long when dropping off the host. Individuals restricted to female medusae remained ectoparasitic for about 39·8 days, ate an average of 13·6 gonads, and had a mean length of only 3·7 mm when becoming free-living (Spaulding, 1972).

The adult stage of *Peachia quinquecapitata* has been described by McMurrich (1913) who also observed a larval anemone parasitizing *Aequorea forskålea* in North American Pacific waters. It probably belongs to the same species. However, since he could not raise it to the adult, non-parasitic stage, he described it as a new species, *Bicidium aequoreae*. The latter genus was created by Agassiz (1859) for a parasite of a scyphozoan medusa on the Atlantic coast of North America.

Further immature actinians have been reported from a number of species of medusae. The majority of these mostly inadequately described forms have been assigned—sometimes erroneously—to the genera *Peachia, Halcampa, Edwardsia* or *Bicidium* (Müller, 1860; Wright, 1861; Graeffe, 1884; Haddon, 1887, 1888; McIntosh, 1887; Dendy, 1888; Browne, 1896; Panikkar, 1938; Nyholm, 1949).

Agents: Trematoda

Marine hydromedusae have frequently been reported as intermediate hosts for Trematoda. Lebour (1916) describes the metacercaria of *Opechona bacillaris* from *Obelia* sp., *Cosmetira pilosella, Turris pileata* and *Phialidium hemisphaericum* from Plymouth (England). Unencysted metacercariae were generally found clinging to the manubrium or stomach wall of the medusae, but sometimes also occurred underneath the umbrella wall. Frequently, every medusa in a haul was infested. *O. bacillaris* occurred most abundantly in Plymouth medusae in early summer and was rare in winter. Franc (1951) observed the metacercariae in spring and summer plankton off Dinard–St.-Malo (France).

The life cycle of *Opechona bacillaris* has been elucidated by Køie (1975). Ophthalmotrichocercous cercariae develop in rediae in prosobranch snails *Nassarius pygmaeus* (Fig. 6-16). Hydromedusae of *Eutonina indicans* proved to be suitable second intermediate hosts. After attachment to the medusa, the cercariae were seen to penetrate the host's epidermis by alternating contractions and relaxations of the oral sucker. As soon as the cercarial body became firmly embedded in the mesogloea, the tail was shed by violent lashing. The entire process of penetration took about 15 to 30 min. A few days after penetration, the pigment of the cercarial eye-spots faded away, as development of the metacercaria progressed.

Nassarius pygmaeus harbouring the rediae of *Opechona bacillaris* frequently carried the hydroid generation of *Podocoryne carnea* on their shells (Fig. 6-17, b). In some experiments, all cercariae emerging from isolated snails were ingested by the hydranths; a single

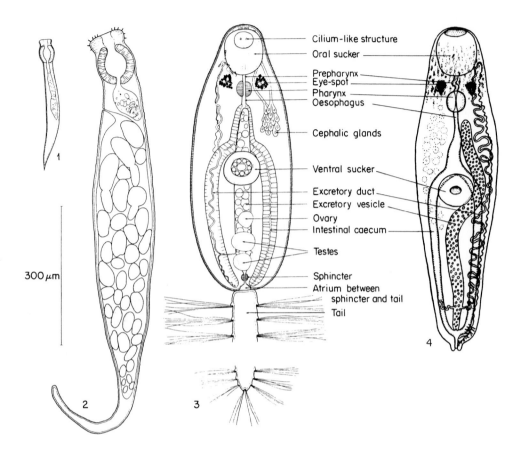

Fig. 6-16: *Opechona bacillaris*. Immature (1) and mature (2) redia from first intermediate host,
Nassarius pygmaeus; free-swimming cercaria (3) and metacercaria (4) from cnidarian or
ctenophoran second intermediate host. (1–3: After Køie, 1975; reproduced by permission of
Ophelia. 4: After Stunkard, 1932; reproduced by permission of Cambridge University Press.)

individual contained up to 5 cercariae. Hydranths examined immediately after
collecting an infested free-living snail nearly always had at least a few cercariae in the
stomach. Free-swimming medusae likewise ingested large numbers of emerged
cercariae (Fig. 6-17, c). On the other hand, *P. carnea* medusae were attacked and
penetrated by *O. bacillaris* cercariae. Up to 4 larvae were seen in individual medusae
which were then seriously affected and hardly able to swim. *P. carnea* may, thus,
simultaneously function as second intermediate host and predator of *O. bacillaris*.
However, the small *P. carnea* medusae may not serve as a normal second intermediate
host in nature. Whether cercariae ingested by medusae can survive and establish
themselves in the host's mesogloea by boring their way through the wall of the
gastrovascular system has not been established.

   Køie (1975) made another interesting and apparently unique observation on the
behaviour of the cercariae of *Opechona bacillaris* which may be interpreted as 'tail
cleaning'. The slightly photopositive cercaria is capable of relatively fast locomotion by
vigorous movements of its muscular tail. It swims tail forward and with the body bent so
that the anterior end points in the swimming direction (Fig. 6-17, a,1). At regular

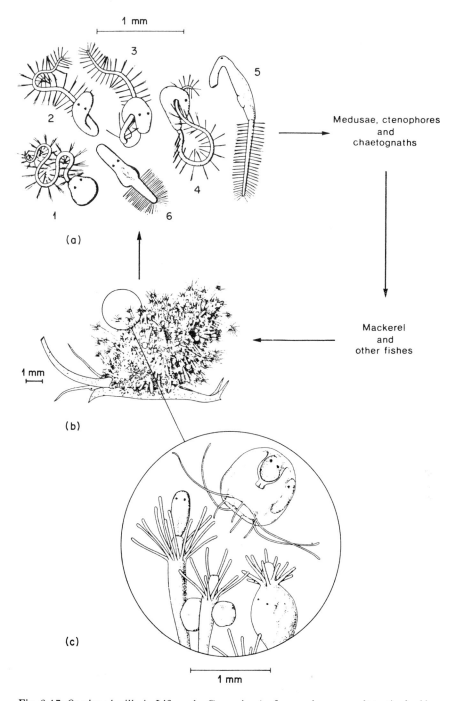

Fig. 6-17: *Opechona bacillaris*. Life cycle. Cercariae (a; for numbers consult text), shed by
first intermediate host *Nassarius pygmaeus* (b), are ingested by polyp and medusal
stage of *Podocoryne carnea* (c). Polpys are epiphoretic on *N. pygmaeus* shells (b);
medusae may also serve as second intermediate host (c). (After Køie, 1975;
modified; reproduced by permission of Ophelia.)

intervals, the tail is straightened out, followed by a rapid bending of the anterior body end towards the base of the tail (2). In a quick movement, the tail is then passed between the two suckers (3,4). Afterwards, body and tail become stiff and the cercaria remains quivering for a while with its anterior end bent (5). A few seconds later, the cercaria resumes normal swimming (1). Sometimes cercariae may crawl on the bottom. The tail is then contracted and shorter than the body (6). Adult *O. bacillaris* are intestinal parasites of the mackerel *Scomber scombrus* and the lumpsucker *Cyclopterus lumpus* (Dawes, 1947), and a dozen or more species of *Opechona* have been described from various fishes in different parts of the world (Stunkard, 1967).

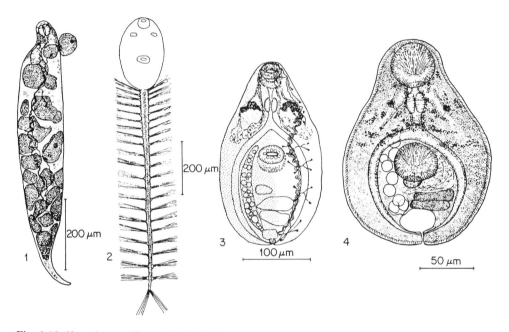

Fig. 6-18: *Neopechona pyriforme*. (1) Redia from *Anachis avara*; individual flattened under cover-glass pressure, cercarial germ-ball emerging at birth pore; (2) general outline of cercaria showing morphology of tail; (3) morphology of cercaria (without tail); (4) metacercaria. (After Stunkard, 1969; modified; reproduced by permission of Marine Biological Laboratory, Woods Hole.)

Metacercariae of the lepocreadiid trematode *Neopechona pyriforme* (Fig. 6-18) occur in the marine hydromedusae *Bougainvillia carolinensis*, *Aequorea forskålea* and *Gonionemus vertens*. The full life cycle of the parasite has been elucidated experimentally by Stunkard (1967, 1968, 1969). Ophthalmotrichocercous cercariae develop in rediae in the digestive gland of the columbellid snail *Anachis avara*. Upon liberation, they penetrate, but do not encyst in, the above-mentioned hydromedusae. *G. vertens*, experimentally exposed to cercariae of *N. pyriforme*, are vigorously attacked (Fig. 6-19). Only little growth occurs in the intermediate hosts. Metacercariae are infective immediately; hence, the medusae are hardly more than paratenic hosts. In experiments, the metacercariae developed into adults in the scup *Stenotomus chrysops*. The species was first described as *Distomum pyriforme* from the rudderfish *Palinurichthys perciformis* by Linton (1900).

Hydromedusae *Aequorea pensilis* from Waltair (Bay of Bengal, India) are hosts for hemiurid metacercariae, about 0·4 mm in length and 0·11 mm in width. The larvae were not identified but it was believed that they may belong to the genus *Aponurus*, adults of which occur in fishes of that region (Rao, 1958). The occurrence of larval hemiurids (which normally have copepods as second intermediate hosts) in medusae is not uncommon (Russell, 1953). Probably, the cnidarians merely act as paratenic hosts for these trematodes.

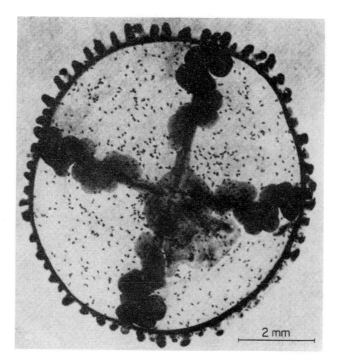

Fig. 6-19: *Gonionemus vertens*. Experimental infestation with *Neopechona pyriforme* after 1-day exposure to cercariae. (After Stunkard, 1969; reproduced by permission of Marine Biological Laboratory, Woods Hole.)

Large numbers of siphonophores *Physalia utricula* from Japanese waters harboured larval distome trematodes. The parasites measured about 1·5 mm in length and were brownish in colour; they appeared to be members of the family Accacoeliidae (Okada, 1932). Adult accacoeliids are intestinal parasites of pelagic fishes.

Long arrays of Cnidaria, harbouring a great variety of larval trematodes, have been listed by Dollfus (1963) and Rebecq (1965). It should be emphasized that, despite the large body of literature existing on the occurrence of metacercariae in medusae, the life cycles of only a few species have, so far, been worked out completely (Rebecq, 1965).

Agents: Cestoda

Larval cestodes of the type *Scolex polymorphus*, 100 μm long, were recovered from deep-sea siphonophores *Agalma* sp. captured in the open Atlantic Ocean. From the description given by Studer (1878) no conclusions can be drawn with respect to the specific identity of the parasite.

Agents: Mollusca

A 'dome-shaped appendix' on the body wall of the nudibranch *Phyllirrhoë bucephala*, described by Krohn (1853) and Müller and Gegenbaur (1853–54), was interpreted as parasitic medusa and consequently named *Mnestra parasites*. The studies on the relationship between the pelagic mollusc and the medusa have a long and fascinating history. Important histological investigations on the association have been contributed by Claus (1875), Vessichelli (1906) and others. Günther (1903) described *M. parasites* as a 'blood-sucking vampire', and Costa (1863) regarded the medusa as part of the nudibranch's body, representing 'a secondary sex character!'

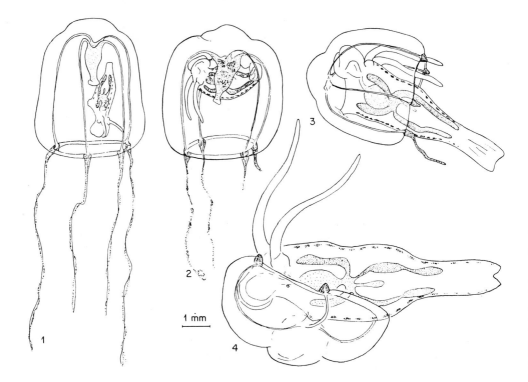

Fig. 6-20: *Phyllirrhoë bucephala* parasitizing *Zanclea costata*. 1: Nudibranch clinging to body wall of medusa; 2: resting and feeding attitude of nudibranch; 3: *P. bucephala* considerably increased in size and deforming host medusa; 4: *P. bucephala* shortly before detachment from host. (After Martin and Brinckmann, 1963; reproduced by permission of Stazione Zoologica di Napoli.)

Vessichelli (1910) and Ankel (1952a, b) assumed that the medusa is not parasitic on the mollusc but that *Mnestra parasites* is attacked by *Phyllirrhoë bucephala*. It remained to Martin and Brinckmann (1963) to identify '*M. parasites*' as the anthomedusa *Zanclea costata* and to establish, by laboratory observations on the development of both partners, the mollusc but that *Mnestra parasites* is attacked by *Phyllirrhoë bucephala*. It remained to attaches to the umbrella of the host medusa, feeding parasitically by suction on the manubrium and on the contents of ring and radial canals. *P. bucephala* grows rapidly, soon exceeding the host in body size. Finally, the nudibranch devours the entire manubrium and the tentacles of the medusa (Fig. 6-20).

Another parasitic nudibranch, *Cephalopyge trematoides*, lives attached to siphonophores *Nanomia bijuga* (formerly *Halistemma tergestinum*), on which it feeds. The mollusc apparently displays host-specificity since it has, thus far, never been found on other cnidarians. Its life cycle is similar to that described for *Phyllirrhoë bucephala*. Whether the adult nudibranch is capable of leading an independent existence, or whether it depends nutritionally on *N. bijuga* or another cnidarian host, remains unknown (Sentz-Braconnot and Carré, 1966). *N. bijuga* has previously been recorded by several authors under various names (Pierantoni, 1923; Baba, 1933; Palombi, 1939; and others) which, according to Steinberg (1956), are all synonyms for *N. bijuga*.

Prosobranchs of the family Janthinidae—which is closely related to the sea anemone-attacking Epitoniidae (see 'Anthozoa')—are highly specialized, pelagic gastropods which associate with, and feed on, siphonophores of the genera *Velella*, *Physalia* and *Porpita*, and probably others. Relatively little is known about their ecology and host–parasite interrelations (Laursen, 1953; Risbec, 1953; Wilson and Wilson, 1956; Ganapati and Rao, 1960).

Agents: Copepoda

Several copepods of the lichomolgid genus *Macrochiron* have been reported as associates of plumulariid hydrozoans from Madagascar by Humes (1966). *M. lytocarpi* and *M. valgum* occurred on *Lytocarpus philippinus*, and *M. rostratum* on *L. philippinus* and *L. spectabilis*. Additional species from the same region—*M. lobatum* from *L. phoeniceus* and *M. vervoorti* from *Aglaophenia cupressina*—have been described by Humes and de Maria (1969). Both papers are taxonomic and contain no information on pathology (Fig. 6-21).

Agents: Amphipoda

Hyperia galba mostly parasitizes scyphomedusae; however, it has also been recorded from a number of hydromedusae. Buchholz (1953) found *Melicertum octocostatum*, *Halitholus cirratus* and *Sarsia tubulosa* in the western Baltic Sea to be infested, and Künne (1952) observed the amphipod on *Phialidium hemisphaericum* from North Sea plankton. The relationship between *H. galba* and hydromedusae has never been examined closely. According to Buchholz (1953), this amphipod shows a distinct preference for scyphomedusae. Possibly, hydromedusae serve merely as transport hosts.

The Mediterranean *Hyperia schizogeneios*, on the other hand, is definitely a parasite of hydromedusae during its developmental phase, attacking primarily species of *Phialidium* (Laval, 1968, 1972). The females deposit up to 5 (normally 1 to 3) larvae in the manubrium or the gonads of the medusa. Immediately after deposition, the larvae start feeding on the host's gonadal tissues. Loss of body substance is easily compensated by well-fed medusae whose body volume, in an individual 5 mm in diameter, is actually about 600 times that of a larva, and the gonads regenerate readily. If, however, the parasite burden is augmented experimentally to, say, 20 times its normal level, the damage becomes critical: within 2 days the manubrium and gonads disappear, and within a few more days the medusa—now unable to feed—decreases in size and is eventually completely devoured by the larval amphipods (Fig. 6-22).

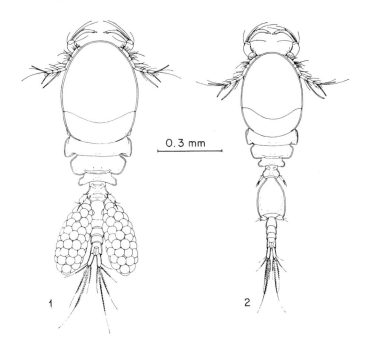

Fig. 6-21: *Macrochiron lobatum* from *Lytocarpus phoeniceus*. Dorsal aspect of female (1) and male (2). (After Humes and de Maria, 1969; reproduced by permission of Zoological Museum, Amsterdam.)

Larvae fed umbrellar tissue developed and metamorphosed normally with only a slight time lag in their development. Hence, *Hyperia schizogeneios* does not depend on substances produced by or present in the host gonads and manubrium. Normal development also occurred in larvae experimentally transferred to *Obelia* sp.

At water temperatures prevailing in the Mediterranean Sea, development of *Hyperia schizogeneios* to the adult stage requires 15 to 30 days and is normally completed on the same host individual. At metamorphosis, the juveniles leave the gonad and attach to the subumbrellar surface or the manubrium (Fig. 6-23). At this stage there is also a change in diet. The young amphipods no longer—or only exceptionally—feed on the host's gonads but ingest food materials collected by the medusa. Only at times of food deficiency (rarely to be expected in nature) do they devour host tissue.

At a sampling station off Villefranche-sur-Mer (French Mediterranean coast), *Hyperia schizogeneios* displayed distinct lunar periodicity (Laval, 1972). Laval reports observations on the ecology of this amphipod and lists hydromedusae *Leuckartiara nobilis* and *Liriope tetraphylla* as additional (although rare) hosts. In general, *H. schizogeneios* leaves its medusa when caught in a plankton net. Riedl (1963) reported the species as

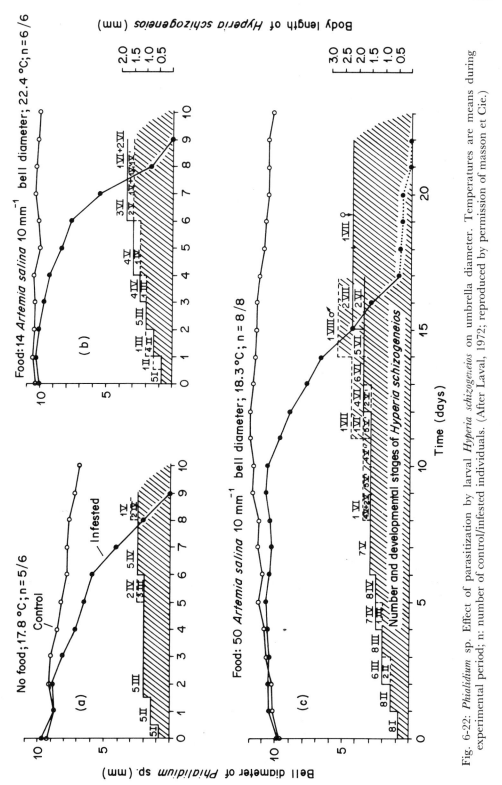

Fig. 6-22: *Phalidium* sp. Effect of parasitization by larval *Hyperia schizogeneios* on umbrella diameter. Temperatures are means during experimental period; n: number of control/infested individuals. (After Laval, 1972; reproduced by permission of masson et Cie.)

occurring rather frequently near the surface in the open sea and particularly in coastal waters but did not mention its apparent obligatory association with hydromedusae.

A single juvenile amphipod, about 1 mm in length and still unidentifiable, was found attached to an individual of *Phialidium* sp. taken off Villefranche-sur-Mer (French Mediterranean coast). When kept in the laboratory with a medusa, the amphipod resembled *Hyperia schizogeneios* in its behaviour. As long as the medusa was adequately fed, the crustacean participated commensalistically in its food (*Artemia salina*) whereas, in the undernourished host, it attacked the gonads. The amphipod lived attached to the medusa for about 1 month, moulted once, but eventually died of a bacterial infection. Nevertheless, its development was sufficiently advanced for it to be identified as a new genus and species, *Bougisia ornata*. It appears to be of rare occurrence in this part of the Mediterranean. Subsequently, only 2 adult males and 1 ovigerous female were obtained from plankton hauls (Laval, 1966).

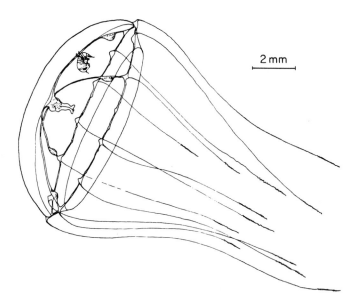

2 mm

Fig. 6-23: *Phialidium* sp. with juvenile male *Hyperia schizogeneios* attached to subumbrellar body surface of host. (After Laval, 1972; reproduced by permission of Masson et Cie.)

Another hyperiid amphipod, *Hyperoche medusarum*, associates externally with hydromedusae *Tima formosa* in Narragansett Bay, Rhode Island, USA (Bowman and co-authors, 1963), as well as with hydromedusae of the genera *Tiaropsis*, *Sarsia*, **Phialidium** and *Polyorchis* in waters off Nanaimo, British Columbia, Canada (von Westernhagen, 1976). Although adult *H. medusarum* were usually found free-swimming, juveniles were frequently encountered close to the surface sitting on the exumbrellae of the medusae. From these observations, as well as from the fact that at Nanaimo *H. medusarum* feeds primarily on *Clupea harengus pallasi* larvae, it may be concluded that associations between this amphipod and hydromedusae are merely accidental, or that hydromedusae serve as transport hosts for *H. medusarum*.

Sheader and Evans (1975) studied feeding in hyperiideans *Parathemisto gaudichaudi*. In the open ocean, these amphipods feed on a wide range of zooplankton, chiefly copepods and chaetognaths. Under laboratory conditions, however, hydromedusae *Aglantha digitale*, *Aequorea vitrina*, *A. forskålea*, *Phialidium hemisphaericum*, *Leuckartiara octona*, *Staurophora mertensi*, *Bougainvillia principes* and *Sarsia tubulosa* were readily accepted. Attempts to use scyphomedusae *Aurelia aurita* and *Cyanea capillata* as food source failed.

Parathemisto gaudichaudi fed mostly on the exumbrellar surface but occasionally in the subumbrellar region, or within the gastric cavity, attaching in a forward position (i.e. with the ventral surface in contact with the host) using all its pereiopods. In previously starved amphipods, feeding usually took 15 to 30 min at 5° to 12° C. After feeding, the amphipods either detached and swam away or, more frequently, remained attached, usually in the backward position, using only the posterior 3 pairs of pereiopods held over the dorsal surface of the pleon. The large hydromedusa then provided a means of transport for the resting amphipods. From Sheader and Evans' (1975) findings it is obvious that *P. gaudichaudi* is a facultative parasite of hydromedusae.

Parathemisto pacifica have been found clinging to the manubrium of 13 of 40 North Pacific anthomedusae *Calycopsis nematophora*. No nematocysts were present in the stomach contents of 5 amphipods examined, and there is no evidence that the amphipods were feeding on the medusae. Interspecific relationships are suggested but their nature is not known (Renshaw, 1965).

In a brief note, Laval (1965) reported on the occurrence of larval hyperiids *Lycaeopsis themistoides* on siphonophores *Chelophyes appendiculata* at Villefranche-sur-Mer (French Mediterranean coast).

There are a few reports on associations between gammaridean amphipods and hydromedusae. *Metopa alderii* is found on *Tima bairdii*; *M. borealis* occurs on *Phialidium* sp., both in European waters (Elmhirst, 1925; Vader, 1972). Both amphipods also often occur on athecate tubularian hydroids (Pirlot, 1932). There is little evidence for parasitism in these associations, the amphipods feeding apparently on secretions from their hosts.

Agents: Pantopoda

Pantopoda—or Pycnogonida, as the sea spiders are more commonly called—associate with hydroid polyps. Little is known about their biology but most, if not all, appear to be parasitic, at least during their larval development. The adults are free-living.

The sea spider *Anoplodactylus erectus*, which occurs in high population densities among clusters of the hydroid *Tubularia crocea* in California (USA), is a true parasite. Its eggs are produced in summer; they release larvae which later pierce the body wall of *T. crocea*, and enter the digestive tract, where they grow parasitically (Hilton, 1916; Ricketts and Calvin, 1968; Fig. 6-24).

In European waters, larval *Phloxichilidium femoratum* and *P. virescens* have been reported from cysts in *Syncoryne eximia*. *P. tubulariae* inhabits the gastric cavity of *Tubularia larynx*; *Anoplodactylus pygmaeus* occupies the gastric cavity of *Obelia* sp. polyps, and *A. petiolatus* the manubrium of *Obelia* sp. medusae (Dogiel, 1913; Lebour, 1945). Okuda (1940) described the development and metamorphosis of *Ammothea alaskensis* in the anthomedusa *Polyorchis karafutoensis* in Japanese waters. Lists of Pycnogonida associated with Hydrozoa have been published by Schlottke (1932), Hedgpeth (1941), Lebour (1945), Ziegler (1960), King (1973, 1974), Wyer and King (1974), Wolff (1976) and others.

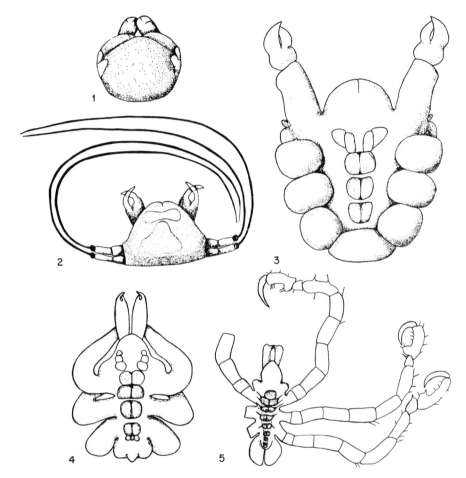

Fig. 6-24: *Anoplodactylus erectus* from *Tubularia crocea*. 1: Embryo exercised from female (×
350); 2: freshly hatched larva, with appendages straightened (× 350); 3: young larva
taken from gastrovascular cavity of *T. crocea* (× 350); 4: older larva from gastrovascular
cavity of *T. crocea* (× 75); 5: free-living individual from surface of a mass of hydroids (×
25). After Hilton, 1916; reproduced by permission of Pomona College.)

DISEASES CAUSED BY METAZOANS: ANTHOZOA

Invertebrates of various phyla associate with anthozoans, in particular with stony corals (Madreporaria). In many of these associations the distinction between 'facultative predators' and 'temporary parasites' is difficult on the basis of the existing information. In fact, such distinction is often a matter of definition.

Agents: Porifera

Sponges of the genus *Cliona* are known for their capacity to bore into calcareous substrates. During penetration, the substrate is gradually destroyed as the sponge hollows out an extensive system of cavities and tunnels.

Clionid sponges penetrate into dead and living coral skeletons. Although not attacking living coral tissue, they contribute to the destruction of solitary and reef-building corals and, hence, will be considered here briefly.

Boring sponges are extremely abundant on the reefs off Hurghada (Egyptian Red Sea coast), invading mainly dead coral but to a lesser extent also living Madreporaria. Among the living corals studied, *Pocillopora* sp. was most prone to attack, the sponges forming series of cavities up to the stems, their basal parts becoming riddled. Occasionally massive living colonies of various genera were subject to sponge boring to a remarkable degree. Thus, a large colony of *Hydnophora exesa*, apparently perfectly healthy, suffered boring from *Cliona onussae* so that the corallum under the surface layer consisted merely of walls and struts between close-set cavities up to 3 cm in diameter (Bertram, 1936).

In shallow water, the effects of boring are frequently masked by rapid biological calcification and energetic wave attrition. The base of shallow-water corals is usually skirted by a layer of living polyps, so that the attachment grows in proportion to the bulk of the corallum. The larger the corals, the better cemented they are to their substrate. Moreover, skeleton parts covered by a layer of living coral polyps are not normally attacked by clionids. In deep water, however, only the upper surfaces of the flattened, horizontally extended colonies are alive, and the holdfast is not covered by living coral tissue. The growth of such colonies, therefore, is not accompanied by a proportional increase in thickness and strength of the base, so that large individuals are often precariously perched on a thin neck which is easily broken.

Under such conditions, calcium carbonate deposition is not as fast as near the surface and the effect of wave turbulence is normally negligible; hence, boring sponges become the main factor of reef erosion. Deep-water corals, with their thinner skeletons, slower growth rates, and large dead areas around the base, are more riddled with sponge burrows than are shallow-water colonies of the same size. At depths below 50 m on the fore-reef slope on the north coast of Jamaica, the loosening of corals—mainly *Agaricia* spp.—through destruction of their basal parts is so marked that large living colonies can be collected easily by hand without the use of tools. Colonies often break off under their own weight and fall into deep water, where they are killed by burial in soft sediments. Hence, clionid sponges may act, to a considerable extent, as controlling factors in the formation and maintenance of coral reefs by modifying the shape of coral formations, weakening coral structures, and supplying coarse fore-reef rubble along the deep fronts of reefs (Goreau and Hartman, 1963).

Boring sponges also attack fossil coral reefs and limestone rock. Measured profiles of the submerged portion of steep cliffs in Harrington Sound (Bermuda) indicate that they are undercut as much as 4 to 5 m by a notch whose flat roof coincides closely with the level of extreme low tides. Bioerosion, mainly due to *Cliona lampa*, was proposed as the mechanism of undercutting (Neumann, 1966). Seven species of *Cliona*, as well as

Cliothosa hancocki and *Thoosa mollis*, which erode limestone in the Adriatic Sea near Rovinj (Yugoslavia), were found to exhibit distinct ecological niche differentiation (Hartman, 1957).

The mechanism of clionid sponges for penetrating calcium carbonate substrates has been studied repeatedly. Nassonov (1883), Letellier (1894) and Cotte (1902) were the first to demonstrate that *Cliona* spp. produce fine calcareous debris in the course of their boring activities. In contrast, more recent authors (Ginsburg, 1957; Revelle and Fairbridge, 1957; Cloud, 1959) maintained that these sponges bore by chemical action, erroneously implying that all the excavated calcium carbonate is removed by solution. However, Warburton (1958), Cobb (1969), Rützler and Rieger (1973) and others have shown that penetration involves mainly a chemical liberation of small pieces of substrate, aided by chemical dissolution of material. Cells of archeocyte origin carve out chips of calcium carbonate (conchyolin in molluscan shells) by means of filopodial extensions and etching secretions. During the process, the cells undergo plasmolysis. The chips are expelled through the exhalant canal system. Only about 2 to 3% of the eroded material is removed in solution. Rützler and Rieger (1973) studied the burrowing in *Cliona lampa* by means of scanning and transmission electron microscopy.

Coral and limestone destruction due to *Cliona* spp. invasion may reach considerable proportions. Laboratory experiments and field observations indicate that *C. lampa* is capable of removing as much as 6 to 7 kg of material from 1 m² of carbonate substrate in 100 days (Neumann, 1966). Numerous papers have been published during the past century on systematics, distribution, ecology and physiology of marine borers including *Cliona* spp. (for references see Clapp and Kenk, 1963; Carriker and co-authors, 1969; Rützler and Rieger, 1973).

The non-burrowing sponge *Mycale laevis* influences the shape of reef corals. When encrusting the lower surfaces of *Montastrea annularis* and other madreporarians, the corals assume a typical shape characterized by aberrant peripheral folding. This relationship, however, appears to be advantageous for both partners: The sponge enjoys a continuously enlarging substrate that is free from competitive sessile organisms; the coral benefits from increased feeding efficiency as a result of water currents produced by *M. laevis*, and is protected from invasion by boring forms, notably clionid sponges (Goreau and Hartman, 1966).

Agents: Trematoda

Carlgren (1924) described and figured a metacercaria of unknown specific identity from the sea anemone *Bunodactis mortenseni* from Auckland (New Zealand). It was seen in the sphincter muscle and in the mesenteries of the anemone (Fig. 6-25). He believed that the presence of the parasite had some influence on the structure of the sphincter. Jungersen (1904; *in*: Dollfus, 1963) observed an unidentified metacercaria in the pennatulid *Virgularia mirabilis*, collected during the Danish Ingolf Expedition.

Agents: Mollusca

Wentletraps–small snails of the family Epitoniidae—are known to be associated with sea anemones in various parts of the world. Thorson (1957) found *Opalia crenimarginata* attached to the column of intertidal anemones *Anthopleura xanthogrammica* in Californian waters. The snails had their long proboscis everted, piercing the anemone's body wall and sucking out the host's body fluids. Normally only the distal end of the proboscis was involved in penetration, but sometimes the entire organ was inserted, the snail being partially embedded in the soft base of the anemone which, however, showed no visible reaction. Once proboscis penetration is accomplished, *O. crenimarginata* remain attached in the same position on *A. xanthogrammica*, sucking for hours or even days.

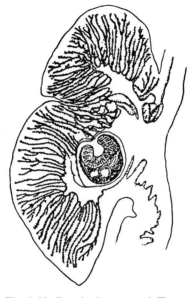

Fig. 6-25: *Bunodactis mortenseni*. Transverse section through sphincter (tentacle side downwards), showing encysted trematode metacercaria *in situ*. (After Carlgren, 1924; reproduced by permission of Dansk naturhistorisk Forening.)

Evidence for a parasitic interrelationship between epitoniids and sea anemones had previously been obtained by Ankel (1936, 1938) who observed nematocysts (probably of *Metridium dianthus* and *Sagartia elegans*) together with zooxanthellae originating from actinians, in the stomach and intestines of *Epitonium (Clathrus) clathrus* from Naples, Italy, and from the west coast of Sweden. Ankel suggested, without making observations, that young anemones are swallowed whole. In Bahamian waters, *E. albidum* has been seen to feed on *Stoichactis helianthus*. In Delaware Bay (New Jersey, USA), *E. rupicola* was found to live side by side with sea anemones *Paranthus rapiformis* and *Haliplanella (Diadumene) luciae*, but did not appear to be associated with them. Experimentally, however, *E. rupicola* fed readily on either species (Robertson, 1963). In Japanese waters, *Habea inazawai*, a primitive epitoniid, has been reported as 'semi-parasitic' on *H. (Diadumene) luciae* (Habe, 1943). Root (1958, cited by Robertson, 1963) found an unidentified species of *Epitonium* from the Philippines to be associated with, and apparently feeding on, mushroom corals of the genus *Fungia*. Thorson (1957) suggested that the entire family 'Scalidae' (=Epitoniidae) may be more or less adapted to a parasitic mode of life, living in association with, and feeding on, Anthozoa.

At least 8 species of *Heliacus*—'sundials' of the family Architectonicidae, which is remote from the Epitoniidae—are ectoparasitic on colonial zoanthid sea anemones of the genera *Zoanthus* and *Palythoa* in Atlantic and Pacific tropical or warm temperate waters. The snails are fairly sedentary and usually attached to their hosts with remarkably sturdy but elastic mucous threads. Feeding occurs only at night, the very long, invaginable proboscis of *Heliacus* spp. producing 3- to 4-mm deep holes in the surface of the host colonies (Robertson, 1967).

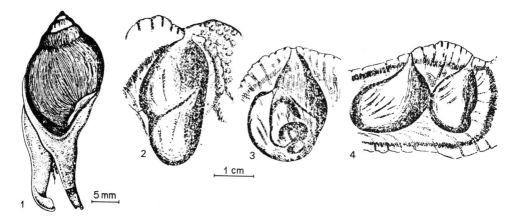

Fig. 6-26: *Leptoconchus cumingii*. 1: Adult individual; 2 and 3: single burrows of adult individuals in corals of genera *Favia* and *Goniopora*; 4: communicating burrows inhabited by *L. cumingii*. (After Gohar and Soliman, 1963b; reproduced by permission of Cairo University Press.)

Many species of gastropods live associated with stony corals. Detailed information is lacking or must be inferred from their modes of life. The array of mollusc relationships to corals reaches from predation over commensalism to facultative and obligate parasitism. Only associations believed to be truly parasitic will be discussed here.

Members of the gastropod family Coralliophilidae are all obligately associated with corals. They invariably lack jaws and radulae. A few species of *Coralliophila* live with gorgonians and zoanthids, *Rhizochilus* with antipatharians, *Latiaxis* with gorgonians, and *Rapa* is embedded in alcyonarians. All other coralliophilids are associated with stony corals; the genera *Quoyula*, *Magilopsis*, *Leptoconchus* and *Magilus*, as well as several species of *Coralliophila*, exhibit marked host-specificity (Fig. 6-26).

The 4 coral-specific genera are restricted to the Indo-Pacific and are derived from *Coralliophila*-like ancestors which lived externally on corals and had regularly coiled shells, while the recent species exhibit progressive morphological adaptation to their parasitic way of life. Thus, *Quoyula* has a limpet-like shell, adapting it for external life on corals; *Magilopsis* and *Leptoconchus* are ovoid, and bore holes into corals, while *Magilus* even became uncoiled and sessile inside corals (Gohar and Soliman, 1963b; Robertson, 1970). *Magilus antiquus* (the only species of this genus) is the most specialized coral symbiote among prosobranchs. While the juvenile shell is still coiled, the adult shell changes into an uncoiled, irregular tube, deeply imbedded in a living coral skeleton, but with the aperture at the surface. The latter keeps pace with the growth of the surrounding coral. There is some disagreement in the literature with respect to the food and mode of feeding in *Leptoconchus* sp. and *Magilus antiquus*. While some investigators believe these gastropods to be ciliary feeders, Gohar and Soliman did not observe feeding, could detect neither animal nor plant remains in the digestive tracts, and thus, conclude that these species are probably not ciliary feeders.

The coral-dwelling species of *Coralliophila* inhabit external host structures (Robertson, 1970). In *C. abbreviata*, the saliva aids in penetrating the coral epidermis, and the muscular proboscis is used as a pump to ingest the zooxanthellae-containing soft tissue of the host coral (Ward, 1965). *C. violacea* depends nutritionally on living corals (Demond, 1957). Ward believes that *C. abbreviata* contributes to the destruction of the *Montastrea annularis* at Barbados.

Phyllidia bourgini, a porostomatous doridoid nudibranch, occurs commonly on *Acropora* spp. (Vicente, 1966); it is probably parasitic. The Phyllidiidae have a large, muscular pharynx, but neither jaws nor a radula.

Further associations between gastropod molluscs and Anthozoa—mainly Madreporaria—have been described and discussed by Demond (1957), Robertson (1963, 1966, 1967, 1970), Bosch (1965), Vicente (1966), Taylor (1968), and others. Their publications contain numerous references to previous pertinent work. Most of the studies, however, do not contain sufficient substance for defining exactly the kind of interrelationship involved. Parasitism cannot be ruled out in many cases.

Numerous bivalve molluscs—representatives of the superfamilies Myacea, Adesmacea, Veneracea, Saxicavacea, Gastrochaenacea, Cardiacea and Mytilacea—bore into calcareous substrates including living and dead coral. As emphasized by Yonge (1963), the basic structure of these animals ideally fits them for this mode of life. While none of them obtains food from the substrate, boring bivalves are discussed here briefly because of their detrimental effect on living coral.

Their shell valves are always the prime tools of penetration, although the manner in which they operate differs greatly among the members of the various superfamilies, and even among closely related forms. Usually the entire bivalve is sunk into the substrate, only the siphon tips protruding slightly from the rock or coral surface. Hence, it may be difficult to recognize their presence in spite of sometimes high population densities.

A striking feature of the gastrochaenacean *Rocellaria cuneiformis*, on the other hand, is the capacity of its siphonal tissues to secrete calcium carbonate, enabling the bivalve to line its burrow and extending it beyond the substrate surface into 2 separate tubes formed by the ends of the distally bifurcated siphon (Otter, 1937; Purchon, 1954). Other members of the genus, and indeed of the entire superfamily Gastrochaenacea, exhibit similar protective mechanisms.

Boring mechanisms in bivalves have been discussed in detail by Yonge (1963). Substrate penetration is primarily mechanical. Only in some representatives of the Mytilacea is the mechanical abrasion of the shell valves assisted by chemical erosion. Thus, the mytilid bivalve *Fungiacava eilatensis* described from the Red Sea by Goreau and co-authors (1969) lives in chemically excavated cavities in the fungiid coral *Fungia scutaria*. Its long siphons open into the coelenteron, where they collect food, probably consisting, to a significant extent, of symbiotic zooxanthellae discharged from the coral tissues. However, *F. eilatensis* is believed to be merely a commensal (Fig. 6-27).

Mytilids of the genus *Lithophaga* commonly attack Red Sea corals. *L. cumingiana, L. hanleyana, L. lima, L. teres* and *L. obesa* have been reported from living Madreporaria at Hurghada (Egypt) and elsewhere (Bertram, 1936; Gohar and Soliman, 1963a). Species such as *Montipora* sp., *Favia stelligera, Cyphastraea* sp. and *Stylophora* sp. hardly escape infestation with high numbers of these borers. Bertram (1936) estimates the amount of primary break-offs of coral colonies near Hurghada due to boring bivalve invasion to be about 20%. Two other mytilids, *Modiolus cinnamoneus* and *Lithophaga laevigata* have been found to bore into dead coral at Hurghada (Gohar and Soliman, 1963c).

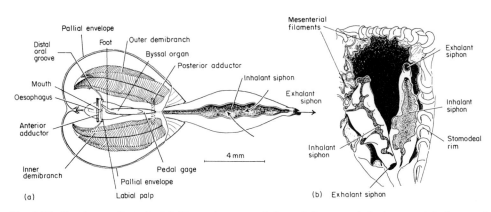

Fig. 6-27: *Fungiacava eilatensis*. (a) Ventral aspect, siphons fully extended. Arrows: inhalent and exhalent currents. (b) Siphons of *F. eilatensis* protruding into coelenteron of *Fungia scutaria*. Viewed from above, i.e. through open stomodaeum. (After Goreau and co-authors, 1969; reproduced by permission of The Zoological Society of London.)

Agents: Annelida

The number of polychaetes and other worms obtained from a block of coral by extraction is often astonishing. Many of the polychaetes—among them *Eunice siciliensis* and *Lysidice collaris*—occupy tunnels apparently excavated by them (Bertram, 1936). Others are probably secondary inquilines living in burrows made by other organisms (Ebbs, 1966).

The coral-eating amphinomid *Hermodice carunculata* has been studied in greater detail (Marsden, 1962, 1963a,b). This polychaete was seen to devour polyps of madreporarians *Porites porites* in Barbados waters. A considerable fraction of these corals had damaged tips apparently eaten away by *H. carunculata*. The contents of the digestive tract of *H. carunculata* taken from the reef were rich in nematocysts and masses of small, spherical, greenish-brown cells resembling zooxanthellae liberated from the coral tissue. However, regarding its free existence, *H. carunculata* should be considered a predator rather than a parasite (or semiparasite).

Syllids *Haplosyllis depressa chamaeleon* have been identified as ectoparasites of gorgonians *Paramuricea chamaeleon* at Banyuls (France). The polychaetes occurred firmly attached to the host, the setae of their parapodia piercing the delicate epidermis covering the coenenchyme. Contact with the gorgonian's tentacles did not obviously harm the worms. On one occasion an individual was seen which had its prostomium and anterior body segments deeply inserted into the gastric cavity of a polyp. Feeding was not observed and examination of the annelid's intestinal contents remained inconclusive. However, the intense colouration of the epidermis, proventriculus and pharynx wall, observed in some individuals, appeared to be derived from the red pigmentation of the gorgonian, and was taken as indicative of a parasitic way of life of *H. depressa chamaeleon* (Laubier, 1960).

Agents: Copepoda

The overwhelming majority of crustacean associates of Anthozoa appear to be copepods; they probably constitute the most important group of all known symbiotes of anthozoans.

The harpacticoid copepod *Paramphiascopsis pallidus*, found in the gorgonian *Eunicella stricta* from Banyuls in the Mediterranean Sea (Soyer, 1963), inhabits 'pocket-like' structures, obviously formed by the host in response to the parasite, and without communicating with the surrounding water. Adults, as well as nauplii and copepodites, of *P. pallidus* were seen side by side in these pockets. The copepod has never been found in free water.

Acontiophorus bracatus, a cyclopoid siphonostome copepod, has been described as an ectoparasite of *Eunicella* sp. and other octocorals of the genera *Parerythropodium* and *Leptogorgia* from Banyuls (Stock and Kleeton, 1963). A curiously transformed siphonostome, *Cholomyzon palpiferum*, lives endoparasitically in *Dendrophyllia nigrescens* and *D. micranthus* in Madagascan waters (Stock and Humes, 1969). Mediterranean *Anemonia sulcata* have been reported as host for *Dinopontius acuticauda* (Stock, 1960). *Asteropontius corallophilus* parasitizes corals of the genera *Pocillopora*, *Montipora*, *Stylophora* and *Porites* from Mauritius, and *Asterocheres scutatus* has been found associated with *Rhodactis rhodostoma* in the Red Sea (Stock, 1966a, b; Schirl, 1973).

A great variety of poecilostome cyclopoid copepods lives associated with Anthozoa. The scale of relationships extends from merely commensal to facultative and even obligately parasitic forms, the mode of life being reflected by morphological characteristics. Ectoparasites are typically cyclopiform or only slightly transformed, whereas endoparasitic species are more or less modified. Only a few of the most recent publications are mentioned here. They contain further references which provide access to the immense body of older literature.

The sabelliphilid *Paranthessius anemoniae* (Bocquet and Stock, 1959), a 'semiparasite' from the sea anemone *Anemonia sulcata* from Roscoff, France, appears to be fairly host-specific. It rests semi-attached on the column of the anemone, apparently feeding on mucus. *P. anemoniae* showed a marked preference for *A. sulcata*, although artificial transfer to *Actinia equina* resulted in some degree of non-genetic adaptation. After a few days on *A. equina* the copepods' colour changed to that of the new host. Colour change appeared to be unrelated to background colouration.

In spite of several studies on *Paranthessius anemoniae* (Gotto and Briggs, 1972; Briggs and Gotto, 1973, Briggs, 1974), the exact nature of the food utilized by this anemone associate is open to speculation. Evidence from histochemical tests indicates the gut contents to be of a mucopolysaccharide nature, as would be expected for a mucus feeder. Probably *P. anemoniae* represents an evolutionary stage between a free-living and parasitic existence (Briggs, 1977).

There was evidence that *Paranthessius anemoniae* possesses a certain degree of immunity to the toxins from the tentacular nematocysts of the sea anemones. Monthly samples taken over a 2-year period in Northern Ireland showed a seasonal fluctuation in infestation level (Briggs, 1976). *Lichomolgus anemoniae*, another species found on *A. sulcata*, clings to the anemone's tentacles. Apparently, *L. anemoniae* is less well-adapted to *A. sulcata* than *P. anemoniae*, since Carton (1963) observed a rather high mortality in the former copepod species under experimental conditions. It appears that the position on the tentacles is a rather 'dangerous' site, and that many of the parasites are actually killed by the nematocysts of the host. Moreover, Carton was able to demonstrate differences in the mortality of Atlantic (Roscoff) and Mediterranean (Banyuls) specimens of *L. anemoniae*, suggesting a varying degree of adaptation to the same species of sea anemone. *L. anemoniae* occurs, according to Carton, also on Mediterranean *Actinia equina*, but never on Atlantic specimens of the same host.

A great number of lichomolgoid cyclopoid copepods occur on and in Anthozoa, most of them are host-specific, and some structurally modified. Almost all of the papers cited below are merely taxonomic, containing only a few ecological notes and no information on pathology. *Aspidomolgus stoichactinus* lives in the gastrovascular cavity of actinians of the genus *Stoichactis* in the West Indies. *Lichomolgus gemmatus*, *L. magnificus* and *L. cuspis* are associated with *S. giganteum* and *Radianthus ritteri* in Madagascan waters, and *L. constrictus* and *L. insectus* inhabit species of *Antipathes* from Madagascar (Humes, 1963, 1969a). Six species belonging to 5 genera of Lichomolgidae have been found for the first time, associated with octocorals at Eniwetok Atoll; 3 species (3 genera) of the same family occur on New Caledonian fungiid corals; 4 species of *Acanthomolgus* on Bermudian gorgonians (Humes, 1973a, b, c); and 7 lichomolgids on alcyonarians and madreporarians in Madagascar (Humes and Frost, 1963).

Further members of the family Lichomolgidae associate with Hexacorallia (Humes and Ho, 1966; 1967a, b; 1968a): 5 species (3 genera) with zoanthids of the genus *Palythoa*, 2 *Lichomolgus* with the small sea anemone *Rhodactis rhodostoma*, a *Lichomolgus* and a *Monomolgus* with the coral *Psammocora contigua*, and 10 lichomolgids from 4 genera with various species of stony corals, all from Madagascar. In addition, 22 new *Lichomolgus* species have been reported from Madagascan Octocorallia by Humes and Ho (1967c; 1968b, c, d). Most lichomolgids are either typically cyclopoid or slightly modified, and live on the body surface of their hosts.

Since most descriptions have been made from preserved material, little is known about the exact location of the parasites on the cnidarians; most drop off their hosts during narcotization and fixation. Thus, *Doridicola trispinosa* and *Pennatulicola pteroidis* have been collected from magnesium sulphate washings of sea-feathers *Pennatula rubra* and *Pteroeides spinosum*, respectively, from the Gulf of Naples (Stock, 1959).

In spite of the loose association between these ectoparasites and their hosts, lichomolgids exhibit varying degrees of host-preference. In 12 species of lichomolgids of the genus *Acanthomolgus* reported from West Indian octocorals, host-specificity was found to be strongly pronounced (Stock, 1975). In Californian waters, *A. eminulus* and *A. pollicaris* are consistent members of the epifaunal community of gorgonians *Muricea californica*. Like most other lichomolgids they are cryptically coloured and may feed on mucus present on the host polyps (Humes and Lewbel, 1977).

The family Lichomolgidae Kossmann, 1877, was revised by Humes and Stock (1973), and a new superfamily, the Lichomolgoidea, has been created. The voluminous publication comprises numerous familiar and generic diagnoses and specific keys, as well as a host list and many references.

Madagascan cyclopoid copepods belonging to other families have been described by Humes and his colleagues. Vahiniids occur in the gastrovascular system of Antipatharia (Humes, 1967) and xarifiids on or within Madreporaria. Some 20 new species have been recorded by Humes (1960, 1962a) and Humes and Ho (1967b, 1968e).

Other cyclopoid copepods from madreporarians include pseudanthessiids (Humes, 1962b) and rhynchomolgids (Humes and Ho, 1967b). All representatives of the above-mentioned families are largely modified with more or less vermiform bodies, characterizing them as true parasites.

Stock and Humes (1970) reported 4 notodelphyids (belonging to 4 different genera), distinctly modified, from the Madagascan octocoral *Parerythropodium fulvum*. This is the first record of notodelphyids from Anthozoa. All other representatives of the family were associated with Tunicata.

Numerous investigations have been devoted to copepods of the family Lamippidae whose structurally strongly modified members live in the gastrovascular cavity of several genera of Octocorallia (Fig. 6-28). About 22 species are known, some of them occurring in deep-sea gorgonians (Joliet, 1882; Versluys, 1902; de Zulueta, 1908, 1910, 1912; Leigh-Sharpe, 1934; Heegaard, 1949; Gotto, 1954; Humes 1957; Bouligand and Delamare Deboutteville, 1959a, b; Bouligand, 1960a, b, 1961, 1965, 1966; Bresciani and Lützen, 1962; Laubier, 1972). Most of the species previously referred to the genus *Lamippe* are now placed in *Enalcyonium* (Bouligand, 1960b).

Lamippids are highly preferential in their choice of a host. Only a few species are known to parasitize more than a single species of cnidarian. Living in their hosts' gastrovascular cavity, these copepods are true endoparasites. Individuals have been seen to ingest host eggs and tissue. They are probably also capable of uptake of dissolved nutrients via their tegument (Bouligand, 1960b, 1966).

Linaresia mammillifera, an aberrant lamippid parasitizing Mediterranean gorgonians *Paramuricea chamaeleon*, exhibits sex dimorphism, as well as peculiar morphological and behavioural adaptations to its parasitic way of life. The male, about 1000 μm long and 200 μm wide, and very much like a normal lamippid in gross morphology, lives endoparasitically in the host's gastrovascular system. The female, 1000 μm long and 750 μm wide, and strikingly resembling a host polyp in shape (Figs. 6-29 and 6-30), lives ectoparasitically in dead calices of *P. chamaeleon* (Bouligand and Delamare Deboutteville, 1959a; Bouligand, 1960a).

Bouligand (1966) was struck by the resemblance, at first sight, of burrowed female *Linaresia mammillifera* with aberrant polyps of *Paramuricea chamaeleon*. Such resemblance might explain the fact that, although the male of *L. mammillifera* had been described as early as 1908 by de Zulueta, the female remained unknown for more than 50 years until Bouligand and Delamare Deboutteville (1959a) discovered it on gorgonians dredged off Cape Creus (Spanish Mediterranean coast). Adult females are cream coloured with yellow specks on their dorsal sides and are capable of displaying mimicry.

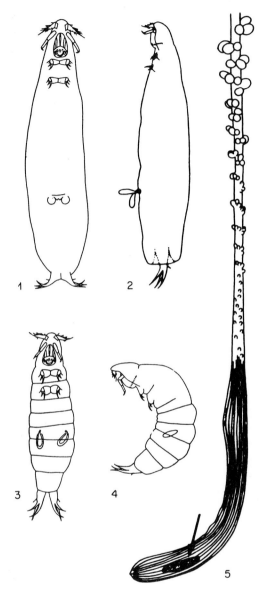

Fig. 6-29: ▶
Linaresia mammillifera. Adult female, ventral (1) and lateral (2) aspects. (After Bouligand, 1960a; reproduced by permission of Masson et Cie.)

Fig. 6-30: ▶
Linaresia mammillifera. Adult female *in situ* in polyp of *Paramuricea chamaeleon.* Top right: closed host polyp. (After Bouligand, 1960a; reproduced by permission of Masson et Cie.)

◀ Fig. 6-28:
Lamippe concinna, parasitic in gastrovascular cavity of *Virgularia schultzei.* Ventral and lateral view of female (1,2) and male (3,4); 5: individual of undetermined sex *in situ* (arrow). (After Humes, 1957; modified; reproduced by permission of Cambridge University Press.)

When dislodged from their host or disturbed, the copepods' appendages become covered with red spots characteristic of the tentacle colouration of *P. chamaeleon* (Bouligand, 1960a, 1966).

Lamippella faurei—a copepod morphologically similar to, although not as strongly transformed as, *Linaresia mammillifera*— has been found to parasitize octocorals *Eunicella verrucosa* and, to a lesser extent, *Alcyonium palmatum, Parerythropodium coralloides* and *Rolandia coralloides* at Banyuls-sur-Mer, French Mediterranean coast (Bouligand and Delamare Deboutteville, 1959b).

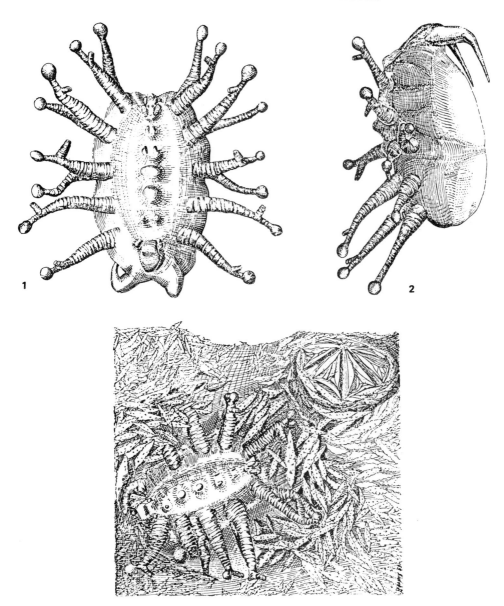

Sea anemones *Bolocera tuediae* from Korsfjorden (Norway) harbour a gall-forming copepod, the antheacherid *Antheacheres duebeni* (Vader, 1970b). These exceptionally large copepods—the male may reach 10 mm, the female even 25 mm—live in conspicuous, roundish galls, formed by the host's mesentery walls, and connected to it by a constricted base. Usually, several galls are present in a single host, concentrated in a large clump resembling a bunch of grapes. The galls are entirely closed, and contain a clear liquid in which the copepods lie loose, the males fixed to the females. They are devoid of a digestive system and hence, must derive their food entirely by diffusion through the body wall, which is exceptionally thin (Bresciani, 1968). The number of

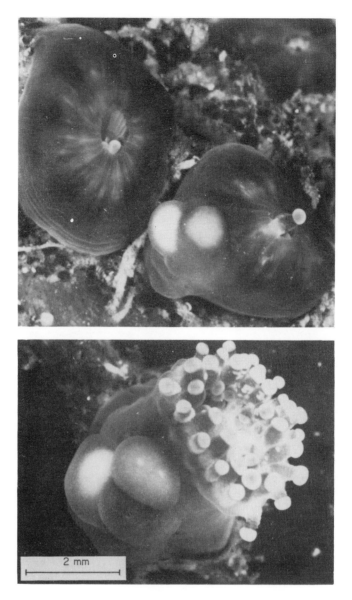

Fig. 6-31: Gall-like protrusions in body wall of *Corynactis viridis*, caused by parasitic copepods *Mesoglicola delagei*. (After Haefelfinger and Laubier, 1965; reproduced by permission of E. J. Brill.)

copepods per gall varies; in larger galls, up to 12 have been counted. In such cases, several adult females with attached males may be present, as well as a few immature specimens. Nothing is known yet about the life cycle of *A. duebeni*. In Korsfjorden, the incidence of infestation of *B. tuediae* with *A. duebeni* was between 43% and 63%, the number of parasites per host being quite variable. The maximum count was 310 in an ovigerous *Bolocera* of 200 g. The presence of *A. duebeni*, even in very high numbers, apparently does not interfere with the reproduction of the host, the incidence of infestation being about the same in ovigerous female *B. tuediae* as in non-ovigerous females or males. The presence of several specimens of *A. duebeni* within a single gall and the grouping of galls in clumps suggests propagation of the parasite within the host. Initial infestation, however, must occur from the surrounding water (Vader, 1970b). *Antheacheres*-like copepods, named *Gastroecus arcticus*, have been recorded from sea anemones *Actinostola intermedia* and *A. spetsbergensis* (Vader, 1970c).

Caullery and Mesnil (1902) and Okada (1927) described gall-inducing copepods *Staurosoma parasiticum* from French Mediterranean and Atlantic *Anemonia sulcata*, and *S. caulleryi* from Japanese *Sagartia nitida*. *S. parasiticum* induces the formation of hazel-nut-sized galls in the mesenteries of *A. sulcata*. Inside the completely closed structure a single large female, up to 25 mm in length, lies curled up with its ventral aspect contacting the inner gall wall. The dwarfed, strongly transformed and degenerate male is attached by means of its mouthparts to the dorsal side of the female's 7th body segment. Sometimes two males, measuring about 2 mm in length, occur on a single female. In galls harbouring mature individuals the long egg-strings which contain light to dark brown ova may be found wound several times around the copepod's body.

The mode of transmission of *Staurosoma parasiticum* to new hosts has not been studied. However, it was observed that the eggs develop into nauplii inside the gall. Hence, liberation of the larvae requires gall rupture. On one occasion a very small, but nevertheless entirely closed gall was observed. Although the enclosed parasite was only slightly larger than a nauplius, it had already lost the morphological features characteristic of the nauplius stage.

Mesoglicola delagei, a copepod 6 to 7 mm in length without sex dimorphism, induces gall formation in *Corynactis viridis* from Roscoff (France). The whitish tumours (Fig. 6-31) can become pedunculate and fall off the host together with the enclosed parasite (Quidor, 1922; Bouligand, 1966). Taton (1934) described several developmental stages of *M. delagei*. Their resemblance to lamippid copepods parasitic in Octocorallia is very striking. Haefelfinger and Laubier (1965) observed *M. delagei* in *C. viridis* from Banyuls (France). About 15% of the actinians had infestations. Of 10 tumours dissected, 6 harboured 1 male and 1 female, 3 contained 2 males and 1 female, and the last tumour yielded 3 males and 1 female.

Agents: Cirripedia

Certain rock barnacles live in association with Madreporaria. Whereas some of these fouling organisms gradually become engulfed and eventually overgrown by the coral, others are specifically modified for this mode of life by having adapted morphologically and physiologically to the growth pattern of the coral. These filter-feeding crustaceans depend on the coral for habitat but not for food.

Lepadomorph barnacles of the genus *Lithotrya* are common borers in Atlantic and Indo-Pacific coral reefs. The cirripeds penetrate the calcareous substratum by means of their contractile peduncle which bears a chitinous covering equipped with 'nail-like bodies'. The boring process is believed to be purely mechanical. Like other barnacles, *Lithotrya* spp. feed on plankton organisms and nutritionally are in no way dependent on the coral (Seymour Sewell, 1926; Cannon, 1935; Yonge, 1963).

Pyrgoma monticulariae from the Indian Ocean is the only known balanomorph cirriped associated with madreporarians that depends on the coral for both habitat and food. It has gained control of certain metabolic activities of its host, including calcification, proliferation of coenenchyme and nematocyst discharge (Ross and Newman, 1969). The distinguishing characteristics of *P. monticulariae* are: an extraordinarily irregular outline and an extremely small aperture—relative to the size of the shell. The shell has been studied in detail by Hiro (1935, 1938). In specimens available from Mauritius (Indian Ocean), a layer of tissue was found growing over the entire external shell surface and the aperture, apparently sealing the barnacle off from the exterior. Squash preparations of this tissue revealed numerous nematocysts, indicating that the overgrowing tissue is an extension of the coral coenenchyme.

Dissection revealed *Pyrgoma monticulariae* to have an aberrant morphology, with but a single pair of biramous cirri, and mandibles and maxillae I modified into sawlike blades. Obviously, these appendages were no longer suited for gathering food by filter-feeding. Although no observations on living individuals were made, details of the feeding process could be inferred. The cirriped had apparently gained metabolic control of the host, preventing skeletal material formed by the coral coenenchyme from overgrowing it, while simultaneously inducing rapid coenenchyme proliferation in the apertural area. The host coenenchyme extends not only over but also into the aperture, and is probably rasped away by means of the structurally modified sawlike mouth parts of the barnacle.

Stomach analyses of *Pyrgoma monticulariae* revealed the presence of macerated tissue and an abundance of undischarged nematocysts. Absence of crustacean, molluscan and protozoan fragments normally encountered in barnacle stomachs, when considered along with the morphological modifications of the mouth parts and food-collecting apparatus, indicates that *P. monticulariae* feeds exclusively on coral tissue. Metabolic activities such as O_2/CO_2 exchange and excretion of soluble nitrogenous wastes evidently takes place through simple diffusion across the investing host structures. Voiding solid wastes, mating and releasing larvae simply require clearing a passage to the exterior (Ross and Newman, 1969).

Agents: Amphipoda

There are only a few published records of associations between amphipods and Anthozoa, and these have not been studied in great detail. Some of the crustaceans involved spend at least part of their life cycle in the gastrovascular cavity of their hosts. Several lysianassid amphipods associate with sea anemones in a more intimate and parasitic or semi-parasitic mode.

Bolocera tuediae from Korsfjorden (Norway) is host for 2 lysianassid amphipods, *Onisimus normani* and *Aristias neglectus* (Vader, 1970a). Nothing is known about the physiological relationship between the amphipods and the sea anemone; it appears, however, to be rather loose. *A. neglectus* has been found in association with sponges from the same area. *O. normani*, on the other hand, appears to be more specialized for a life in the gastrovascular cavity of the anemone. Some degree of adaptation must be present, since the amphipod is not affected by the digestive enzymes or by the nematocysts of the host.

A small fraction of the *Onisimus normani* collected near Bergen (Norway) by Vader

(1967) turned out to be infested with cryptoniscid isopods, probably members of the little known family Podasconidae. This is an interesting case of hyperparasitism in a parasite of cnidarians.

Lysianassids *Allogausia recondita* have been described from within the gastrovascular cavity of sea anemones *Anthopleura elegantissima*; *Cereactis aurantiaca* and *Peachia hastata* have been reported as hosts for *Acidostoma neglectum* and *A. nodiferum* occurs together with *Actinostola callosa* (Stasek, 1958; Vader, 1967; Ansell, 1969). Dahl (1964), in a revision of the genus *Acidostoma*, pointed out that *A. neglectum*, and probably other members of the genus as well, live ectoparasitically on anthozoans. Dahl's morphological investigations led him to the conclusion that the genus *Acidostoma* is one of the few amphipod genera having mouthparts adapted for sucking.

An apparently commensal association between gammarids *Melita obtusata* and *Anemonia sulcata* has been described by Hartnoll (1971). The amphipods crawled on and between the tentacles of the anemones without being swallowed. In contrast, individuals of *Marinogammarus* sp. used as controls were covered by tentacles and swallowed as soon as they touched the anemone. The apparent immunity of *M. obtusata* against the toxin of *A. sulcata* was also effective against *Tealia felina*.

Agents: Mysidacea

Clarke (1955) discussed the known associations between mysids of the genus *Heteromysis* and sea anemones. Most if not all of these represent cases of commensalism. Bahamian *H. actiniae*, for instance, feed on ejected wastes of the sea anemone *Bartholomea annulata*.

Agents: Decapoda

Associations between Anthozoa—particularly Actiniaria— and Decapoda seem to be frequent, especially in tropical waters (Davenport, 1962; Holthuis and Eibl-Eibesfeldt, 1964; Patton, 1967a, b; Hartnoll, 1971; Bruce, 1977). Many of these represent cases of commensalism or mutualism (cleaning symbioses). Mediterranean anemone shrimps *Periclimenes amethysteus* and *P. sagittifer*, however, were seen both in the laboratory and in the field to nip off and devour their hosts' tentacle tips, behaviour indicating an intermediate stage between commensalism and parasitism (Svoboda and Svoboda, 1975).

Several decapod crabs are known to be associated with stony corals. *Hapalocarcinus marsupialis* induces gall formation in branching corals of the family Pocilloporidae. The mechanism (Figs. 6-32 to 6-35) has been studied in great detail in species of *Seriatopora*, *Sideropora* and *Pocillopora* by Potts (1915).

Only female *Hapalocarcinus marsupialis* live burrowed in the coral, while males are free-living. The coral grows around the crab, eventually enclosing it, except for several small openings in the top of the gall. Both corallites and polyps on the inside of the gall exhibit structural malformations in response to the presence of the crab (Potts, 1915). Other members of the Hapalocarcinidae form pits and crevices in the various stony corals (Fize and Seréne, 1957). Some of them are highly modified in structure, and are

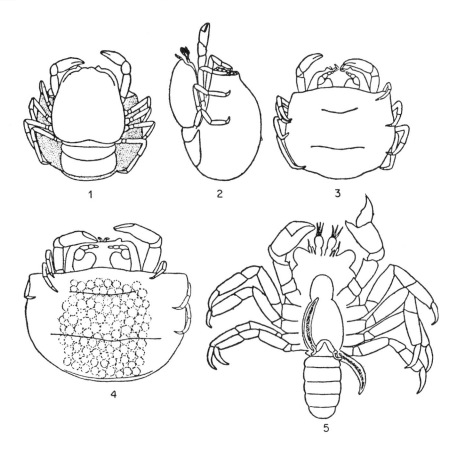

Fig. 6-32: *Hapalocarcinus marsupialis*. Dorsal (1), lateral (2) and ventral (3) aspects of
mature females; × 4. Note bulging abdomen which is wider than carapace. Dotted
circles in (4): eggs seen through semi-transparent abdomen of ovigerous female;
× 4. 5: Ventral view of male with abdomen extended to show copulatory stylets;
× 18. (After Potts, 1915; not copyrighted.)

seemingly unable to survive outside their galls for any length of time. The decapod
xanthid crab *Domecia acanthophora*, living in association with the branching corals
Acropora prolifera, *A palmata* and *A. cervicornis* in the Caribbean Sea, is merely
commensal. Although looking much like any free-living xanthid, *D. acanthophora* move
very little in nature. They inhabit typical 'resting places' on the coral, the mechanical
contact stimulating the build-up of characteristic structural deformities in the coral
(Patton, 1967a, b).

Knudsen (1967) described xanthid crabs of the genera *Trapezia* and *Tetralia* as
obligate ectoparasites of pocilloporid and acroporid corals. Numerous brachyurans and
anomurans collected off Eniwetok (Marshall Islands) and Queensland (Australia) have
been classified as 'obligate commensals' of branching corals (Garth, 1964; Patton, 1966).
Most of these associations require further and closer inspection in order to reveal their
true nature.

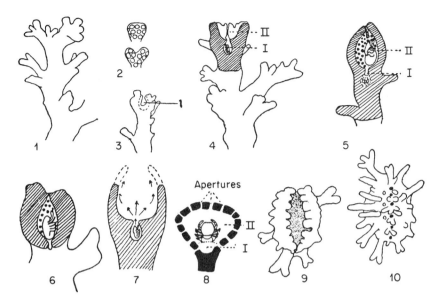

Fig. 6-33: *Pocillopora caespitosa*. Stages of gall-formation caused by *Hapalocarcinus marsupialis*. 1: Normal colony branch; 2: coral tip showing dichotomous branching; 3: first stage of gall-formation (dotted line: extent of Chamber I); 4: typical 'open'gall (Chamber I inhabited by crab, Chamber II being formed); 5: 'closed' gall (Chamber II completed and occupied by crab; Chamber I deserted and partially filled with spongy coenenchyme; black spots: position of coral thecae); 6: older 'closed' gall with increased wall thickness and restriction of interior space; 7: 'open' gall (crab's respiratory current influencing coral growth); 8: 'closed' gall showing relation of inhabitant to remaining apertures; 9: 'open' gall showing converging laminar branches (border consisting of a series of short processes; few twigs having been formed on outer surface); 10: 'closed' gall from above; apertures seen as black spots and numerous twigs arising from outer gall surface. (After Potts, 1915; not copyrighted.)

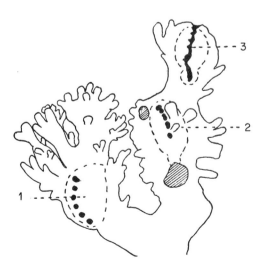

Fig. 6-34: *Pocillopora caespitosa*. Old established galls induced by *Hapalocarcinus marsupialis*. Black spots in '1' and '2' or black line in '3': respiratory apertures or fissure; dotted lines: internal shape of gall cavity. '1' and '2' are old galls, with well-developed coral branches arising from their surface. (After Potts, 1915; not copyrighted.)

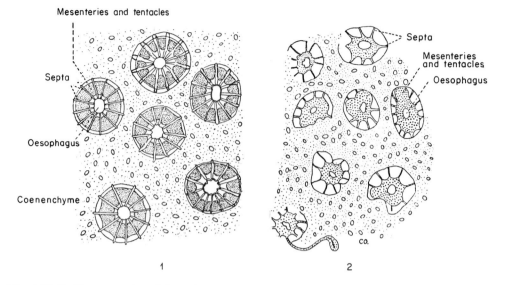

Fig. 6-35: *Pocillopora caespitosa.* Effect of *Hapalocarcinus marsupialis* on colony growth. Outside (1) and inside (2) of gall; ×20; preparation after prolonged decalcification. 1: Polyps regularly developed; tentacles and mesenteries composed of thick, deeply staining tissue; septa normal in number and symmetrically arranged. 2: Polyps stunted and irregular; tentacles and mesenteries not well developed and septa often placed asymmetrically and sometimes reduced in number. (After Potts, 1915; not copyrighted.)

Agents: Pantopoda

Pycnogonids have been reported from a variety of sea anemones. Although sound evidence is lacking in most cases, the sea spiders probably feed on the body fluids of their hosts (Schlottke, 1932; Schmitt, 1934; Fry, 1965; King, 1973, 1974; Wyer and King, 1974).

Pycnogonum rickettsi and *P. stearnsi* from Californian waters were seen feeding on *Anthopleura xanthogrammica* and *Metridium senile.* Some of the pycnogonids found at the bases of *A. xanthogrammica* had the proboscis shallowly inserted into a small hole in the side of the host's column and were apparently feeding upon body juices or bits of the anemone (Ziegler, 1960). In European waters, *Actinia equina, Metridium senile* and *Tealia felina* have been reported as hosts for *P. littorale* (Schmidt and Bückmann, 1971; Wyer and King, 1974).

TUMOURS AND ABNORMALITIES: SCYPHOZOA

During diving operations in the Baltic Sea, numerous *Aurelia aurita* were observed with 3, 5 or 6 gonad 'rings', instead of the normal number of 4 (Lauckner, unpublished). While the loss of one or more 'rings' may be due to parasitism by *Hyperia galba*, additional gonadal structures must be regarded as abnormal. Similar tri-, penta- and hexamerous *A. aurita* (Fig. 6-36) have been described by Zak (1971).

No other abnormalities or tumours of scyphozoans have come to the reviewer's attention.

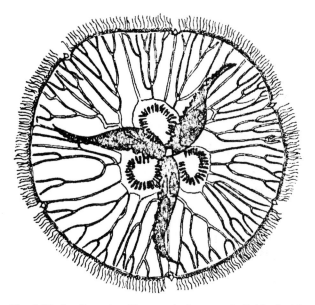

Fig. 6-36: *Aurelia aurita*. Abnormal trimerous individual with 3 gonads and 3 oral lappets. (After Zak, 1971; reproduced by permission of Instytut Zoologiczny Uniwersytetu.)

TUMOURS AND ABNORMALITIES: HYDROZOA

Studies on tumours and other structural abnormalities in Hydrozoa have mostly been confined to freshwater species, particularly *Hydra* spp. (Koch, 1912; Chang and co-authors, 1952). Korschelt (1924) describes strange 'neoplasms' in polyps of the marine hydroid *Syncoryne decipiens*. These abnormalities are assumed to be related to senescence. Polyp hypertrophy, as an expression of aging, has also been observed in the colonial marine hydroid *Hydractinia echinata* (Toth, 1966). Turner (1952) gave a detailed account of the regulation of spontaneous structural abnormalities in *Hydra oligactis*.

Reports on true neoplasms in cnidarians are infrequent in the literature, and their authenticity has often been questioned (Sparks, 1969). Attempts to induce neoplastic growths in cnidarians experimentally did not result in changes comparable to those found in mammals treated with carcinogenic substances (Kaiser, 1965).

TUMOURS AND ABNORMALITIES: ANTHOZOA

Although malformed corals are relatively common, most abnormalities can be directly attributed to the effects of predation, reaction to injury or response to parasites and commensals. These aspects will not be considered further here. Squires (1965a), however, described anomalous growth of the only known specimen of the oculinid, deep-water coral *Madrepora kauaiensis*, dredged off the Island of Kauai, Hawaii (USA) in 1902 by the research vessel '*Albatross*'. Squires suggested the anomalies observed in 3 of the 239 corallites of the sample to be neoplastic, although an earlier investigator interpreted them as individuals of another genus and superfamily of coral which had grown upon the *M. kauaiensis*, probably a species of *Mussa*. Squires disagreed with that interpretation because the skeletal elements of the abnormal corralites were organically connected to the colony and hence, were formed asexually by polyps lower on the branch. Since the coral specimen is unique and is a holotype, dissection of the skeleton was restricted. The 3 individuals of *M. kauaiensis* considered to be pathological, differed from normal corallites in several important features: the largest was about 9 times normal size. Departure from normal symmetry was obvious, septa being inserted in an almost meaningless fashion. Structurally, the corallites showed features indicative of rapid growth of both polyp and skeleton.

The arrangement of skeletal elements led Squires (1965a) to the conclusion that the normal division and insertion of mesenteries was followed until a stage of growth beyond that of a normal polyp was reached, and that then mesentery formation and hence, septal insertion became disordered and chaotic. The author assumes that disorders of the observed magnitude could neither be ascribed to unusual environmental factors nor to incomplete or abnormal repair after injury, and he concluded 'that the 3 anomalous growths of *M. kauaiensis* resulted from processes similar to those of neoplastic change in higher animals' (Squires, 1965a, p. 505). He admits, however, that complications arose with respect to his diagnosis, because the evidence for neoplasia was indirect, owing to the absence of soft tissues, precluding cytological and histological studies.

In a critique of the article by Squires (1965a), White (1965) draws attention to the fact that the abnormalities in question bear extraordinary resemblances, both in apparent structure and in distribution, to galls resulting from continued presence of sedentary predators. Abnormal growth of such galls is stimulated through the activity of 'growth hormones' secreted by the resident symbiote. Soule (1965) offered another explanation, assuming that the 3 abnormal corallites of *Madrepora kauaiensis* were actually colonies of a cyclostomate ectoproct belonging to the genus *Lichenopora*. He pointed out that many members of this genus had been referred to *Madrepora*, which would be a good indication of the superficial resemblance of the mineralized parts of these two animals. In a rebuttal, Squires (1965b) could not entirely rule out the explanations given by White and Soule. The question of whether neoplasia occurs in Anthozoa remains, hence, unanswered.

Literature Cited (Chapter 6)

Agassiz, L. (1859). On some new actinoid polyps of the United States. *Proc. Boston Soc. nat. Hist.*, **7**, 23–24.

Agrawal, V. P. (1963). The digestive system of some British amphipods. Part II (Description of mouth parts). *Proc. natn. Inst. Sci. India*, **33 B**, 631–644.

Agrawal, V. P. (1967). The feeding habit and the digestive system of *Hyperia galba*. *Symp. mar. biol. Ass. India (Ser. 2)*, **1967**, 545–548.

Ankel, W. E. (1936). Prosobranchia. *Tierwelt Nord. Ostsee*, **9b**, 1–240.

Ankel, W. E. (1938). Beobachtungen an Prosobranchiern der schwedischen Westküste. *Arkiv Zool.*, **30A**, 1–27.

Ankel, W. E. (1952a). *Phyllirrhoë, Mnestra* und die Probleme der Gemeinschaften des ozeanischen Pleustals. *Zool. Anz.*, **15** (Suppl.), 396–404.

Ankel, W. E. (1952b). *Phyllirrhoë bucephala* Per. & Les. und die Meduse *Mnestra parasites* Krohn. *Pubbl. Staz. zool. Napoli*, **23**, 91–140.

Ansell, A. D. (1969). Association of the amphipod *Acidostoma neglectum* Dahl with the sea anemone *Peachia hastata* Gosse. *J. nat. Hist.*, **3**, 345–347.

Ansell, A. D. and Trueman, E. R. (1968). The mechanism of burrowing in the anemone, *Peachia hastata* Gosse. *J. exp. mar. Biol. Ecol.*, **2**, 124–134.

Baba, K. (1933). A pelagic nudibranch, *Cephalopyge orientalis*, nov.sp. from Japan. *Annotnes zool. jap.*, **14**, 157–160.

Băcescu, M. (1973). A new case of commensalism in the Red Sea: the mysid *Idiomysis tsurnamali* n.sp. with the Coelenterata *Megalactis* and *Cassiopea*. *Rev. roum. Biol. (Zool.)*, **18**, 3–7.

Badham, C. (1917). On a larval actinian parasitic in a *Rhizostoma*. *Q. Jl microsc. Sci.*, **62**, 221–230.

Ball, G. H. and Moebius, R. E. (1955). A foettingeriid (Apostomea) from the sea anemone *Anthopleura xanthogrammica*. *J. Protozool.*, **2** (Suppl.), 2.

Barham, E. G. and Pickwell, G. V. (1969). The giant isopod, *Anuropus*: a scyphozoan symbiont. *Deep Sea Res.*, **16**, 525–529.

Beers, C. D. (1963). Lack of evidence for encystment in the parasitic amoeba *Hydramoeba hydroxena* (Entz). *J. Protozool.*, **10**, 495–501.

Bertram, G. C. L. (1936). Some aspects of the breakdown of coral at Ghardaqa, Red Sea. *Proc. zool. Soc. Lond.*, **106**, 1011–1026.

Blackburn, M. (1948). Notes on some parasitic actinian larvae, and one of their host medusae, in Australian waters. *J. Coun. scient. ind. Res. Aust.*, **21**, 183–189.

Bocquet, C. and Stock, J. H. (1959). IV. Copépodes parasites d'invertébrés des côtes de la Manche. VI. Rédescription de *Paranthessius anemoniae* Claus (Copepoda Cyclopoida), parasite d'*Anemonia sulcata* (Pennant). *Archs Zool. exp. gén.*, **98**, 43–53.

Bosch, H. F. (1965). A gastropod parasite of solitary corals in Hawaii. *Pacif. Sci.*, **19**, 267–268.

Bouligand, Y. (1960a). Sur l'organisation des lamippides, copépodes parasites des octocoralliaires. *Vie Milieu*, **11**, 335–380.

Bouligand, Y. (1960b). Notes sur la famille des Lamippidae, première partie. *Crustaceana*, **1**, 258–278.

Bouligand, Y. (1961). Notes sur la famille des Lamippidae, 2. *Crustaceana*, **2**, 40–52.

Bouligand, Y. (1965). Notes sur la famille des Lamippidae, troisième partie. *Crustacean*, **8**, 1–24.

Bouligand, Y. (1966). Recherches récentes sur les copépodes associés aux anthozoaires. *Symp. zool. Soc. Lond.*, **16**, 267–306.

Bouligand, Y. and Delamare Deboutteville, C. (1959a). Le dimorphisme sexuel de *Linaresia mammillifera* Zulueta 1908, copépode parasite de l'octocoralliaire *Muricea chamaeleon* von Koch. *C.r. hebd. Séanc. Acad. Sci., Paris*, **248**, 286–288.

Bouligand, Y. and Delamare Deboutteville, C. (1959b). *Lamippella faurei* n.g., n.sp., considérations morphologiques sur la famille des lamippides, copépodes parasites des octocoralliaires. *C.r. hebd. Séanc. Acad. Sci., Paris*, **249**, 1807–1809.

Bowman, T. E., Meyers, C. D. and Hicks, S. D. (1963). Notes on associations between hyperiid amphipods and medusae in Chesapeake and Narragansett Bays and the Niantic River. *Chesapeake Sci.*, **4**, 141–146.

Bresciani, J. (1968). Den cuticulare struktur hos parasitiske crustaceer. *Tiedoksianto*, **9**, 32.

Bresciani, J. and Lützen, J. (1962). Parasitic copepods from the west coast of Sweden including some new or little known species. *Vidensk. Meddr dansk naturh. Foren.*, **124**, 367–408.

Briggs, R. P. (1974). Aspects of the biology, and structure of the associated copepod *Paranthessius anemoniae* Claus. Ph.D. Thesis, The Queens University of Belfast.

Briggs, R. P. (1976). Biology of *Paranthessius anemoniae* in association with anemone hosts. *J. mar. biol. Ass. U.K.*, **56**, 917–924.

Briggs, R. P. (1977). Structural observations on the alimentary canal of *Paranthessius anemoniae*, a copepod associate of the snakelocks anemone *Anemonia sulcata*. *J. Zool.*, **182**, 353–368.

Briggs, R. P. and Gotto, R. V. (1973). A first record of *Lichomolgus actiniae* Della Valle, 1880 (Copepoda, Cyclopoida) in British waters. *Crustaceana*, **24**, 336–337.

Browne, E. T. (1896). On British hydroids and medusae. *Proc. zool. Soc. Lond.*, **1891**, 459–500.

Bruce, A. J. (1977). The possible identity of *Coralliocaris macrophthalma* (H. Milne Edwards, 1837) (Decapoda Natantia, Pontoniinae). *Crustaceana*, **32**, 203–205.

Brusca, G. J. (1967a). The ecology of pelagic Amphipoda. I. Species accounts, vertical zonation and migration of Amphipoda from the waters off southern California. *Pacif. Sci.*, **21**, 382–392.

Brusca, G. J. (1967b). The ecology of pelagic Amphipoda. II. Observations on the reproductive cycles of several pelagic amphipods from the waters off southern California. *Pacif. Sci.*, **21**, 449–456.

Bryden, R. R. (1952). Ecology of *Pelmatohydra oligactis* in Kirkpatricks Lake, Tennessee. *Ecol. Monogr.*, **22**, 45–68.

Buchholz, H. A. (1953). Die Wirtstiere des Amphipoden *Hyperia galba* in der Kieler Bucht. *Faun. Mitt. Norddeutsch.*, **1**, 5–6.

Burkholder, P. R. and Burkholder, L. W. (1958). Antimicrobial activity of horny corals. *Science, N.Y.*, **127**, 1174–1175.

Cachon, J. (1953). Morphologie et cycle évolutif de *Diplomorpha paradoxa* (Rose et Cachon), péridinien parasite des siphonophores. *Bull. Soc. zool. Fr.*, **78**, 408–414.

Cachon, J. (1964). Contribution à l'étude des péridiniens parasites. Cytologie. Cycles évolutifs. *Annls Sci. nat., Zool.* (Ser. 12), **6**, 1–158.

Cachon, J. and Cachon, M. (1971). *Protoodinium chattoni* Hovasse. Manifestations ultrastructurales des rapports entre le péridinien et la méduse-hôte: fixation, phagocytose. *Arch. Protistenk.*, **113**, 293–305.

Cachon, J., Cachon, M. and Bouquaheux, F. (1965). *Stylodinium gastrophilum* Cachon, péridinien dinococcide parasite de siphonophores. *Bull. Inst. océanogr. Monaco*, **65** (1359), 3–8.

Cachon, J., Cachon, M. and Charnier, M. (1972). Ultrastructure du bodonidé, *Trypanophis grobbeni* Poche, parasite de siphonophores. *Protistologica*, **8**, 223–236.

Cannon, H. G. (1935). On the rock-boring barnacle, *Lithotrya valentiana. Scient. Rep. Gt Barrier Reef Exped.*, **5**, 1–17.

Carlgren, O. (1924). Papers from Dr. Mortensen's Pacific Expedition 1914–1916. XXI. Actiniaria from New Zealand and its subantarctic islands. *Vidensk. Meddr dansk naturh. Foren.*, **77**, 179–261.

Carriker, M. R., Smith, E. H. and Wilce, R. T. (Eds) (1969). Penetration of calcium carbonate substrates by lower plants and invertebrates. *Am. Zool.*, **9**, 629–1020.

Carton, Y. (1963). Étude de la spécificité parasitaire chez *Lichomolgus actiniae* D. V. (copépode cyclopoide). *C.r. hebd. Séanc. Acad. Sci., Paris*, **256**, 1148–1150.

Caullery, M. and Mesnil, F. (1902). Sur *Staurosoma parasiticum* Will, copépode gallicole parasite d'une actinie. *C.r. hebd. Séanc. Acad. Sci., Paris*, **134**, 1314–1317.

Chang, J. T., Hsieh, H. H. and Liu, D. D. (1952). Observations on *Hydra*, with special reference to abnormal forms and bud formation. *Physiol. Zoöl.*, **25**, 1–10.

Chatton, É. (1906). Les blastodinides, ordre nouveau de dinoflagellés parasites. *C.r. hebd. Séanc. Acad. Sci., Paris*, **143**, 981–983.

Chatton, É. (1920). Les péridiniens parasites. *Archs Zool. exp. gén.*, **59**, 1–475.

Chatton, É. and Lwoff, A. (1924). Sur un infusoire marin astome, *Spirophrya subparasitica* n.g., n.sp., à deux hôtes, copépode et hydraire. *C.r. hebd. Séanc. Acad. Sci., Paris*, **178**, 1642

Chatton, É. and Lwoff, A. (1935). Les ciliés apostomes. Morphologie, cytologie, éthologie, évolution, systématique. I. Aperçu historique et général; étude monographique des genres et des espèces. *Archs Zool. exp. gén.*, **77**, 1–453.

Clapp, W. F. and Kenk, R. (1963). Marine borers. An annotated bibliography. Washington, D.C., Office of Naval Research, Dept. of the Navy.

Clarke, W. D. (1955). A new species of the genus *Heteromysis* (Crustacea, Mysidacea) from the Bahama Islands, commensal with a sea-anemone. *Am. Mus. Novit.*, **1716**, 11–13.

Claus, C. (1875). Über die Struktur der Muskelzellen und über den Körperbau von *Mnestra parasitica* Krohn. *Verh. zool. -bot. Ges. Wien*, **25**, 9–11.

Cloud, P. E. (1959). Geology of Saipan, Mariana Islands. Part 4. Topography and shoal water ecology. *Bull. U.S. geol. Surv.*, 280–284, 361–445.

Cobb, W. R. (1969). Penetration of calcium carbonate substrates by the boring sponge, *Cliona. Am. Zool.*, **9**, 783–790.

Coleman, D. C. (1966). The laboratory population ecology of *Kerona pediculus* (O.F.M.) epizoic on *Hydra* spp. *Ecology*, **47**, 705–711.

Corrington, J. L. (1927). Commensal association of a spider crab and a medusa. *Biol. Bull. mar. biol. Lab., Woods Hole*, **53**, 346–350.

Costa, A. (1863). Sulla *Filliroe bucephala*. *Rend. Accad. Sci. Fis. Mat. Soc. reale, Napoli*, **2**, 110–112.

Cotte, J. (1902). Note sur le mode de perforation des clionides. *C.r. Séanc. Soc. Biol.*, **54**, 626–637.

Dahl, E. (1959a). The hyperiid amphipod, *Hyperia galba*, a true ectoparasite on jellyfish. *Univ. Bergen Årb. 1959, Naturvitensk. rekke*, **9**, 1–8.

Dahl, E. (1959b). The amphipod, *Hyperia galba*, an ectoparasite of the jelly-fish, *Cyanea capillata*. *Nature, Lond.*, **183**, 1749.

Dahl, E. (1961). The association between young whiting, *Gadus merlangus*, and the jelly-fish *Cyanea capillata*. *Sarsia*, **3**, 47–55.

Dahl, E. (1964). The amphipod genus *Acidostoma*. *Zool. Meded. Leiden*, **39**, 48–58.

Danielsen, D. C. (1890). Actinida. *Norske Nordhavs Exped. (1876–1878)*, **19**, 133.

Davenport, D. (1962). Physiological notes on actinians and their associated commensals. *Bull. Inst. océanogr., Monaco*, **1237**, 1–15.

Dawes, B. (1947). *The Trematoda of British Fishes*, Ray Society, London.

Deckart, M. and Löfflath, K. (1954). Ein Parasit auf *Hydra*. *Mikrokosmos*, **43**, 202–203.

Demond, J. (1957). Micronesian reef-associated gastropods. *Pacif. Sci.*, **11**, 275–341.

Dendy, A. (1888). Note on some actinian larvae parasitic upon a medusa from Port Philip. *Proc. R. Soc. Vict.*

Dogiel, V. (1913). Embryologische Studien an Pantopoden. *Z. wiss. Zool.*, **107**, 576–741.

Dollfus, R. P. (1923). Énumération des cestodes du plancton et des invertébrés marins. *Annls Parasit. hum. comp.*, **1**, 276–300 and 363–394.

Dollfus, R. P. (1926). Sur l'état actuel de la classification des Didymozoonidae Monticelli, 1888 (= Didymozoidae Franz Poche, 1907). *Annls Parasit. hum. comp.*, **4**, 148–161.

Dollfus, R. P. (1931). Nouvelle addendum à mon "Énumération des cestodes du plancton et des invertébrés marins". *Annls Parasit. hum. comp.*, **9**, 552–560.

Dollfus, R. P. (1960). Critique de récentes innovations apportées à la classification des Accacoeliidae (Trematoda-Digenea). Observations sur des métacercaires de cette famille. *Annls Parasit. hum. comp.*, **23**, 648–671.

Dollfus, R. P. (1963). Liste des coelentères marins, paléarctiques et indiens, où ont été trouvés des trématodes digénétiques. *Bull. Inst. Pêch. marit. Maroc*, **9/10**, 33–57.

Duboscq, O. and Rose, M. (1926). *Trypanophis major* n.sp., parasite d'*Abylopsis pentagona*. *Bull. Soc. zool. Fr.*, **51**, 372–376.

Duboscq, O. and Rose, M. (1927). Les stades gregariniens et les kystes de *Tryphanophis major* Duboscq et Rose. *Bull. Soc. Hist. nat. Afr. N.*, **18**, 94.

Duboscq, O. and Rose, M. (1933). *Trypanophis grobbeni* Poche et *Trypanophis major* Duboscq et Rose. *Archs Zool. exp. gén.*, **74**, 411–435.

Ebbs, N. K. (1966). The coral-inhabiting polychaetes of the northern Florida reef tract. Part I. Aphroditidae, Polynoidae, Amphinomidae, Eunicidae, and Lysaretidae. *Bull. mar. Sci.*, **16**, 485–555.

Elmhirst, R. (1925). Associations between the amphipod genus *Metopa* and coelenterates. *Scott. Nat.*, **1925**, 149–150.

Entz, G. (1912). Über eine Amöbe auf Süsswasser-Polypen (*Hydra oligactis* Pall.). *Arch. Protistenk.*, **27**, 19–47.

Fize, A. and Seréne, R. (1957). Les hapalocarcinidés du Viet-Nam. *Archs Mus. natn. Hist. nat. Paris* (Ser. 7), **5**, 3–202.

Floyd, J. F. (1916). Note on *Trypanophis grobbeni*, a protozoan parasite of Siphonophora. *Proc. R. Soc. Edinb.* (A), **20**, 62–64.

Franc, A. (1951). Le zooplancton de la région de Dinard-St-Malo. *Bull. Lab. marit. Dinard*, **24**, 25–40.

Fry, W. G. (1965). The feeding mechanism and preferred foods of three species of Pycnogonida. *Bull. Br. Mus. nat. Hist. (Zool.)*, **12**, 195–224.

Fulton, J. F. (1923). *Trichodina pediculus* and a new closely related species. *Proc. Boston Soc. nat. Hist.*, **37**, 1–30.

Ganapati, P. N. and Rao, D. V. S. (1960). Notes on the feeding habits of *Ianthina janthina* Linnaeus. *J. mar. biol. Ass. India*, **1**, 251–252.

Garth, J. S. (1964). The Crustacea Decapoda (Brachyura and Anomura) of Eniwetok, Marshall Islands, with special reference to the obligate commensals of branching corals. *Micronesica*, **1**, 137–144.

Ginsburg, R. N. (1957). Early diagenesis and lithification of shallow-water carbonate sediments in South Florida. *Spec. Publs Soc. econ. Paleont. Miner., Tulsa*, **5**, 80–100.

Gohar, H. A. F. and Soliman, G. (1963a). On three mytilid species boring in living corals. *Publs mar. biol. Stn Ghardaqa*, **12**, 65–98.

Gohar, H. A. F. and Soliman, G. N. (1963b). On the biology of three coralliophilids boring in living corals. *Publs mar. biol. Stn Ghardaqa*, **12**, 99–126.

Gohar, H. A. F. and Soliman, G. (1963c). On two mytilids boring in dead coral. *Publs mar. biol. Stn Ghardaqa*, **12**, 205–218.

Goormaghtigh, E. and Parmentier, M. (1973). Le crustacé amphipode *Hyperia galba*, parasite de la méduse *Rhizostoma octopus*. *Naturalistes belg.*, **54**, 131–135.

Goreau, T. F., Goreau, N. I., Soot-Ryen, T. and Yonge, C. M. (1969). On a new commensal mytilid (Mollusca: Bivalvia) opening into the coelenteron of *Fungia scutaria* (Coelenterata). *J. Zool. Lond.*, **158**, 171–195.

Goreau, T. F. and Hartman, W. D. (1963). Boring sponges as controlling factors in the formation and maintenance of coral reefs. In R. F. Sognnaes (Ed.), *Mechanisms of Hard Tissue Destruction. Am. Ass. adv. Sci.*, **75**, 25–54.

Goreau, T. F. and Hartman, W. D. (1966). Sponge: effect on the form of reef corals. *Science, N.Y.*, **151**, 343–344.

Gosse, P. H. (1855). Description of *Peachia hastata*. *Trans. Linn. Soc.*, **21**.

Gotto, R. V. (1954). A copepod new to the British Isles, and others hitherto unrecorded from Irish coastal waters. *Ir. Nat. J.*, **11**, 133–135.

Gotto, R. V. and Briggs, R. P. (1972). *Paranthessius anemoniae* Claus: An associated copepod new to British and Irish waters. *Ir. Nat. J.*, **17**, 243–244.

Graeffe, E. (1884). Übersicht der Seethierfauna des Golfes von Triest. III. Coelenteraten. *Arb. zool. Inst. Univ. Wien*, **5**.

Günther, R. T. (1903). On the structure and affinities of *Mnestra parasites* Krohn with a revision. *Mitt. zool. Stn Neapel*, **16**, 35–62.

Gutsell, J. S. (1928). The spider crab, *Libinia dubia*, and the jelly-fish, *Stomolophus meleagris*, found associated at Beaufort, North Carolina. *Ecology*, **9**, 358–359.

Haahtela, I. and Lassig, J. (1967). Records of *Cyanea capillata* (Scyphozoa) and *Hyperia galba* (Amphipoda) from the Gulf of Finland and the northern Baltic. *Ann. zool. Fenn.*, **4**, 469–471.

Habe, T. (1943). Observation on *Habea inazawai*, with special reference to its development. (Jap.; Engl. summary.) *Jap. J. Malac.*, **13**, 65–67.

Haddon, A. C. (1887). A note on the arrangement of the mesenteries in the parasitic larva of *Halcampa chrysanthellum*. *Scient. Proc. R. Dubl. Soc.*, **5**, 473–481.

Haddon, A. C. (1888). On larval Actiniae parasitic in Hydromedusae at St. Andrews. *Ann. Mag. nat. Hist.* (Ser. 6), **2**.

Haedrich, R. L. (1967). The stromateoid fishes: Systematics and a classification. *Bull. Mus. comp. Zool. Harv.*, **135**, 31–139.

Haefelfinger, H. R. and Laubier, L. (1965). Découverte en Méditerranée occidentale de *Mesoglicola delagei* Quidor, copépode parasite d'actinies. *Crustaceana*, **9**, 210–212.

Hartman, W. D. (1957). Ecological niche differentiation in the boring sponges (Clionidae). *Evolution*, **11**, 294–297.

Hartnoll, R. G. (1971). The relationship of an amphipod and a spider crab with the snakelocks anemone. *Rep. mar. biol. Stn Port Erin*, **83**, 37–42.

Hayashi, K. I. and Miyake, S. (1968). Three caridean shrimps associated with a medusa from Tanabe Bay, Japan. *Publs Seto mar. biol. Lab.*, **16**, 11-19.

Hedgpeth, J. W. (1941). A key to the Pycnogonida of the Pacific coast of North America. *Trans. San Diego Soc. nat. Hist.*, **9**, 253–264.

Heegaard, P. (1949). Notes on parasitic copepods. *Vidensk. Meddr. dansk. naturh. Foren.*, **111**, 235–245.

Hilton, W. A. (1916). Life history of *Anoplodactylus erectus* Cole. *J. Ent. Zool.*, **8**, 25–34.

Hiro, F. (1935). A study of cirripeds associated with corals occurring in Tanabe Bay. *Rec. oceanogr. Works Japan*, **7**, 1–28.

Hiro, F. (1938). Studies on animals inhabiting reef corals. II. Cirripeds of the genera *Creusia* and *Pyrgoma*. *Palao trop. biol. Stn Stud.*, **3**, 391–416.

Hollowday, E. D. (1946). On the commensal relationship between the amphipod *Hyperia galba* (Mont.) and the scyphomedusa *Rhizostoma pulmo* Agassiz var. *octopus* Oken. *J. Quekett microsc. Club*, **4**, 187–190.

Holmes, S. J. (1905). The Amphipoda of southern New England. *Bull. Bur. Fish., Wash.*, **24**, 459.

Holthuis, L. B. and Eibl-Eibesfeldt, I. (1964). A new species of the genus *Periclimenes* from Bermuda (Crustacea, Decapoda, Palaemonidae). *Senckenberg. biol.*, **45**, 185–192.

Hovasse, R. (1922). Sur un péridinien, parasite intracellulaire des vélelles. *C. r. hebd. Séanc. Acad. Sci., Paris*, **174**, 1745–1747.

Hovasse, R. (1923). *Endodinium chattoni* (nov. gen., nov. sp.), parasite des vélelles. Un type exceptionnel de variation du nombre des chromosomes. *Bull. biol. Fr. Belg.*, **57**, 107–130.

Hovasse, R. (1924). '*Zooxanthella chattonii*' (*Endodinium chattonii*). *Bull. biol. Fr. Belg.*, **58**, 34–38.

Hovasse, R. (1935). Deux péridiniens parasites convergents: *Oodinium poucheti* (Lemm.), *Protoodinium chattoni* gen. nov. sp. nov. *Bull. biol. Fr. Belg.*, **69**, 59–86.

Humes, A. G. (1953). Two new semiparasitic harpacticoid copepods from the coast of New Hampshire. *J. Wash. Acad. Sci.*, **43**, 360–373.

Humes, A. G. (1957). *Lamippe concinna* sp. n., a copepod parasitic in a West African pennatulid coelenterate. *Parasitology*, **47**, 447–451.

Humes, A. G. (1960). New copepods from madreporarian corals. *Kieler Meeresforsch.*, **16**, 229–235.

Humes, A. G. (1962a). Eight new species of *Xarifia* (Copepoda, Cyclopoida), parasites of corals in Madagascar. *Bull. Mus. comp. Zool. Harv.*, **128**, 36–63.

Humes, A. G. (1962b). *Kombia angulata* n.gen., n.sp. (Copepoda, Cyclopoida) parasitic in a coral in Madagascar. *Crustaceana*, **4**, 47–56.

Humes, A. G. (1963). New species of *Lichomolgus* (Copepoda, Cyclopoida) from sea anemones and nudibranchs in Madagascar. *Cah. O.R.S.T.O.M.* (Ser. Océanogr.), **6**, 59–129.

Humes, A. G. (1966). New species of *Macrochiron* (Copepoda, Cyclopoida) associated with hydroids in Madagascar. *Beaufortia*, **14**, 5–28.

Humes, A. G. (1967). *Vahinius petax* n.gen., n.sp., a cyclopoid copepod parasitic in an antipatharian coelenterate in Madagascar. *Crustaceana*, **12**, 235–242.

Humes, A. G. (1969a). Cyclopoid copepods associated with antipatharian coelenterates in Madagascar. *Zool. Meded., Leiden*, **44**, 1–30.

Humes, A. G. (1969b). *Aspidomolgus stoichactinus* n.gen., n.sp. (Copepoda, Cyclopoida) associated with an actiniarian in the West Indies. *Crustaceana*, **16**, 225–242.

Humes, A. G. (1969c). A cyclopoid copepod, *Sewellochiron fidens* n.gen., n.sp., associated with a medusa in Puerto Rico. *Beaufortia*, **16**, 171–183.

Humes, A. G. (1970). *Paramacrochiron japonicum* n.sp., a cyclopoid copepod associated with a medusa in Japan. *Publ. Seto mar. biol. Lab.*, **18**, 223–232.

Humes, A. G. (1973a). Cyclopoid copepods (Lichomolgidae) from octocorals at Eniwetok Atoll. *Beaufortia*, **21**, 135–151.

Humes, A. G. (1973b). Cyclopoid copepods (Lichomolgidae) from fungiid corals in New Caledonia. *Zool. Anz.*, **190**, 312–333.

Humes, A. G. (1973c). Cyclopoid copepods of the genus *Acanthomolgus* (Lichomolgidae) associated with gorgonians in Bermuda. *J. nat. Hist.*, **7**, 85–115.

Humes, A. G. and Frost, B. W. (1963). New lichomolgid copepods (Cyclopoida) associated with alcyonarians and madreporarians in Madagascar. *Cah. O.R.S.T.O.M.* (Ser. Oceanogr.), **6**, 131–212.

Humes, A. G. and Ho, J. -S. (1966). New lichomolgid copepods (Cyclopoida) from zoanthid coelenterates in Madagascar. *Cah. O.R.S.T.O.M.* (Ser. Oceanogr.), **4**, 3–47.

Humes, A. G. and Ho, J. -S. (1967a). Two new species of *Lichomolgus* (Copepoda, Cyclopoida) from an actiniarian in Madagascar. *Cah. O.R.S.T.O.M.* (Ser. Oceanogr.), **5**, 3–21.

Humes, A. G. and Ho, J. -S. (1967b). New cyclopoid copepods associated with the alcyonarian coral *Tubipora musica* (Linnaeus) in Madagascar. *Proc. U.S. natn. Mus.*, **121**, 1–24.

Humes, A. G. and Ho, J. -S. (1967c). New cyclopoid copepods associated with the coral *Psammocora contigua* (Esper) in Madagascar. *Proc. U.S. natn. Mus.*, **122**, 1–32.

Humes, A. G. and Ho, J. -S. (1968a). Cyclopoid copepods of the genus *Lichomolgus* associated with octocorals of the family Nephtheidae in Madagascar. *Proc. U.S. natn. Mus.*, **125**, 1–41.

Humes, A. G. and Ho, J. -S. (1968b). Cyclopoid copepods of the genus *Lichomolgus* associated with octocorals of the family Alcyoniidae in Madagascar. *Proc. biol. Soc. Wash.*, **81**, 635–691.

Humes, A. G. and Ho, J. -S. (1968c). Cyclopoid copepods of the genus *Lichomolgus* associated with octocorals of the families Xeniidae, Nidaliidae, and Telestidae in Madagascar. *Proc. biol. Soc. Wash.*, **81**, 693–749.

Humes, A. G. and Ho, J. -S. (1968d). Lichomolgid copepods (Cyclopoida) associated with corals in Madagascar. *Bull. Mus. comp. Zool. Harv.*, **136**, 353–413.

Humes, A. G. and Ho, J. -S. (1968e). Xarifiid copepods (Cyclopoida) parasitic in corals in Madagascar. *Bull. Mus. comp. Zool. Harv.*, **136**, 415–459.

Humes, A. G. and Lewbel, G. S. (1977). Cyclopoid copepods of the genus *Acanthomolgus* (Lichomolgidae) associated with a gorgonian in California. *Trans. Am. microsc. Soc.*, **96**, 1–12.

Humes, A. G. and Maria, A. de (1969). The cyclopoid copepod genus *Macrochiron* from hydroids in Madagascar. *Beaufortia*, **16**, 137–155.

Humes, A. G. and Stock, J. H. (1973). A revision of the family Lichomolgidae Kossmann, 1877, cyclopoid copepods mainly associated with marine invertebrates. *Smithson. Contr. Zool.*, **127**, 1–368.

Hyman, L. H. (1940). *The Invertebrates*, Vol. 1, Protozoa through Ctenophora, McGraw-Hill, New York.

Jachowski, R. (1963). Observations on the moon-jelly, *Aurelia aurita*, and the spider crab, *Libinia dubia*. *Chesapeake Sci.*, **4**, 195.

Joliet, L. (1882). Observations sur quelques crustacés de la Méditerranée. Sur une troisième espèce du genre *Lamippe*, *Lamippe duthiersii*, parasite du *Paralcyonium elegans* M.-Edw. *Archs Zool. exp. gén.* (Ser. 1), **10**, 101–111.

Kaiser, H. E. (1965). Artspezifische Untersuchungen über die Carcinogenese. 1. Mitteilung: Untersuchungen über die Reaktion nach Injektion, Implantation and Verfütterung von polycyclischen Kohlenwasserstoffen bei Coelenteraten und Echinodermen. *Arch. Geschwulstforsch.*, **25**, 118–121.

Keysselitz, G. (1904). Über *Trypanophis grobbeni (Trypanosoma grobbeni* Poche). *Arch. Prostistenk.*, **3**, 367–375.

King, P. E. (1973). *Pycnogonids*, Hutchinson, London.

King, P. E. (1974). British sea spiders. *Synopses Br. Fauna*, **5**, 1–68.

Kinne, O. (1977). Cultivation of animals. Research cultivation. In O. Kinne (Ed.), *Marine Ecology*, Vol. III, Cultivation, Part 2. Wiley, Chichester. pp. 579–1293.

Knudsen, J. W. (1967). *Trapezia* and *Tetralia* (Decapoda, Brachyura, Xanthidae) as obligate ectoparasites of pocilloporid and acroporid corals. *Pacif. Sci.*, **21**, 51–57.

Koch, W. (1912). Missbildungen bei *Hydra. Zool. Anz.*, **39**, 8–13.

Køie, M. (1975). On the morphology and life-history of *Opechona bacillaris* (Molin, 1859) Looss, 1907 (Trematoda, Lepocreadiidae). *Ophelia,* **13**, 63–86.

Kölliker, A. (1860). Über das ausgebreitete Vorkommen von pflanzlichen Parasiten in den Hartgebilden niederer Thiere. *Z. wiss. Zool.*, **10**, 215–232.

Kohlmeyer, J. (1972). Marine fungi deteriorating chitin of Hydrozoa and keratin-like annelid tubes. *Mar. Biol.*, **12**, 277–284.

Korschelt, E. (1924). *Lebensdauer, Altern und Tod*, G. Fischer, Jena.

Krohn, A. (1853). Über die Natur des kuppelförmigen Anhanges am Leibe von *Phyllirrhoë bucephalum. Arch. Naturgesch.*, **19**, 278–281.

Künne, C. (1948). Medusen als Transportmittel für Aktinienlarven. *Natur Volk*, **78**, 174–176.

Künne, C. (1952). Untersuchungen über das Großplankton in der Deutschen Bucht und im Nordsylter Wattenmeer. *Helgoländer wiss. Meeresunters.*, **4**, 1–54.

Kuskop, M. (1921). Uber die Symbiose von Siphonophoren und Zooxanthellen. *Zool. Anz.*, **52**, 257–266.

Lambert, F. J. (1936). Observations on the scyphomedusae of the Thames estuary and their metamorphoses. *Trav. Stn zool. Wimereux*, **12** (Mém. 3), 281–307.

Laubier, L. (1960). Une nouvelle sous-espèce de syllidien: *Haplosyllis depressa* Augener ssp. nov. *chamaeleon*, ectoparasite sur l'octocoralliaire *Muricea chamaeleon* von Koch. *Vie Milieu*, **11**, 75–87.

Laubier, L. (1972). *Lamippe (Lamippe) bouligandi* sp. nov., copépode parasite d'octocoralliaire de la mer du Labrador. *Crustaceana*, **22**, 285–293.

Laursen, D. (1953). The genus *Ianthina*; a monograph. *Dana Rep.*, **6**, 1–40.

Laval, P. (1965). Présence d'une période larvaire au début du développement de certains hypériides parasites (Crustacés Amphipodes). *C.r. hebd. Séanc. Acad. Sci., Paris*, **260**, 6195–6198.

Laval, P. (1966). *Bougisia ornata*, genre et espèce nouveaux de la famille des Hyperiidae (Amphipoda, Hyperiidea). *Crustaceana*, **10**, 210–218.

Laval, P. (1968). Développement en élevage et systématique d'*Hyperia schizogeneios* Stebb. (Amphipode hypériide). *Archs Zool. exp. gén.*, **109**, 25–67.

Laval, P. (1972). Comportement, parasitisme et écologie d'*Hyperia schizogeneios* Stebb. (Amphipode hypériide) dans le plancton de Villefranche-sur-Mer. *Annls Inst. océanogr., Monaco*, **48**, 49–74.

Lebour, M. V. (1916). Medusae as hosts for larval trematodes. *J. mar. biol. Ass. U.K.*, **11**, 57–59.

Lebour, M. V. (1945). Notes on the Pycnogonida of Plymouth. *J. mar. biol. Ass. U.K.*, **26**, 139–165.

Leigh-Sharpe, W. H. (1934). The Copepoda of the Siboga Expedition. Part II. Commensal and parasitic Copepoda. *Siboga Exped.*, **24b**, 1–43.

Letellier, A. (1894). Une action purement mécanique suffit aux cliones pour creuser leurs galeries dans les valves des huîtres. *C.r. hebd. Séanc. Adac. Sci., Paris.* **118**, 986–989.

Li, Y.-Y. F., Baker, F. D. and Andrew, W. (1963). A method for tissue culture of *Hydra* cells. *Proc. Soc. exp. Biol. Med.*, **113**, 259–262.

Linton, E. (1900). Fish parasites collected at Woods Hole in 1898. *Bull. U.S. Fish. Commn*, **19**, 267–304.

McIntosh, W. C. (1887). Notes from the St. Andrews Marine Laboratory. 3. On the commensalistic habits of the larval forms of *Peachia*. *Ann. Mag. nat. Hist.* (Ser. 5), **20**, 97–104.

McMurrich, J. P. (1913). On two new actinians from the coast of British Columbia. *Proc. zool. Soc. Lond.*, **1913**, 963–972.

Mansueti, R. (1963). Symbiotic behavior between small fishes and jellyfishes, with new data on that between the stromateid, *Peprilus alepidotus*, and the scyphomedusa, *Chrysaora quinquecirrha*. *Copeia*, **1963**, 40–80.

Marsden, J. R. (1962). A coral-eating polychaete. *Nature, Lond.*, **193**, 598.

Marsden, J. R. (1963a). A preliminary report on digestive enzymes of *Hermodice carunculata*. *Can. J. Zool.*, **41**, 159–164.

Marsden, J. R. (1963b). The digestive tract of *Hermodice carunculata* (Pallas), Polychaeta: Amphinomidae. *Can. J. Zool.*, **41**, 165–184.

Martin, R. and Brinckmann, A. (1963). Zum Brutparasitismus von *Phyllirrhoë bucephala* Per. and Les. (Gastropoda, Nudibranchia) auf der Meduse *Zanclea costata* Gegenb. (Hydrozoa, Anthomedusae). *Pubbl. Staz. zool. Napoli*, **33**, 206–223.

Martin, W. E. (1938). Studies on trematodes of Woods Hole: The life cycle of *Lepocreadium setiferoides* (Miller and Northup), Allocreadiidae, and the description of *Cercaria cumingiae* n.sp. *Biol. Bull. mar. biol. Lab., Woods Hole*, **75**, 463–473.

Menzies, R. J. and Dow, T. (1958). The largest known bathypelagic isopod, *Anuropus bathypelagicus* n.sp. *Ann. Mag. nat. Hist.* (Ser. 13), **1**, 1–6.

Metz, P. (1967). On the relations between *Hyperia galba* Montagu (Amphipoda, Hyperiidae) and its host *Aurelia aurita* in the Isefjord area (Sjaelland, Denmark). *Vidensk. Meddr dansk naturh. Foren.*, **130**, 85–108.

Miller, H. M. and Northup, F. E. (1926). The seasonal infestation of *Nassa obsoleta* (Say) with larval trematodes. *Biol. Bull. mar. biol. Lab., Woods Hole*, **50**, 490–508.

Moestafa, S. H. and McConnaughey, B. H. (1966). *Catostylus ouwensi* (Rhizostomeae, Catostylidae), a new jellyfish from Irian (New Guinea) and *Ouwensia catostyli* n.gen., n.sp., parasitic in *C. ouwensi*. *Treubia*, **27**, 1–9.

Morgan, W. de (1925). *Foettingeria actiniarum* (parasitic in anemones). *Q. Jl microsc. Sci.*, **68**, 343–360.

Müller, F. (1860). On *Philomedusa vogtii*, a parasite on medusae. *Ann. Mag. nat. Hist.* (Ser. 3), **6**, 432–436.

Müller, H. and Gegenbaur, C. (1853–54). Über *Phyllirrhoë bucephalum. Z.wiss. Zool.*, **5**, 355–371.

Nassonov, N. (1883). Zur Biologie und Anatomie der *Clione. Z. wiss. Zool.*, **39**, 295–308.

Neumann, A. C. (1966). Observations on coastal erosion in Bermuda and measurements of the boring rate of the sponge, *Cliona lampa. Limnol. Oceanogr.*, **11**, 92–108.

Nyholm, K. -G. (1949). On the development and dispersal of *Athenaria actinia* with special reference to *Halcampa duodecimcirrata* M. Sars. *Zool. Bidr. Upps.*, **27**, 465–505.

Nyholm, K. -G. (1963). A sporozoan parasite of *Boreohydra simplex. Zool. Bidr. Upps.*, **35**, 289–292.

Okada, Y. K. (1927). *Staurosoma caulleryi*, copépode parasite d'une actinie. Description de *Staurosoma caulleryi* sp.n. *Annotnes zool. jap.*, **11**, 173–182.

Okada, Y. K. (1932). Développement post-embryonnaire de la physalie pacifique. Appendice: le parasite de la physalie. *Mem. Coll. Sci. Kyoto Univ.* (Ser. B), **8**, 1–26.

Okuda, S. (1940). Metamorphosis of a pycnogonid parasitic in a hydromedusa. *J. Fac. Sci. Hokkaido Univ.* (Ser. 6), **7**, 73–86.

Orton, J. H. (1922). The mode of feeding of the jelly-fish, *Aurelia aurita*, on the smaller organisms in the plankton. *Nature, Lond.*, **110**, 178–179.

Otter, G. W. (1937). Rock-destroying organisms in relation to coral reefs. *Scient. Rep. Gt Barrier Reef Exped.*, **1**, 323–352.

Palombi, A. (1939). *Boopsis mediterranea* Pierantoni= *Cephalopyge trematoides* (Chun). Contributo allo studio della morfologia, sistematica e biologia del genere *Cephalopyge* (Gastropoda: fam. Phyllirrhoidae). *Boll. Zool. Torino*, **10**, 65–73.

Panikkar, N. K. (1938). Studies on *Peachia* from Madras. *Proc. Indian Acad. Sci.* (Section B), **7**, 182–205.

Patton, W. K. (1966). Decapod Crustacea commensal with Queensland branching corals. *Crustaceana*, **10**, 271–295.

Patton, W. K. (1967a). Commensal Crustacea. *Proc. Symp. Crust.*, **3**, 1228–1244.

Patton, W. K. (1967b). Studies on *Domecia acanthophora*, a commensal crab from Puerto Rico, with particular reference to modifications of the coral host and feeding habits. *Biol. Bull. mar. biol. Lab., Woods Hole*, **132**, 56–67.

Phillips, J. H. (1963). Immune mechanism in the phylum Coelenterata. In E. C. Dougherty (Ed.), *The Lower Metazoa, Comparative Biolgy and Physiology*. Univ. Calif. Press, Berkeley. pp. 425–431.

Phillips, J. H. and Yardley, B. J. (1960). Detection in invertebrates of inducible, reactive materials resembling antibody. *Nature, Lond.*, **188**, 728–730.

Phillips, P. J. (1973). The occurrence of the remarkable scyphozoan, *Deepstaria enigmatica*, in the Gulf of Mexico and some observations on cnidarian symbionts. *Gulf Res. Rep.*, **4**, 166–168.

Phillips, P. J. and Levin, N. L. (1973). Cestode larvae from scyphomedusae of the Gulf of Mexico. *Bull. mar. Sci.*, **23**, 574–584.

Phillips, P. J., Burke, W. D. and Keener, E. J. (1969). Observations on the trophic significance of jellyfishes in Mississippi Sound with quantitative data on the associative behaviour of small fishes with medusae. *Trans. Am. Fish. Soc.*, **98**, 703–712.

Pierantoni, U. (1923). Sopra un nuovo Phyllirrhoidae del Golfo di Napoli *(Boopsis mediterranea* n.g., n.sp.). *Pubbl. Staz. zool. Napoli*, **5**, 83–96.

Pirlot, J. -M. (1932). Sur quelques amphipodes associés aux colonies de tubulaires dans la région de Bergen. *Bull. Soc. r. Sci. Liège*, **1932**, 21–27.

Poche, F. (1903). Über zwei neue in Siphonophoren vorkommende Flagellen nebst Bemerkungen über die Nomenclatur einiger verwandter Formen. *Arb. zool. Inst. Univ. Wien*, **14**, 307–358.

Poche, F. (1911). Über die wahre Natur der von Will und Busch in Siphonophoren beobachteten "Eingeweidewürmer". *Zool. Anz.*, **38**, 369–373.

Potts, F. A. (1915). *Hapalocarcinus*, the gall-forming crab with some notes on the related genus *Cryptochirus. Pap. Dep. mar. Biol. Carnegie Instn Wash.*, **8**, 33–69.

Purchon, R. D. (1954). A note on the biology of the lamellibranch *Rocellaria (Gastrochaena) cuneiformis* Spengler. *Proc. zool. Soc. Lond.*, **124**, 859–911.

Quidor, A. (1922). Sur *Mesoglicola delagei* Quidor et son hôte. *Annls Sci. nat. Zool.* (Ser. 10), **5**, 77–81.

Rao, K. H. (1958). Hemiurid larvae (Trematoda) in the medusa *Aequorea pensilis* (Haeckel) from the Bay of Bengal. *Ann. Mag. nat. Hist.*, **1**, 702–704.

Rasmussen, E. (1973). Systematics and ecology of the Isefjord marine fauna (Denmark). *Ophelia*, **11**, 1–495.

Rebecq, J. (1965). Considérations sur la place des trématodes dans le zooplancton marin. *Annls Fac. Sci. Marseille*, **38**, 61–84.

Reddiah, K. (1968). Three new species of *Paramacrochiron* (Lichomolgidae) associated with medusae. *Crustaceana*, **1** (Suppl.), 193–209.

Reddiah, K. (1969). *Pseudomacrochiron stocki* n.g., n.sp., a cyclopoid copepod associated with a medusa. *Crustaceana*, **16**, 43–50.

Rees, W. J. (1966). *Cyanea lamarcki* Péron and Lesueur (Scyphozoa) and its association with young *Gadus merlangus* L. (Pisces). *Ann. Mag. nat. Hist.* (Ser. 13), **9**, 285–287.

Renshaw, R. W. (1965). Distribution and morphology of the medusa, *Calycopsis nematophora*, from the North Pacific Ocean. *J. Fish. Res. Bd Can.*, **22**, 841–847.

Revelle, R. and Fairbridge, R. (1957). Carbonates and carbon dioxide. In J. W. Hedgpeth (Ed.), *Treatise on Marine Ecology and Palaeoecology*, Vol. I, Ecology. *Mem. geol. Soc. Am.*, **67**, 239–296.

Reynolds, B. D. and Looper, J. B. (1928). Infection experiments with *Hydramoeba hydroxena* nov. gen. *J. Parasit.*, **15**, 23–30.

Rice, N. E. (1960). *Hydramoeba hydroxena* (Entz), a parasite on the freshwater medusa, *Craspedacusta sowerbii* Lankester, and its pathogenicity for *Hydra cauliculata* Hyman. *J. Protozool.*, **7**, 151–156.

Ricketts, E. F. and Calvin, J. (1968). *Between Pacific Tides*, Stanford Univ. Press, Stanford, Calif.

Riedl, R. (Ed.) (1963). *Fauna und Flora der Adria*, Parey, Hamburg.

Risbec, J. (1953). Note sur la biologie et l'anatomie de *Janthina globosa* (Gast. prosobranches). *Bull. Soc. zool. Fr.*, **78**, 194–201.

Robertson, R. (1963). Wentletraps (Epitoniidae) feeding on sea anemones and corals. *Proc. malac. Soc. Lond.*, **35**, 51–63.

Robertson, R. (1966). Coelenterate-associated prosobranch gastropods. *Am. malac. Un. a. Reps*, **1966**, 6–8.

Robertson, R. (1967). *Heliacus* (Gastropoda: Architectonicidae) symbiotic with Zoanthiniaria (Coelenterata). *Science, N.Y.*, **156**, 246–248.

Robertson, R. (1970). Review of the predators and parasites of stony corals, with special reference to symbiotic prosobranch gastropods. *Pacif. Sci.*, **24**, 43–54.

Romanes, G. J. (1877). An account of some new species, varieties and monstrous forms of medusae. II. *J. Linn. Soc. Zool.*, **13**, 190–194.

Rose, M. (1933). Sur un infusoire foettingéridé parasite des siphonophores. *C.r. hebd. Séanc. Acad. Sci., Paris*, **197**, 868–869.

Rose, M. (1939a) Sur le passage de la forme flagellée à la forme grégarinienne chez *Trypanophis grobbeni* Poche. *Archs Zool. exp. gén.*, **80**, 39–48.

Rose, M. (1939b). Sur la physiologie de l'appareil parabasal de *Trypanophis grobbeni* Poche. *C.r. hebd. Séanc. Acad. Sci., Paris*, **208**, 939–941.

Rose, M. (1947). Sur le cycle évolutif de *Trypanophis grobbeni* Poche. *Bull. biol. Fr. Belg.*, **81**, 6–32.

Rose, M. and Cachon, J. (1951). *Diplomorpha paradoxa*, n.g., n.sp. protiste de l'ectoderme des siphonophores. *C.r. hebd. Séanc. Acad. Sci., Paris*, **233**, 451–452.

Rose, M. and Cachon, J. (1952a). Le mouvement chez *Diplomorpha paradoxa*, parasite des siphonophores. *C.r. hebd. Séanc. Acad. Sci., Paris*, **234**, 669–671.

Rose, M. and Cachon, J. (1952b). L'émission des bras du *Diplomorpha paradoxa*. *C.r. hebd. Séanc. Acad. Sci., Paris*, **234**, 2306–2308.

Ross, A. and Newman. W. A. (1969). A coral-eating barnacle. *Pacif. Sci.*, **23**, 252–256.

Rützler, K. and Rieger, G. (1973). Sponge burrowing: Fine structure of *Cliona lampa* penetrating calcareous substrata. *Mar. Biol.*, **21**, 144–162.

Russell, F. S. (1953). *The Medusae of the British Isles*, Cambridge University Press.

Russell, F. S. (1967). On a remarkable new scyphomedusan. *J. mar. biol. Ass. U.K.*, **47**, 469–473.

Sars, G. O. (1895). Amphipoda. An account of the Crustacea of Norway. *Cammermeyer, Christiania*, **1**, 1-711.

Scheuring, L. (1915). Beobachtungen über den Parasitismus pelagischer Jungfische. *Biol. Zbl.*, **35**, 181–190.

Schirl, K. (1973). Cyclopoida Siphonostomata (Crustacea) von Banyuls (Frankreich, Pyrénées orientales) mit besonderer Berücksichtigung des Gast-Wirtverhältnisses. *Bijdr. Dierk.*, **43**, 64–92.

Schlichter, D. (1975). Produktion oder Übernahme von Schutzstoffen als Ursache des Nesselschutzes von Anemonenfischen? *J. exp. mar. Biol. Ecol.*, **20**, 49–61.

Schlottke, E. (1932). Die Pantopoden der deutschen Küsten. *Wiss. Meeresunters. (Helgoland)*, **18**, 1–10.

Schmidt, H. W. and Bückmann, D. (1971). Beobachtungen zur Lebensweise von *Pycnogonum littorale* (Ström) (Pantopoda). *Oecologia (Berl.)*, **7**, 242–248.

Schmitt, W. L. (1934). Notes on certain pycnogonids. *J. Wash. Acad. Sci.*, **24**, 61–70.

Schriever, G. (1975). In situ-Beobachtungen an *Hyperia galba* Montagu (Amphipoda, Hyperiidae) in der westlichen Ostsee. *Kieler Meeresforsch.*, **31**, 107–110.

Schulze, P. (1913). Hypertrophie der Tentakeln von *Hydra oligactis* Pall. infolge massenhaften Befalls mit *Kerona pediculus* O.F.M. *Zool. Anz.*, **42**, 19–20.

Sentz-Braconnot, E. and Carré, C. (1966). Sur la biologie du nudibranche pélagique *Cephalopyge trematoides*. Parasitisme sur le siphonophore *Nahomia bijuga*, nutrition, développement. *Cah. Biol. mar.*, **7**, 31–38.

Seymour Sewell, R. B. (1926). A study of *Lithotrya nicobarica* Reinhardt. *Rec. Indian Mus.*, **28**, 269–330.

Sheader, M. and Evans, F. (1975). Feeding and gut structure of *Parathemisto gaudichaudi* (Guerin) (Amphipoda, Hyperiidae). *J. mar. biol. Ass. U.K.*, **55**, 641–656.

Shojima, Y. (1963). Scyllarid phyllosomas' habit of accompanying the jellyfish. *Bull. Jap. Soc. scient. Fish.*, **29**, 349–353.

Sims, H. W. and Brown, C. L. (1968). A giant scyllarid phyllosoma larva taken north of Bermuda (Palinuridea). *Crustaceana*, **1968** (Suppl. 2), 80–82.

Soule, J. D. (1965). Abnormal corallites. *Science, N.Y.*, **150**, 78.

Sournia, A., Cachon, J. and Cachon, M. (1975). Catalogue des espèces et taxons infraspécifiques de dinoflagellés marins actuels publiés depuis la révision de J. Schiller. II. Dinoflagellés parasites ou symbiotiques. *Arch. Protistenk.*, **117**, 1–19.

Southwell, T. (1921). On a larval cestode from the umbrella of a jelly-fish. *Mem. Indian Mus.*, **5**, 561–562.

Soyer, J. (1963). Copépodes harpacticoides de Banyuls-sur-Mer. 2. *Paramphiascopsis pallidus* (Sars), espèce nouvelle pour la Méditerranée. *Vie Milieu*, **14**, 571–578.

Spangenberg, D. B. and Claybrook, D. L. (1961). Infection of *Hydra* by Microsporidia. *J. Protozool.*, **8**, 151–152.

Sparks, A. K. (1969). Review of tumors and tumor-like conditions in Protozoa, Coelenterata, Platyhelminthes, Annelida, Sipunculida, and Arthropoda, excluding insects. *Natn. Cancer Inst. Monogr.*, **31**, 671–682.

Spaulding, J. G. (1972). The life cycle of *Peachia quinquecapitata*, an anemone parasitic on medusae during its larval development. *Biol. Bull. mar. biol. Lab., Woods Hole*, **143**, 440–453.

Squires, D. F. (1965a). Neoplasia in a coral? *Science, N.Y.*, **148**, 503–505.

Squires, D. F. (1965b). Abnormal corallites. *Science, N.Y.*, **150**, 78.

Stasek, C. R. (1958). A new species of *Allogausia* (Amphipoda, Lysianassidae) found living within the gastrovascular cavity of the sea-anemone *Anthopleura elegantissima. J. Wash. Acad. Sci.*, **48**, 119–127.

Steinberg, J. E. (1956). The pelagic nudibranch *Cephalopyge trematoides* (Chun, 1889) in New South Wales, with a note on other species in this genus. *Proc. Linn. Soc. N.S.W.*, **81**, 184–192.

Stephensen, K. (1923). Crustacea Malacostraca V. Amphipoda I. *Dan. Ingolf Exped.*, **3**, 1–102.

Stiven, A. E. (1964a). Experimental studies on the epidemiology of the host-parasite system, *Hydra*, and *Hydramoeba hydroxena* (Entz). I. The effect of the parasite on the individual host. *Physiol. Zool.*, **35**, 166–178.

Stiven, A. E. (1964a). Experimental studies on the epidemiology of the host-parasite system, *Hydra*, and *Hydramoeba hydroxena* (Entz). II. The components of a simple epidemic. *Ecol. Monogr.*, **34**, 119–142.

Stiven, A. E. (1964b). The effect of the pathogenic rhizopod *Hydramoeba hydroxena* (Entz) on reproduction in *Chlorohydra viridissima* under various levels of temperature. *Biol. Bull. mar. biol. Lab., Woods Hole,* **126**, 319–331.

Stiven, A. E. (1965). The association of symbiotic algae with the resistance of *Chlorohydra viridissima* (Pallas) to *Hydramoeba hydroxena* (Entz). *J. Invertebr. Pathol.,* **7**, 356–367.

Stock, J. H. (1959). Copepoda associated with Neapolitan invertebrates. *Pubbl. Staz. zool. Napoli,* **31**, 59–75.

Stock, J. H. (1960). Sur quelques copépodes associés aux invertébrés des côtes du Roussillon. *Crustaceana,* **1**, 218–257.

Stock, J. H. (1966a). Cyclopoida Siphonostoma from Mauritius (Crustacea, Copepoda). *Beaufortia,* **13**, 145–194.

Stock, J. H. (1966b). Copepoda associated with invertebrates from the Gulf of Aqaba. *Proc. K. ned. Akad. Wet.,* **69**, 204–216.

Stock, J. H. (1975). On twelve species of the genus *Acanthomolgus* (Copepoda Cyclopoida: Lichomolgidae) associated with West Indian octocorals. *Bijdr. Dierk.,* **45**, 237–269.

Stock, J. H. and Humes, A. G. (1969). *Cholomyzon palpiferum* n. gen., n.sp., a siphonostome cyclopoid copepod parasitic in the coral *Dendrophyllia* from Madagascar. *Crustaceana,* **16**, 57–64.

Stock, J. H. and Humes, A. G. (1970). On four new notodelphyid copepods, associated with an octocoral, *Parerythropodium fulvum* (Forskål), in Madagascar. *Zool. Anz.,* **184**, 194–212.

Stock, J. H. and Kleeton, G. (1963). Copépodes associés aux invertébrés des côtes du Roussillon. 3. *Acontiophorus bracatus* n.sp., un cyclopoide siphonostome associé aux octocoralliaires. *Vie Milieu,* **14**, 551–559.

Studer, T. (1878). Über Siphonophoren des Tiefenwassers. *Z. Zool.,* **31**, 1–24.

Stunkard, H. W. (1932). Some larval trematodes from the coast in the region of Roscoff, Finistère. *Parasitology,* **24**, 321–343.

Stunkard, H. W. (1967). The life-cycle and developmental stages of a digenetic trematode whose unencysted metacercarial stages occur in medusae. *Biol. Bull. mar. biol. Lab., Woods Hole,* **133**, 488.

Stunkard, H. W. (1968). Studies on the life-history of *Distomum pyriforme* Linton, 1900. *Biol. Bull. mar. biol. Lab., Woods Hole,* **135**, 439.

Stunkard, H. W. (1969). The morphology and life-history of *Neopechona pyriforme* (Linton, 1900) n.gen., n.comb. (Trematoda: Lepocreadiidae). *Biol. Bull. mar. biol. Lab., Woods Hole,* **136**, 96–113.

Stunkard, H. W. (1972). Observations on the morphology and life-history of the digenetic trematode, *Lepocreadium setiferoides* (Miller and Northup, 1926) Martin, 1938. *Biol. Bull. mar. biol. Lab., Woods Hole,* **142**, 326–334.

Svoboda, A. and Svoboda, B. (1975). The Mediterranean anemone shrimps of the genus *Periclimenes*, Costa (Decapoda: Palaemonidae). *Pubbl. Staz. zool. Napoli,* **39**, 345–346.

Taton, H. (1934). Contribution à l'étude du copépode *Mesoglicola delagei* Quidor. *Trav. Stn biol. Roscoff,* **12**, 51–65.

Taylor, D. L. (1971). Ultrastructure of the 'Zooxanthella' *Endodinium chattonii* in situ. *J. mar. biol. Ass. U.K.,* **51**, 227–234.

Taylor, J. D. (1968). Coral reef and associated invertebrate communities (mainly molluscan) around Mahé, Seychelles. *Philos. Trans. R. Soc* (Ser. B), **254**, 129–206.

Thapar, G. S. (1964). A new cercaria from ephyrula larvae of *Aurelia* sp. from Indian waters. *Indian J. Helminth.,* **16**, 75–81.

Thiel, H. (1970). Scyphozoa. In *The Encyclopedia of the Biological Science.* Van Nostrand-Reinhold, New York. pp. 830–836.

Thiel, M. E. (1970). Das Zusammenleben von Jung- und Kleinfischen mit Rhizostomeen (Scyphomedusae). *Ber. dt. wiss. Kommn Meeresforsch.,* **21**, 444–473.

Thiel, M. E. (1976). Wirbellose Meerestiere als Parasiten, Kommensalen oder Symbionten in oder an Scyphomedusen. *Helgoländer wiss. Meeresunters.,* **28**, 417–446.

Thomas, L. R. (1963). Phyllosoma larvae associated with medusae. *Nature, Lond.,* **198**, 208.

Thorson, G. (1957). Parasitism in the marine gastropod family Scalidae. *Vidensk. Meddr dansk naturh. Foren.,* **119**, 55–58.

Threlkeld, W. L. and Reynolds, B. D. (1929). The pathogenicity of *Hydramoeba hydroxena* in different hydrogen ion concentrations. *Arch. Protistenk.*, **68**, 409–414.

Toth, S. E. (1966). Polyp hypertrophy as an expression of ageing in the colonial marine hydroid *Hydractinia echinata*. *J. Geront.*, **21**, 221–229.

Turner, C. L. (1952). The regulation of spontaneous structural anomalies in *Pelmatohydra oligactis*. *Biol. Bull. mar. biol. Lab., Woods Hole*, **103**, 104–119.

Uchida, T. (1963). The systematic position of the Hydrozoa. *Jap. J. Zool.*, **14**, 1–14.

Uhlemeyer, B. L. (1922). Some preliminary observations on *Kerona pediculus*. *Wash. Univ. Stud. scient. Ser.*, **9**, 237–271.

Vader, W. (1967). Notes on Norwegian marine amphipods. *Sarsia*, **29**, 283–294.

Vader, W. (1970a). Amphipods associated with the sea anemone, *Bolocera tuediae*, in Western Norway. *Sarsia*, **43**, 87–98.

Vader, W. (1970b). *Antheacheres duebeni* M. Sars, a copepod parasitic in the sea anemone, *Bolocera tuediae* (Johnston). *Sarsia*, **43**, 99–106.

Vader, W. (1970c). On the occurrence of a gall-forming copepod in *Actinostola* spp. (Anthozoa). *Sarsia*, **43**, 107–110.

Vader, W. (1972). Associations between gammarid and caprellid amphipods and medusae. *Sarsia*, **50**, 51–56.

Vallentin, R. (1888). *Psoropsermium lucernariae*. *Zool. Anz.*, **11**, 622–623.

Vannucci Mendes, M. (1944). Sobre a larva de *Dibothriorhynchus dinoi*, n.sp. parasita dos Rhizostomata (Cest. Tetrarhynchidea). *Archs Mus. parana*, **4**, 47–82.

Versluys, J. (1902). Voorkomen van parasiten in de polypen van eenige diepzee gorgoniden (Siboga-Exped.). *Tijdschr. ned. dierk. Ver.* (2), **7**, III-IV.

Vessichelli, N. (1906). Contribuzioni allo studio della *Phyllirrhoë bucephala* Peron & Lésueur. *Mitth. zool. Sta. Neapel*, **18**, 105–135.

Vessichelli, N. (1910). Nuove contribuzioni allo studio della *Phyllirrhoë bucephala* Peron & Lésueur. *Mitth. zool. Sta. Neapel*, **20**, 108–128.

Vicente, N. (1966). Contribution à l'étude des gastéropodes opisthobranches de la région de Tuléar. *Trav. Stn mar. Endoume-Marseille*, **5** (Suppl.), 87–131.

Warburton, F. E. (1958). The manner in which the sponge *Cliona* bores in calcareous objects. *Can. J. Zool.*, **36**, 555–562.

Ward, J. (1965). The digestive tract and its relation to feeding habits in the stenoglossan prosobranch *Coralliophila abbreviata* (Lamarck). *Can. J. Zool.*, **43**, 447–464.

Weill, R. (1935). Revue des protistes commensaux ou parasites des cnidaires. Observations sur des formes peu connues ou nouvelles. *Archs Zool. exp. gén.*, **77**, 47–70.

Werner, B. (1959). The hydromedusae of Port Erin Bay in May and June, 1957. *Rep. mar. biol. Sta. Port Erin*, **71**, 32–38.

Werner, B. (1973). New investigations on systematics and evolution of the class Scyphozoa and the phylum Cnidaria. *Publs Seto mar. biol. Lab.*, **20**, 35–61.

Werner, B. (1976). Die neue Cnidarierklasse Cubozoa. *Verh. dt. zool. Ges.*, **69**, 230.

Westernhagen, H. von (1976). Some aspects of the biology of the hyperiid amphipod *Hyperoche medusarum*. *Helgoländer wiss. Meeresunters.*, **28**, 43–50.

White, M. G. and Bone, D. G. (1972). The interrelationship of *Hyperia galba* (Crustacea, Amphipoda) and *Desmonema gaudichaudi* (Scyphomedusae, Semaeostomae) from the Antarctic. *Br. Antarct. Surv. Bull.*, **27**, 39–49.

White, P. R. (1965). Abnormal corallites. *Science, N.Y.*, **150**, 77–78.

Wilson, D. P. and Wilson, M. A. (1956). A contribution to the biology of *Ianthina janthina* (L.). *J. mar. biol. Ass. U.K.* (Ser. 2), **35**, 291–305.

Wolff, W. J. (1976). Distribution of Pantopoda in the estuarine area in the southwestern part of the Netherlands. *Neth. J. Sea Res.*, **10**, 472–478.

Wright, T. S. (1861). Observations on British zoophytes. On *Halcampa fultoni*, a parasitic Actinia. *Proc. R. phys. Soc. Edinb.*, **2**.

Wyer, D. and King, P. E. (1974). Feeding in British littoral pycnogonids. *Estuar. coast. mar. Sci.*, **2**, 177–184.

Yonge, C. M. (1963). Rock-boring organisms. In R. F. Sognnaes (Ed.), *Mechanisms of Hard Tissue Destruction*. (*Am. Ass. Adv. Sci.*, **75**, 1–24.)

Zak, B. (1971). Anomalies in body structure of jelly-fish *Aurelia aurita* L. in Southern Baltic. (Pol.) *Przeglad Zool.*, **15**, 57–66.

Ziegler, A. C. (1960). Annotated list of Pycnogonida collected near Bolinas, California. *Veliger, 3*, 19–22.

Zulueta, A. de (1908). Note préliminaire sur la famille des Lamippidae, copépodes parasites des alcyonnaires. *Archs Zool. exp. gén. (4)*, **9**, 1–30.

Zulueta, A. de (1910). Deuxième note sur la famille des Lamippidae, copépodes parasites des alcyonnaires. *Archs Zool. exp. gén. (5)*, **6**, 137–148.

Zulueta, A. de (1912). Los copépodos parásitos de los celentéreos. *Mems R. Soc. esp. Hist. nat.*, **7**, 5–58.

7. DISEASES OF CTENOPHORA

G. LAUCKNER

The Ctenophora, particularly the Tentaculata, occupy an important position in the marine food web. The ecology of *Pleurobrachia pileus* has been studied in detail (consult Fraser, 1970, and Greve, 1971, for references). Feeding voraciously on zooplankton, this comb jelly competes for food with many fish species. Fish larvae are also attacked, while adult fishes feed on *P. pileus* and other ctenophores even to gorging. The importance of *P. pileus* as a link in the marine food web is reflected by the fact that it serves as intermediate or paratenic host for a number of larval helminths.

DISEASES CAUSED BY MICRO-ORGANISMS

So far, no microbial diseases have been reported from ctenophores. From acquarium observations, it appears, however, that *Pleurobrachia pileus* may acquire bacterial infections. Under adverse conditions of stress, i.e. crowding in containers and starvation, the epidermis may acquire a greyish tinge, from which unidentified bacteria have been isolated. Specimens with progressing discolouration eventually succumb (Lauckner, unpublished).

DISEASES CAUSED BY PROTOZOANS

Agents: Ciliata

Trophonts of *Pericaryon cesticola*, an apostome foettingeriid ciliate, occur in *Cestus veneris* off Villefranche-sur-Mer (France). The trophonts, which resemble *Foettingeria actiniarum* reported from various actinians, attach to the wall of the ctenophore's gastrovascular cavity with their ventral sides by means of an apical stylet and increase considerably in size during their development. The fate of trophonts expelled from the ctenophore remains unknown but they probably encyst in sea water and develop into tomonts which, in turn, produce numerous tomites. These presumably attach to pelagic copepods and become phoronts. *C. veneris* acquires an infestation by ingesting phoront-bearing copepods (Chatton, 1911; Chatton and Lwoff, 1935; see Chapter 6).

Pericaryon cesticola trophonts were sometimes hyperparasitized by an enigmatic protistan parasite which bears some resemblance to peridineans *Amoebophrya stycholonchae* found in radiolarians *Sticholonche zanclea* (Chatton and Lwoff, 1935; see Chapter 3).

Unidentified apostomes, probably foettingeriids, have also been observed in the digestive tract of *Pleurobrachia pileus* from Helgoland (German North Sea coast). In the ctenophore, the protozoans grew rapidly. Their life cycle remained unknown but probably involves copepods which are preyed upon by *P. pileus* (Greve, 1971).

DISEASES CAUSED BY METAZOANS

Agents: Cnidaria and Ctenophora

As briefly mentioned by Mayer (1912), the mesogloea of *Mnemiopsis leidyi* from the Atlantic coast of North America is often infested by pink, worm-shaped, parasitic, larval actinians, *Edwardsia leidyi*. These cnidarian larvae have also been found among the stomach contents of butterfishes *Peprilus triacanthus* and harvestfishes *P. paru* from the North American Atlantic coast, which indicates that these teleosts feed to a large extent on *M. leidyi* (Dunnington and Mansueti, 1955; Oviatt and Nixon, 1973; Oviatt and Kremer, 1977).

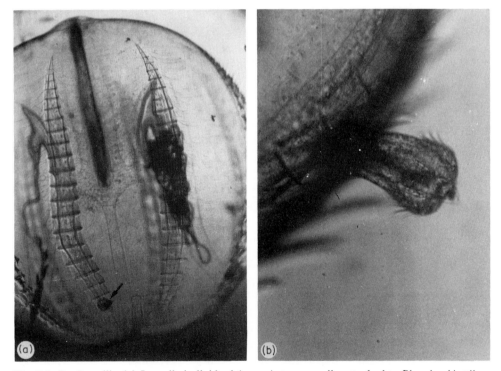

Fig. 7-1: *Beroë gracilis.* (a) Juvenile individual (arrow), temporarily attached to *Pleurobrachia pileus*; (b) same, enlarged side view. (Photographs courtesy Dr. Wulf Greve.)

Juvenile ctenophores *Beroë gracilis* may sometimes be found temporarily attached to the body and tentacles of *Pleurobrachia pileus* (Fig. 7-1), feeding on tissue pieces, eggs and larvae of the 'host'. In this phase, *B. gracilis* may be regarded as a temporary ectoparasite of *P. pileus* (Greve, 1971).

Agents: Trematoda

A considerable number of larval trematodes have been reported from Ctenophora. Lebour (1916) described the metacercaria of the lepocreadiid *Opechona bacillaris* clinging to the inside of the stomach of *Pleurobrachia pileus*. The adult stage is a common parasite of the mackerel *Scomber scombrus* and the lumpsucker *Cyclopterus lumpus*. *O. bacillaris* metacercariae (Fig. 6-16) have also been found in the same ctenophore host from waters off Roscoff, France, and from Øresund, Denmark (Stunkard, 1932; Køie, 1975). The unidentified 'small trematodes' found, sometimes in considerable numbers, in *P. pileus* collected during the Danish Ingolf Expedition (Mortensen, 1912), may possibly belong to the same species.

Lebour (1916) mistook the tailless metacercaria of *Opechona bacillaris* for a cercaria, and reported it to occur also free in the plankton, as did Franc (1951). It appears more likely that the unencysted freely moving metacercariae have been passively pressed out of the body cavities of their jellyfish hosts during the catch. *O. bacillaris* also infests a number of hydromedusae (Lebour, 1916). On the other hand, it has been suspected that, for still unknown reasons, some trematodes of plankton animals leave their hosts and occur free in the water (Rebecq, 1965).

Infestation of Ctenophora by metacercariae appears to undergo marked seasonal and annual fluctuations. Fraser (1970) recorded the following numbers of larval *Opechona retractilis* per 1000 *Pleurobrachia pileus* from Scottish waters:

	March to August	September to February
1966	17	3230
1967	33	450
1968	25	4720

This change from low (summer) to high (winter) infestation intensity was quite sudden, and occurred about the end of August. Although November was the month with the highest mean—more than 4 metacercariae per *Pleurobrachia pileus*——very high individual numbers were also found in September. Particularly high figures were 140 and 120 *Opechona retractilis* (in individuals of 12- and 11-mm height) in September, and 104 in one of 14 mm in November. *O. retractilis* is a parasite of the whiting *Gadus merlangus* (Dawes, 1947), and the abundance fluctuations of this parasite by no means reflect the population dynamics of the final host. Fraser (1970) suggested that the rapid increase in parasitism was due to a sudden cercarial invasion, rather than to a cumulative build-up of numbers with the increasing age of the host. Fraser's data are paralleled by the findings of Franc (1951), who observed *O. bacillaris* metacercariae free in the plankton off Dinar–St Malo on the Atlantic coast of France, only from July until the end of September. Ward and Fillingham (1934) maintain—as have several previous authors—that *O. retractilis* is identical to *O. bacillaris*.

Experimental penetration of *Mnemiopsis leidyi* by cercariae of *Neopechona pyriforme* (Fig. 6-18) was accomplished by Stunkard (1969). The ctenophore proved to be a favourable intermediate host for this trematode which was also found to attack a number of scyphomedusae and hydromedusae (Stunkard, 1967, 1968, 1970; see also Chapter 6).

Derogenes varicus is another larval trematode reported from *Pleurobrachia pileus* from the German Bight (Künne, 1952). It has also been described as a progenetic metacercaria from *Lernaeocera lusci*, a parasitic copepod of the bib *Gadus luscus* (Dollfus, 1954). The reviewer has also observed progenesis in *D. varicus* metacercariae from *P. pileus*. The ctenophore appears, therefore, to act merely as a paratenic host in this case, acquiring its parasite burden by digesting infested copepods. *D. varicus* is a common intestinal parasite of fishes. Dawes (1947) quoted the names of 42 teleostean hosts. The metacercaria of *D. varicus* (Fig. 7-2) was first described as *Distoma beroës* from *Beroë rufescens*. More than 12 metacercariae were recovered from individual hosts (Will, 1844).

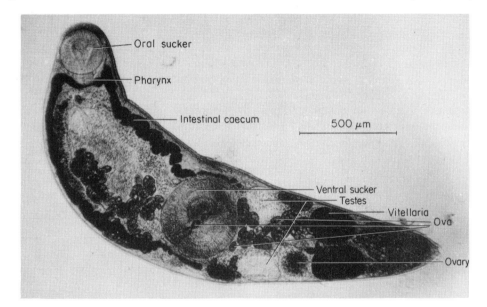

Fig. 7-2: *Derogenes varicus*. Progenetic metacercaria from *Pleurobrachia pileus*. (Original.)

Although *Pleurobrachia pileus* is a cosmopolitan, populations from the northern and southern hemispheres apparently do not share a common trematode fauna. Boyle (1966) described 3 larval digeneans from *P. pileus* in New Zealand waters. The first, a member of the Fellodistomatidae, was identified as *Tergestia agnostomi* (Fig. 7-3). Adult worms occur in the intestinal tract of yellow-eyed mullets *Agnostomus forsteri* (Manter, 1954) which are known to feed on ctenophores. The second trematode (Fig. 7-3) was believed to be the larval stage of the hemiurid *Lecithocladium excisum*, an intestinal parasite of red perch *Caesioperca lepidoptera* and blue cod *Paraperca colias*. The third larval digenean was an unidentified member of the family Allocreadiidae, possibly *Pseudocreadium* sp. All trematodes were constantly associated with the gastrovascular system of *P. pileus*. The majority occurred inside the pharynx or with the oral sucker embedded in pharyngeal tissue. On a few occasions, however, the parasites were observed in the mesogloea beside a horizontal or tentacular canal.

Pleurobrachia globosa from Madras has been reported as a host for another, yet undetermined allocreadiid metacercaria, which occurred at a high infestation rate, 8 out

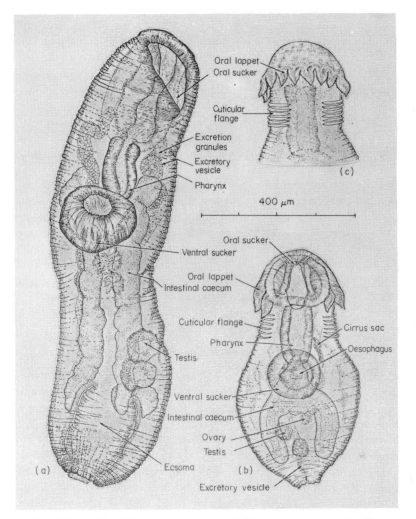

Fig. 7-3: *Lecithocladium excisum* (a) and *Tergestia agnostomi* (b) from
Pleurobrachia pileus. (a,b: Ventral aspects of metacercariae; c: dorsal
view of anterior body region of *T. agnostomi*). (After Boyle, 1966;
reproduced by permission of Royal Society of New Zealand.)

of the 14 ctenophores examined carrying 1 to 3 metacercariae (Anantaraman, 1959).
Unencysted metacercariae of *Cercaria laevicardium* were found in ctenophores *Mnemiopsis
leidyi* from the North American Atlantic coast. Cercariae of this species emerged from
sporocysts in the bivalve *Laevicardium mortoni*; the adult stage is unknown (Martin, 1945;
Stunkard, 1970). However, since a number of teleosts, including *Peprilus triacanthus, P.
paru* and *Mola mola*, are known to feed on ctenophores (Bigelow and Schroeder, 1953;
Dunnington and Mansueti, 1955; Oviatt and Nixon, 1973; Oviatt and Kremer, 1977),
the adult stage of *C. laevicardium* may be found in these hosts or related species.

Dollfus (1960) discussed the presence of larval forms of the trematode family
Accacoeliidae in planktonic cnidarians and ctenophores *Beroë ovata*. Dollfus (1963) and
Rebecq (1965), in their host–parasite reference lists, recorded several further, mostly

undetermined or inadequately described larval trematodes from a great number of Ctenophora. Their publications aptly summarize the widely scattered information concerning the relationship between Coelenterata and larval Trematoda.

Nothing definite is known about the effects of metacercarial invasion on Ctenophora. Larval trematodes reported from *Pleurobrachia pileus* are well equipped with large, strong oral and ventral suckers and a muscular pharynx, and thus, may be capable of direct ingestion of host tissue. Lumps of what appears to be tissue debris can frequently be seen in the intestinal caeca. Pathological effects could, therefore, be direct (feeding on the host's expenses) or indirect (secondary bacterial infections due to destruction of the host's tender epidermis by the action of the suckers). Clusters of bacteria are sometimes seen protruding from the depression of the ventral sucker of *Derogenes varicus*, isolated from its host, and pressed under a cover glass. If secondary wound infections by bacteria would be of any significance, even a few metacercariae could contribute to increased mortality of infested *P. pileus*. Despite such inferred mechanism, it seems very improbable that small and fragile animals, such as ctenophores, would be capable of tolerating a parasite burden of some hundred individuals for long periods of time. Without presenting conclusive evidence, Boyle (1966) assumes that the growth rate of parasitized ctenophores may be less than that of unparasitized individuals.

Agents: Cestoda

Larval tetraphyllidean cestodes have frequently been recovered from the digestive tract of ctenophores in various parts of the world. Most of these have been designated *Scolex polymorphus* or *S. pleuronectis* (Fig. 7-4). Their further fate and the adult stages remain unknown. Larvae of this type, named *S. acalepharum*, occur in *Bolinopsis infundibulum* in Norway. *S. polymorphus* has accidentally been discovered in *Pleurobrachia pileus* from Woods Hole, Massachusetts, USA (van Cleave, 1927). Another larval tetraphyllid, named *Tetrastoma playfairi*, has been reported from *Cydippe densa* in the Mediterranean and from *P. pileus* in the English Channel and adjacent Atlantic waters. Some authors assume *T. playfairi* to be the larval form of *Acanthobothrium crassicolle* (Dollfus, 1936).

Unspecified cestodes have been reported from the digestive tract of *Pleurobrachia pileus* from the German Bight by Künne (1950, 1952), and larval Tetraphyllidea of the type *Scolex pleuronectis* have been found in material from the waters around the Isle of Sylt by the reviewer. *P. pileus* acquires infestations by ingestion of copepods serving as first intermediate hosts for these cestodes. Apstein (1911) described and figured *Scolices pleuronectis* dissected from copepods *Calanus finmarchicus*, and Anantaraman and Krishnaswamy (1958) reported the presence of unidentified tetraphyllidean larvae in the copepod *Eucalanus pseudattenuatus*. Wundsch (1912) established the names *Plerocercoides aequoreus* and *P. armatus* for 2 tetraphyllidean larvae from marine copepods.

Van Cleave (1927), who reported *Scolex polymorphus* from preserved *Pleurobrachia pileus* collected near Woods Hole, offered another explanation regarding the presence of larval cestodes in the ctenophore: Since both crustaceans and small fishes are common food for *P. pileus*, and since both are normal hosts to marine tapeworms, the worms may have been introduced into the ctenophores' digestive tracts along with either fish or copepod and survived after the earlier host had been digested.

The scolices found in *Calanus finmarchicus* by Apstein (1911) and in *Pleurobrachia pileus* by the reviewer are virtually identical in size and shape. Thus, little development takes place in the ctenophore, suggesting that it merely acts as a paratenic host. Further growth and development probably occur in clupeids and other fishes. Anantaraman (1963) described larval tetraphyllids from the gastric cavity of *P. globosa* as well as from decapod crustaceans, bivalves, gastropods and fishes from the Madras coast (India).

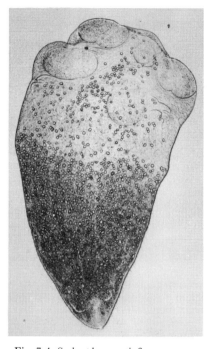

Fig. 7-4: *Scolex pleuronectis* from gastro-vascular system of *Pleurobrachia pileus*. (Original.)

The entire life cycles of these larval cestodes remain unknown, but Reichenbach-Klinke (1956, 1957), who experimentally infected rough hounds *Scyliorhinus canicula* with scolices from clupeids, obtained adult *Acanthobothrium coronatum* and *Calliobothrium* sp., respectively. Tetraphyllids have exclusively elasmobranchs as final hosts. The possible specific identities and adult stages of cestode larvae occurring in ctenophores have been discussed further by Williams (1968). Nothing is known about pathological effects of larval cestodes on ctenophores.

Agents: Nematoda

Larval nematodes, probably members of the genus *Thynnascaris (Contracaecum)*, are known to parasitize ctenophores (Künne, 1952) which probably play the role of paratenic hosts. First intermediate hosts are copepods, and ctenophores become infested by digesting nematode-invaded specimens. Liberated worms penetrate the stomach wall, and enter the mesogloea, where further growth occurs. Larger specimens can frequently be seen with the naked eye in *Pleurobrachia pileus* (Fig. 7-5).

The first record of a nematode in a ctenophore is probably that of Forbes (1839, p. 148). He noted from material taken at St. Andrews (Scotland) that 'Imbedded in the substance of one of these animals, near the stomach, is a remarkable parasitic worm, in shape resembling a *Filaria*'. Mortensen (1912) observed larval nematodes in *Pleurobrachia pileus* believed to be *Agamonema capsularia*, a species reported as adult from *Cyclopterus lumpus* and *Squalus fernandinus*, both of which are known to prey upon *P. pileus*. Probably,

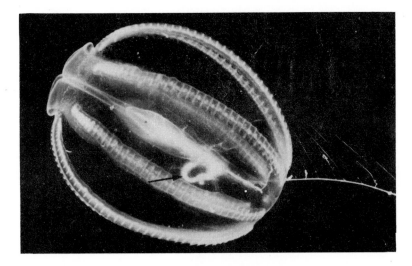

Fig. 7-5: *Pleurobrachia pileus*. Larval nematode (*Thynnascaris* sp.?) extending from stomach into mesogloea of ctenophore. (Photograph courtesy M. Söhl.)

all these authors dealt with third-stage larvae of the same species, *Thynnascaris gadi* (Fig. 7-6), an intestinal parasite mainly of Gadiformes. In most reports on this nematode the erroneous designation *Contracaecum aduncum* has been employed (for discussion of the problem see Hartwich, 1975). Larval nematodes from ctenophores and other marine invertebrates have also been misidentified as *Anisakis* sp. or *Ascaris* sp. Boyle (1966) observed two distinct species of larval nematodes in *P. pileus* from New Zealand waters, one of which was believed to be *Contracaecum aduncum* (=probably *Thynnascaris gadi*).

Nematode infestation of Ctenophora apparently shows wide geographic and annual variation. While, according to Greve (1971), nematodes are the dominating parasites of *P. pileus* at Helgoland, especially during the winter months, they are of rare occurrence in Scottish waters, and were found singly only in September (Fraser, 1970). Peak infestations appear to be higher in inshore waters of the German Bight, although considerable variation occurs (Table 7-1).

As evidenced by the table, larval nematodes by far outnumber the trematodes as parasites of *Pleurobrachia pileus* in German coastal waters. The opposite is true for Scottish waters (Fraser, 1970). Boyle (1966) recorded three times as many trematodes as nematodes in *P. pileus* from New Zealand.

With respect to the pathogenicity, Greve (personal communication) observed no detectable effect of nematode parasitism on *P. pileus*. In aquarium experiments, infested

Table 7-1

Pleurobrachia pileus. Infestation with larval nematodes (number of larvae individual^{-1} and infestation rates), trematodes and cestodes (number of larvae individual^{-1}). Isle of Sylt, North Sea (Original)

Date of collection	*P. pileus* (number of individuals examined)	Nematodes (total number recovered)	*P. pileus* infested with nematodes (%)	Infestation rate with nematodes		Trematodes *Derogenes varicus*	Cestodes *Scolex pleuronectis*
				(mean)	(range)		
March 1972	10	29	100	2·90	1–5	0	0
April 1972	8	30	100	3·75	1–11	0	0
May 1972	37	85	76	2·30	1–11	8	5
May 1973	112	26	17	0·23	1–2	4	0
July 1974	96	4	4	0·04	1	0	0

ctenophores exhibited the same growth rate as uninfested specimens. In contrast, Lauckner (unpublished) found reduced longevity of heavily infested *P. pileus* under conditions of semi-starvation. It should be remembered that certain nematodes are capable of elaborating substances which interfere with the host's physiology, by inducing allergic and other responses. 'Ascaron', a toxin produced by *Ascaris*, for instance, is believed to be responsible for pathological reactions in the central nervous

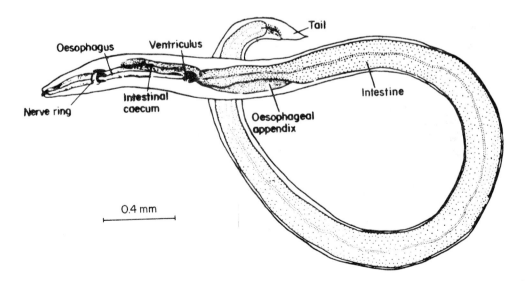

Fig. 7-6: *Thynnascaris (Contracaecum)* sp. Type IV larva from *Pleurobrachia pileus*. (After Boyle, 1966; reproduced by permission of the Royal Society of New Zealand.)

system of vertebrates (Noble and Noble, 1964). Whether larval nematodes parasitizing ctenophores are able to produce such substances is unknown, but appears likely.

Agents: Amphipoda

Hyperoche mediterranea, a hyperiid amphipod, parasitizes *Pleurobrachia bachei* in Californian waters. Larvae and early juveniles live endoparasitically in ctenophores whereas late juveniles and adults are free-living. The appearance of *H. mediterranea* in the plankton was found to be associated with *P. bachei* when the abundance of hosts exceeded about 100 individuals m^{-3} (May/June to November). Larger amphipods were present in highest abundance when most post-larval ctenophores had reached a diameter of 6 to 8 mm. Mostly *H. mediterranea* occurred singly but occasionally up to 8 crustaceans per ctenophore host were recorded. The *P. bachei–H. mediterranea* association has not been studied in depth but there appears to be some detrimental effect on the host. No other parasites have been recorded from *P. bachei* in La Jolla Bight (Hirota, 1974).

Farther to the north, *Hyperoche mediterranea* is replaced by *H. medusarum*. As is the case with *H. mediterranea*, little information is available on the biology of this species. Of 135 *Pleurobrachia bachei* collected from coastal waters off northern California, 20 housed *H. medusarum*. Four of these were inhabited by 2 amphipods; all others contained single individuals. Twenty-one were juveniles, ranging from 0·75 to 1·5 mm in length. Three were adults—1 male, 2·5 mm long, and 2 females, 2·75 and 3·0 mm in length. The smaller of the 2 females was carrying ova in the brood pouch (Brusca, 1970).

All these individuals were embedded in the mesogloea of *Pleurobrachia bachei* but were never very closely associated with organs such as the tentacular sheaths or gut. In all cases, except one, there appeared to be no direct communication between the position of the amphipods and the outside, that is, the crustaceans were completely encased within the host (Fig. 7-7, 1). Apparently the amphipods did not prefer any particular spot or spatial orientation; they were found in various parts of the hosts' bodies. The single adult male had the anterior part of its head, including the antennae, stuck out of the ctenophore's body through an orifice (Fig. 7-7, 2). Brusca (1970), who based his observation on formalin-preserved material, assumes that the amphipods enter the ctenophores as juveniles and that they feed upon the mesogloeal contents.

In contrast to Brusca (1970), who stated that *Hyperoche medusarum* lives endoparasitically in *Pleurobrachia bachei* in Californian waters, Evans and Sheader (1972) recorded *H. medusarum* as an ectoparasite of *P. pileus* in the North Sea. Scyphomedusae *Aurelia aurita* and *Cyanea capillata*, ctenophores *Pleurobrachia pileus* and the two hyperiid amphipods *Hyperoche medusarum* and *Hyperia galba* were all fairly common in inshore plankton samples taken off Blyth (England). Many of the *A. aurita* and *C. capillata* harboured *H. galba* but none contained *H. medusarum*.

Bowman and co-authors (1963), on the other hand, recorded *Hyperoche medusarum* in plankton hauls from Connecticut and Chesapeake Bay (USA) waters which also yielded several individuals of *Cyanea capillata*. They concluded that the amphipods had been associated with these scyphomedusae.

In laboratory experiments, when given a choice between either of these potential jellyfish hosts, *Hyperoche medusarum* invariably attacked *Pleurobrachia pileus* but neither of the scyphomedusae (Evans and Sheader, 1972). The amphipods attached themselves to the external surface of *P. pileus*, usually to one of the comb rows, but did not enter the internal cavities of the host as reported by Brusca (1970) and Hirota (1974) and as known for *Hyperia galba* in *Aurelia aurita* and other scyphomedusae (see Chapter 6). For holding on to its ctenophore host, *H. medusarum* uses Pereiopods 3 and 4, whose terminal segments are posteriorly directed, and pereiopods 5, 6 and 7, whose terminal segments are anteriorly directed, to give a means of firm attachment to the moving comb of the host.

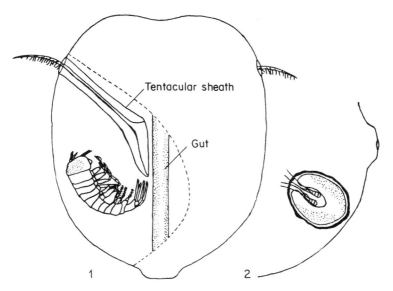

Fig. 7-7: *Hyperoche medusarum*. 1: Position of adult female (2·75 mm in length) in mesogloea of host, *Pleurobrachia bachei*; 2: external view of portion of *P. bachei* near oral region, showing head of male *H. medusarum* protruding from orifice in body wall of host. (After Brusca, 1970; reproduced by permission of Southern California Academy of Sciences.)

The observations conducted by Evans and Sheader (1972) suggest that feeding normally takes place on the oral half of the ctenophore. The host's epidermis is initially pierced by the mouth parts, but the wound produced is usually small. The tissue obtained is conveyed to the mouth parts using the chelate Pereiopods 1 and 2. After feeding, the parasite may leave its host or may remain attached. In the latter case, it fixes itself backwards to a comb-plate using its posterior pereiopods, held over the pleon, and by assuming an inactive curled position with the urus in contact with the anterior pereiopods, so that the head and urus face away from the host.

Bowman and co-authors (1963) who described a similar posture for *Hyperia galba* on scyphomedusae *Cyanea capillata* (Fig. 6-11) obviously observed these amphipods during their inactive, that is, non-feeding phase. They took this behaviour to be indicative of a non-parasitic mode of life.

An examination of the gut of large numbers of *Hyperoche medusarum* revealed completely unidentifiable contents, suggesting that only soft food, presumably *Pleurobrachia pileus* tissue, was taken (Evans and Sheader, 1972). However, according to von Westernhagen (1976), stomachs of *H. medusarum* fed live herring larvae exhibit similarly unidentifiable contents.

Based on field observations and laboratory experiments, Evans and Sheader (1972)—in accordance with Sars (1895)—concluded that *Hyperoche medusarum* is wholly parasitic and that, in the North Sea, *Pleurobrachia pileus* is utilized as host.

These findings contrast with Brusca's (1970) observations. The discrepancies are difficult to explain. Adult *Hyperoche medusarum*, possibly present on the body surface of ctenophores in Brusca's material prior to collection, could have abandoned their hosts during collection (Brusca reports neither on the method of collection nor on the associated fauna in his plankton hauls). On the other hand, Evans and Sheader (1972) do not give the body lengths of the amphipods studied. Possibly they dealt with large adult *H. medusarum*, while the body lengths reported by Brusca for adults endoparasitic in *Pleurobrachia bachei*—male: 2·5 mm, females: 2·75 and 3·0 mm—may be taken as indicative of an adolescent stage or—in the case of the 2·75-mm ovigerous female—of a dwarfed form. In rearing experiments conducted by von Westernhagen (1976), juvenile *H. medusarum* fed exclusively on herring larvae attained sexual maturity after 69 days at a body length of about 6·5 mm.

It appears likely that *Hyperoche medusarum*, in the absence of other prey, can live as a facultative endoparasite in ctenophores during early development and then shift to an ectobiotic (ectoparasitic) or a free-living phase after reaching a certain developmental stage. A similar shift from obligate endoparasitism to facultative ectoparasitism has been reported for the *Hyperia schizogeneios–Phialidium* sp. association (Laval, 1968, 1972; see also Chapter 6). Hirota (1974) reported *H. mediterranea* to be endoparasitic in *Pleurobrachia bachei* during its larval and early juvenile phase, and free living in its late juvenile and adult stage.

The fact that Brusca (1970) did not report ectobiotic stages and that, in turn, Evans and Sheader (1972) observed no endoparasitic stages of *Hyperoche medusarum* associated with *Pleurobrachia pileus* and *P. bachei* could be explained by seasonal (and also spatial) variations. Brusca made his collections during spring 1969, whereas the latter authors conducted their observations and experiments in September and October, 1970.

Differences in behaviour between Atlantic and Pacific populations of *Hyperoche medusarum*, as suggested by von Westernhagen (1976), appear unlikely, as do differences in host species *(Pleurobrachia pileus, P. bachei)*. More likely, *H. medusarum* is an opportunistic predator feeding on a wide spectrum of planktonic organisms. *H. medusarum* can (but must not) spend its early life phase endoparasitically in ctenophores. As demonstrated by von Westernhagen, this association is not obligatory—not even for newly born individuals. When offered yolk-sac herring larvae, amphipods freshly released from the marsupium immediately start to feed on them. *H. medusarum* can easily be raised in the laboratory from larva to adult on a diet consisting exclusively of larval *Clupea harengus pallasi*.

When given a choice between several teleost larvae such as *Clupea harengus pallasi*, *Pholis laeta*, *Anoplarchus purpurescens* and *Artadius lateralis* and crustaceans such as zoeae and megalopae of decapods and various copepod species, *Hyperoche medusarum* usually attacks and devours *C. harengus pallasi*.

Although *Hyperoche medusarum* has a distinct preference for fishes, interactions between hyperiids and ctenophores—even at the population level—cannot be ruled out. Thus,

Hirota (1974) found that in La Jolla Bight (California, USA) maximal abundance of *H. mediterranea* occurred about a week after the *Pleurobrachia bachei* maximum. This may represent an 'overshoot' phenomenon in a density-dependent parasite–host system.

In conclusion, then, *Hyperoche* spp. apparently can easily switch from one prey organism to another, thus exerting varying impact on one or more links in the marine food web. The ecology of *Hyperoche* spp. and their parasite–host relationships should be studied more thoroughly in the future, not least because of their potential effect on commercial fisheries. Von Westernhagen and Rosenthal (1976) suggested that the abundant occurrence of *H. medusarum* in Departure Bay (British Columbia, Canada) during the spawning season of Pacific herring *Clupea harengus pallasi* and its feeding on herring larvae might have some bearing on the recruitment of herring stocks in British Columbia waters.

In addition to *Pleurobrachia pileus* and *P. bachei*, ctenophores *Beroë* sp. have been reported as hosts for *Hyperoche medusarum* (Stephensen, 1923). *Hyperia galba* parasitizes *P. pileus* and *Beroë cucumis* in the North and Baltic Seas, although these hyperiids are usually associated with scyphomedusae (Buchholz, 1953).

TUMOURS AND ABNORMALITIES

Abnormalities of the locomotory apparatus of *Pleurobrachia pileus* have been reported by Greve (1971). In some specimens, the ciliary plates were degenerated and entirely devoid of cilia. Abnormal animals dominated in surface samples, sometimes up to 100%. A correlation with low water temperatures (3° C) was obvious.

Tumours have, so far, not been reported from Ctenophora.

Literature Cited (Chapter 7)

Anantaraman, S. (1959). Metacercaria (Allocreadioidea) in the planktonic ctenophore, *Pleurobrachia globosa* Moser 1903, from the Madras coast. *Nature, Lond.*, **183**, 1407–1408.

Anantaraman, S. (1963). Larval cestodes in marine invertebrates and fishes with a discussion of the life cycles of the Tetraphyllidea and the Trypanorhyncha. *Z. ParasitKde*, **23**, 309–314.

Anantaraman, S. and Krishnaswamy, S. (1958). Tetraphyllidean larvae in the marine copepod, *Eucalanus pseudattenuatus* Sewell, from the Madras coast. *J. zool. Soc. India*, **10**, 1–3.

Apstein, C. (1911). Parasiten von *Calanus finmarchicus*. *Wiss Meeresunters. (Kiel)*, **13**, 205–222.

Bigelow, H. B. and Schroeder, W. C. (1953). Fishes of the Gulf of Maine. *Fish. Bull. Fish. Wildl. Serv. U.S.*, **53**, 1–577.

Bowman, T. E., Meyers, C. D. and Hicks, S. D. (1963). Notes on associations between hyperiid amphipods and medusae in Chesapeake and Narragansett Bays and the Niantic River. *Chesapeake Sci.*, **4**, 141–146.

Boyle, M. S. (1966). Trematode and nematode parasites of *Pleurobrachia pileus* O. F. Müller in New Zealand waters. *Trans. R. Soc. N. Z. (Zool.)*, **8**, 51–62.

Brusca, G. J. (1970). Notes on the association between *Hyperoche medusarum* A. Agassiz (Amphipoda, Hyperiidea) and the ctenophore, *Pleurobrachia bachei* (Müller). *Bull. S. Calif. Acad. Sci.*, **69**, 179–181.

Buchholz, H. A. (1953). Die Wirtstiere des Amphipoden *Hyperia galba* in der Kieler Bucht. *Faun. Mitt. Norddeutsch.*, **1**, 5–6.

Chatton, É. (1911). Ciliés parasites des cestes et des pyrosomes. *Perikaryon cesticola* n.g., n.sp. et *Conchophrys davidoffi*, n.g., n.sp. *Archs Zool. exp. gén.* (Ser. 5), **8**, 13.

Chatton, É. and Lwoff, A. (1935). Les ciliés apostomes. Morphologie, cytologie, éthologie, évolution, systématiques. I. Aperçu historique et général; étude monographique des genres et des espèces. *Archs Zool. exp. gén.*, **77**, 1–453.

Cleave, H. J. van (1927). Ctenophores as the host of a cestode. *Trans Am. microsc. Soc.*, **46**, 214–215.

Dawes, B. (1947). *The Trematoda of British Fishes*, Ray Society, London.

Dollfus, R. P. (1936). Invertébrés marins et thalassoides. In C. Joyeux & J. Baer (Eds), *Cestodes*. Paul Lechevalier, Paris. (*Faune de France*, **30**, 509–539.)

Dollfus, R. P. (1954). Métacercaire progénétique de *Derogenes* (Trematoda Hemiuroidea) chez un copépode parasite de poisson. *Vie Milieu*, **5**, 565–568.

Dollfus, R. P. (1960). Critique de récentes innovations apportées à la classification des Accacoeliidae (Trematoda Digenea). Observations sur des métacercaires de cette famille. *Annls Parasit. hum. comp.*, **23**, 648–671.

Dollfus, R. P. (1963). Liste des coelentères marins, paléarctiques et indiens, où ont été trouvés des trématodes digénétiques. *Bull. Inst. Pêch. marit. Maroc*, **9/10**, 33–57.

Dunnington, E. and Mansueti, R. (1955). School harvest fish feeds on sea walnuts. *Md. Tidewat. News*, **5**, 3–4.

Evans, F. and Sheader, M. (1972). Host species of the hyperiid amphipod *Hyperoche medusarum* (Krøyer) in the North Sea. *Crustaceana*, **3** (Suppl.), 275–276.

Forbes, E. (1839). On two British species of *Cydippe*. *Ann. Mag. nat. Hist.*, **1839**, III.

Franc, A. (1951). Le zooplancton de la région de Dinard-St.-Malo. *Bull. Lab. marit. Dinard*, **24**, 25–40.

Fraser, J. H. (1970). The ecology of the ctenophore *Pleurobrachia pileus* in Scottish waters. *J. Cons. perm. int. Explor. Mer*, **33**, 149–168.

Greve, W. (1971). Ökologische Untersuchungen an *Pleurobrachia pileus*. 1. Freilanduntersuchungen. *Helgoländer wiss. Meeresunters.*, **22**, 303–325.

Hartwich, G. (1975). I. Rhabditida und Ascaridida. *Tierwelt Dtl.*, **62**, 1–256.

Hirota, J. (1974). Quantitative natural history of *Pleurobrachia bachei* in La Jolla Bight. *Fish. Bull. Calif.*, **72**, 295–335.

Køie, M. (1975). On the morphology and life-history of *Opechona bacillaris* (Molin, 1859) Looss, 1907 (Trematoda, Lepocreadiidae). *Ophelia*, **13**, 63–86.

Künne, C. (1950). Das Plankton. In F. Ehrenbaum, H. Lübbert, A. Willer (Eds), *Handbuch der Seefischerei Nordeuropas*, Vol. 1. Schweizerbart, Stuttgart. pp. 10–85.

Künne, C. (1952). Untersuchungen über das Großplankton in der Deutschen Bucht und im Nordsylter Wattenmeer. *Helgoländer wiss. Meeresunters.*, **4**, 1–54.

Laval, P. (1968). Développement en élevage et systématique d'*Hyperia schizogeneios* Stebb. (Amphipode hypéride). *Archs Zool. exp. gén.*, **109**, 25–67.

Laval, P. (1972). Comportement, parasitisme et écologie d'*Hyperia schizogeneios* Stebb. (Amphipode hypéride) dans le plancton de Villefranche-sur-Mer. *Annls Inst. océanogr., Monaco*, **48**, 49–74.

Lebour, M. V. (1916). Medusae as hosts for larval trematodes. *J. mar. biol. Ass. U.K.*, **11**, 57–59.

Manter, H. W. (1954). Some digenetic trematodes from fishes of New Zealand. *Trans. R. Soc. N.Z.*, **82**, 475–568.

Martin, W. E. (1945). Two new species of marine cercariae. *Trans. Am. microsc. Soc.*, **64**, 203–212.

Mayer, A. G. (1912). Ctenophores of the Atlantic coast of North America. *Carnegie Inst. Wash., Publ. No.* **162**, 1–58.

Mortensen, T. (1912). Ctenophora. *Dan. Ingolf-Exped.*, **5**, 1–95.

Noble, E. R. and Noble, G. A. (1964). *Parasitology. The Biology of Animal Parasites*, Lea and Febiger, Philadelphia.

Oviatt, C. A. and Kremer, P. M. (1977). Predation on the ctenophore, *Mnemiopsis leidyi*, by butterfish, *Peprilus triacanthus*, in Narragansett Bay, Rhode Island. *Chesapeake Sci.*, **18**, 236–240.

Oviatt, C. A. and Nixon, S. W. (1973). The demersal fish of Narragansett Bay: an analysis of community structure, distribution and abundance. *Estuar. coastal mar. Sci.*, **1**, 361–378.

Rebecq, J. (1965). Considérations sur la place des trématodes dans le zooplancton marin. *Annls Fac. Sci. Marseille*, **38**, 61–84.

Reichenbach-Klinke, H.-H. (1956). Die Larvenentwicklung bei der Bandwurmordnung Tetraphyllidea Braun, 1900. *Abh. braunschw. wiss. Ges.*, **8**, 61–73.

Reichenbach-Klinke, H.-H. (1957). Artzugehörigkeit und Entwicklung der als *Scolex pleuronectis* Müller bekannten Cestodenlarven (Cestoidea, Tetraphyllidea). *Zool. Anz.*, **20** (Suppl.), 317–324.

Sars, G. O. (1895). Amphipoda. An account of the Crustacea of Norway. *Cammermeyer, Christiania*, **1**, 1–711.

Stephensen, K. (1923). Crustacea Malacostraca V. Amphipoda I. *Dan. Ingolf-Exped.*, **3**, 1–102.

Stunkard, H. W. (1932). Some larval trematodes from the coast in the region of Roscoff, Finistère. *Parasitology*, **24**, 321–343.

Stunkard, H. W. (1967). The life-cycle and developmental stages of a digenetic trematode whose unencysted metacercarial stages occur in medusae. *Biol. Bull. mar. biol. Lab., Woods Hole*, **133**, 488.

Stunkard, H. W. (1968). Studies on the life-history of *Distomum pyriforme* Linton, 1900. *Biol. Bull. mar. biol. Lab., Woods Hole*, **135**, 439.

Stunkard, H. W. (1969). The morphology and life-history of *Neopechona pyriforme* (Linton, 1900) n. gen., n. comb. (Trematoda: Lepocreadiidae). *Biol. Bull. mar. biol. Lab., Woods Hole*, **136**, 96–113.

Stunkard, H. W. (1970). The marine cercariae of the Woods Hole, Massachusetts, region. *Biol. Bull. mar. biol. Lab., Woods Hole*, **138**, 66–76.

Ward, H. B. and Fillingham, J. (1934). A new trematode in a toadfish from southeastern Alaska. *Proc. helminth. Soc. Wash.*, **1**, 25–31.

Westernhagen, H. von (1976). Some aspects of the biology of the hyperiid amphipod *Hyperoche medusarum. Helgoländer wiss. Meeresunters.*, **28**, 43–50.

Westernhagen, H. von and Rosenthal, H. (1976). Predator-prey relationship between Pacific herring, *Clupea harengus pallasi* larvae and a predatory hyperiid amphipod *Hyperoche medusarum. Fish. Bull. U.S.*, **74**, 669–674.

Will, F. (1844). Über *Distoma beroës. Arch. Naturgeschichte*, **10**, 343–344.

Williams, H. H. (1968). The taxonomy, ecology and host specificity of some Phyllobothriidae (Cestoda: Tetraphyllidea), a critical revision of *Phyllobothrium*, Beneden, 1849 and comments on some allied genera. *Philos. Trans. R. Soc.* (Ser. B.), **253**, 231–307.

Wundsch, H. H. (1912). Neue Plerocercoide aus marinen Copepoden. *Arch. Naturgesch.*, **78**, 1–20.

8. DISEASES OF TENTACULATA

G. LAUCKNER

The Phoronida, Bryozoa and Brachiopoda are usually treated as independent although closely related phyla (Hyman, 1940). For convenience—i.e. scarcity of information concerning their diseases—we shall follow Kaestner (1954–1963) in regarding them as classes in the phylum Tentaculata.

8.1 PHORONIDA

The Phoronida comprise only some 20 exclusively marine species. Next to nothing is known about their parasites and diseases. Unidentified gregarines, 100 μm in diameter, were found attached to the epithelial cells of the intestinal wall of *Phoronis hippocrepia* and *P. sabatieri* from Wimereux, France, and *P. psammophila* from Naples, Italy. The parasites, which strikingly resembled the host's ova, occurred most frequently in specimens with well-developed ovaries. Cysts filled with spores were seen floating in close contact with the host's ova in the perivisceral fluid of *P. sabatieri*. The spores are presumably discharged together with the ova, permitting infestation of host embryos while they are still within the lophophore (de Selys-Longchamps, 1907).

Kozloff (1945) described *Heterocineta phoronopsidis*, a thigmotrich ancistrocomid ciliate parasitic on the tentacles of *Phoronopsis viridis* from Bodega Bay, California, USA. The parasite feeds on the epithelial cells of the host's tentacles by means of its suctorial organ. Ingested nuclei or fragments of nuclei from *P. viridis* were frequently seen in the food-vacuoles. Other members of the genus *Heterocineta* are ectoparasitic on freshwater mussels, prosobranchs and pulmonates (Jarocki, 1934, 1935). Although Kozloff (1945) stated that the ancistrocomid from *P. viridis* differs fundamentally from other species of *Heterocineta* in having a groove-like depression originating on the left side of the body near the anterior end, and extending posteriorly along the dorsal surface close to the left margin, and despite the fact that other *Heterocineta* species occur in fresh water, the author included the ancistrocomid from *P. viridis* in the same genus (Fig. 8-1).

Unidentified progenetic trematode metacercariae were found in the lopophoral coelom of *Phoronis psammophila* from Naples, Italy. The unencysted larval worms, which were quite transparent and measured approximately 250 μm in length, were attached to the epithelial lining of the coelom by means of their ventral sucker. The metacercariae were observed several times within autotomized tentacle crowns of *P. psammophila*. Whether the parasites stimulate the host to autotomize was not determined (de Selys-Longchamps, 1907).

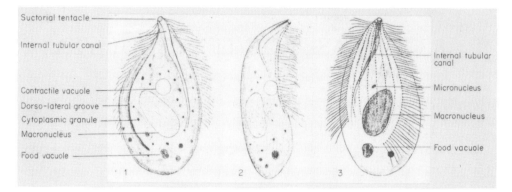

Fig. 8-1: *Heterocineta phoronopsidis* from the tentacles of *Phoronopsis viridis*. 1: Dorsal aspect; 2: lateral view from right side, both from life; 3: ventral aspect, Schaudinn's fixative—iron haematoxylin. × 1940. (After Kozloff, 1945; reproduced by permission of the Marine Biological Laboratory, Woods Hole.)

8.2 BRYOZOA

The Bryozoa are almost entirely marine; only a few of the some 3000 known recent species have penetrated into brackish and freshwater habitats. Reports on parasites of bryozoans, however, are almost entirely confined to freshwater species. Modern methods of cultivation (Kinne, 1976, 1977) now facilitate critical research on disease-causing symbioses in a number of marine bryozoans.

Filamentous structures, composed of slightly curved rods, believed to be bacteria, were found associated with hypertrophy of the vestibular glands of the chilostome bryozoan *Palmicellaria skenei*. The organisms were situated in the mucous contents of the main pouch of the gland. The association is permanent in the collecting area, Roscoff, France, and apparently, does not cause harm to the host (Lutaud, 1965).

Microsporidans *Nosema bryozoides* have repeatedly been reported from freshwater bryozoans *Plumatella fungosa*, *P. casmiana*, *P. repens*, *Stolella evelinae* and *Lophopus crystallinus* (Korotneff, 1892; Schröder, 1910a; Braem, 1911; Marcus, 1934, 1941; Wiebach, 1959, 1963). The parasite attacks the spermatogonia, coelomocytes, peritoneum and statoblast of the host, causing hypertrophy and destruction of affected cells, and occasionally, death of individual polypides or entire colonies. Another unnamed sporozoan caused pathological changes in the gut epithelium of *P. fungosa* (Schröder, 1913).

Wiebach (1959) mentions further protozoans associated with freshwater bryozoans, including holotrich ciliates *Kerona polyporum* and peritrichs *Trichodina pediculus*.

Capsulated organisms, forming 'brown bodies' in the septa between the zooecia, and believed to be parasitic protozoans or algae, occur in marine bryozoans *Alcyonidium gelatinosum* from Dutch waters (Lacourt, 1949).

Peculiar vermiform bodies have repeatedly been reported from the coelom of *Carbasea papyrea*, *C. pisciformis* and other marine Bryozoa. The nature of these objects, which are variable in shape, coiled, looped and sometimes constricted, is uncertain. They probably comprise more than one type of structure, and in some cases, they may be parasitic protozoans (Palk, 1911; Hastings, 1943).

Another organism frequently found in the coelom of freshwater bryozoans *Plumatella repens* and *P. fungosa* is *Buddenbrockia plumatellae*. Its vermiform body is composed of two cell layers with a hollow, coelom-like space inside, and measures from 50 μm to 1500 μm in length. Braem (1911) believed the organism to be a trematode sporocyst, but Schröder (1910a, b) assigned it to the Mesozoa and discussed similarities and differences between *B. plumatellae* and Dicyemida and Orthonectida. Early developmental stages are found attached to the inner wall of the host coelom, while older stages occur free in the coelom of the bryozoans. *B. plumatellae* probably lives at the expense of its host with heavy infestations causing emaciation and death of individual polypids (Braem, 1911).

Although Schröder (1910a, b) identified the parasite as a mesozoan, he later (1912a, b) revised his earlier findings, and assumed the organism was a degenerate nematode. He further noted that sometimes the spermatozoa of *Plumatella* sp. penetrate and kill the eggs of the parasite. *Buddenbrockia plumatellae* also occurs in the coelom of bryozoans *Stolella evelinae* from Brazil (Marcus, 1941). The latter author concluded that *B. plumatellae* cannot be assigned to any group of known organisms.

Encysted trematode metacercariae have been observed in freshwater bryozoans *Lophopus crystallinus* (Marcus, 1934), and occasionally, oligochaete annelids, probably *Chaetogaster diaphanus* and *C. diastrophus*, occur within bryozoan cystids. Their relationship to the bryozoans is not clear; possibly, they absorb coelomic fluid (Wiebach, 1959, 1963).

Minute polychaetes *Serpula oblita* were found to build their tubes within zooecia of bryozoans *Onychocella cyclostoma* and *O. subpiriformis*, causing degeneration of the affected individuals (Annoscia, 1968).

Tumours or neoplastic formations have not been recorded from the Bryozoa. It is interesting, in this respect, to note that antineoplastic substances have been isolated from bryozoans *Nugula nerita*, *Amathia convoluta* and *Thalamaporella gothica floridana*. Injection of extracts from these animals into leukaemic mice resulted in a 168% to 200% life extension, as compared to untreated controls (Pettit and co-authors, 1970).

Monstrous double zooecia have been observed in *Membranipora reticulatum* and *Cryptosula pallasiana* (Lacourt, 1949; Jebram, 1977). Jebram and Voigt (1977) reviewed the literature on the occurrence of monster zooids and double polypids in fossil and recent Cheilostomata Anasca.

8.3 BRACHIOPODA

The Brachiopoda, comprising a group of some 280 exclusively marine species, are remarkably free of metazoan parasites and other associates (Vader, 1970a), and microbial disease agents have, so far, not been reported from members of this phylum.

Trematodes are the only true parasites hitherto recorded from brachiopods. Paine (1962) described unencysted gymnophallid metacercariae from the coelomic spaces of the inarticulate brachiopod *Glottidia pyramidata,* collected from intertidal waters of the west coast of Florida, USA. Usually, the larval trematodes were found in close association with the host's gonad, which in heavy infestations often was noticeably reduced or even destroyed. The metacercariae then appeared to attack secondarily the digestive gland and mantle sinuses. The maximum number of metacercariae per host was 12, multiple infestations not being uncommon. The incidence of infestation varied seasonally, 60% to 90% of all *G. pyramidata* longer than 6·0 mm, examined in August and November, being parasitized, while samples taken in March and April gave no evidence of infestation, and specimens collected in December, January and late May gave intermediate values. The specific identity of the metacercaria remained unknown. The author suspected, however, that it might be related to a gymnophallid furcocercous cercaria, described as *Cercaria pusilla* from the bivalve *Chione cancellata* by Holliman (1961). The pelecypod was observed to be locally abundant, and aggregated in the vegetation covering the brachiopods. The adult parasites are likely to occur in avian predators of *G. pyramidata*. This is the first record of trematodes from brachiopods.

Vader (1970a) reported an association between the lysianassid amphipod *Aristias neglectus* and the brachiopods *Terebratulina caputserpentis* and *Macandrewia cranium* from Kosterfjorden, Sweden, and Bergen, Norway. The amphipods, which were all immature, occurred in the branchial cavity of the brachiopods. Members of the genus *Aristias* are usually found associated with Porifera, Tunicata, Echinodermata, and with the sea-anemone *Bolocera tuediae* (Vader, 1970b). The only other record of an association between an amphipod and Brachiopoda is one observed by Walker (1909), a single ovigerous female of *Leucothoë spinicarpa* from Suakin Harbour, Red Sea, occurring in an unidentified brachiopod. The nature of the association between these two amphipods and their various hosts is still unknown. As has been pointed out by Vader (1970a), both species show a clear tendency towards inquilinism, together with a very low degree of host-specificity. Their occasional occurrence in Brachiopoda—sedentary, microphagous animals which afford excellent protection—is, therefore, not altogether unexpected.

Diorygma atrypophilia, believed to be an annelid-like parasite, was described from fossil *Atrypa zonata* from Poland merely on the basis of the structure of peculiar boring holes observed in the valves of the brachiopods (Biernat, 1961).

Literature Cited (Chapter 8)

Annoscia, E. (1968). *Briozoi. Introduzione allo studio con particolare riguardo ai briozoi italiani e mediterranei*, Palaeontographia Italica, Pisa.

Biernat, G. (1961). *Diorygma atrypophilia* n.gen., n.sp.—a parasitic organism of *Atrypa zonata* Schnur. *Acta palaeont. pol.*, **6**, 17–28.

Braem, F. (1911). Beiträge zur Kenntnis der Fauna Turkestans. Auf Grund des von D. D. Pedaschenko gesammelten Materials. VII. Bryozoen und deren Parasiten. *Trudy imp. S-petersb. Obshch. Estest.*, **42**, 3–35.

Hastings, A. B. (1943). Polyzoa (Bryozoa). I. Scrupocellariidae, Epistomiidae, Farciminariidae, Bicellariellidae, Aeteidae, Scrupariidae. *'Discovery' Rep.*, **22**, 301–510.

Holliman, R. B. (1961). Larval trematodes from the Apalachee Bay area, Florida, with a checklist of known marine cercariae arranged in a key to their superfamilies. *Tulane Stud. Zool.*, **9**, 1–74.

Hyman, L. H. (1940). *The Invertebrates*, Vol. 1, Protozoa through Ctenophora, McGraw-Hill, New York.

Jarocki, J. (1934). Two new hypocomid ciliates, *Heterocineta janickii* sp.n. and *H. lwoffi* sp.n., ectoparasites of *Physa fontinalis* (L.) and *Viviparus fasciatus* Müller. *Mem. Acad. Cracovie, Cl. Sci. math. nat.* (Ser. B II), **1934**, 167.

Jarocki, J. (1935). Studies on ciliates from fresh-water molluscs. I. General remarks on protozoan parasites of Pulmonata. Transfer experiments with species of *Heterocineta* and *Chaetogaster limnaei*, their additional host. Some new hypocomid ciliates. *Bull. int. Acad. pol. Sci. Lett., Cl. Sci. math. nat.* (Ser. B II), **1935**, 201.

Jebram, D. (1977). Monster zooids in *Cryptosula pallasiana* (Bryozoa, Cheilostomata Ascophora). *Helgoländer wiss. Meeresunters.*, **29**, 404–413.

Jebram, D. and Voigt, E. (1977). Monsterzooide und Doppelpolypide bei fossilen und rezenten Cheilostomata Anasca (Bryozoa). *Abh. Verh. naturwiss. Ver. Hamburg*, **20**, 151–183.

Kaestner, A. (1954-1963). *Lehrbuch der Speziellen Zoologie*, VEB Fischer, Jena.

Kinne, O. (1976). Cultivation of marine organisms: water-quality management and technology. In O. Kinne (Ed.), *Marine Ecology*, Vol. III, Cultivation, Part 1. Wiley, London. pp. 19-300.

Kinne, O. (1977). Cultivation of animals. Research cultivation. In O. Kinne (Ed.), *Marine Ecology*, Vol. III, Cultivation, Part 2. Wiley, Chichester. pp. 579-1293.

Korotneff, A. (1892). *Myxosporidium bryozoides. Z. wiss. Zool.*, **53**, 591–596.

Kozloff, E. N. (1945). *Heterocineta phoronopsidis* sp.nov., a ciliate from the tentacles of *Phoronopsis viridis* Hilton. *Biol. Bull. mar. biol. Lab., Woods Hole*, **89**, 180–183.

Lacourt, A. W. (1949). Bryozoa of the Netherlands. *Archs néerl. Zool.*, **8**, 289–321.

Lutaud, G. (1965). Sur la présence de micro-organismes spécifiques dans les glandes vestibulaires et dans l'aviculaire de *Palmicellaria skenei* (Ellis et Solander), bryozoaire chilostome. *Cah. Biol. Mar.*, **6**, 181–190.

Marcus, E. (1934). *Über Lophopus crystallinus* (Pall.). *Zool. Jb. (Anat. Ontogenie Tiere)*, **58**, 501–606.

Marcus, E. (1941). Sobre Bryozoa do Brasil. (Eng. summary.) *Bolm. Fac. Filos. Cienc. Univ. S. Paolo (Zool.)*, **5**, 3–169.

Paine, R. T. (1962). Ecological notes on a gymnophalline metacercaria from the brachiopod *Glottidia pyramidata. J. Parasit.*, **48**, 509.

Palk, M. (1911). On an enigmatic body in certain Bryozoa. *Zool. Anz.*, **38**, 209–212.

Pettit, G. R., Day, J. F., Hartwell, J. L. and Wood, H. B. (1970). Antineoplastic components of marine animals. *Nature, Lond.*, **227**, 962–963.

Schröder, O. (1910a). Eine neue Mesozoenart (*Buddenbrockia plumatellae* n.g., n.sp.) aus *Plumatella repens* L. und *Pl. fungosa* Pall. *Sitz.-ber. Heidelb. Akad. Wiss.* (Math.-Naturw. Kl.), **6**, 1–8.

Schröder, O. (1910b). *Buddenbrockia plumatellae*, eine neue Mesozoenart aus *Plumatella repens* L. und *Pl. fungosa* Pall. *Z. wiss. Zool.*, **96**, 525–537.

Schröder, O. (1912a). Zur Kenntnis der *Buddenbrockia plumatellae* O. Schröder. *Z. wiss. Zool.*, **102**, 79–91.

Schröder, O. (1912b). Weitere Mitteilungen zur Kenntnis der *Buddenbrockia plumatellae. Verh. naturh.-med. Ver. Heidelb.*, **11**, 230–237.

Schröder, O. (1913). Über einen einzelligen Parasiten des Darmepithels von *Plumatella fungosa* Pallas. *Zool. Anz.*, **43**, 220–223.

Selys-Longchamps, M. de (1907). Phoronis. *Fauna Flora Golf Neapel*, **30**, 1–280.

Vader, W. (1970a). The amphipod, *Aristias neglectus* Hansen, found in association with Brachiopoda. *Sarsia*, **43**, 13–14.

Vader, W. (1970b). *Antheacheres duebeni* M. Sars, a copepod parasitic in the sea anemone, *Bolocera tuediae* (Johnston). *Sarsia*, **43**, 99–106.

Walker, A. O. (1909). Amphipoda Gammaridea from the Indian Ocean, British East Africa, and the Red Sea. *Trans. Linn. Soc. Lond.* (Ser. 2, Zool.), **12**, 323–344.

Wiebach, F. (1959). Kommensalen, Feinde und Parasiten der Süsswasser-Moostierchen. *Mikrokosmos*, **48**, 168–172.

Wiebach, F. (1963). Studien über *Plumatella casmiana* Oka (Bryozoa). *Vie Milieu*, **14**, 579–596.

9. DISEASES OF SIPUNCULIDA, PRIAPULIDA AND ECHIURIDA

G. LAUCKNER

These small phyla of exclusively marine animals contain only a few species, namely about 240, 5 and 70, respectively (Kaestner, 1954–63). Next to nothing is known about parasites and diseases of priapulids and echiurids. Sipunculids have been primarily studied with respect to their internal defense mechanisms and the antibacterial activity of the coelomic fluid. An annotated bibliography (Johnson, 1968) contains a number of pertinent references. The taxonomy in these phyla is somewhat obsolete. Although the sipunculan genus *Golfingia*—the largest in its phylum—has recently been revised (Cutler and Murina, 1977), mostly the designations of the original authors have been used here.

DISEASES CAUSED BY MICRO-ORGANISMS

Agents: Bacteria

Apparently, no natural bacterial infections have been observed in sipunculids, priapulids or echiurids. Thomas (1931) studied the fate of *Sipunculus nudus*, experimentally infected with *Bacterium tumefaciens*. Five days after the injection of 0·5 ml of a virulent bacterial suspension, the sipunculids became sluggish, and no longer buried in the sediment. Death occurred 6 days after injection. Four days after infection, blood was taken from a contaminated sipuncle, and inoculated into a healthy specimen. After 3 successive passages, the pathogen became so virulent, as to kill previously healthy sipuncles within 15 h. Upon inoculation, *B. tumefaciens* multiplied rapidly, although, due to phagocytosis, free bacteria were still low in numbers on the second day. They immediately infected the red blood cells of the coelomic fluid, eventually causing lysis of the cells, which assumed considerable proportions within 4 days after inoculation.

On the other hand, Bang and Krassner (1958) found that several strains of marine bacteria were destroyed within 24 h when more than 100 million organisms were injected into healthy *Phascolosoma (Golfingia) gouldi*. Only an occasional infection was produced which eventually killed the sipunculid. Blood removed from healthy worms proved to be sterile when cultured on ZoBell's sea-water agar at room temperature. When incubated with varying concentrations of different bacteria, *P. gouldi* blood became sterile again after 5 to 24 h at room temperature. Consistent sterility was obtained within the same time intervals, when a combination of bacteria and blood was kept at 0° C, while control preparations of bacteria remained viable for several days at this temperature. Destruction of 1 million organisms was achieved with 0·2 ml of whole blood within 24 h. *P. gouldi* blood also inhibited a *Vibrio* sp. from the horseshoe crab *Limulus polyphemus* and *Aerococcus viridans* var. *homari* from lobsters *Homarus americanus in vitro*. Heating the blood for 10 min at 70° C, or allowing it to stand at room temperature for 24 h, as well as freezing and thawing, destroyed the antibacterial activity. In contrast, heated or frozen blood showed growth-promoting activity. Dialysis of blood against sea water at 4° C caused some loss of activity. It was found that the antibacterial activity occurred in both the cellular and fluid portions of the blood, but was stronger in the latter (Krassner, 1963). Vaccination of *P. gouldi* with dead or living *Vibrio* sp. from *L. polyphemus* did not change the antibacterial activity of the sipunculid serum *in vitro*. No evidence of development of resistance in the vibrio was found (Rabin and Bang, 1963, 1964).

Blitz (1966), on the other hand, reports a lessened resistance of *Phascolosoma agassizi* inoculated with killed or living bacteria, or with carbon particles, to subsequent infection with bacteria. Normal serum contains an agglutinin active against Gram-negative bacteria and a lysozyme-like enzyme digesting Gram-positive pathogens.

Sipunculids *Dendrostoma zostericola* and echiurids *Urechis caupo*—experimentally fed exclusively on bacteria *Rhodococcus agilis, Flavobacterium boreale* and *Bacillus marinus*—suffered no ill effects from their bacterial diet and could be maintained in the laboratory without losing weight. Some even gained weight, whereas unfed controls either lost weight or died of starvation (ZoBell and Feltham, 1938).

DISEASES CAUSED BY PROTOZOANS

Agents: Flagellata

Abnormal *Golfingia capensis* from South African waters have been described by Wesenberg-Lund (1963). The abnormality consisted of a 'corky' skin at each body end in some individuals, while others were corky all over. Several specimens seemed to be sloughing, leaving a clean, clear skin underneath. The abnormal condition, which was possibly due to an unknown disease, occurred in *G. capensis* of all sizes from Lambert's Bay, and was not known from other areas. Bang (1966) reported on a similar ulcerative skin disease of *Sipunculus nudus* from the French Atlantic coast at Loquemeau, which appeared to be caused by a parasitic flagellate.

Agents: Sporozoa

Sipunculids, priapulids and echiurids are frequently parasitized by sporozoans. Ikeda (1912) described two species of Myxospora, *Tetractinomyxon intermedium* and *T. irregulare*, from the sipunculid *Petalostoma minutum (= Phascolosoma johnstoni)* from Plymouth, England (Fig. 9-1). A detailed account of the morphology, ecology and development of the little studied Actinomyxida has been published by Janiszewska (1955).

Gregarines are the most frequently reported sporozoans parasitizing sipunculids and echiurids. Unnamed gregarines, believed to be members of the family Selenidiidae, occurred abundantly in *Phascolosoma vulgare* and *P. elongatum* from the French Atlantic and English Channel coasts. Stages of the parasites were seen in the lumen of the digestive tract or free in the body cavity of the sipunculids. The gregarines were sometimes hyperparasitized by another sporozoan (Brasil and Fantham, 1907). Dogiel (1907) described what could have been the same or a closely related schizogregarine from *Sipunculus nudus* which he named *Schizocystis sipunculi*. Pixell-Goodrich (1950) identified gregarines from the same host, formerly known as *Gregarina sipunculi*, as members of the genera *Urospora* and *Lithocystis* and named them *U. legeri*, *U. hardyi* and *L. lankesteri* (Fig. 9-2). *Filipodium ozakii* and *Selenidium folium* are intestinal and coelomic parasites of *Siphonosoma cumanense* in Japanese waters (Hukui, 1939).

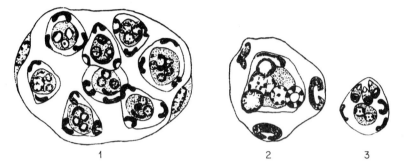

Fig. 9-1: *Tetractinomyxon intermedium* from body cavity of *Petalostoma minutum*. 1: Pansporocyst with 8 mature spores; 2: end view of single spore, showing exo- and endospore, 3 nuclei of polar capsules, 1 binucleated sporozoite and 3 nuclei of envelope; 3: same spore, side view. (After Janiszewska, 1955; reproduced by permission of Polish Academy of Sciences.)

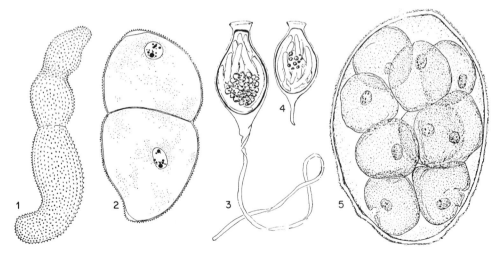

Fig. 9-2: Gregarines from *Sipunculus nudus*. 1: *Lithocystis lankesteri*. Associated pairs, alive, showing cuticular processes after removal of many coelomic corpuscles; 2: fixed and stained specimens; 3: spore containing 8 sporozoites and large residual body; 4: spore of *Urospora hardyi*; 5: *Urospora sipunculi*. Capsule containing 9 trophozoites. (After Pixell-Goodrich, 1950; reproduced by permission of Oxford University Press.)

Sipunculids *Phascolion strombi* from the French Atlantic coast are hosts for gregarines *Lecudina franciana*. Initial stages of the parasite are intra-epithelial in the host's intestine. Young growing trophozoites migrate into the intestinal lumen. Freely moving trophozoites, pointed at one end, constantly change their shape (Fig. 9-3). Associations of two trophozoites were never seen in material comprising 300 *P. strombi*. In rare instances, *L. franciana* was found to be hyperparasitized by microsporidans, *Metchnikovella berliozi* (Arvy, 1952).

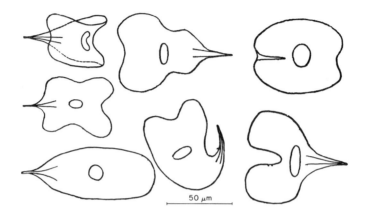

Fig. 9-3: *Lecudina franciana* from intestine of *Phascolion strombi*. Variations in body shape attained during gliding movement of trophozoite. (After Arvy, 1952; reproduced by permission of the Laboratoire Maritime du Dinard.)

Three species of 'blood sporozoans' parasitizing *Phascolosoma minutum* from England, *P. varians* from Florida (USA) and *Themiste hennahi* from Chile and Peru appeared to be host-specific. The stages observed in these sipunculids—merozoites, trophozoites and schizonts—gave rise to cysts and represented the schizogonic phase of the life cycle only. The sexual phase remains unknown (Jones, 1974). Because nematodes, probably members of the Mermithidea also occurred in the samples, Jones speculated that these worms might be involved in the life cycle of the protozoans.

Gregarina bonelliae has been described by Frenzel (1885) from the gut of Mediterranean echiurids *Bonellia viridis*, and Seitz (1907) briefly mentioned another, as yet unnamed gregarine from the intestine of *Urechis chilensis*. Mackinnon and Ray (1931a) described 2 gregarines from *Thalassema neptuni* from Plymouth (England), namely *Hentschelia thalassemae* and *Lecythion thalassemae* (Figs 9-4 and 9-5). In these species, syzygy was frequently observed. Gametocytes did not develop further until they had been passed out with the fæces. In sea water, a cyst formed and spores developed.

A third gregarine from the same host, *Hyperidion thalassemae*, considerably puzzled its discoverers, Mackinnon and Ray (1931b). Host cells parasitized by young intracellular stages not only became strongly hypertrophied but simultaneously protruded from the intestinal wall, hanging almost free in the gut lumen and being connected to the wall by 4 or 5 rooting cytoplasmic threads (Fig. 9-6).

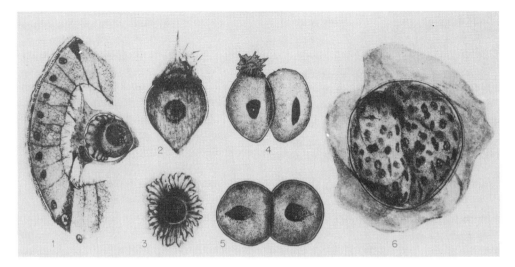

Fig. 9-4: *Hentschelia thalassemae* from intestine of *Thalassema neptuni*. 1: Young intracellular trophozoite; note hypertrophy of host cell and its projection into gut lumen (× 1000); 2: mature trophozoite; note intracellular epimerite (× 350); 3: end view of epimerite (× 933); 4: two individuals during onset of syzygy (one individual still retains its intracellular epimerite; nuclei are elongating); 5: two individuals in complete syzygy (× 500); 6: fixed and stained gametocyst showing nuclei in process of division. From smear of faecal balls of *T. neptuni* (× 500). (After Mackinnon and Ray, 1931a; reproduced by permission of Oxford University Press.)

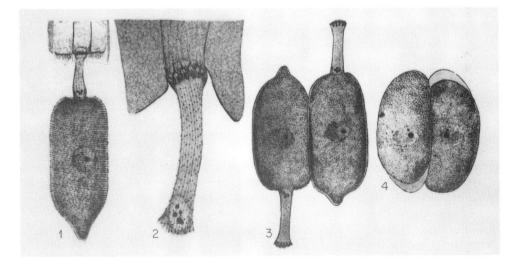

Fig. 9-5: *Lecythion thalassemae* from intestine of *Thalassema neptuni*. 1: Mature trophozoite, attached to host intestinal epithelium (× 400); 2: epimerite of fully grown gregarine (× 1400); 3: two individuals initiating syzygy (× 500); 4: slightly later stage in which epimerites have folded over and are being resorbed (× 500). In 3 and 4 the pellicular striations of the gregarines' body have been omitted. (After Mackinnon and Ray, 1931a; reproduced by permission of Oxford University Press.)

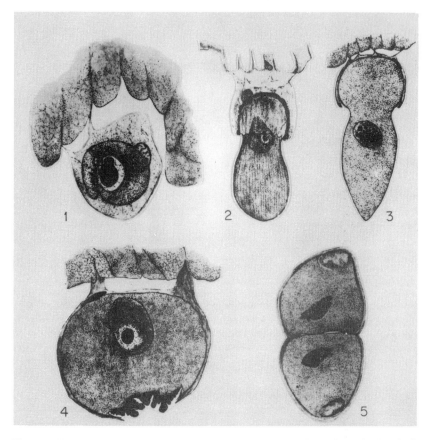

Fig. 9-6: *Hyperidion thalassemae*. 1: Young intracellular parasite in intestinal cell of
Thalassema neptuni. Note hypertrophy of host cell. 2: Half-grown trophozoite. 3:
Older trophozoite in longitudinal section. Note rooting processes of host cell
which is reduced to a mere skin around parasite. 4: Individual completely
retracted into host cell. Note folded, sucker-like mucron (bottom). 5: Association
of two individuals. (After Mackinnon and Ray, 1931b; reproduced by permission
of Oxford University Press.)

A gregarine exhibiting a similar mode of attachment, and possibly related to
Hyperidion thalassemae is *Zygosoma globosum* parasitizing in the mid-gut of *Urechis caupo* from
Drake's Bay, California (Noble, 1938a). The first gregarine of this genus, originally
described by Greeff (1880) as *Chonorhynchus gibbosus*, but later renamed *Zygosoma
gibbosum*, was recovered from *Echiurus pallasii* in Norwegian waters.

Urechis unicinctus from Hiroshima (Japan) waters is host for *Enterocystis yumushii* and
Lecudina fluctus (Iitsuka, 1933). Noble (1938a) disagreed with Iitsuka in referring the
latter gregarine to the genus *Lecudina* and placed it in genus *Zygosoma*. *E. bullis*, a
gregarine very similar to *E. yumushii* was found in *Urechis caupo* from Drake's Bay (Noble,
1938b).

Coccidians parasitize representatives of all 3 phyla of this group. Some have been
mistaken for gregarines by the original investigators.

Priapulids *Halicryptus spinulosus* and *Priapulus caudatus* have been reported to harbour a
coccidian parasite in the gut. The observed effect on the host was merely mechanical in

this infestation; no cell changes were involved. Lüling (1942) studied the parasite in great detail but did not name it.

Among the little known sporozoans inhabiting the gut and coelom of *Petalostoma minutum* (= *Phascolosoma johnstoni*), Ikeda (1914) observed a coccidian, which he named *Dobellia binucleata*. This sporozoan was present in 8 to 10% of the sipunculids dissected. Intracellular macroschizonts arising from sporozoites produced 16 fusiform macromerozoites. These develop into a spherical form which grows *in situ*. Some or most of them fall off into the gut lumen and attack neighbouring epithelial cells. Autoinfestation is thus effected, and the entire life cycle may be completed in a single host individual. Transfer of the parasite to other hosts is by oocysts expelled with the faeces and swallowed by another *P. minutum*. The various life-cycle stages of *Dobellia binucleata* have been described in great detail by Ikeda (1914).

A curious protozoan, *Exoschizon siphonosomae*, parasitizes sipunculids *Siphonosoma cumanense* in Japanese waters (Hukui, 1939). The parasite was believed to be a gregarine but is probably a coccidian.

Similarly, Lankester (1881) reported on what he believed to be a gregarine in the echiurid *Thalassema neptuni*. Mackinnon and Ray (1929, 1937), however, showed the agent to be a coccidian parasite, which they named *Ovivora thalassemae*. The organism infested the eggs of *T. neptuni*, which were killed.

Ovivora thalassemae (Figs 9-7 and 9-8) has a one-host life cycle, both schizogony and sporogony occurring in *Thalassema neptuni*. Sporozoites, representing the earliest (infective) stage in the life cycle of the parasite, were not seen at all and schizogonic stages, resulting from sporozoite penetration into host eggs, were encountered on only a few occasions. Schizonts, which measured 50 to 80 μm in diameter, were always at an advanced stage of development (Fig. 9-7, 1). Merozoites (2,3), about 10 μm long, develop immediately below the pellicle. The merozoites escape from the sipunculid's egg in which they develop and invade adjacent ones in their vicinity. A single schizont produces such a large number of merozoites that only 2 or 3 asexual parasites within one genital pouch of *T. neptuni* would be sufficient to account for the heavy infestation with the sexual forms commonly observed. The smallest trophozoites (5) found in an egg measured about 19 × 5 μm. Growth in length is much more rapid than in width, and hence a worm-like form is eventually assumed, the body lying curved within the host egg, exceeding by far the egg's diameter. In life, when seen in transmitted light, these trophozoites look like greyish streaks within the egg; in reflected light they appear glistening white (4). The parasites never move within the egg, and when artificially released they remain quite immobile.

By the time the parasites are fully grown, the host egg shows clear signs of degeneration, but its contents are usually not completely used up until the spores have been formed. The maturing parasites shorten, thicken and eventually round off to form the (female) macrogametocyte, about 50 μm in diameter, and the (male) microgametocyte, approximately 30 μm in diameter (6). The macrogametocyte develops into a single macrogamete whereas the microgametocyte gives rise to numerous microgametes about 20 μm in length (Fig. 9-8, 1–3). Normally, there are at least 2 parasites in a single ovum but sometimes there may be as many as 4. Occasionally, all may be of the same sex (2). Male and female parasites lying within the same host egg are seldom mature at the same time. Generally, the microgametes have to penetrate other eggs in order to effect fertilization.

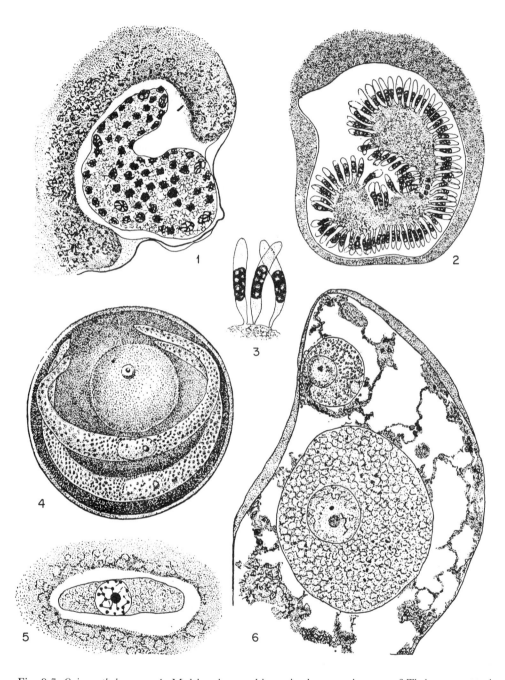

Fig. 9-7: *Ovivora thalassemae*. 1: Multinucleate schizont in degenerating egg of *Thalassema neptuni*. × 870; 2: schizont with merozoites forming at periphery. × 870; 3: merozoites on schizont surface. × 2175; 4: host egg with 2 fully grown vermiform trophozoites. × 435; 5: young vermiform trophozoite, probably a sexual form. × 1830; 6: degenerating host egg with large female and small male gametocyte. × 870. (After Mackinnon and Ray, 1937; reproduced by permission of Cambridge University Press.)

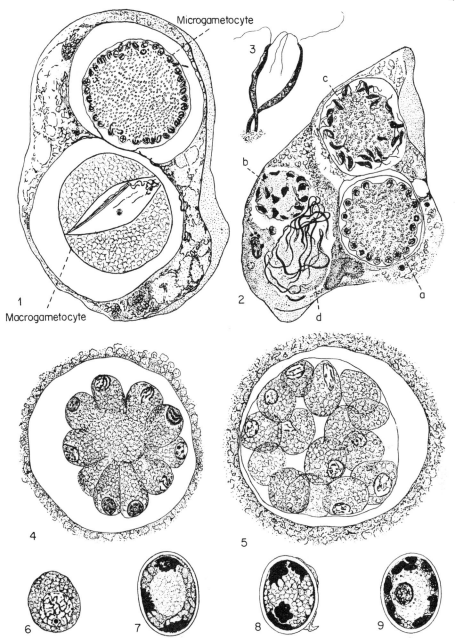

Fig. 9-8: *Ovivora thalassemae*. 1: Male and female gametocyte side by side in egg of *Thalassema neptuni*. Female with fertilization spindle, male with microgametes forming at periphery. × 720. 2: Four male parasites in 1 host egg; a: nuclei at periphery; b: microgametes with compact nuclei and flagella; c: slightly later stage; d: microgametes breaking from cytoplasmic residuum. × 720. 3: Two maturing microgametes still attached to cytoplasmic residuum. × 1540. 4: Uninucleate sporoblasts in process of differentiation. × 720. 5: Oocyst with sporoblasts surrounded by delicate oocyst membrane. × 720. 6: Sporoblast with resting nucleus. × 1000. 7–9: Spores with 3, 4 and 10 nuclei, some of which are dividing. × 1300. (After Mackinnon and Ray, 1937; reproduced by permission of Cambridge University Press.)

Zygote formation initiates sporogony. Nuclear divisions ensue, followed by cytoplasmic divisions which cut centripetal furrows into the cytoplasm (4). Eventually, numerous sporoblasts are delimited within the previously formed oocyst (5), leaving no residuum. The number of sporoblasts varies with the size of the zygote. It is common to find 50. The sporoblasts (6) develop into sporocysts, about $15 \cdot 5 \times 13 \cdot 5$ μm in dimension, which may contain as many as 12 nuclei (7–9). Fully developed sporozoites, the infective stage, have never been seen. They probably differentiate after the sporocyst has been expelled from the genital pouch of a spawning host.

How *Thalassema neptuni* acquires an *Ovivora thalassemae* infestation has not been established. The gonads were never infested and presumably the sporozoites—which in all probability hatch from ingested sporocysts in the host's gut—enter a nephridial sac either through its coelomic funnel or by burrowing through its wall after the eggs have been assembled within it. Judging from the scarcity of schizogonic stages, the number of sporozoites reaching their destination appears to be small. Incidences of *O. thalassemae* infestation seem to fluctuate appreciably. On one occasion, 8 out of 12 mature female *T. neptuni* from Plymouth (England) were found infested, whereas during a subsequent survey only 25 mature females out of 935 worms had the parasite. However, once established, infestations may be heavy in individual hosts (Mackinnon and Ray, 1937).

Agents: Ciliata

Holotrichous ciliates *Ptyssostoma thalassemae* occur in the alimentary tract of echiurids *Thalassema neptuni*, and holotrichs *Cryptochilus cuenoti* live in the gut of sipunculids *Phascolosoma vulgare* in European waters (Mackinnon and Ray, 1931a; Tétry, 1959). Peritrichs *Urceolaria korschelti* have been reported from the end-gut of *Urechis unicinctus* in Japanese waters (Iitsuka, 1933), and *Trichodina urechi* from the mid-gut of *U. caupo* in California, USA (Noble, 1940). Both authors say nothing on pathology. The method of infestation of young worms by the presumed commensals was not determined, but small, very young *U. caupo* were found to be without *T. urechi*; this indicates that primary infestation is correlated with a certain size or stage in the life cycle of the host.

The response of Sipunculida to protozoal infestation has been studied by several authors. The very effective internal defense mechanisms of sipunculids are not only capable of destroying bacteria. Pixell-Goodrich (1950) observed the destruction of gregarines by the host, *Sipunculus nudus*, with the formation of brwonish masses of phagocytes engulfing the parasites. Ikeda (1912) described phagocytosis of freed spores of the actinomyxidan *Tetractinomyxon intermedium* and a microsporidan, *Nosema* sp., by the coelomic cells of sipunculids. Many of the ingested spores were partly or fully digested, but others appeared normal. Bang (1962) studied the response of *S. nudus* to injections of *Anophrys maggi*, a ciliate pathogenic to shore crabs *Carcinus maenas*. A lysin, produced by the worm after inoculation with ciliates, caused *in vitro* lysis in *A. maggi*. No disease was induced in the worms. Production of the lysin could likewise be stimulated by inoculation with heavy suspensions of live or heat-killed *Vibrio* sp. The substance was also present in sipunculids having a disease which was apparently caused by a flagellate burrowing into the surface epithelium of *S. nudus*, producing ulcerations and papules. Ciliates other than *A. maggi* were attacked likewise by the lysin which appeared shortly after the worms had been inoculated, then was lost, and reappeared after one or two days (Bang and Bang, 1962; Bang, 1966).

Phascolosoma agassizi, on the other hand, proved to be susceptible to lethal invasion by protozoans (and bacteria) normally present in sea water. Stress such as increased water temperature, decreased aeration or debilitation due to previous treatment or exposure to an infectious agent resulted in increased disease susceptibility. Signs of stress were loss of contractibility, flaccidness, disturbed osmotic control resulting in water uptake and destruction of normal cellular coelom constituents.

A ciliate isolated from *Phascolosoma agassizi* and maintained in axenic culture failed to stimulate observable lysins when injected into healthy worms. The protozoan caused a lethal infestation, however, in a laboratory population of *P. agassizi*. Transmission occurred via the ambient sea water. Test worms were able to eliminate up to $2·65 \times 10^3$ ciliates injected into their coelom (Blitz, 1966).

DISEASES CAUSED BY METAZOANS

Agents: Trematoda

Stehle (1954) studied the effect of cercarial invasion on sipunculids *Phascolosoma vulgare*, *P. elongatum*, *Phascolion strombi* and *Sipunculus nudus* from Roscoff, France. As revealed by histological examination, cercariae penetrating the brain of worms left a path of tissue destruction behind them which was characterized by abnormal connective

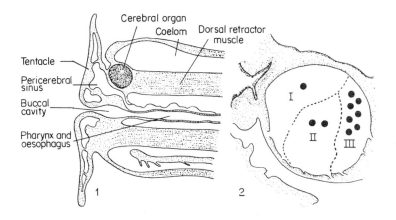

Fig. 9-9: *Phascolosoma vulgare*. 1: Longitudinal section through anterior part of proboscis showing position of cerebral organ; 2: longitudinal section through cerebral organ showing relative frequency of cercarial attack of different sectors. (After Stehle, 1954; reproduced by permission of Springer-Verlag.)

tissue, various degenerative processes in cells and nerve fibres, and atrophy. The brains of 16 out of 22 individuals were found to harbour encysted metacercariae which exhibited a marked preference for the posterior giant cell sector. Heavy infestations almost entirely destroyed the posterior brain sector; this destruction resulted in malfunction of the neurosecretory processes of the worms (Figs 9-9 and 9-10).

Encysted metacercariae were also found, but less frequently, at the basis of tentacles, in the connective tissue of the pharynx and between the fibres of the anterior retractor muscle, about 40% of the worms being infested. Lesions produced in these body parts were less severe than those in the brain. Metacercariae penetrating the body became surrounded by a cyst consisting of host-connective tissue, while those in the brain did not become encapsulated.

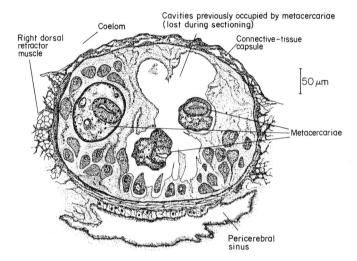

Fig. 9-10: *Phascolosoma elongatum*. Transverse section through cerebral organ at level of posterior sector, showing 3 metacercariae *in situ*. (After Stehle, 1954; reproduced by permission of Springer-Verlag.)

A parasite which resembled a larval distome trematode in the musculature of echiurids *Urechis chilensis* was found by Seitz (1907). Kozloff (1953) described a rhabdocoel turbellarian, *Collastoma pacifica*, from the gut of the sipunculid *Dendrostoma pyroides*, and Tétry (1959) mentioned *C. monorchis* from the intestine of *Golfingia vulgare*.

Agents: Cestoda

Unidentified larval tetraphyllidean tapeworms, 0·25 to 0·32 mm in length, have been found free in the proximal siphonal lumen of *Urechis caupo* from the North American Pacific coast. The worms were also seen in hernia-like swellings of the siphon wall, which appeared to be caused by them. Although no life-cycle studies have been conducted, stingrays *Myliobatus californicus*—the only animals in the area known to prey upon echiurids—were believed to harbour the adult stage (Fisher, 1946).

Agents: Mollusca

The fauna associated with sipunculids *Phascolion strombi* from the Swedish west coast was studied in detail by Hylleberg Kristensen (1970). The author identified some 17 species of associates, but careful ecological and experimental work revealed only the pyramidellid gastropod *Menestho diaphana* as a true parasite. The species had previously been described as *Odostomia perezi* from gastropod shells inhabited by *P. strombi* off Finistère, France (Dautzenberg and Fischer, 1925; Fig. 9-11).

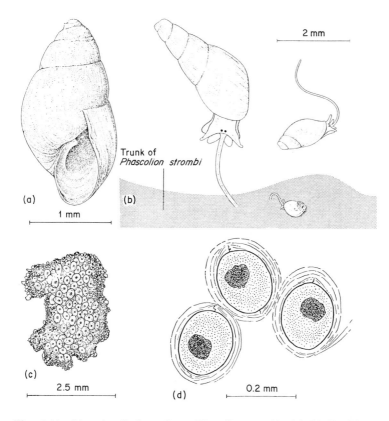

Fig. 9-11: *Menestho diaphana* from *Phascolion strombi*. (a) Shell; (b) two individuals in feeding position on host; third snail with everted proboscis, searching for host; (c) egg mass of *M. diaphana* from siphonal canal of *Nassarius* sp. shell inhabited by *P. strombi*. Eggs are embedded in colourless, sticky mucus with adhering mud particles; (d) eggs at higher magnification. (After Hylleberg Kristensen, 1970; reproduced by permission of Ophelia.)

Menestho diaphana feeds on the coelomic fluid and blood cells of its host by means of a long suctorial proboscis, which is injected into the coelomic cavity. Puncturing of the host's body wall is accomplished by a protrusible stylet, and feeding occurs by an alternation of sucking and stylet movement (Fig. 9-12). *M. diaphana* is an obligate ectoparasite, being chemotactically attracted to *P. strombi*. Its strict host-specificity has been ascertained by a number of choice experiments. The smallest snails collected from sipunculid habitations measured about 380×270 μm (dimensions of larval shell in juveniles), indicating that *M. diaphana* becomes associated with *P. strombi* at an early stage (Hylleberg Kristensen, 1970).

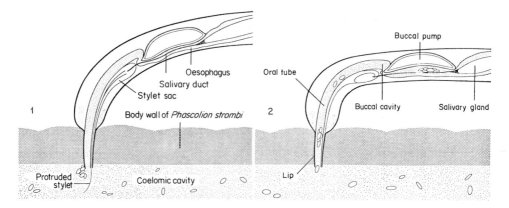

Fig. 9–12: *Menestho diaphana*. Feeding mechanism. 1: Protrusion of stylet into coelomic cavity of *Phascolion strombi;* no sucking occurs during piercing process. 2: After a few seconds, the stylet is withdrawn into the stylet sac; host blood and lumps of coelomic cells are sucked through the proboscis due to vigorous pumping of the buccal pump. (After Hylleberg Kristensen, 1970; reproduced by permission of Ophelia.)

Agents: Copepoda

A single female *Heliogabalus pulvauratus*, about 3·6 mm long, was described briefly from *Aspidosiphon levis* collected during the Siboga Expedition (Leigh-Sharpe, 1934). The structurally strongly modified copepod whose 3 pairs of pereiopods were reduced to stout chitinous stumps (Fig. 9-13) was recovered from the body surface of the sipunculid.

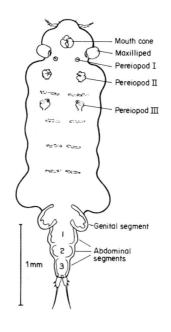

Fig. 9-13: *Heliogabalus pulvauratus*. Female, ventral aspect. (After Leigh-Sharpe, 1934; reproduced by permission of E. J. Brill.)

Åkessonia occulata (Fig. 9-14) lives in the coelomic cavity of sipunculids *Golfingia minuta* off the west coast of Sweden (Bresciani and Lützen, 1962). The large females, up to 1·6 mm in length, are readily discernible through the host's transparent body wall and are conspicuous by their violent pulsatory movements. The egg sacs are enormously long and lie curled up in the coelomic cavity, sometimes filling it entirely. Two males, 400 to 500 μm long, are normally attached to the female's abdomen. In the female, the labrum and labium are well developed and highly chitinized. In the male, no mouth opening was observed.

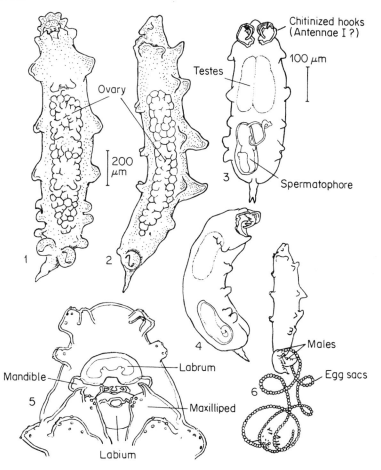

Fig. 9-14: *Åkessonia occulata*. Female (1, ventral view; 2, lateral aspect) and male (3, ventral view; 4, lateral view); 5: buccal area of female; 6: female with attached males and egg sacs. (After Bresciani and Lützen, 1962; reproduced by permission of Dansk naturhistorisk Forening.)

Almost all *Golfingia minuta* from Gullmar Fjord (Sweden) were parasitized. Each host harboured a single female (with attached males). Infested sipunculids exhibited parasitic castration (Bresciani and Lützen, 1962). The only other internal parasitic copepod known to invade sipunculids is *Siphonobius gephyreicola*, reported from *Aspidosiphon brocki* and incompletely described by Augener (1903).

TUMOURS AND ABNORMALITIES

Reports on tumours and abnormalities are rare among sipunculids, priapulids and echiurids. Tumours have been reported only on two occasions, both from *Sipunculus nudus* (Hérubel, 1906; Ladreyt, 1922a, b). In the light of modern science, it appears, however, doubtful that these abnormal growths represent true malignancy (Scharrer and Lochhead, 1950). The above-mentioned reports have been analyzed in detail by Sparks (1969, 1972) and the interpretation given below is essentially his.

Hérubel (1906) gave the first description of a tumour on the right posterior third of a specimen of *S. nudus* from Roscoff, France. The growth appeared to be of particular interest, since it was the first observed among the more than 1000 sipunculids the author had dissected over a number of years. It had an oval base, approximately 1 cm in diameter, and an elevated hump, projecting outward for about 5 mm, and consisted of numerous cells compressed into a hollow cavity within the skin, extending from the epidermis and cuticle on the top to the circular muscles of the integument on the bottom. Microscopical sections showed degenerating muscle fibres, some of which were in the process of being phagocytized by amoebocytes. Hérubel diagnosed the structure as a muscle tumour, presumably induced by parasites. Since no illustrations are given in the paper, it is impossible to decide whether the abnormal growth actually represented a tumour or, as seems more likely, a heavy leukocytic response to an injury. A hollow cavity filled with cells is a more convincing description of an abscess than a tumour (Sparks, 1969, 1972).

Abnormal growth of the dorsal Poli canal in *Sipunculus nudus*, described in detail by Ladreyt (1922a), was considered to be neoplastic. The tumour originated from the endothelium of the anterior third of the oesophageal tube, and appeared at the opening of the coelom like a voluminous, reddish-grey and brownish pea, projecting into the coelomic cavity. Normally, the cells forming the external and internal linings of the Poli canals are either nonciliated, flattened elements or ciliated cells of undulating shape, giving rise to the formation of blood elements, such as urn cells and haemocytes. In the diseased sipunculid, all cells of the vascular endothelium were of the simple, flattened type, with no sign of differentiation into blood cells. This 'precancerous' stage of dedifferentiation was accompanied by hypertrophy, amitosis, frequent multipolar mitoses and nuclear fragmentation in cells of the Poli canal walls. Fully grown cancerous cells were greatly elongated with free extremities more or less inflated and containing voluminous nuclei, irregular or globular in shape and rich in chromatin. The entire tumour consisted of a massive aggregate of one or more layers of these atypical, hypertrophied cells. According to the author, the dedifferentiation of the Poli canal cells was accompanied by a progressive loss of functional capacity, no traces of respiratory pigment or excretory activity being left in the fully transformed cells.

Ladreyt (1922a) emphasized that hyperplastic growths associated with inflammation are common in invertebrates, and are most frequently granulomas induced by parasitic activities. He states, however, that the abnormal growth in question was obviously quite different from that type of hyperplasia, and thus, considered it a complex malignant tumour which he called an endoperithelioma. In a consecutive publication (Ladreyt, 1922b), he posed the question of whether the formation of endothelial neoplasms in the sipunculids might be induced by protozoans (*Urospora* sp.?) or foreign matter, such as sponge spicules or sea-urchin spines ingested with the sand in which the animals live.

Despite the lengthy descriptions and discussions, no illustrations accompany Ladreyt's (1922a, b) papers. Other authors have not considered the evidence sufficient for a positive diagnosis of malignancy of the sipunculid tumour in question and, as has been pointed out by Scharrer and Lochhead (1950), the lack of photomicrographs or any illustrations makes conclusive interpretations difficult, if not impossible. Sparks (1969) could not help wondering how Ladreyt (1922a) could ascertain so much about the origin and development of the tumour in *Sipunculus nudus* when only one specimen, and that apparently fully developed, was available for study.

Literature Cited (Chapter 9)

Arvy, L. (1952). Sur deux parasites de *Phascolion strombi* Montagu. *Bull. Lab. marit. Dinard*, **36**, 7–13.

Augener, H. (1903). Zur Kenntnis der Gephyreen. *Arch. Naturgesch.*, **69**.

Bang, F. B. (1962). Serological aspects of immunity in invertebrates. *Nature, Lond.*, **196**, 88–89.

Bang, F. B. (1966). Serologic response in a marine worm, *Sipunculus nudus*. *J. Immun.*, **96**, 960–972.

Bang, F. B. and Bang, B. G. (1962). Studies on sipunculid blood: Immunologic properties of coelomic fluid and morphology of 'urn cells'. *Cah. Biol. mar.*, **3**, 363–374.

Bang, F. B. and Krassner, S. M. (1958). Antibacterial activity of *Phascolosoma gouldii* blood. *Biol. Bull. mar. biol. Lab., Woods Hole*, **115**, 343.

Blitz, R. R. (1966). The clearance of foreign material from the coelom of *Phascolosoma agassizi*. *Diss. Abstr.*, **26**, 3584.

Brasil, L. and Fantham, H. B. (1907). Sur l'existence chez les sipunculides de schizogrégarines appartenant à la famille des Selenidiidae. *C. r. hebd. Séanc. Acad. Sci., Paris*, **144**, 518–520.

Bresciani, J. and Lützen, J. (1962). Parasitic copepods from the west coast of Sweden including some new or little known species. *Vidensk. Meddr dansk naturh. Foren.*, **124**, 367–408.

Cutler, E. B. and Murina, V. V. (1977). On the sipunculan genus *Golfingia* Lankester, 1885. *Zool. J. linn. Soc.*, **60**, 173–187.

Dautzenberg, Ph. and Fischer, P. H. (1925). Les mollusques marins du Finistère. *Trav. Stn biol. Roscoff*, **3**, 1–180.

Dogiel, V. (1907). Beiträge zur Kenntnis der Gregarinen. II. *Schizocystis sipunculi* n.sp. *Arch. Protistenk.*, **8**, 203–215.

Fisher, W. K. (1946). Echiuroid worms of the North Pacific Ocean. *Proc. U.S. natn. Mus.*, **96**, 215–292.

Frenzel, J. (1885). Über einige in Seethieren lebende Gregarinen. *Arch. mikrosk. Anat. EntwMech.*, **24**, 545–588.

Greeff, R. (1880). Die Echiuren. VII. Parasiten der Echiuren. *Nova Acta Acad. Caesar. Leop. Carol.*, **41**, 128–131.

Hérubel, M. A. (1906). Sur une tumeur chez un invertébré (*Sipunculus nudus*). *C. r. hebd. Séanc. Acad. Sci., Paris*, **143**, 979–981.

Hukui, T. (1939). On the gregarines from *Siphonosoma cumanense* (Keferstein) Spengel. *J. Sci. Hiroshima Univ.* (Ser. 3), **7**, 1–23.

Hylleberg Kristensen, J. (1970). Fauna associated with the sipunculid *Phascolion strombi* (Montagu), especially the parasitic gastropod *Menestho diaphana* (Jeffreys). *Ophelia*, **7**, 257–276.

Iitsuka, S. (1933). Two new gregarines from *Urechis unicinctus* von Drasch. *J. Sci. Hiroshima Univ.* (Ser. B), **2**, 193–204.

Ikeda, I. (1912). Studies on some sporozoan parasites of sipunculoids. I. The life-history of a new actinomyxidian, *Tetractinomyxon intermedium* g. et sp. nov. *Arch. Protistenk.*, **25**, 240–275.

Ikeda, I. (1914). Studies on some sporozoan parasites of sipunculoids. II. *Dobellia binucleata*, n.g., n.sp.; a new coccidian from the gut of *Petalostoma minutum* Keferst. *Arch. Protistenk.*, **33**, 205–246.

Janiszewska, J. (1955). Actinomyxidia. Morphology, ecology, history of investigations, systematics, development. *Acta parasit. pol.*, **2**, 405–437.

Johnson, P. T. (1968). *An Annotated Bibliography of Pathology in Invertebrates other than Insects*, Burgess, Minneapolis.

Jones, I. (1974). Comparative observations on blood sporozoa of sipunculids. In *Proceedings of the 3rd International Congress of Parasitology, Munich*, **3**, 1722–1723.

Kaestner, A. (1954–1963). *Lehrbuch der Speziellen Zoologie*, VEB Fischer, Jena.

Kozloff, E. N. (1953). *Collastoma pacifica* sp. nov., a rhabdocoel turbellarian from the gut of *Dendrostoma pyroides* Chamberlin. *J. Parasit.*, **39**, 336–339.

Krassner, S. M. (1963). Further studies on an antibacterial factor in the blood of *Phascolosoma gouldii*. *Biol. Bull. mar. biol. Lab., Woods Hole*, **125**, 382–383.

Ladreyt, F. (1922a). Sur une tumeur cancéreuse du siponcle (*Sipunculus nudus* L.). *Bull. Inst. océanogr. Monaco*, **405**, 1–8.

Ladreyt, F. (1922b). Unicité évolutive et pluralité étiologique des tumeurs cancéreuses chez quelques animaux marins (rousettes, raies, tortues, siponcles). Faits et théories. *Bull. Inst. océanogr. Monaco*, **414**, 1–16.

Lankester, E. R. (1881). On *Thalassema neptuni* Gaertner. *Zool. Anz.*, **4**, 350–356.

Leigh-Sharpe, W. H. (1934). The Copepoda of the Siboga Expedition. Part II. Commensal and parasitic Copepoda. *Siboga Exped.*, **24b**, 1–43.

Lüling, K. H. (1942). Über eine neue Coccidie im Darm der Priapuliden: *Priapulus caudatus* (Lam.) und *Halicryptus spinulosus* (v. Sieb.). *Arch. Protistenk.*, **96**, 39–74.

Mackinnon, D. L. and Ray, H. N. (1929). Lankester's 'gregarine' from the eggs of *Thalassema neptuni*. *Nature, Lond.*, **124**, 877.

Mackinnon, D. L. and Ray, H. N. (1931a). Observations on dicystid gregarines from marine worms. *Q. Jl microsc. Sci.* (Ser. 2), **74**, 439–466.

Mackinnon, D. L. and Ray, H. N. (1931b). A new protozoon, *Hyperidion thalassemae* n.gen., n.sp., from the intestine of *Thalassema neptuni* Gärtner. *Q. Jl microsc. Sci.*, **74**, 467–475.

Mackinnon, D. L. and Ray, H. N. (1937). A coccidian from the eggs of *Thalassema neptuni* Gaertner. *Parasitology*, **29**, 457–468.

Noble, E. R. (1938a). The life cycle of *Zygosoma globosum* sp.nov., a gregarine parasite of *Urechis caupo*. *Univ. Calif. Publs Zool.*, **43**, 41–65.

Noble, E. R. (1938b). A new gregarine from *Urechis caupo*. *Trans. Am. microsc. Soc.*, **57**, 142–146.

Noble, G. (1940). *Trichodina urechi* n.sp., an entozoic ciliate from the echiuroid worm, *Urechis caupo*. *J. Parasit.*, **26**, 387–405.

Pixell-Goodrich, H. L. (1950). Sporozoa of *Sipunculus*. *Q. Jl microsc. Sci.* (Ser. 2), **91**, 469–476.

Rabin, H. and Bang, F. B. (1963). Studies on the antibacterial activity of *Golfingia gouldi* coelomic fluid. *Biol. Bull. mar. biol. Lab., Woods Hole*, **125**, 388.

Rabin, H. and Bang, F. B. (1964). In vitro studies of the antibacterial activity of *Golfingia gouldi* (Pourtalès) coelomic fluid. *J. Insect Pathol.*, **6**, 457–465.

Scharrer, B. and Lochhead, M. S. (1950). Tumors in the invertebrates: a review. *Cancer Res.*, **10**, 403–419.

Seitz, P. (1907). Der Bau von *Echiurus chilensis* (*Urechis* n.g. *chilensis*). *Zool. Jb.* (Anat. Ontogenie Tiere), **24**, 323–356.

Sparks, A. K. (1969). Review of tumors and tumor-like conditions in Protozoa, Coelenterata, Platyhelminthes, Annelida, Sipunculida, and Arthropoda, excluding insects. *Natn. Cancer Inst. Monogr.*, **31**, 671–682.

Sparks, A. K. (1972). *Invertebrate Pathology, Noncommunicable Diseases*, Academic Press, New York and London.

Stehle, G. (1954). Die gewebezerstörende Wirkung von Cercarien in Rüssel und Gehirn verschiedener Sipunculiden. *Z. ParasitKde*, **16**, 353–362.

Tétry, A. (1959). Classe des sipunculiens. In P.-P. Grassé (Ed.), *Traité de Zoologie*, Vol. V. Masson et Cie, Paris. pp. 785–854.

Thomas, J.-A. (1931). Sur l'infection du géphyrien *Sipunculus nudus* par le *Bacterium tumefaciens* Sm. *C. r. Séanc. Soc. Biol.*, **108**, 772–774.

Wesenberg-Lund, E. (1963). South African sipunculids and echiuroids from coastal waters. *Vidensk. Meddr dansk naturh. Foren.*, **125**, 101–146.

ZoBell, C. E. and Feltham, C. B. (1938). Bacteria as food for certain marine invertebrates. *J. mar. Res.*, **1**, 312–327.

10. DISEASES OF PLATYHELMINTHES

G. LAUCKNER

The phylum Platyhelminthes comprises the classes Turbellaria, Trematoda and Cestoda. Most of the Turbellaria are free-living; only a few are parasitic. The two other classes consist entirely of parasitic forms. Trematodes and cestodes are frequently attacked by Protozoa, particularly sporozoans. Parasitism in parasites has been termed 'hyperparasitism'. Experimental hyperparasitism has been repeatedly suggested as a means of biological control. Many kinds of abnormalities in Platyhelminthes, both larval and adult, have also been reported. In this section, some information has been included on parasites and structural abnormalities of non-marine platyhelminths. We hope that this will stimulate comparable research on marine flatworms and expect that such investigations will reveal parallelisms in non-marine and marine platyhelminths.

A general review of the physiology, life cycles and phylogeny of parasitic flatworms has been presented by Stunkard (1937). Dollfus (1946) authored a lengthy treatment of the literature on parasites of helminths, and Johnson (1968) assembled an annotated list of references on diseases and abnormalities in Platyhelminthes.

DISEASES CAUSED BY MICRO-ORGANISMS

Agents: Viruses

Endonuclear inclusions, which appear to be viruses, have been described from cells of laboratory-cultivated, acoelous marine turbellarians *Convoluta roscoffensis* (Oschman, 1969). The inclusion structures are approximately 1000 Å in diameter and hexagonal in shape. Many of the particles were found to be arranged in parallel rows. If accepted provisionally as a virus, the structures described seem to be the first of their kind found in platyhelminths.

Flatworms may act as vectors for viral diseases of higher animals, without being affected by the agents themselves. Thus, *Neorickettsia helminthoeca*, responsible for the usually fatal disease of dogs referred to in America as 'salmon poisoning disease', is transmitted by the metacercariae of *Nanophyetus salmincola* found encysted in salmonid fishes. The canids acquire the virus infection by eating contaminated salmon (Philip, 1955). The role of helminths in the transmission of viruses and bacteria has been briefly reviewed by Stefanski (1959).

Agents: Bacteria

A bacterial disease of the acoelous marine turbellarian *Archaphanostoma agile*, occurring in a laboratory-cultivated population, has been described by Apelt (1969). Infected *A.*

agile left a trace of mucus behind them; finally, disintegration occurred, starting at the tip of the tail. Succumbed specimens became purple-red in colour, and were overrun with bacteria. The disease, which was termed 'red pest', sometimes killed the entire population of a culture dish within a day. Addition of 0·25 g p-Amino-benzene-sulphonacetamide ('Albucid') per litre sea water prevented outbreaks of the disease without affecting the turbellarians.

Apelt (1969) also observed another disease of unknown, but presumably non-bacterial etiology in cultivated *A. agile* and *Pseudaphanostoma psammophilum*, which he termed 'bubble disease'. Affected individuals developed large vacuoles in the peripheral parenchyma which sometimes became filled with diatoms. These, however, were not digested, but even multiplied. Bubble-diseased turbellarians ceased to produce eggs; they were unable to take up food during an advanced stage of the disease. Bubble formation and death could not be attributed to senescence (Fig. 10-1).

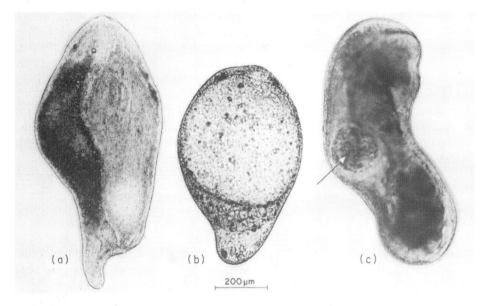

Fig. 10-1: 'Bubble disease' in turbellarians. (a) *Pseudaphanostoma psammophilum* with bubbles in peripheral parenchyma constricting central parenchyma. (b) Advanced stage of 'bubble disease'. Affected individuals stop feeding, become smaller and eventually die. (c) *Archaphanostoma agile* with vacuole in peripheral parenchyma containing undigested diatoms (arrow). (After Apelt, 1969; reproduced by permission of Springer-Verlag.)

Agents: Fungi

Fungus diseases have, thus far, only been found in freshwater platyhelminths, where they appear to be of frequent occurrence. Buckley and Clapham's (1929) paper is of particular interest because it discusses experimental fungus infection of helminth eggs as a possible means of biological control of helminthiases. Liver fluke *Fasciola hepatica* and tapeworm *Hymenolepis diminuta* and *Dibothriocephalus latus* ova were experimentally infected with and destroyed by the two chytrid fungi *Catenaria anguillulae* and

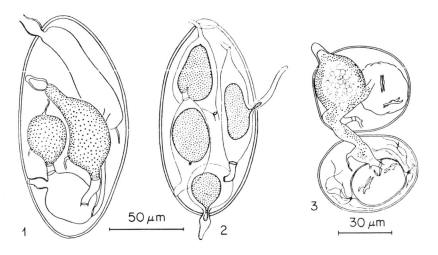

Fig. 10-2: *Catenaria anguillulae*. 1: *Fasciola hepatica* ovum with typical infection; 2: ovum with 4 resting spores; 3: two infected *Hymenolepis diminuta* eggs in which the mycelium has penetrated the thin shell and attacked another adjacent ovum. (After Buckley and Clapham, 1929; reproduced by permission of London School of Hygiene and Tropical Medicine.)

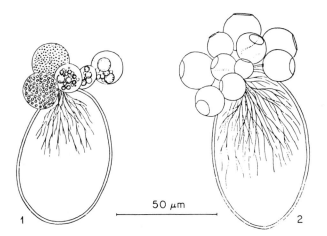

Fig. 10-3: *Rhizophydium carpophilum*. 1: *Dibothriocephalus latus* ovum with sporangia in different stages of development; 2: egg with a bunch of dehisced sporangia. Note internal mycelium. (After Buckley and Clapham, 1929; reproduced by permission of London School of Hygiene and Tropical Medicine.)

Rhizophydium carpophilum (Figs 10-2 and 10-3). Laboratory tap water appeared to be the vehicle for the fungi. Butler and Humphries (1932) succeeded in cultivating *C. anguillulae* in artificial media containing aqueous extracts of *F. hepatica* ova. Growth in the cultivated fungus was much more extensive than when the agent was growing as a parasite (Fig. 10-4).

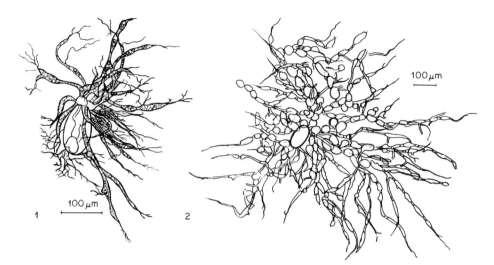

Fig. 10-4: *Catenaria anguillulae*. Outgrowth of mycelium from *Fasciola hepatica* ova in artificial medium. 1: Outgrowth from single thallus showing 21 hyphal strands; 2: outgrowth of mycelium from infected ovum showing over 270 sporangia in which dehiscence and discharge of spores had occurred. (After Butler and Humphries, 1932; reproduced by permission of Proceedings of the Royal Dublin Society.)

DISEASES CAUSED BY PROTOZOANS

Agents: Flagellata

A mastigophoran of the genus *Hexamita* has been found hyperparasitic in the reproductive system of *Deropristis inflata,* a trematode living in the digestive tract of *Anguilla chrysypa* and other marine fishes (Hunninen and Wichterman, 1938). The flagellate lives in the eggs and uterus of the flatworm. Heavily infested eggs harboured 20 or even more parasites and did not give rise to the development of miracidia. The pyriform organism (Fig. 10-5) measured from 7·7 to 14·3 μm in length and 3·3 to 6·7 μm in width. The cytoplasm of affected ova was found to be destroyed or used up by the protozoans in their metabolic activities, thus showing their parasitic nature. Eggs containing developed miracidia never harboured *Hexamita* sp.

Examination of 124 *Deropristis inflata* from 35 *Anguilla chrysypa* revealed infestations in trematodes from 20 of the eels; the other 15 harboured non-infested flukes. The worms in 14, 2, 2 and 2 of these eels were 100, 75, 50 and 33% infested, respectively. In hosts where the trematodes were heavily infested with the protozoans, every single individual harboured the flagellates in large numbers. *Hexamita* sp. appeared to be host-specific. The organism was not found in 23 *Zoogonus rubellus* or in 16 hemiurids that also live in *A. chrysypa.* The flagellates were also conspicuously absent from the intestinal contents of eels harbouring infested trematodes. Moreover, a total of 88 *A. chrysypa,* free of *D. inflata,* were examined and none of them harboured flagellates in the intestinal contents or in the mucosa. How *D. inflata* acquired the *Hexamita* sp. infestation remained, therefore, unexplained. It was suspected that the eels (which at the time they were examined were negative for *Hexamita* sp.) may have harboured the agent at an earlier stage of their life and later were freed of these protozoans whereas the trematodes acquired their hyperparasites via their hosts' intestinal route.

Flagellated protozoans, actively moving and resembling *Chilomastix* species, occurred within the intestinal caeca of trematodes *Lepocreadium trulla* living in the digestive tract of marine teleosts *Ocyurus chrysurus* at Tortugas, Gulf of Mexico (Manter, 1930). The protozoans were not found free among the intestinal contents of the fish host.

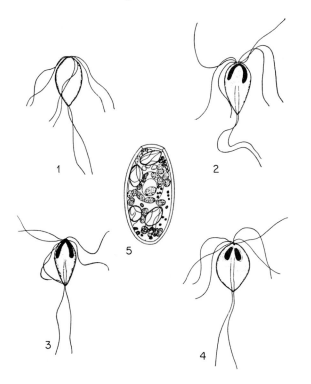

Fig. 10-5: *Hexamita* sp. from reproductive system of *Deropristis inflata*. 1: Typical view of living individual showing 6 anterior and 2 posterior flagella; 2, 3, 4: fixed and stained specimens showing flagella, nuclei and axostyles; 5: egg of *D. inflata* as seen in uterus, containing 4 living *Hexamita* sp. in addition to yolk material and other inclusions. (After Hunninen and Wichterman, 1938; reproduced by permission of Journal of Parasitology.)

Agents: Sporozoa

Several species of gregarines, mostly members of the genus *Monocystella*, have been reported from a number of freshwater turbellarians (Vandel, 1921; see Valkanov, 1935, and de Puytorac and Grain, 1960, for references).

Freshwater planarians *Otomesostoma auditivum* harboured coccidians *Eucoccidium monoti* in their gut epithelium and adjacent parenchyma. Macrogamonts were oval, up to 30 × 45 μm in size, and microgamonts were spherical, measuring 19 to 22 μm in diameter. Autoinfestation may lead to the accumulation of considerable numbers of parasites in individual hosts (Reisinger, 1959).

Most of the Protozoa infesting Platyhelminthes belong to the subphylum Microspora (Sprague, 1969). They particularly invade larval trematodes. Léger (1897) described

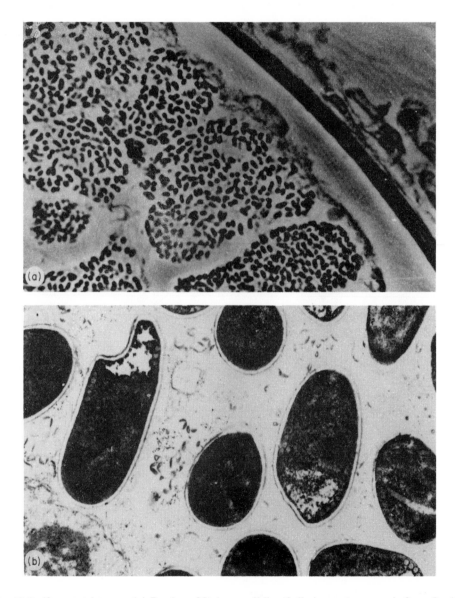

Fig. 10-6: *Nosema spelotremae*. (a) Portion of *Spelotrema (Microphallus)* sp. metacercaria from *Carcinus maenas* containing clusters of *N. spelotremae* spores. Stained toluidine blue. × 720. (b) Electron micrograph of *N. spelotremae* spores. At posterior ends are cross sections of coiled polar filaments. × 15650. (After Stanier and co-authors, 1968; reproduced by permission of Academic Press.)

microsporidans (which he referred to the genus *Glugea*) from the trematode *Brachycoelium* sp., parasitic in *Donax vittatus, Tellina fabula* and other marine pelecypods. The trematode, first reported by Giard (1897), is probably a gymnophallid metacercaria (see Chapter 12). Infested metacercariae were opaque, somewhat larger and less active than normal ones. Restudied by Dollfus (1912) and named *Nosema legeri*, the parasite was found to infest metacercariae of *Gymnophallus gibberosus* (erroneously described as *G. somateriae strigatus* in the original paper) occurring in *Donax vittatus* from the French Atlantic coast. The spores of *N. legeri* are ovoidal, $2 \cdot 5 \times 5$ μm, and have a conspicuous posterior vacuole. They appear in parenchyma and other tissues of the host, infesting and killing essentially all metacercariae in a particular pelecypod, while not affecting the host. Dubois (1907) found spores in gymnophallid metacercariae, recovered from the pearl oyster *Margaritifera margaritifera*, which he considered to be close to or identical with those described by Léger from other marine bivalves. Dollfus pointed out that Jameson (1902), assuming that he was figuring normal *G. gibberosus* in *Mytilus edulis*, apparently dealt with metacercariae infested with *Nosema* sp.

Bucephalus cuculus, parasitic in oysters *Crassostrea virginica*, has been found infested by *Nosema dollfusi* (Sprague, 1964). The spores of this species are smaller than those of *N. legeri*, measuring 3×2 μm. *N. dollfusi* develops in the cytoplasm of cells in the sporocyst wall. The cytoplasm of infested cells may be greatly hypertrophied. Eventually, lysis occurs. A species of *Nosema* infested metacercariae of *Meiogymnophallus minutus* in cockles *Cardium edule* from South Wales (Bowers and James, 1967). The incidence of infestation varied irregularly from month to month, from 5% to 26% of all cockles harbouring the hyperparasite. Cockles under three years old very rarely contained hyperparasitized metacercariae. Whenever infestation occurred, most of the metacercariae within a particular host were affected. The spores of the microsporidan caused the body to enlarge (sometimes to almost twice the normal size) and to become opaque and greyish white. The authors believe that the hyperparasite kills the larval trematodes.

A microsporidan hyperparasite of larval trematodes in marine Crustacea is *Nosema spelotremae*, which occurs in the encysted metacercariae of *Microphallus similis* in shore crabs *Carcinus maenas* (Guyénot and co-authors, 1925; Stunkard, 1957). Infested metacercariae become enlarged, and are completely destroyed. Stanier and co-authors (1968) studied the ultrastructure of *N. spelotremae* by means of electron microscopy (Fig. 10-6).

How larval trematodes occurring in marine hosts become infested with microsporidans has not been investigated. Cort and co-authors (1960a, b) achieved experimental transmission of a *Nosema* hyperparasite in 12 species of larval freshwater strigeoid trematodes by feeding its spores to the snail hosts. The microsporidan—later described as a new species, *Nosema strigeoideae*—and its pathogenicity have been studied in detail by Hussey (1971). In contrast to the above-mentioned microsporidans infesting metacercariae, this species attacks the sporocyst and cercarial stages of the host. Primary infestation appears to be in the sporocyst wall, spreading from there to the developing cercarial embryos. In living *N. strigeoideae*-infested sporocysts, masses of developing stages and mature spores filled the enlarged cuticular-wall cells and protruded into the sporocyst cavity. Attack of germinal masses and embryos at various stages of development appeared to destroy cells and to cause bloating; in mature, heavy infestations the sporocysts finally contained only spores, loose cells, masses of disorganized material and some greatly injured cercarial embryos. Even though heavily infested with mature spores and sometimes grossly distorted, nearly mature and mature cercariae remained alive and showed considerable movement, although little coordination and thus little locomotion.

Trematodes may carry over their hyperparasites from the cercarial to the metacercarial stage. Thus, cercariae of several species emerging from freshwater snails in the Woods Hole region (Massachusetts, USA) were found to harbour a (not further specified but apparently microsporidan) sporozoan parasite. In crushed snails, the sporozoan was observed in both snail and trematode tissues. One of the species of cercariae, an echinostome, encysted in the host snails and retained the sporozoan in the metacercarial stage (Martin, 1936).

Microsporidan infestations of Cestoda are known only from nonmarine species. Guyénot and co-authors (1922) reported a microsporidan infestation of a larval cestode, parasitic in the snake *Tropidonotus natrix*. The larvae were eventually killed by the hyperparasite, leaving only a granular pulp. Dollfus (1923) described a microsporidan, probably a species of *Pleistophora*, from a fish cestode, and Dissanaike (1955, 1957a, b, 1958) recorded *Nosema helminthorum*, a hyperparasite of anoplocephalid cestodes of the genus *Monieza*.

Little is known about the host-specificity of Microsporida parasitic in Platyhelminthes. Martin (1936), for instance, reported a microsporidan found in cercariae emerging from *Succinea* sp. It was not limited to a single trematode species, and was also observed in the tissues of the snail host. Brumpt (1936), on the other hand, mentioned *Nosema echinostomi*, which frequently parasitizes the cercariae and rediae of freshwater echinostome trematodes. The hyperparasite, in this instance, showed some host-specificity, for it did not attack other species of trematodes inhabiting the same mollusc.

Although, in most cases discussed above, virtually all trematodes are killed in microsporidan hyperinfestation, this is not invariably the case. Cort and co-authors (1960a) reported *Nosema* infestation of sporocysts and cercariae of various strigeoid trematodes from freshwater snails. Only a small portion of the naturally occurring hyperinfestations were found to be spore-producing, and only a fraction of the total number of larval trematodes were infested. In most cases, the injury was slight, and did not greatly decrease cercarial production. Emerging cercariae were always free of *Nosema* infestation. The authors' field observations were markedly contrasted to experimental infestations carried out by Cort and co-authors (1960b). Experimental transmission of the hyperparasite was achieved by feeding spores to snails. Very large spore doses were used, and almost all of the experimental infestations were extraordinarily heavy, affecting most of the larval trematodes. Development was rapid, spores being produced within about 2 weeks of exposure; after 3 weeks, they were present in enormous numbers. The authors suggested that the difference might be due to some type of resistance, evolving in natural infestations by ingestion of only a few spores within a given time interval. In contrast, with the enormous numbers of spores ingested by the snails within a very short time, such resistance may have been prevented from developing. Since the *Nosema* used in the study infested 12 different species of strigeoids in the same area, it obviously lacks host-specificity. Moderate development may, thus, also be the expression of poor adaptation by the hyperparasite to a comparably new host.

A review summarizing information on 15 species of Microsporida reported as hyperparasites of trematodes (12) and cestodes (3) has been presented by Canning (1975). It contains a bibliography with 35 titles.

In addition to the Microsporida mentioned, a number of Haplosporida have been reported as hyperparasites of larval trematodes from marine pelecypods and crustaceans. *Urosporidium pelseneeri* parasitizes the sporocysts of *Cercaria pectinata* in clams *Donax vittatus* from Boulogne, French Atlantic coast. This haplosporidan was originally described by Caullery and Chappellier (1906) who failed to observe the delicate 'tails' on the spores (Fig. 10-7) and hence established the genus *Anurosporidium*. Cépède (1911)

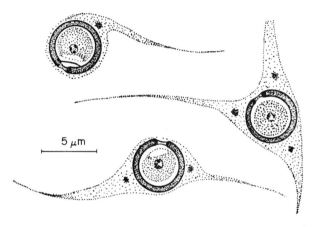

Fig. 10-7: *Urosporidium pelseneeri*, haplosporidan hyperparasite of *Cercaria pectinata* from *Donax vittatus* and
Barnea candida. Spores reveal structural details and
variable number of tails. (After Sprague, 1970b;
reproduced by permission of American Fisheries Society.)

further discussed the affinities of the parasite. Finally, Dollfus (1925, 1946) made a new study, found tails and abolished the genus *Anurosporidium*. The host of *U. pelseneeri*, *Cercaria pectinata*, had previously been studied by Pelseneer (1895) who mistook parasitized sporocysts for normal ones. However, according to Dollfus (1925), normal sporocysts are white or yellowish whereas parasitized ones are deep violet or blackish. Caullery and Chappellier (1906) observed intracellular schizogonic stages of *U. pelseneeri* within the sporocyst wall of *C. pectinata*. Advanced stages and spores accumulate in vast numbers in the sporocyst cavity. Development of the parasite is fast. In recently infested host sporocysts, germinal masses and cercariae in various stages of development occur side by side with the pathogen. In advanced infestations, however, the sporocyst lumen is completely overwhelmed by haplosporidan spores which measure about 5 to 5·5 μm in diameter and possess a variable number of protoplasmic processes (Fig. 10-7). If an infestation occurs, all sporocysts in a given pelecypod host are affected. Apparently, establishment of the haplosporidan occurs at a very early stage in the life history of the trematode host, possibly in the miracidium.

A haplosporidan, similar to, or identical with, the organism found in *Donax vittatus*, has been observed to parasitize the sporocysts of an undetermined trematode in *Barnea candida* from Wimereux, French Atlantic coast (Guyénot, 1943; Fig. 10-8). While the author comments on the absence of spore tails, Dollfus (1946), who restudied the parasite, found tails. He identified the sporocysts from *B. candida* as *Cercaria pectinata* and concluded that the sporozoan is very probably *Urosporidium pelseneeri*.

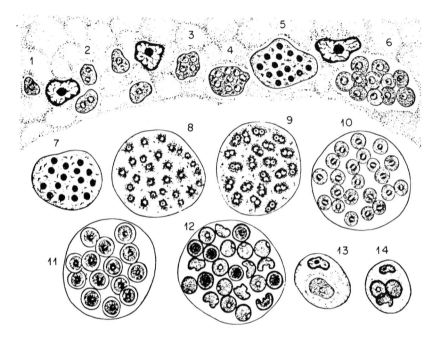

Fig. 10-8: *Urosporidium* (?) sp. Developmental stages of haplosporidan from trematode sporocysts in *Barnea candida*. 1–6: Schizogonic stages occurring in sporocyst wall. 1: Uninucleate schizont; 2 binucleate schizont; 3–5: plasmodia with 4, 8 and 16 nuclei; 6: decomposition of residual plasmodium and formation of new schizont generation. 7–12: Sporogonic stages occurring in sporocyst lumen. 7: Gametocyte; 8: gametes; 9: copulation; 10: zygotes; 11: sporoblasts; 12: spores. 13–14: Haemocyte of molluscan host phagocytizing schizont (13) and spores (14). (After Guyenot, 1943; reproduced by permission of Revue suisse de Zoologie.)

Urosporidium constantae parasitizes sporocysts of *Bucephalus longicornutus* in New Zealand mud oysters *Ostrea lutaria*, causing complete destruction of the cercarial embryos (Howell, 1967). The author discussed the hyperparasite's use in the biological control of *B. longicornutus*. However, the prevailing ecological situation as well as collection difficulties seem to preclude effective control.

Ormières and co-authors (1972, 1973) described *Urosporidium jiroveci*, another haplosporidan hyperparasite in sporocysts of *Gymnophallus nereicola* found in clams *Abra ovata* from Camargue, French Mediterranean coast. The sporozoan appeared to exhibit some degree of host-specificity since it did not occur in sporocysts of *Gymnophallus fossarum* in *Scrobicularia plana* living side by side with trematode-infested and hyperparasitized *A. ovata*. On the other hand, *U. jiroveci* attacked sporocysts of *Paratimonia gobii* but not those of *Cercaria plumosa* (Bartoli, 1974).

The number of *Gymnophallus nereicola* sporocysts affected by *Urosporidium jiroveci* in any one host varies considerably; only in extreme cases do all sporocysts harbour the sporozoan. Germinal masses are more easily infested than mature cercariae. As the number of parasites increases, the cercariae gradually disappear from the sporocyst lumen. Sporocysts overwhelmed by *U. jiroveci* are black in colour. The abundance of *U. jiroveci* infestations varies considerably with the season. During September/October, up to 75% of the trematode-infested *Abra ovata* were found to be hyperparasitized by the haplosporidan (Fig. 10-9). *U. jiroveci* infestations may be a limiting factor to *G. nereicola* parasitization in *A. ovata* (Bartoli, 1974).

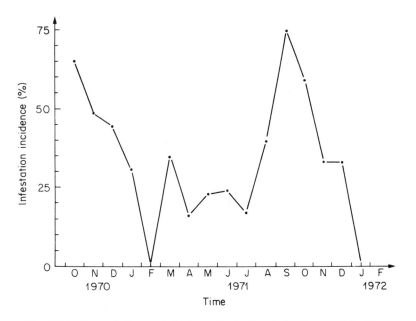

Fig. 10-9: *Gymnophallus nereicola* from *Nereis diversicolor*. Seasonal incidence of hyperparasitization by *Urosporidium jiroveci*. (After Bartoli, 1974; reproduced by permission of the author.)

Another, as yet unidentified, haplosporidan in sporocysts of *Bucephalus cuculus* from American oysters *Crassostrea virginica* was briefly described by Mackin and Loesch (1955). The spores of this species were large, 3 to 5 × 5 to 7 μm, and ovate. Sporocysts were destroyed by the hyperparasite, resulting in an intense cellular reaction by the oyster. According to Sprague (1970b), who reexamined slides obtained from the above-mentioned authors, the spores of this haplosporidan bore no resemblance to those of *Urosporidium*. Haplosporida with plasmodial stages like those described by Mackin and Loesch (1955) have been found in a few cases as hyperparasites of *B. cuculus* in oysters from Maryland, USA, but there were no spores. Plasmodia were most frequently seen in the sporocyst lumen but also appeared intracellularly in the sporocyst wall. Plasmodia varied greatly in size and shape. The smaller ones were almost spherical with minimum diameters of 2·5 μm. Large ones were irregular in shape, measured up to 30 × 50 μm, and often had distinct pseudopodia (Sprague, 1970b).

The occurrence of a haplosporidan hyperparasite in *Donax variabilis* from the Texas coast has been briefly mentioned by Mackin and Loesch (1955). They believed that this hyperparasite was neither identical with that in *Bucephalus cuculus* from *Crassostrea virginica* in America nor with *Urosporidium pelseneeri* in *Cercaria pectinata* from *D. vittatus* in France.

A single haplosporidan hyperparasite has been reported from larval trematodes invading marine crustaceans. Thirty-two percent of 120 *Callinectes sapidus* at Beaufort (North Carolina, USA) harboured metacercariae of the microphallid *Megalophallus* sp., hyperparasitized by *Urosporidium crescens* (DeTurk, 1940). Spores are about 5 μm in diameter and possess and epispore prolonged into one tail (Fig. 10-10).

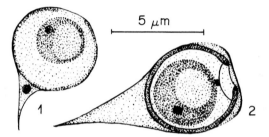

Fig. 10-10: *Urosporidium crescens*, haplosporidan hyperparasite of *Megalophallus* sp. from *Callinectes sapidus*. Immature (1) and mature (2) spore. (After Sprague, 1970a; reproduced by permission of American Fisheries Society.)

The brief description of DeTurk (1940), which misidentified the trematode host as *Spelotrema nicolli*, has been supplemented by a number of ecological observations summarized by Sprague (1970a). Perkins (1971) made a detailed study on the sporulation of *Urosporidium crescens* by means of electron microscopy. Earliest recognizable stages of the parasite are amoeboid-shaped plasmodia found between the connective-tissue cells of *Megalophallus* sp. While extensive lesions with many plasmodia were not found, these were distributed individually between host cells. The plasmodia did not appear to cause damage to the neighbouring connective-tissue cells. When sporulation occurred, large lacunae were established between the host cells accompanied by host-tissue lysis. Each lacuna contained a single sporont or group of spores. Parasitized metacercarial cysts were markedly hypertrophied, measuring up to 1 mm in diameter as compared with uninfested cysts of about 0·2 mm in diameter (Fig. 10-11). However, even though the metacercariae were overwhelmed by *U. crescens*, motility could still be observed in the encysted worms. Since the sporozoans were never observed in crab tissues and since dead infested metacercariae were not observed in living crabs, it was assumed that the haplosporidan is released from the trematode only upon death of the crab and subsequent release of the cyst from crab tissues. Spore liberation requires rupture of the worm cyst.

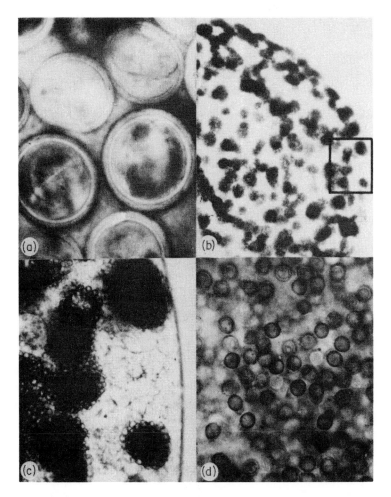

Fig. 10-11: *Urosporidium crescens*, hyperparasitic in metacercariae of *Megalophallus* sp. in *Callinectes sapidus*. (a) Normal metacercariae. × 130. (b) Margin of infested metacercaria at same magnification, demonstrating advance of hypertrophy. (c) Portion of same metacercaria as in b, magnified to 600 × and showing clusters of spores. (d) Spores magnified to 1300 ×. (After Sprague, 1970a; reproduced by permission of American Fisheries Society.)

Although *Urosporidium crescens* drastically alters the metacercariae of *Megalophallus* sp., it has no known effect on the crab host. Moreover, there is no evidence that the trematode causes mortalities in *Callinectes sapidus* even though large cyst numbers may be found in the musculature, hepatopancreas and gills. Infested metacercariae appear as conspicuous black specks, scattered throughout the body and at the bases of the host's gills. Crabs in which such black specks occur are commonly known as 'pepper crabs'. Meat from such diseased blue crabs is not readily marketable. Therefore, the *U. crescens—Megalophallus* sp. complex is commercially significant even though mortalities of *C. sapidus* are not involved.

Urosporidium sp., similar to or identical with *U. crescens*, was present in microphallid metacercariae in several shrimp *Palaemonetes pugio* from Sapelo Island, Georgia, USA (Sprague, 1970a).

Agents: Ciliata

Astomatous ciliates *Sieboldiellina planariarum* parasitize in the gut of freshwater triclads *Planaria torva* (Bishop, 1926). More remarkable is the occurrence of ciliates within the enteron of freshwater rhabdocoels *Stenostoma leucops*. Up to 50 individuals, measuring 40 to 50 μm in length, were seen in a single host. Undisturbed parasites settled down on the outer wall of the enteron but when disturbed they moved actively through the worm's mesenchymal tissue. The ciliates, named *Holophrya virginia*, did not appear to destroy the mesenchyme but apparently fed on nutrients carried by the host's body fluids (Kepner and Carroll, 1923). There are several other reports on ciliates from non-marine turbellarians.

DISEASES CAUSED BY METAZOANS

Agents: Mesozoa

Orthonectid mesozoans *Rhopalura paraphanostomae* occurred in the parenchyma of acoelous turbellarians *Paraphanostoma macroposthium* and *P. brachyposthium* in Scandinavian waters, the former species apparently being the favourite host. Adult *R. paraphanostomae* measured about 120 μm in length and 30 μm in width; juvenile individuals were 50 μm long. Frequently, virtually all *P. macroposthium* from a particular sampling station harboured the mesozoans which sometimes occupied the entire parenchyma. Thirty or even more parasites were recovered from individual turbellarians. Despite such intense infestation, the host was apparently little affected. No parasitic castration of male *Paraphanostoma* spp. occurred and spermatozoa were always produced in considerable quantities. In females, however, the gonad development was entirely suppressed (Westblad, 1942).

Agents: Turbellaria

There are some reports on helminth parasites of Platyhelminthes, both marine and non-marine. Two interesting cases, concerning the occurrence of turbellarians in turbellarians, are considered below.

One of several alloeocoelous turbellarians *Plagiostomum* sp. collected from deep waters in Godthaabfjord (Greenland), which appeared very sluggish, exhibited convex projections of its body surface as well as several yellowish oval bodies in its parenchyma. Examination of sectioned material revealed that the body distortions of the alloeocoel were caused by the presence, in the parenchyma, of 2 parasitic graffillid (provorticid) turbellarians, one 0·55 mm and the other 0·3 mm long. The yellowish bodies turned out to be egg capsules of the parasite at various stages of development (Fig. 10-12). The parasite, named *Oekiocolax plagiostomorum*, caused partial castration of the host, destroying its ovary. Testes and vitellaria were left unaffected (Reisinger, 1930). Unidentified rhabdocoels were found to parasitize acoels *Paraphanostoma crassum* (Westblad, 1942).

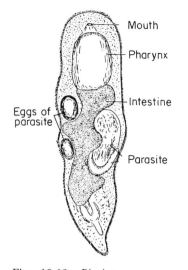

Fig. 10-12: *Plagiostomum* sp. parasitized by *Oekiocolax plagiostomorum*. × 70. (After Reisinger, 1930; reproduced by permission of Springer-Verlag.)

Agents: Trematoda

Frankenberg (1935) observed great numbers of encysted metacercariae in turbellarians *Planaria polychroa* kept in aquaria. Echinostomatid cercariae emerged from snails *Planorbis corneus*, and penetrated the planarians, which, in some cases, became paved with metacercariae. According to the author, even heavy infestations appeared to have no visible effect on the flatworms. The cercariae also penetrated other planarians, *Bdellocephala punctata* and *Polycelis nigra*, as well as the rhabdocoel turbellarian *Microstomum lineare*.

Martin (1938) found unencysted metacercariae of the marine trematode *Lepocreadium setiferoides* in the triclad turbellarian *Procerodes warreni*. Stunkard (1972) obtained experimental infestations with the same trematode in acoelous turbellarians *Childia* sp. and in the polyclads *Euplana gracilis* and *Stylochus ellipticus*. The ophthalmotrichocercous distome cercariae of *L. setiferoides* develop in rediae in the haemocoel of the snail *Nassarius obsoletus*, and the adults occur in various marine fish species, particularly in flatfishes.

Polyclad turbellarians *Planocera* sp. from Port Phillip Bay (Victoria, Australia) harboured unencysted larval trematodes lying free in the lumen of their main gut, as well as in the posterior intestinal branches. The worms measured 780 to 900 μm in length and 310 to 340 μm in width; they appeared to belong to the Allocreadiidae and were tentatively identified as *Peracreadium* sp. Their further life-cycle stages are not known (Prudhoe, 1945).

'*Cercariaeum lintoni*', the metacercarial stage of *Zoogonus lasius*, has been reported from triclad turbellarians *Bdelloura candida* from the Woods Hole area (Massachussetts, USA). The flatworms were used in infestation experiments, and metacercariae dissected from their tissues did not exhibit the developmental changes that characterize metacercariae dissected from cysts in the normal second intermediate host, *Nereis virens* (Shaw, 1933).

Experimental encystation of *Renicola parvicaudata* cercariae in polyclads *Euplana gracilis* has been obtained by Stunkard (1950). However, the cysts were extruded after a few days, indicating that the turbellarian was not an adequate second intermediate host.

An interesting case of a trematode–trematode association has been reported by Manter (1943). Of 300 adult *Neorenifer grandispinus* (a snake trematode), 13 harboured in their parenchyma unencysted individuals of *Mesocercaria marcianae*. The metacercariae had invaded the other trematode by direct penetration of its cuticula and body wall. The penetration area was considerably damaged: loss of cuticula and body-wall muscles left the parenchyma exposed. Internal damage occurred in the reproductive organs.

Without doubt, the most interesting example of hyperparasitism is that discovered by Cort and co-authors (1941), in which the cercariae of the strigeid *Cotylurus flabelliformis* develop inside the rediae and sporocysts of other trematodes in snails which are antagonistic to the strigeid larvae. This is true of planorbid and physid snails, the normal hosts being species of the genus *Lymnaea*. Very remarkably, under such conditions of hyperparasitism, the tetracotyle stage is reached more rapidly than in the normal host. Cort and co-authors suggest the reason to be the protection afforded against the immunizing reactions of the abnormal host, as well as the utilization of nutrient substances which the other trematodes have absorbed for the nourishment of their own progeny.

Hyperparasitism in the Helminthes in general has been exhaustively reviewed by Dollfus (1946). Sprague (1970a, b) and Sprague and Couch (1971) reviewed and revised the literature concerned with protozoan parasites and hyperparasites of marine molluscs and crustaceans, including microsporidan parasites of trematodes.

Agents: Cestoda

An individual of *Stylochus castaneus* from Rufisque (Senegal) was found to harbour an unidentified tetraphyllidean plerocercoid of the type *Scolex polymorphus*. The larva, which was provided with a large apical sucker, occurred in the terminal body portion of the turbellarian (Palombi, 1939).

Agents: Aschelminthes

Larvae of a *Gordius* species were found by Cort (1915) in the trematode *Brachycoelium hospitale*, itself a parasite in the intestine of the green newt *Diemictylus viridescens*. This was apparently not a case of accidental parasitism because 8 out of 16 trematodes from several hosts were infested, 2 with 2 larvae each, and the others with 1 a piece. Fischthal (1942) described a larval *Paragordius* which occurred free in the parenchyma of a trematode closely related to *Plagiorchis sinitsini*.

Agents: Copepoda

Lichomolgoid copepods *Pseudanthessius latus* have been found in association with the polyclad turbellarian *Kaburakia excelsa* (reported as *Cryptophallus magnus* by Illg, 1950) from San Juan Island, Washington (USA), and from unidentified turbellarians in Washington and California (USA). Lebour (1908) briefly mentions a parasitic copepod which was found clinging to the side of *Derogenes varicus*, a trematode living on the gill filaments of a long rough dab *Hippoglossoides platessoides*. Although Lebour suggests the copepod to be closely related to the genus *Ergasilus*, it is possible that she was dealing with a species of *Pseudanthessius*. Judging from her rough sketches, the anterior 'hooks' could well be the second antennae of a pseudanthessiid.

TUMOURS AND ABNORMALITIES

Tumours among the flatworms have been reported only from freshwater representatives of the class Turbellaria (Sparks, 1969). Spontaneous tumours have been observed in the planarian *Dugesia tigrina* (Stéphan, 1960). They appear as a massive infiltration of the parenchyma with glandular cells. Lange (1966) described tumours from planarians *D. etrusca* and *D. ilvana*. The growths, found in laboratory-cultivated planarians, multiplied rapidly by transverse fission. Most began at the posterior tip, and development was progressive, eventually leading to lysis of both tumour and host. No recurrence was observed in anterior parts of animals that had been divided away from the tumorous posterior parts. The author believed that tumours in the planarians might be the result of differentiation error, rather than neoplasia. Foster (1963), on the other hand, suggests abnormal growths induced in *D. dorotocephala* by application of carcinogens to be true neoplasia. The observed growths were nodular, increased rapidly in size, became necrotic and eventually, caused death of the animals. For further discussions and references to experimental tumour production in turbellarians consult Seilern-Aspang (1960a, b).

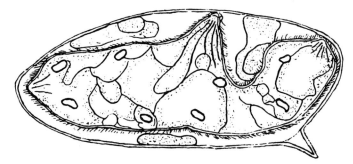

Fig. 10-13: *Schistosoma mansoni*. Abnormal partial twinning of miracidium. (After Janer, 1941; reproduced by permission of Journal of Parasitology.)

Considerable abnormalities have been observed in trematodes. Mostly nonmarine forms are involved. Miracidial twinning in *Schistosoma mansoni* was reported by Hoffman and Janer (1936). The double organisms were fused anteriorly along approximately one-third of their length, and they did not penetrate snail hosts, as did a number of simultaneously used normal miracidia. A similar case of miracidial twinning was seen by Janer (1941; Fig. 10-13). A case of conjoined twin rediae, with the oral openings diametrically opposed, occurred in *Notocotylus quinqueserialis* (Fig. 10-14). Each twin contained a fully developed muscular pharynx and an intestine. The body cavity, containing numerous cercarial embryos at different stages of development, was shared by the conjoined pair (Schell, 1960).

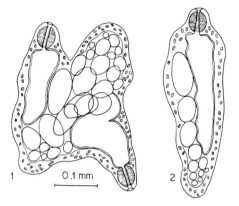

Fig. 10-14: *Notocotylus quinqueserialis* from freshwater snails *Physa gyrina*. 1: Abnormal partial twinning of redia; 2: normal redia. (After Schell, 1960; reproduced by permission of Journal of Parasitology.)

Partial twinning of a cercaria of *Alloglossidium corti* was described by Hussey (1941; Fig. 10-15), and Hussey and Stahl (1961) described and figured extensive abnormalities found in unidentified stylet-bearing trematode larvae. In this latter case, all cercariae were recovered from one single snail, *Stagnicola emarginata canadensis*, from Alanson, Michigan (USA). Abnormal metacercariae, as well as precocious metacercarial development in sporocysts, have been reported by McMullen (1938). Further abnormalities in developing trematodes and cestodes have been described by Kuntz (1948), whose paper includes a discussion of earlier literature, as well as a bibliography. Reports on abnormalities in adult Platyhelminthes include those by Hoffman (1936), concerning an abnormal ovary in *Fasciola hepatica*, and Honigberg (1944), who described a proglottid of the cestode *Dipylidium canicum* which had one complete extra set of reproductive organs. As has been shown by Voge (1961), high-temperature stress may lead to the development of abnormalities in cysticercoids of *Hymenolepis diminuta*. In some tissues, growth and differentiation were inhibited; in others, they were enhanced; a few tissues appeared unaffected.

Records of anomalies in marine platyhelminths are apparently scarce. Pelseneer (1906) figured a specimen of *Cercaria setifera* with a trifid instead of a normal straight tail. A similar case of abnormal tail bifurcation was observed by Rothschild (1936) in a microphallid cercaria from *Hydrobia ulvae*. The same author described various deviations from normal pigmentation in notocotylid cercariae from *H. ulvae*. In normal cercariae, the brown pigment is evenly dispersed over the entire dorsal and ventral body surfaces. The most common type of abnormal pigmentation was a more or less complete absence of pigment in the posterior third of the body, with unusually dense scattered aggregations in the region of the bifurcation of the oesophagus. In a second common variation the body below the oesophagus was unpigmented, except for nerve paths, which were clearly outlined by aggregations of pigment granules. Several other abnormalities, mostly comprising unusual pigment concentrations in certain body regions of the cercariae, were noted. The total amount of pigment variation in cercariae from a single snail host was so great that, unless the origin of the cercariae had been known, several different species would have appeared to be under inspection.

Margolis (1956) reported on an anomalous development of vitellaria of *Hemiurus levinseni*, a common parasite of marine fishes. The specimen had an extra vitelline mass, i.e. 3 rather than 2 vitellaria. According to Manter (1931), local and general disorganization of the vitelline glands may be observed in some trematodes.

Disturbances in testicular development are probably the most common structural abnormality among trematodes. Monorchism—development of only one testis instead of two—has been described for at least 9 species belonging to 6 different families. One specimen of *Podocotyle atomon* had both testes lacking, a very unusual condition which also occurs in *Helicometra execta*. A mutilated and regenerated specimen of *H. torta* exhibited loss of one testis apparently due to mechanical injury. Malformations probably caused by injury and subsequent regeneration frequently occur in the head spines of *Stephanochasmus* spp. Several small spines appear to replace a large one.

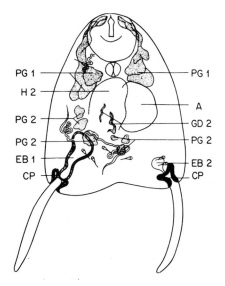

Fig. 10-15: *Alloglossidium corti*. Abnormal partial twinning of cercaria (A = ventral sucker; CP = caudal pockets; EB = excretory vesicle; GD = penetration-gland duct; H = head region; PG = penetration gland). (After Hussey, 1941; reproduced by permission of Journal of Parasitology.)

A metacercarial disease which might be, at least in part, responsible for pearl-formation in marine pelecypods, has been observed by Lauckner (unpublished). Healthy metacercariae of *Meiogymnophallus minutus* from cockles *Cardium edule* have their excretory vesicles filled with small, spherical granules, consisting mostly of calcium carbonate (Fig. 10-16, 1). In a few out of several hundred specimens, these granules had coalesced, forming one or more large, conspicuous clumps within the body of the metacercariae. Precipitation was apparently progressive, starting in one limb of the excretory vesicle, and finally involving the whole granular contents of the organ. In the diseased specimen shown (Fig. 10-16, 2) concretions have already formed in the left anterior portion of the vesicle, while the right limb is still unaffected and contains normally shaped excretion granules.

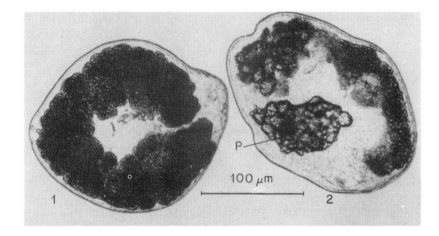

Fig. 10-16: *Meiogymnophallus minutus*. 1: Normal metacercaria, with its excretory vesicle densely packed with highly refractive excretion granules; 2: abnormal metacercaria exhibiting crystalline precipitation (P) and condensation of granules within left limb of vesicle. (Original.)

The disease, whose etiology remains unknown, eventually causes the death of affected metacercariae. Their tissue remains are partly resorbed by the host's haemocytes, while the chalky concretions persist within the connective tissue surrounding the bulk of *Meiogymnophallus minutus* metacercariae situated below the hinge of the bivalve (see Vol. II).

Meiogymnophallus minutus definitely does not cause pearl-formation in *Cardium edule*, although this has repeatedly been suspected (e.g. Cheng and Rifkin, 1970). It has been shown by Lauckner (1971) that pearl-formation in *C. edule*, *C. lamarcki*, *Mytilus edulis* and other marine pelecypods is stimulated by *Gymnophallus gibberosus*, a larval trematode, closely related and morphologically similar to *Meiogymnophallus minutus*. Unencysted, mobile metacercariae of this species live between mantle and shell of bivalves, particularly in the region of the posterior adductor muscle. Excretion granules from the excretory pore, probably expelled under pressure of the host's adductor muscle, give rise to the formation of calcium carbonate concretions which are found loose between the muscle fibres. Nuclei of large concretions sometimes contain fibrous structures resembling dead metacercariae. In contrast to speculations made by a number of investigators, it has been ascertained that viable metacercariae never become encapsulated by host tissue. On the other hand, it is possible that pearl-formation occurs around *G. gibberosus* metacercariae that had been killed either by microsporidan hyperparasites or by the above-described build-up of calcium carbonate concretions within the metacercarial body, although this phenomenon has, so far, only been observed in *M. minutus* metacercariae.

Literature Cited (Chapter 10)

Apelt, G. (1969). Fortpflanzungsbiologie, Entwicklungszyklen und vergleichende Frühentwicklung acoeler Turbellarien. *Mar Biol.*, **4**, 267–325.

Bartoli, P. (1974). Recherches sur les Gymnophallidae F. N. Morozov, 1955 (Digenea), parasites d'oiseaux des côtes de Camargue: Systématique, biologie et écologie. Thesis, Univ. de droit, d'économie et des sciences, Aix-Marseille.

Bishop, A. (1926). Notes upon *Sieboldiellina planariarum* (Siebold), a ciliate parasite of *Planaria torva*. *Parasitology*, **18**, 187–194.

Bowers, E. A. and James, B. L. (1967). Studies on the morphology, ecology and life-cycle of *Meiogymnophallus minutus* (Cobbold, 1859), comb.nov. (Trematoda: Gymnophallidae). *Parasitology*, **57**, 281–300.

Brumpt, E. (1936). *Précis de Parasitologie*, 5th ed., Masson et Cie., Paris.

Buckley, J. J. C. and Clapham, P. A. (1929). The invasion of helminth eggs by chytridiacean fungi. *J. Helminth.*, **7**, 1–14.

Butler, J. B. and Humphries, A. (1932). On the cultivation in artificial media of *Catenaria anguillulae*, a chytridiacean parasite of the ova of the liver fluke, *Fasciola hepatica*. *Scient. Proc. R. Dubl. Soc.*, **20**, 301–324.

Canning, E. U. (1975). The microsporidian parasites of Platyhelminthes: Their morphology, development, transmission and pathogenicity. Commonwealth Inst. Helminth. Commonwealth Agricultural Bureaux, St. Albans, Herts., England. *Misc. Publs*, **2**, 1–32.

Caullery, M. and Chappellier, A. (1906). *Anurosporidium pelseneeri*, n.g. n.sp., haplosporidie infectant les sporocystes d'un trématode parasite de *Donax trunculus* L. *C. r. Séanc. Soc. Biol.*, **60**, 325–328.

Cépède, C. (1911). Le cycle évolutif et les affinités systématiques de l'haplosporidie des *Donax*. *C.r. hebd. Séanc. Acad. Sci., Paris*, **153**, 507–509.

Cheng, T. C. and Rifkin, E. (1970). Cellular reactions in marine molluscs in response to helminth parasitism. In S. F. Snieszko (Ed.), *Symp. Diseases Fish. Shellfish. Am. Fish. Soc., Wash., Spec. Publ.*, **5**, 443–496.

Cort, W. W. (1915). *Gordius* larvae parasitic in a trematode. *J. Parasit.*, **1**, 198–199.

Cort, W. W., Hussey, K. L. and Ameel, D. J. (1960a). Studies on a microsporidian hyperparasite of strigeoid trematodes. I. Prevalence and effect on the parasitized larval trematodes. *J. Parasit.*, **46**, 317–325.

Cort, W. W., Hussey, K. L. and Ameel, D. J. (1960b). Studies on a microsporidian hyperparasite of strigeoid trematodes. II. Experimental transmission. *J. Parasit.*, **46**, 327–336.

Cort, W. W., Olivier, L. and Brackett, S. (1941). The relation of physid and planorbid snails to the life cycle of the strigeid trematode, *Cotylurus flabelliformis* (Faust, 1917). *J. Parasit.*, **27**, 437–448.

DeTurk, W. E. (1940). The occurrence and development of a hyperparasite, *Urosporidium crescens* sp.nov. (Sporozoa, Haplosporidia), which infests the metacercariae of *Spelotrema nicolli*, parasitic in *Callinectes sapidus*. *J. Elisha Mitchell Sci. Soc.*, **56**, 231–232.

Dissanaike, A. S. (1955). Microsporidian infections in tapeworms: instances of hyperparasitism. *Trans. R. Soc. trop. Med. Hyg.*, **49**, 294–295.

Dissanaike, A. S. (1957a). On Protozoa hyperparasitic in helminths, with some observations on *Nosema helminthorum* Moniez, 1887. *J. Helminth.*, **31**, 47–64.

Dissanaike, A. S. (1957b). The morphology and life cycle of *Nosema helminthorum* Moniez, 1887. *Parasitology*, **47**, 335–346.

Dissanaike, A. S. (1958). Experimental infection of tapeworms and oribatid mites with *Nosema helminthorum*. *Expl Parasit.*, **7**, 306–318.

Dollfus, R. P. (1912). Contribution à l'étude des trématodes marins des côtes du Boulonnais. Une méta-cercaire margaritigène parasite de *Donax vittatus* da Costa. *Mém. Soc. zool. Fr.*, **25**, 85–144.

Dollfus, R. P. (1923). Sur un sporozoaire parasite de cestode. *Annls Parasit. hum. comp.*, **1**, 201–202.

Dollfus, R. P. (1925). Liste critique des cercaires marines à queue sétigère signalées jusqu'à présent. *Trav. Stn zool. Wimereux*, **9**, 43–65.

Dollfus, R. P. (1946). Parasites (animaux et végétaux) des helminthes. Hyperparasites, ennemis et prédateurs des helminthes parasites et des helminthes libres. *Encyclopédie Biologique*, **27**, 1–482.

Dubois, R. (1907). Sur un sporozoaire parasite de l'huître perlière, *Margaritifera vulgaris* Jam. Son rôle dans la formation des perles fines. *C. r. Séanc. Soc. Biol.*, **62**, 310–313.

Fischthal, J. H. (1942). A *Paragordius* larva (Gordiacea) in a trematode. *J. Parasit.*, **28**, 167.

Foster, J. A. (1963). Induction of neoplasms in planarians with carcinogens. *Cancer Res.*, **23**, 300–303.

Frankenberg, G. v. (1935). Trematodencysten in Turbellarien. *Zool. Anz.*, **112**, 237–242.

Giard, A. (1897). Sur un distome (*Brachycoelium* sp.) parasite des pélécypodes. *C. r. Séanc. Soc. Biol.*, **49**, 956–957.

Guyénot, E. (1943). Sur une haplosporidie, parasite dans un sporocyste de la pholade, *Barnea candida* L. *Revue suisse Zool.*, **50**, 283–286.

Guyénot, E., Naville, A. and Ponse, K. (1922). Une larve de cestode parasitée par une microsporidie. *C. r. Séanc. Soc. Biol.*, **87**, 635–637.

Guyénot, E., Naville, A. and Ponse, K. (1925). Deux microsporidies parasites de trématodes. *Revue suisse Zool.*, **31**, 399–422.

Hoffman, W. A. (1936). An abnormal ovary in *Fasciola hepatica* (Trematoda: Fasciolidae). *Proc. helminth. Soc. Wash.*, **3**, 62.

Hoffman, W. A. and Janer, J. L. (1936). Miracidial twinning in *Schistosoma mansoni* (Trematoda: Schistosomatidae). *Proc. helminth. Soc. Wash.*, **3**, 62.

Honigberg, B. (1944). A morphological abnormality in the cestode, *Dipylidium caninum. Trans. Am. microsc. Soc.*, **63**, 342–344.

Howell, M. (1967). The trematode, *Bucephalus longicornutus* (Manter, 1954) in the New Zealand mud-oyster, *O. rea lutaria. Trans. R. Soc. N.Z.*, **8**, 221–237.

Hunninen, A. V. and Wichterman, R. (1938). Hyperparasitism: a species of *Hexamita* (Protozoa, Mastigophora) found in the reproductive systems of *Deropristis inflata* (Trematoda) from marine eels. *J. Parasit.*, **24**, 95–101.

Hussey, K. L. (1941). Partial twinning in a stylet cercaria. *J. Parasit.*, **27**, 92–93.

Hussey, K. L. (1971). A microsporidan hyperparasite of strigeoid trematodes, *Nosema strigeoideae* sp. n. *J. Protozool.*, **18**, 676–679.

Hussey, K. L. and Stahl, W. B. (1961). Extensive abnormalities in larval trematode infection. *J. Parasit.*, **47**, 445–446.

Illg, P. L. (1950). A new copepod, *Pseudanthessius latus* (Cyclopoida: Lichomolgidae), commensal with a marine flatworm. *J. Wash. Acad. Sci.*, **40**, 129–133.

Jameson, H. L. (1902). On the origin of pearls. *Proc. zool. Soc. Lond.*, **1**, 140–166.

Janer, J. L. (1941). Miracidial twinning in *Schistosoma mansoni. J. Parasit.*, **27**, 93.

Johnson, P. T. (1968). *An Annotated Bibliography of Pathology in Invertebrates other than Insects*, Burgess, Minneapolis.

Kepner, W. A. and Carroll, R. P. (1923). A ciliate endoparasitic in *Stenostoma leucops. J. Parasit.*, **10**, 99–100.

Kuntz, R. E. (1948). Abnormalities in development of helminth parasites with a description of several anomalies in cercariae of digenetic trematodes. *Proc. helminth. Soc. Wash.*, **15**, 73–77.

Lange, C. S. (1966). Observations on some tumours found in two species of planaria—*Dugesia etrusca* and *D. ilvana. J. Embryol. exp. Morph.*, **15**, 125–130.

Lauckner, G. (1971). Zur Trematodenfauna der Herzmuscheln *Cardium edule* und *Cardium lamarcki. Helgoländer wiss. Meersunters.*, **22**, 377–400.

Lebour, M. V. (1908). Trematodes of the Northumberland coast. No. II. *Trans. nat. Hist. Soc. Northumb.*, **3**, 28–45.

Léger, L. (1897). Sur la présence de glugéidées chez les distomes parasites des pélécypodes. *C. r. Séanc. Soc. Biol.* (Ser. 10), **49**, 957–958.

Mackin, J. G. and Loesch, H. (1955). A haplosporidian hyperparasite of oysters. *Proc. natn. Shellfish. Ass.*, **45**, 182–183.

McMullen, D. B. (1938). Observations on precocious metacercarial development in the trematode superfamily Plagiorchioidea. *J. Parasit.*, **24**, 273–280.

Manter, H. W. (1930). Studies on the trematodes of Tortugas fishes. *Carnegie Instn Yb.*, **29**, 338–340.

Manter, H. W. (1931). Some abnormalities of trematodes. *J. Parasit.*, **18**, 124.

Manter, H. W. (1943). One species of trematode, *Neorenifer grandispinus* (Caballero, 1938) attacked by another, *Mesocercaria marcianae* (La Rue, 1917). *J. Parasit.*, **29**, 387–392.

Margolis, L. (1956). Anomalous development of vitallaria in *Hemiurus levinseni* (Trematoda). *Can. J. Zool.*, **34**, 207–208.

Martin, W. E. (1936). A sporozoan parasite of larval trematodes. *J. Parasit.*, **22**, 536.

Martin, W. E. (1938). Studies on trematodes of Woods Hole: The life cycle of *Lepocreadium setiferoides* (Miller and Northup), Allocreadiidae, and the description of *Cercaria cumingiae* n.sp. *Biol. Bull. mar. biol. Lab., Woods Hole*, **75**, 463–473.

Ormières, R., Sprague, V. and Bartoli, P. (1972). Light and electron microscope study of *Urosporidium* sp. (Haplosporida), hyperparasite of trematode sporocysts in the clam *Abra ovata* (Philippi). (Abstract.) *J. Protozool.*, **19** (Suppl.), 24.

Ormières, R., Sprague, V. and Bartoli, P. (1973). Light and electron microscope study of a new species of *Urosporidium* (Haplosporida), hyperparasite of trematode sporocysts in the clam *Abra ovata*. *J. Invertebr. Pathol.*, **21**, 71–86.

Oschman, J. L. (1969). Endonuclear viruslike bodies in *Convoluta roscoffensis* (Turbellaria, Acoela). *J. Invertebr. Pathol.*, **13**, 147–148.

Palombi, A. (1939). Turbellaria Polycladidea. In Résultats scientifiques des croisières du navire-école belge 'Mercator'. *Mém. Mus. r. Hist. nat. Belg.* (Ser. 2), **2**, 95–114.

Pelseneer, P. (1895). Un trématode produisant la castration parasitaire chez *Donax trunculus*. *Bull. scient. Fr. Belg.*, **27**, 357–363.

Pelseneer, P. (1906). Trématodes parasites de mollusques marins. *Bull. scient. Fr. Belg.*, **40**, 161–186.

Perkins, F. O. (1971). Sporulation in the trematode hyperparasite *Urosporidium crescens* DeTurk, 1940 (Haplosporida: Haplosporidiidae)—an electron microscope study. *J. Parasit.*, **57**, 9–23.

Philip, C. B. (1955). There's always something new under the 'parasitological' sun (the unique story of helminth-borne salmon poisoning disease). *J. Parasit.*, **41**, 125–148.

Prudhoe, S. (1945). Two notes on trematodes. *Ann. Mag. nat. Hist.* (Ser. 11), **7**, 378–383.

Puytorac, P. de and Grain, J. (1960). Sur deux grégarines du genre *Monocystella* endoparasites des planaires ochridiennes: *Fonticola ochridana* Stankovic et *Neodendrocoelum sancti-naumi* Stankovic. *Annls Parasit. hum. comp.*, **35**, 197–208.

Reisinger, E. (1930). Zum Ductus-genito-intestinalis-Problem. I. Über primäre Geschlechtstrakt-Darmverbindungen bei rhabdocoelen Turbellarien. (Zugleich ein Beitrag zur europäischen und grönländischen Turbellarienfauna). *Z. Morph. Ökol. Tiere*, **16**, 49–73.

Reisinger, E. (1959). Anormogenetische und parasitogene Syncytienbildung bei Turbellarien. *Protoplasma*, **50**, 627–643.

Rothschild, M. (1936). A note on the variation of certain cercariae (Trematoda). *Nov. zool.*, **40**, 170–175.

Schell, S. C. (1960). A case of conjoined twin rediae. *J. Parasit.*, **46**, 448.

Seilern-Aspang, F. (1960a). Experimentelle Beiträge zur Frage der Zusammenhänge Regeneration—Geschwulstbildung. *Arch. EntwMech. Org.*, **152**, 491–516.

Seilern-Aspang, F. (1960b). Syncytiale und differenzierte Tumoren bei Tricladen. *Arch. EntwMech. Org.*, **152**, 517–523.

Shaw, R. C. (1933). Observations on *Cercariaeum lintoni* Miller and Northup and its metacercarial development. *Biol. Bull. mar. biol. Lab., Woods Hole*, **64**, 262–275.

Sparks, A. K. (1969). Review of tumors and tumor-like conditions in Protozoa, Coelenterata, Platyhelminthes, Annelida, Sipunculida, and Arthropoda, excluding insects. *Natn. Cancer Inst. Monogr.*, **31**, 671–682.

Sprague, V. (1964). *Nosema dollfusi* n.sp. (Microsporidia, Nosematidae), a hyperparasite of *Bucephalus cuculus* in *Crassostrea virginica. J. Protozool.*, **11**, 381–385.

Sprague, V. (1969). Microsporida and tumors, with particular reference to the lesion associated with *Ichthyosporidium* sp. Schwartz, 1963. *Natn. Cancer Inst. Monogr.*, **31**, 237–249.

Sprague, V. (1970a). Some protozoan parasites and hyperparasites in marine decapod Crustacea. In S. F. Snieszko (Ed.), *Symp. Diseases Fish. Shellfish. Am. Fish Soc., Wash., Spec. Publ.*, **5**, 416–430.

Sprague, V. (1970b). Some protozoan parasites and hyperparasites in marine bivalve molluscs. In S. F. Snieszko (Ed.), *Symp. Diseases Fish. Shellfish. Am. Fish. Soc., Wash., Spec. Publ.*, **5**, 511–526.

Sprague, V. and Couch, J. (1971). An annotated list of protozoan parasites, hyperparasites, and commensals of decapod Crustacea. *J. Protozool.*, **18**, 526–537.

Stanier, J. E., Woodhouse, M. A. and Griffin, R. L. (1968). The fine structure of the spore of *Nosema spelotremae*, a microsporidian parasite of a *Spelotrema* metacercaria encysted in the crab *Carcinus maenas. J. Invertebr. Pathol.*, **12**, 73–82.

Stefanski, W. (1959). The role of helminths in the transmission of bacteria and viruses. *Proc. Int. Congr. Zool.*, **15**, 697–699.

Stéphan, F. (·1960). Tumeurs spontanées chez la planaire *Dugesia tigrina. C. r. Séanc. Soc. Biol.*, **156**, 920–922.

Stunkard, H. W. (1937). The physiology, life cycles and phylogeny of the parasitic flatworms. *Am. Mus. Novit.*, **908**, 1–27.

Stunkard, H. W. (1950). Further observations on *Cercaria parvicaudata* Stunkard and Shaw, 1931. *Biol. Bull. mar. biol. Lab., Woods Hole*, **99**, 136–142.

Stunkard, H. W. (1957). The morphology and life history of the digenetic trematode, *Microphallus similis* (Jägerskiöld, 1900) Baer, 1943. *Biol. Bull. mar. biol. Lab., Woods Hole*, **112**, 254–266.

Stunkard, H. W. (1972). Observations on the morphology and life-history of the digenetic trematode, *Lepocreadium setiferoides* Miller and Northup, 1926) Martin, 1938. *Biol. Bull. mar. biol. Lab., Woods Hole*, **142**, 326–334.

Valkanov, A. (1935). Untersuchungen über den Entwicklungskreis eines Turbellarienparasiten (*Monocystella arndti*). *Z. ParasitKde*, **7**, 517–538.

Vandel, A. (1921). *Lankesteria planariae*, grégarine parasite des planaires d'eau douce. *C. r. Séanc. Soc. Biol.*, **84**, 718–719.

Voge, M. (1961). Effect of high temperature stress on histogenesis in the cysticercoid of *Hymenolepis diminuta* (Cestoda: Cyclophyllidea). *J. Parasit.*, **47**, 189–195.

Westblad, E. (1942). Studien über skandinavische Turbellaria Acoela II. *Ark. Zool.*, **33A**, 1–48.

11. DISEASES OF NEMERTEA

G. Lauckner

Most of the approximately 750 species of Nemertea or Rhynchocoela are marine. Although they live in easily accessible shallow reaches of coastal regions, their parasites and diseases have rarely been examined. No reports on microbial agents of nemerteans have come to the reviewer's attention.

DISEASES CAUSED BY PROTOZOANS

Agents: Sporozoa

Intestinal gregarines are of common occurrence in nemerteans. Intracellular and coelomic stages have also been observed. When present in large numbers, trophozoites may obstruct almost the entire gut lumen (Kölliker, 1849; Punnett, 1901; Gontcharoff, 1951; Vinckier and co-authors, 1970; Gibson, 1972).

Ovoid bodies observed in the parenchyma of *Lineus sanguineus* from Roscoff (France), initially believed to be eggs, turned out to be the coelomic stage of an acephaline gregarine. Host cells bordering the parasite were found to be deformed and degenerated. Gametocysts of the yet unnamed gregarine have likewise been observed (Fig. 11-1). The parasites were only found in female *L. sanguineus* and possibly castrated their hosts (Gontcharoff, 1951).

Approximately 75% of *Lineus ruber* from Plymouth (England) harboured acephaline gregarines *Urospora nemertes*. Trophozoites, 150 to 180 μm long and 15 to 20 μm wide, with basophil, PAS-positive cytoplasm and prominent nuclei, were observed in all parts of the gut lumen. Intracellular stages were common in the columnar cells of the gut wall. The gregarine did not appear to harm *L. ruber*—except for a few occasions, when infested columnar cells reacted against developing intracellular stages, and caused them to degenerate into masses of yellowish-brown crystals. Such cells then burst, either *in situ* or after being shed into the gut lumen, and the crystals were eliminated with the faeces (Jennings, 1960). Hyperparasitization has been reported by Vinckier and co-authors (1970): Microsporidans, named *Nosema vivieri*, were found to infest undetermined monocystid gregarines parasitic in unspecified nemerteans from Wimereux, France (see Chapter 3).

Nemerteans are frequently attacked by sporozoans which parasitize in the gut lumen or, more commonly, in body tissues (Punnett, 1901; Gibson, 1972). Individuals of *Lineus sanguineus* from Roscoff (France) were sometimes found to be overwhelmed by sporozoan cysts which formed large clusters in the epithelium of the digestive tract (Gontcharoff, 1951). Brinkmann (1917) observed sporozoan-like structures in *Nectonemertes primitiva* ova, as well as in the brain and general parenchyma of *Parabalaenanemertes fusca*.

Individuals of *Lineus bilineatus* from Plymouth (England) are hosts for *Haplosporidium nemertis*; at the time of observation, about 50% of the population were infested. Ovoid operculate spores, measuring 6 to 7 × 3 to 4 μm, occurred in great numbers in the connective tissue which separates the digestive tract from the internal layer of longitudinal muscles. Sometimes also the subcutaneous tissue became affected. Small subspherical binucleate plasmodia were the earliest stages of *H. nemertis* discernible in the host tissues. Growth of the plasmodia to a definite size of 30 to 40 μm is accompanied by synchronous nuclear division. The resulting multinucleate plasmodia resolve into uninucleate sporoblasts which, in turn, develop into spores. The presence of *H. nemertis* appeared to suppress gonad development in *L. bilineatus* (Debaisieux, 1919, 1920).

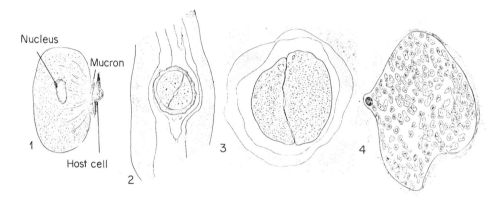

Fig. 11-1: Gregarines from intestine of *Lineus sanguineus*. 1: Trophozoite from coelom attached to host cell; 2: gametocyst attached to intestinal wall; 3: young liberated gametocyst; 4: mature gametocyst with numerous sporozoite-containing oocysts. (After Gontcharoff, 1951; reproduced by permission of Annales de Sciences naturelles.)

Haplosporidium malacobdellae has been found in 2·96% (36 out of 1218) *Malacobdella grossa* from Robin Hood's Bay, Yorkshire, England (Gibson, 1968; Jennings and Gibson, 1968). The most common and most easily recognizable stage in the life history of this haplosporidan parasite is the spore-enclosing resting cyst, which is oval in shape, 20 to 25 μm long and 10 to 15 μm wide. Individual cysts may enclose up to 40 oval to subspherical non-operculate spores, 3 to 3·5 × 2·5 μm in dimension. Plasmodia undergoing schizogony vary in size from 5 × 8 μm to 15 × 25 μm. Plasmodia undergoing schizogony and sporogony, as well as cysts containing mature spores, occur principally in the parenchyma of *M. grossa*. However, as the number of plasmodia increases, they aggregate around the intestine and eventually form a band some 150 μm in depth. At this stage, also the epidermis, proboscis and proboscis sheath, the endothelium of the blood vascular system and the walls of the foregut are invaded.

While healthy *Malacobdella grossa* are cream coloured, heavily infested individuals appear to be pigmented, due to the yellowish-brown colour of the haplosporidan spores, and the dark band of plasmodia encircling the gut and proboscis is clearly visible to the naked eye (Gibson, 1968). Host age, as judged from body size, does not appear to influence the susceptibility to infestation by *Haplosporidium malocobdellae*. Individuals of various sizes (3·5 to 19·5 mm) harboured parasites at all stages of development.

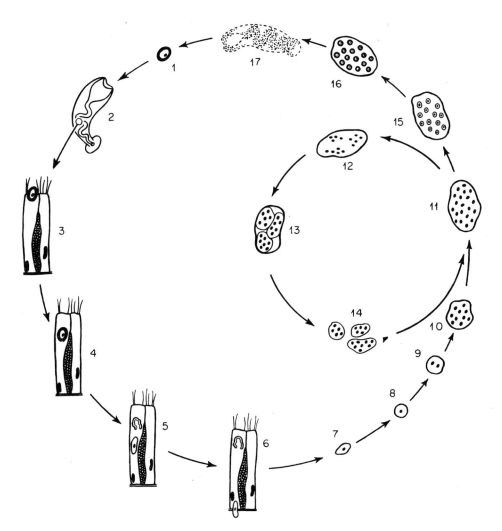

Fig. 11-2: *Haplosporidium malacobdellae* from *Malacobdella grossa*. Life cycle. 1: Free-floating mature spore; 2: ingestion of spore by *M. grossa*; 3, 4: phagocytosis of spore by columnar intestinal cell; 5: hatching of spore; 6: migration of amoebula into parenchyma; 7–10: growth and nuclear multiplication of amoebula to form plasmodium; 11–14: stages of schizogony; 15, 16: sporogony; 17: death of host and release of spores. (After Jennings and Gibson, 1968; reproduced by permission of Archiv für Protistenkunde.)

The life cycle of *Haplosporidium malacobdellae* (Fig. 11-2) reveals typical haplosporidan patterns, except that the spores remain confined within the plasmodial membrane after their formation and do not appear to be released until the host dies. In long established infestations the bulk of the host's body is loaded with spore-containing resting cysts. Heavily infested hosts become quiescent and no longer show the behavioural patterns characteristic of healthy or lightly infested *Malacobdella grossa*. Under laboratory conditions, heavily infested individuals gradually die and disintegrate. Subsequently, the parasite's resting cysts likewise disintegrate, releasing individual spores into the surrounding sea water. A similar process of spore liberation upon death of the host is believed to occur in nature.

Normally, *Malacobdella grossa* reaches maturity at a body length of approximately 10 to 11 mm. Heavily infested individuals of this or larger size, however, never revealed fully developed gonads, mature ova or sperm. In contrast, infested *M. grossa* which had mature gonads carried only a light parasite burden; it seems likely that infestation had occurred after the onset of gonad maturation. On the basis of these observations it was concluded that infestation with *Haplosporidium malacobdellae* causes parasitic castration in both sexes of *M. grossa*, provided the infestation is established early in life before the onset of sexual maturity (Jennings and Gibson, 1968).

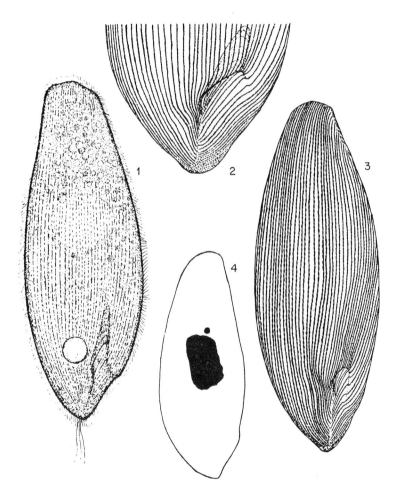

Fig. 11-3: *Thigmophrya annella* from *Malacobdella grossa*. 1: Living individual; 2 and 3: silver-impregnated specimens, ventral view; 4: nuclei stained with borax carmine. (After Fenchel, 1965; reproduced by permission of Ophelia.)

Agents: Ciliata

Two arhynchodinid ciliates are known to occur in the gut of *Malacobdella grossa*. *Thigmophrya annella* (Fig. 11-3) was found in nearly all individuals commensal within the mantle cavity of *Cyprina islandica* and other bivalves from Gullmarfjord (Sweden). The ciliates were always present in large numbers (Fenchel, 1965). *Orchitophrya malocobdellae* (Fig. 11-4) occurred in the intestines of 4·9% of 168 *M. grossa* living within the mantle cavity of *Zirfaea crispata* from Robin Hood's Bay, Yorkshire, England. Low numbers of ciliates appeared to have no adverse effects upon their hosts but it was assumed that in cases in which the nemerteans' intestines were gorged with ciliates there might be a serious interference with their feeding mechanism (Jennings, 1968).

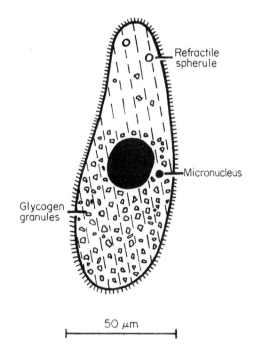

Fig. 11-4: *Orchitophrya malacobdellae* from *Malacobdella grossa*. (After Jennings, 1968; reproduced by permission of Archiv für Protistenkunde.)

DISEASES CAUSED BY METAZOANS

Agents: Mesozoa

Tetrastemma flavidum from Vauville (France) harboured orthonectid mesozoans *Rhopalura pelseneeri* in the parenchyma. Adults measured 120 to 150 × 30 μm (Caullery and Mesnil, 1901). Similar but somewhat smaller parasites (105 × 25 μm), found in

Tetrastemma vermiculus from Wimereux (France), were regarded as a variety and named *R. pelseneeri* var. *vermiculicola* (Caullery, 1914).

Lineus gesserensis from British waters are host for an undetermined orthonectid. Probably a member of the genus *Rhopalura*, the mesozoan was found burying in the body wall, giving the host a perforated and honeycombed appearance (Punnett, 1901).

A single *Amphiporus ochraceus* from Woods Hole (Massachussetts, USA) yielded a number of as yet undetermined individuals of a species of *Rhopalura*, 126 μm in length and 18 μm in diameter. Of 171 *A. ochraceus* examined subsequently, none has been found harbouring the parasite (Meinkoth, 1956).

Agents: Cestoda

About 120 tetraphyllidean plerocercoid larvae were found in a single *Cerebratulus lacteus* from Beaufort (North Carolina, USA). The larvae occurred free in the tissue spaces of the nemertean, with no signs of cysts around them. A few adhered to the outer walls of the digestive tract but the exact location of the parasites could not be determined because the host had fragmented. The cestodes appeared to belong to the genus *Echeneibothrium* but positive identification to the species level was not possible (Hunter, 1950). This is the first record of a nemertean as an intermediate host for larval helminths.

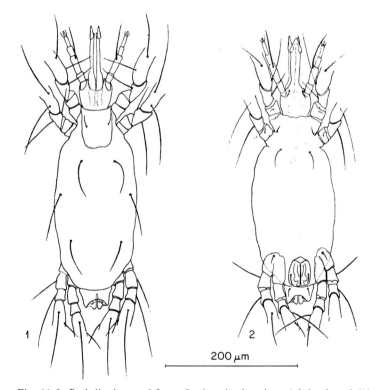

200 μm

Fig. 11-5: *Parhalixodes travei* from *Cerebratulus hepaticus*. Adult, dorsal (1) and ventral (2) aspect. (After Laubier, 1960; reproduced by permission of Acarologia.)

Agents: Arthropoda

Lichomolgoid copepods *Pseudanthessius nemertophilus* lived associated with *Lineus longissimus* collected near Wimereux (France). The relationship is believed to be semiparasitic (Gallien, 1936). Halacarids *Parhalixodes travei* (Fig. 11-5) occur as ectoparasites on *Cerebratulus hepaticus* from the western Mediterranean Sea. Both adults and larvae were firmly attached to the dorsal body surface of a single host 5 cm in length (Laubier, 1960).

Literature Cited (Chapter 11)

Brinkmann, A. (1917). Die pelagischen Nemertinen. *Bergens Mus. Skr.*, **3**, 1–194.

Caullery, M. (1914). *Rhopalura pelseneeri* C. et M., var. *vermiculicola* var.nov., orthonectide parasite de *Tetrastemma vermiculus* Qtfg. *Bull. Soc. zool. Fr.*, **39**, 121–124.

Caullery, M. and Mesnil, F. (1901). Recherches sur les orthonectides. *Archs Anat. microsc.*, **4**, 381–470.

Debaisieux, P. (1919). *Haplosporidium nemertis*, nov.sp. *C. r. Séanc. Soc. Biol., Paris*, **82**, 1399–1400.

Debaisieux, P. (1920). *Haplosporidium (Minchinia) chitonis* Lank., *Haplosporidium nemertis*, nov. sp., et le groupe des haplosporidies. *Cellule*, **30**, 291–313.

Fenchel, T. (1965). Ciliates from Scandinavian molluscs. *Ophelia*, **2**, 71–173.

Gallien, L. (1936). *Pseudanthessius nemertophilus* nov.sp., copépode commensal de *Lineus longissimus* Sowerby. *Bull. Soc. zool. Fr.*, **60**, 451–459.

Gibson, R. (1968). Studies on the biology of the entocommensal rhynchocoelan *Malacobdella grossa*. *J. mar. biol. Ass. U.K.*, **48**, 637–656.

Gibson, R. (1972). *Nemerteans*, Hutchinson, London.

Gontcharoff, M. (1951). Biologie de la régéneration et de la reproduction chez quelques Lineidae de France. *Annls Sci. nat. Hist., Zool.* (Ser. 11), **13**, 149–235.

Hunter, W. S. (1950). The nemertean, *Cerebratulus lacteus*, as an intermediate host for cestode larvae. *J. Parasit.*, **36**, 496.

Jennings, J. B. (1960). Observations on the nutrition of the rhynchocoelan *Lineus ruber* (O. F. Müller). *Biol. Bull. mar. biol. Lab., Woods Hole*, **119**, 189–196.

Jennings, J. B. (1968). A new astomatous ciliate from the entocommensal rhynchocoelan *Malacobdella grossa* (O. F. Müller). *Arch. Protistenk.*, **110**, 422–425.

Jennings, J. B. and Gibson, R. (1968). The structure and life history of *Haplosporidium malacobdellae* sp.nov., a new sporozoan from the entocommensal rhynchocoelan *Malacobdella grossa* (O. F. Müller). *Arch. Protistenk.*, **111**, 31–37.

Kölliker, A. (1849). Beiträge zur Kenntnis niederer Thiere. *Z. wiss. Zool.*, **1**, 1–37.

Laubier, L. (1960). *Parhalixodes travei* n.g., n.sp., un nouvel Halixodinae (halacariens) ectoparasite de némerte en Méditerranée occidentale. *Acarologia*, **2**, 541–551.

Meinkoth, N. A. (1956). A North American record of *Rhopalura* sp. (Orthonectida:Mesozoa), a parasite of the nemertean *Amphiporus ochraceus* (Verrill). *Biol. Bull. mar. biol. Lab., Woods Hole*, **111**, 308.

Punnett, R. C. (1901). Lineus. In W. A. Herdman (Ed.) *L. M. B. C. Memoirs on Typical British Marine Plants and Animals*. William & Norgate, London. (*Lpool mar. biol. Comm.*, **7**, 1–37.)

Vinckier, D., Devauchelle, G. and Prensier, G. (1970). *Nosema vivieri* n.sp. (Microspora, Nosematidae) hyperparasite d'une grégarine vivant dans le coelome d'une némerte. *C.r. hebd. Séanc. Acad. Sci., Paris* (Ser. D), **270**, 821–823.

12. DISEASES OF MOLLUSCA: GASTROPODA

G. Lauckner

Before we review the diseases of the Gastropoda, some introductory comments seem desirable which pertain to the Mollusca as a whole. Space considerations have forced us to subdivide the mollusc review. The chapters devoted to bivalves, amphineurans, placophorans and cephalopods will appear in Volume II of this treatise.

The phylum Mollusca comprises six classes containing some 112,000 known species (Kaestner, 1954–1963): the Monoplacophora, of which the only living genus is *Neopilina*; the Amphineura, with some 1000 exclusively marine species; the Gastropoda with over 85,000 species (55,000 Prosobranchia, mostly marine; 10,000 Opisthobranchia, exclusively marine; 20,000 Pulmonata, mainly terrestrial and freshwater); the Scaphopoda, with some 300 exclusively marine species; the Bivalvia or Pelecypoda, with 25,000 predominantly marine species, and the Cephalopoda, with 600 solely marine species. The Mollusca thus represent the second largest phylum behind the Arthropoda (>810,000 species). Methods for cultivating marine molluscs have been reviewed by Kinne (1977) and Kinne and Rosenthal (1977).

Molluscs constitute an important and often dominant part of the benthos in coastal and estuarine waters. Many species of high economic value, particularly oysters and mussels, have been cultivated all over the world for decades or even centuries, and other species of lesser or no direct commercial value are important as fish food or as intermediate hosts of economically significant trematode parasites. Since early attempts to cultivate marine molluscs, it has been recognized that they may sometimes be subject to devastating diseases. Epizootics among cultivated pelecypods have occurred at more or less irregular time intervals in different parts of the world, often bringing the related industry to a standstill. Despite the fact that much information about some diseases of pelecypods has been accumulated in recent decades, the etiology of other serious maladies still remains insufficiently understood or even entirely unknown.

Wild populations of Mollusca, particularly of bivalves, undergo marked, long-term fluctuations or are subject to sudden and unexpected mass mortalities (Dexter, 1944; Burkenroad, 1946; Coe, 1956; Johnson, 1968). A causal relationship between such fluctuations and disease has repeatedly been suspected, but rarely proven.

Marine molluscs, littoral forms in particular, are generally well adapted to the entirety of physical factors governing their habitats, even to strong fluctuations of these factors. Thus, only extreme deviations from normal ecological conditions may result in occasional mass mortalities of marine organisms, including molluscs (Brongersma-Sanders, 1957).

In other cases, 'red tides' caused by blooms of dinoflagellates, mainly of the genera *Gonyaulax* and *Gymnodinium*, have been found responsible for mass mortalities of marine molluscs (Coe, 1956; Stohler, 1960; Grindley and Nel, 1968). The role of external metabolites in the marine environment is well established (Lucas, 1947, 1949, 1955, 1958), and it has been demonstrated experimentally that metabolites released by dinoflagellates *Prorocentrum triangulatum*, present in extremely high population densities, caused abortions of embryos and immature larvae of laboratory-reared European oysters *Ostrea edulis*. The released larvae soon died (Loosanoff and Davis, 1963; Loosanoff, 1974).

Diseases of microbial and parasitic aetiology are probably the most important, but least studied factors which might be responsible for mass mortalities as well as for at least part of the 'natural mortality' of molluscs. Unfortunately, disease studies concentrate almost entirely on commercially important bivalves such as oysters and mussels. The role of microbial diseases, as well as protozoan infestations, in the life history of these molluscs is now rather well understood, but the importance of parasites—particularly helminths and crustaceans—remains to be ascertained in most cases. There is an obvious lack of experimental attempts to evaluate this factor.

The principal known diseases of commercially important marine bivalve Mollusca have been reviewed by Sindermann and Rosenfield (1967). Sindermann (1970a) extended this synopsis to include diseases of marine Gastropoda and Cephalopoda, and supplemented it with a separate, extended bibliography (Sindermann, 1970b). Another important source of general information is the review by Cheng (1967) on marine molluscs as hosts for symbioses, which includes a list of known parasites of commercially important species.

Next to nothing is known about diseases and parasites of the Monoplacophora, the Amphineura and the Scaphopoda.

Only a few species of marine snails are of direct economic importance. Their utilization as seafood is mainly restricted to the Indopacific, eastern Asia and some coastal regions of North and Central America and Europe, particularly the Mediterranean.

Abalones *Haliotis* spp. are extensively exploited in the Pacific Ocean. Yearly landings of the Californian abalone industry, for instance, averaged some 4·5 million pounds between 1951 and 1969 (Frey, 1971). 'Conchs' *Strombus gigas* are harvested in enormous quantities in the Bahamas and West Indies, where they constitute an important part of the native diet (Randall, 1964; Berg, 1976). Periwinkles *Littorina littorea* and, to a lesser extent, dogwhelks *Buccinum undatum* are fished commercially in England, France and Belgium. In France, *L. littorea* is grown commercially in so-called 'parcs'. This is, so far, the only known example of snail mariculture (Cole, 1956; Pax, 1962). In 1867, for instance, 76,000 baskets of periwinkles, weighing 1900 tons and worth more than £50,000, were consumed in London alone (Zinn, 1964). Limpets of the genus *Patella* are eaten by coastal dwellers all over the world, sometimes in considerable quantities. In Hawaii and other Pacific islands, *Patella hawaiiensis* and related limpets are served in a traditional dish eaten at Polynesian banquets or 'luaus' (Cheng, 1967). Many other marine snails are considered delicacies by various ethnic groups (Palombi and Santarelli, 1953; Pax, 1962).

The indirect economic importance of marine Gastropoda probably even exceeds its commercial value in the negative sense. Oyster drills of the genera *Urosalpinx, Thais,*

Purpura and *Ocenebra* are among the most damaging pests on oyster beds, particularly in the USA and Japan (Baughman, 1947; Quayle, 1969), and slipper-limpets *Crepidula fornicata* have been a serious threat to the European oyster industry (Korringa, 1950; Lambert, 1951; Cole, 1956).

The Gastropoda are hosts for a great variety of helminth parasites, in particular larval digenetic trematodes. A considerable amount of information on the pathogenicity of these parasites in the Mollusca has accumulated during the past decades. However, although innumerable papers on the ecology and physiology of molluscs have been written, the parasitological literature has—with a very few exceptions—not been taken into account. The fact that even in such fundamental publications as the 'Physiology of Mollusca' (Wilbur and Yonge, 1964, 1966) or 'Biology of Intertidal Animals' (Newell, 1970) the interference of helminth parasites with the physiology, morphology and behaviour of molluscs has received no, or at best passing, attention, is a deplorable omission. The coexistence of two important scientific disciplines—ecology and parasitology—almost entirely without interdisciplinary contact is astonishing, if not frustrating.

In his review of the literature on the pathogenesis of helminths in the Mollusca, Wright (1966) has emphasized that studies on host–parasite relationships have concentrated on a relatively narrow field, and that the title of his review should, therefore, more accurately be 'The Pathogenesis of the Digenea in the Basommatophora.' About 75% of the relevant papers cited by Wright (1966) are concerned with the effects of trematodes on freshwater snails, and the influence of economic considerations is demonstrated by the fact that over half of these deal with the larval stages of blood and liver flukes of man and domestic animals. Only comparatively recently have marine mollusc–trematode associations found interest from the patho-physiological point of view.

Several marine snail species are known as carriers of the larval stages of avian schistosomes, whose emerging cercariae are capable of producing dermatitis in humans in various parts of the world (Penner, 1950, 1953a, b; Stunkard, 1951; Stunkard and Hinchliffe, 1951, 1952; Chu, 1952; Hutton, 1952, 1960; Leigh, 1952, 1953, 1955; Orris and Combes, 1952; Sindermann and Gibbs, 1953; Chu and Cutress, 1954; Bearup, 1955, 1956; Sindermann, 1956, 1960; Sindermann and co-authors, 1957; Grodhaus and Keh, 1958; Wagner, 1960; Ewers, 1961; Short and Holliman, 1961; McDaniel and Coggins, 1971, 1972; Murray and Hyland, 1976; and others).

Innumerable marine gastropods act as first intermediate hosts for larval trematodes whose metacercarial stages occur in commercially important bivalve molluscs, crustaceans and fishes. The detrimental effects of these helminth parasites on their second intermediate hosts have been studied only in a few cases, and their influence on the hosts—individually or at the population level—is not adequately understood; it should not be underestimated. A few examples of evident pathogenic effects caused by trematode invasion will be discussed below.

DISEASES CAUSED BY MICRO-ORGANISMS

Despite the substantial direct and indirect economic importance of marine Gastropoda, next to nothing is known about their microbial diseases. This situation, however, appears to reflect a lack of scientific scrutiny rather than absence of such diseases from this class. Moreover, this lack of information is all the more appalling when contrasted to the situation in the well-studied Bivalvia.

Agents: Viruses and Bacteria

No snail diseases of viral or bacterial etiology have, so far, become evident in marine Gastropoda, although such diseases are well documented for the Pelecypoda. A strong possibility exists that viruses are also responsible for mass mortalities of molluscan larvae reared under laboratory conditions as well as in nature (Loosanoff, 1974). Laboratory-reared larval and juvenile bivalves may be affected by bacteria (Loosanoff, 1954; Walne, 1958; Guillard, 1959; Loosanoff and Davis, 1963). Bacterial infections have also been observed in bivalve larvae from plankton samples. Some agents appear to be of a specific nature, affecting the larvae of one particular group only (Loosanoff, 1966). It is beyond doubt that such bacterial diseases exist also in Gastropoda. There is an urgent need for investigations in this area. Acid-fast (mycobacterial) infections have, for example, been reported from freshwater snails (Michelson, 1961).

Agents: Fungi

A fungus infection of ova within the egg capsules was observed in oyster drills *Urosalpinx cinerea* kept in outdoor tidal tanks at Milford, Connecticut, USA (Ganaros, 1957). Experimental transmission of the pathogen (Fig. 12-1) was successful in sterilized sea water at 20° C and a salinity of $21^0/oo$ S. The ova did not have to be moribund for the infection to develop. In one experiment, a flask with 200 ml of sea water and 20 washed egg capsules, containing ova and early gastrulae, was contaminated with 3 ml of inoculum. One hundred per cent infection occurred within 24 days. In the meantime, controls had developed from ova to protoconchs with no sign of infection. In another experiment, 12 egg cases were used, 4 of which contained ova, 4 veliger larvae, and 4 other protoconchs. After 28 days, the capsules which initially harboured protoconchs had released them; the veliger larvae developed into protoconchs, but the egg cases that contained ova turned out to be infected and did not develop. Hence, the infectivity of the fungus appears to be confined to the ova and early developmental stages, but not to older larvae from the protoconch onward.

The fungus, which was isolated and cultured, was believed to be a new form belonging to the Lagenidiales and probably to the Sirolpidiaceae. It resembled *Sirolpidium zoophthorum*, which was found responsible for some epizootic mortalities in cultures of clam larvae (Davis and co-authors, 1954; Vishniac, 1955), and also resembled *Plectospira dubia*, a marine fungus capable of infecting crustacean eggs (Atkins, 1954). Moreover, a pure culture of the fungus from *Urosalpinx cinerea* ova, which was sent to England, was able to provoke infection in eggs of oyster crabs *Pinnotheres pisum*. Vishniac (1958) subsequently reported the isolation and cultivation of the fungus, which he termed *Haliphtorus milfordensis*, from *Urosalpinx cinerea* egg capsules from Long Island Sound (USA). When grown on artifical media, it was distinctly mycelial and composed of much-branched, somewhat irregular, hyphae, 10 to 13 μm in diameter (up to 25 μm in older parts), with strongly vacuolated cytoplasm (Fig. 12-1). Sparrow (1974) made a comparative study on *H. milfordensis* and *Haliphtorus* sp., associated with crustacean eggs. Fuller and co-authors (1964) isolated a similar organism from the surface of *Enteromorpha* sp. and other marine algae.

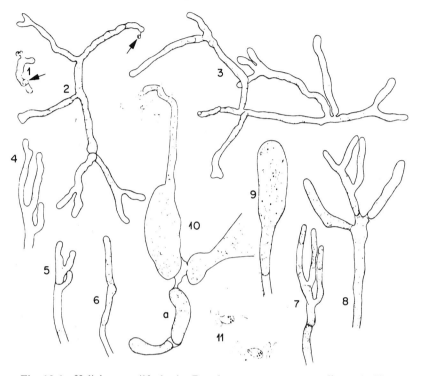

Fig. 12-1: *Haliphtorus milfordensis.* Development on agar medium. 1: Young 24-h-old thallus (arrow: zoospore cyst); 2, 3: 48-h-old thalli (arrow: zoospore cyst); 4–8: 72-h-old thalli with initiation of fragmentation into subthalli by young parts of parent thalli; 9: subthallus undergoing zoosporogenesis; 10: 72-h thallus with 4 adjacent subthalli at a vegetative condition, upper subthalli bearing mature zoospores which escape from discharge tube; 11: biflagellate zoospores. 1–8 and 10: × 150; 9 and 11: × 825. (After Sparrow, 1974; reproduced by permission of Institut für Meeresforschung, Bremerhaven.)

Ganaros (1957) discussed the possible use of the fungus as a biological control for oyster drills. He was, however, pessimistic with respect to the practicability of such control, since any measure in the field would demand the creation of environmental conditions conducive to infection and dissemination. On the other hand, if this fungus could be carried and spread by the drills themselves, it might offer a specific, natural infecting agent capable of efficiently reducing the population density of *Urosalpinx cinerea*.

In the reviewer's opinion, one might well arrive at quite the opposite conclusion. The low degree of host-specificity of this particular pathogen is made evident by the successful experimental infection of crustacean eggs. Since the fungus, on the other hand, resembles the bivalve pathogen *Sirolpidium zoophthorum*, it is possible that it can invade the ova of other economically important molluscan and crustacean species as well.

Large-scale dissemination of the cultured fungus could, therefore, have detrimental effects on commercial shellfisheries. Unfortunately, the studies of this fungus were discontinued. As also emphasized by Sindermann (1970a), its possible use as a biological control for *Urosalpinx cinerea* needs further investigation.

Various fungi have been isolated from both dead and living mollusc shells. Bornet and Flahault (1889) described two organisms, which were believed to be fungi and named *Ostracoblabe implexa* and *Lythopythium gangliiforme*, from shells of living and dead molluscs. Bonar (1936) reported ascomycetes *Didymella conchae* (Fig. 12-2) from small black pits on the outer surface of limpets *Acmaea digitalis*, *A. fenestrata*, *A. limatula*, *A. pelta*, *A. scabra* and *A. scutum*, as well as from winkles *Littorina planaxis* and black turbans *Tegula funebralis* from California, USA.

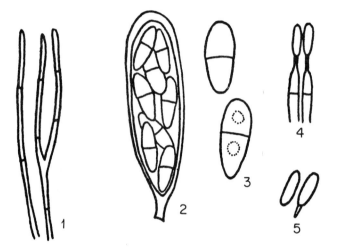

Fig. 12-2: *Didymella conchae*, an ascomycete fungus parasitizing in the shell matrix of marine molluscs. 1: paraphyses; 2: ascus; 3: ascospores; 4: conidiophores; 5: conidia. (After Bonar, 1936; reproduced by permission of The Regents of the University of California Press.)

Fruiting bodies of a pyrenomycetous form were regularly present in a large percentage of the shells of these molluscs. The surface of infected shells appeared roughened—sometimes 'honey-combed'—and greyish, also exhibiting a very evident dissolution of part of the calcareous matrix. In densely invaded areas, the shell material could be dissected away as a crumbling mass. Infections regularly started near the apex, and very often, the younger, marginal part showed no involvement. There was no evidence of any damage to the animal itself. According to Grant (note added to Bonar's 1936 paper), *Didymella conchae* appears to be widespread on the North American Pacific coast, attacking particularly the limpets *Acmaea digitalis* and *A. pelta*, uninfected shells of these two species actually being rare. The damage caused by this fungus has brought about, in part, certain taxonomical problems. In many cases, the external appearance of affected shells may be so changed that classification becomes exceedingly difficult. Misidentification as well as erroneous synonymizations of limpets have thus been the consequence.

Various fungi occur in dead molluscan shells, and probably contribute greatly to the deterioration of such structures (Zebrowski, 1937; Korringa, 1951; Johnson and Anderson, 1962; Höhnk, 1969). These and other records of fungi, as well as micro-organisms believed to be fungi, have been reviewed and summarized by Johnson and Sparrow (1961) and Kohlmeyer (1969).

DISEASES CAUSED BY PROTOZOANS

Agents: Sporozoa

Eugregarines *Nematopsis legeri*, originally described as *Porospora galloprovincialis* by Léger and Duboscq (1925), use a number of European marine bivalves, as well as gastropods *Trochocochlea turbinata*, *T. articulata*, *T. mutabilis*, *Gibbula adamsoni*, *G. divaricata*, *G. rarilineata*, *Pisania maculosa*, *Cerithium rupestre*, *Columbella rustica* and *Conus mediterraneus*, as intermediate hosts (Hatt, 1927a, b, c, 1931). Gymnospores, 7 μm in diameter, and spores, 14 to 15 μm long, have been isolated from the gill tissue and blood sinuses. Infestation of individual molluscs with *N. legeri* can be heavy, with the formation of minor local lesions on the surfaces of the gill lamellae during the penetration of gymnospores, but with only slight general effect on the intermediate host. A related species, *Porospora gigantea*, is known to use *Trochocochlea mutablis* as intermediate host (Hatt, 1931). Both gregarines appear to be restricted to European waters.

Coccidia *Merocystis kathae* parasitize in the renal organ of dogwhelks *Buccinum undatum* from the North and Baltic Seas (Dakin, 1911; Foulon, 1919, Patten, 1935; Køie, 1969). Sporogony occurs intracellularly. Although attacked host kidney cells undergo marked hypertrophy, there appears to be no noticeable general injury to the whelk. Schizogonic stages of the parasite are not known; possibly an additional host is necessary to complete the life cycle of *M. kathae*.

Coccidians *Pseudoklossia patellae* occur intracellularly in the digestive gland, hepatopancreatic ducts, intestine and kidney of limpets *Patella vulgata* from Roscoff, France, and Plymouth, England. Schizogony has not been observed (Debaisieux, 1922; Fig. 12-3).

Piridium sociabile, a protozoan parasite originally believed to be a schizogregarine, occurs in the subepithelial connective tissue on the ventral part of the foot of dogwhelks *Buccinum undatum* from England and Öresund, Denmark (Patten, 1936; Køie, 1969). Hyman (1967) disagreed with Patten's tentative identification, and placed *P. sociabile* among the Coccidia. Crofts (1929) briefly mentioned what he believed to be haplosporidan capsules in the digestive gland and gonads of *Haliotis* sp.

Agents: Ciliata

Several species of arhynchodinid thigmotrich ciliates have been reported from the gill surfaces of marine gastropods: *Ancistrum cylidioides* from *Natica habraea* and *A. barbatum* from *Fusus syracusanus* and *Murex trunculus* from the Gulf of Naples (Issel, 1903); *A. hydrobiae* occurs in the mantle cavity of *Hydrobia ulvae* and *H. ventrosa* in the Baltic Sea (Fenchel, 1965). *Protophrya ovicola* (Fig. 12-4), another arhynchodinid closely related to *Ancistrum*, lives in the mantle cavity of periwinkles *Littorina obtusata*, *L. littorea* and *L. saxatilis*, as well as in the brood pouch of the latter species, where it has been observed penetrating the gelatinous capsule of the host's eggs, and to be entering the embryos. Heavily invaded female *L. saxatilis* produce an offspring with many abnormal individuals (Cépède, 1910). *Ancistrum* and most other Arhynchodina are suspension feeders equipped with ciliary filtering devices. It is not clear whether these organisms

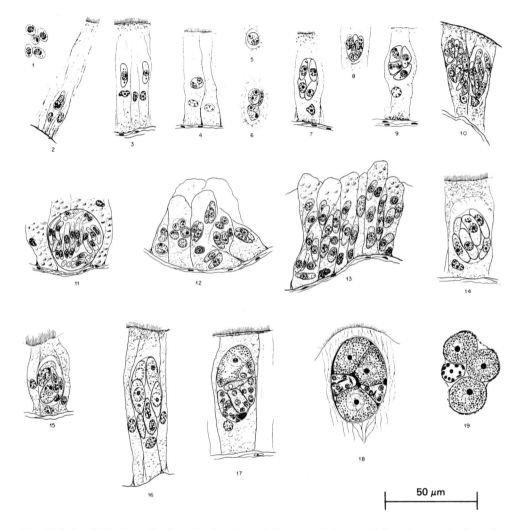

Fig. 12-3: *Pseudoklossia patellae* from *Patella vulgata*. 1: Parasites in lumen of digestive gland acinus; 2: young trophozoite within ciliated intestinal epithelium cell; 3: mature trophozoites; 4, 5: binucleate trophozoites undergoing division; 6: trophozoites in different stages of maturity; 7, 8: 4 trophozoites within host cell; 9: 4 trophozoites undergoing nuclear division within digestive gland cell; 10, 11: multiplication of trophozoites within host cell; 12, 13: intense infestation of cells in digestive gland acinus; 14–18: formation of micro- and macrogamonts; 19: 3 macrogamonts and 1 microgamont containing microgametes, enclosed by membrane and being discharged into lumen of digestive gland tubule. 20, 21: *Pseudoklossia chitonis* from *Acanthochites fascicularis*. 20: Micro- and macrogamonts within secretory cells of digestive gland; 21:2 microgamonts from lumen of posterior intestine of A. fascicularis. (After Debaisieux, 1922; reproduced by permission of La Cellule.)

can cause tissue destruction in the molluscan host. Most of them appear to be non-pathogenic. *Ancistrumina obtusae* from the mantle cavity of *Cerithidea obtusa*, an estuarine snail inhabiting Gangetic mangrove swamps, is believed to be a commensal (Yusuf and Choudhury, 1977).

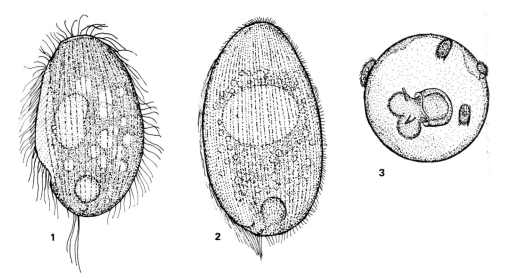

Fig. 12-4: Ciliates associated with marine prosobranchs. 1: *Ancistrum hydrobiae* (left lateral view) from gills of *Hydrobia* spp. 2: *Protophrya ovicola*, parasitic in brood pouch of *Littorina* spp.; living individual seen from left side. 3: Egg of *Littorina saxatilis* invaded by *P. ovicola*. (After Fenchel, 1965; reproduced by permission of Ophelia.)

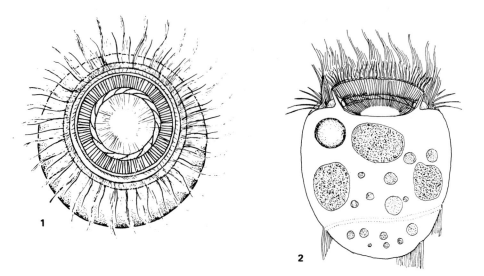

Fig. 12-5: *Leiotrocha patellae* parasitic on the gills of *Patella* spp. 1: scopula of living individual; 2: optical section through living individual. (After Fenchel, 1965; reproduced by permission of Ophelia.)

Leiotrocha patellae (Fig. 12-5), a peritrich ciliate of the family Urceolariidae, occurs on the gills of various species of limpets *Patella* spp. in Europe (Cuénot, 1891; Caullery and Mesnil, 1915). *L. patellae* probably embodies a complex of morphologically very similar forms which exhibit some degree of host-specificity. Thus, Brouardel (1951) could demonstrate experimentally that specimens of *Leiotrocha* were attracted to isolated gill filaments from *Patella* species from which they were obtained, but not to filaments taken from other limpet species. *Trichodina baltica*, another peritrich, occurs on the gills of *Hydrobia ventrosa* in the Baltic Sea (Raabe and Raabe, 1959). Nothing is known about the pathogenicity of peritrich ciliates in molluscan hosts. Trichodinids living on the gill epithelium of fishes, however, are known to feed on the host's blood cells. Since *Trichodina* spp. taken from the gills of molluscs do not survive long outside the host, they are probably parasitic.

Agents: Protophyta

It is well known that blue-green algae can cause corrosion and deterioration of molluscan shells (Bornet and Flahault, 1889). An unidentified threat-forming cyanophycean in corroded periwinkle *Littorina littorea* shells, probably a member of the order Chamaesiphonales, was believed to be responsible for the corrosion and destruction of the calcareous matrix of the shell (Kessel, 1937).

Conducting a detailed study on shell-boring algae, Nielsen (1972) isolated cyanophyceans *Hyella balani*, *Mastigocoelus testarum* and *Plectonema terebrans*, as well as chlorophyceans *Eugomontia sacculata*, *Gomontia polyrhiza*, *Phaeophila dendroides* and *P. tenuis* from corroded *Littorina littorea* shells obtained from Laesø (Kattegat). The occurrence of some of the algae exhibited a distinct correlation with wave exposure.

DISEASES CAUSED BY METAZOANS

Agents: Mesozoa

Lang (1954) reported orthonectid Mesozoa *Rhopalura philinae* from the opisthobranch snail *Philine scabra* dredged in Gullmarfjord, Sweden. Males measured 540 to 700 μm, and females 223 to 314 μm in length. They occupy the mantle cavity, the blood sinuses, the excretory organs and the hermaphroditic gland. The host is not castrated, even in heavy infestations, but there appears to be a certain effect on the eggs, some giving the impression of being aborted. Apparently, *R. philinae* is monoecious, females and males occurring in separate hosts.

Agents: Cnidaria

A number of hydroids and medusae are known to be associated with marine prosobranchs. Most of them are merely epiphoronts, and none of these associations appears to be truly parasitic or disease-causing in nature (Rees, 1967). Thus, they will not be considered further here.

Three athecate hydroids, *Pandea conica*, *P. rubra* and *Kinetocodium danae*, appear to be obligatory associates of nudibranchs (pteropods) *Cleodora clione limacina* and *Diacria trispinosa*, respectively. There is no indication in the *Pandea* spp. of any structural modifications towards parasitism (Rees, 1967). In *K. danae*, however, the long tubular polyps have reduced tentacles and a well-developed suctorial mouth. Although feeding activity was not observed directly, one preserved specimen had its mouth tightly adhering to the surface of the host's foot. The disposition of the nutritive hydrants anterior to the lateral spines of the shell, as well as their close proximity to the pteropod's body, could be taken as indicative of a parasitic way of life in this hydroid (Kramp, 1921, 1957).

Agents: Turbellaria

Polyclad turbellarians *Hoploplana inquilina thaisana* have been reported from the mantle cavity of oyster drills *Thais floridana floridana* from the Gulf of Mexico, as well as from *Urosalpinx cinerea* and *Eupleura caudata* from Delaware Bay, New Jersey, USA. Incidence and intensity of infestation were usually low, and the relationship appeared to be merely commensalistic (Pearse, 1938; Hyman, 1940; Stauber, 1941; Schechter, 1943).

A rhabdocoel turbellarian *Graffilla buccinicola* occurs in dogwhelks *Buccinum undatum* and Neptune whelks *Neptunea antiqua* from the North Sea and the Kattegat. Several dozen specimens may be found in the renal organ and the mantle cavity of individual hosts. In heavily attacked snails the kidney may be somewhat dilated, with local weakening of tissue, and may contain large amounts of mucus. No serious injury has, however, been observed. *G. buccinicola* also occurs in the stomach, the intestine and the tubules of the hepatopancreas of the whelks (Jameson, 1897; von Graff, 1903; Dakin, 1912; Westblad, 1926; Køie, 1969).

Agents: Trematoda

The overwhelming majority of gastropod parasites belongs to the platyhelminth class Trematoda Digenea. Marine snails serve primarily as first intermediate hosts and, to a lesser extent, also as second intermediate hosts. In a few cases, gastropods have been reported as final hosts for digenetic trematodes. Only comparatively few examples of gastropod-trematode associations can be treated here in detail, the emphasis being on economically important and most-studied marine host species.

The specific and even generic names of the trematodes mentioned below are not necessarily those of the original workers. Misidentification, multiple descriptions and tentative synonymizations are the rule rather than the exception in trematodology. The present state of 'Quantitative Helminthology' can thus be characterized by quoting from Stunkard and Uzmann (1958, p. 285): 'The situation is chaotic and one of utter confusion'.

This is mainly due to the total inadequacy of data processing in parasitology. Comparative specific descriptions of trematodes rely to a great extent upon morphometric measurements. Treatment of such data has essentially remained the same today as in the beginnings of parasitology. Usually, only the mean and observed range of body dimensions are reported to demonstrate the variability of a given species. However, the observed range of measurements is 'the poorest of all measures of dispersion' (Simpson and co-authors, 1960, p. 80). Exact morphometric characterization and comparison of trematodes is, therefore, impossible on the basis of available information. Improper treatment of measurement data has frequently led to misconceptions regarding intra- versus interspecific variation in parasitic flatworms (Stunkard, 1957b).

This makes a review of the pertinent literature on trematode parasites of molluscs problematic.

Statistical methods, routinely applied for a considerable time in many fields of research, but apparently unknown to parasitologists, are well-suited to solve taxonomic problems in trematodology (Lauckner, 1971). Helminthologists engaged in systematic work, but inexperienced in statistical handling of descriptive and experimental data should read Simpson and co-authors' (1960) brilliantly written 'Quantitative Zoology' and continue with Snedecor and Cochran (1967). The application of more sophisticated mathematical methods, such as discriminant analysis (Fisher, 1936), or regression analysis (Draper and Smith, 1966), will probably contribute measureably in the future to the solution of taxonomic problems, particularly in studies on trematodes. Regarding the fact that morphometric data are often obscured by allometric growth of parasites (Reimer, 1970), the pursuit of growth problems is to be recommended. The chapter on growth in Simpson and co-authors (1960) might serve as a useful, clear introduction to the solution of growth problems.

Gastropods as First Intermediate Hosts for Digenea

Among the **Archaegastropoda**, members of the suborders Patellacea (limpets) and Trochacea (top shells) have been reported particularly as first intermediate hosts for larval trematodes.

Cercaria patellae, an echinostome philophthalmid larva, develops in rediae in the intertubular spaces within the digestive gland of *Patella vulgata* from Loch Ryan, Scotland (Lebour, 1907b, 1911). Heavy infestations result in profound damage, involving histolysis of the glandular epithelium and, eventually, total atrophy and destruction of the hepatopancreatic and gonadal tissue (Rees, 1934). The parasite has also been reported from 10% of *P. intermedia*, 17% of *P. depressa*, and 4% of *P. vulgata* from various other localities along the British coast (Crewe, 1951), and James (1968c) recorded it from 3·77% of 503 *P. vulgata*, 4·66% of 150 *P. intermedia*, and 3·66% of 328 *P. depressa* in Cardigan Bay, Wales. Although large limpets were mainly infested, there was no evidence for parasite-induced gigantism (Crewe, 1951).

The life cycle of *Cercaria patellae* remains unknown. It is similar to *Parorchis acanthus* whose rediae and cercariae develop in oyster drills *Thais lapillus*, but unlike *P. acanthus*, the cercariae of *C. patellae* do not encyst on solid surfaces; they probably require a second intermediate host. Lysaght (1941) suggested that certain metacercariae found in *Littorina neritoides* may be those of *C. patellae*. The adult stage is possibly identical with *Echinostephilla virgula*, a trematode parasite in the intestine of the turnstone *Arenaria interpres* (Lebour, 1908c, 1911).

Unidentified xiphidiocercariae, provisionally named 'Cercaria B', developing in tightly packed, salmon-coloured masses of sporocysts in the intertubular sinuses of the digestive gland, have been observed in *Patella intermedia* and *P. vulgata*. 'Cercaria B' appears to be a rare parasite, only 22 of more than 5000 limpets being infested (Crewe, 1951). Although its life cycle is not yet known, it is, beyond doubt, a species of *Renicola*, whose adult stage may be found in the kidney of some shore birds. The parasite apparently has no effect on the condition of the gonads, which were never found infested. Degeneration of host tissues was restricted to the space occupied by the sporocysts, the effects induced by the germinal sacs being very similar to those caused by *Cercaria patellae*.

Several cotylocercous xiphidiocercariae—unidentified or given provisional names, and probably all members of the family Opecoelidae—are known to parasitize in sporocysts in top shells *Gibbula cineraria*, *G. divaricata* and *G. umbilicalis* from Millport, England, from Archachon and Roscoff, France, and from the Mediterranean Sea (Lespès, 1857; Pelseneer, 1906; Lebour, 1911; Stunkard, 1932; Palombi, 1934; Dollfus and Euzet, 1964; Graefe, 1971). Crofts (1929) reports on an unidentified larval trematode, presumably a member of the Opecoelidae, which develops in orange-coloured sporocysts in visceral mass, mantle, mucus glands and gills of *Haliotis* sp. from British waters.

Similarly, unidentified cotylocercous opecoelid xiphidiocercariae, as well as cystophorous hemiurid cercariae, have been isolated from other Archaegastropoda—*Phasianella speciosa*, *Calliostoma conulum* and *C. striatum* from the Mediterranean Sea (Palombi, 1938, 1940). Nothing is known about the pathogenicity or the life cycles of these parasites. They appear to be related to or represent members of the genus *Podocotyle*. Small crustaceans probably serve as second intermediate hosts and fishes as final hosts.

Among the **Mesogastropoda**, members of the Hydrobiidae (genus *Hydrobia*), Littorinidae (genus *Littorina*), Turritellidae (genus *Turritella*), Potamididae (genus *Cerithidea*) and Cerithiidae (genera *Cerithium* and *Bittium*) have been particularly reported as first intermediate hosts for a great variety of trematodes.

Despite their small size, snails of the genus *Hydrobia* are favourite hosts for larval trematodes. A vast number of species of Digenea have been recorded from *H. ulvae*, *H. ventrosa* and *H. acuta* in various parts of the North Sea, the Baltic Sea, the European Atlantic coast and the Mediterranean (Lebour 1907a, 1908a, 1911; Markowski, 1936; Rothschild, 1936a, b, 1938a, b, c, d, e, f, 1941a; Rothschild and Rothschild, 1939; Chabaud and Biguet, 1954; Chabaud and Buttner, 1959; Deblock and co-authors, 1961; Honer, 1961a, b; Ankel, 1962; Reimer, 1962, 1963a, b, 1964b, 1970; Rebecq, 1961, 1964a, b; Deblock and Rosé, 1965; Loos-Frank, 1967, 1968a, b; Maillard, 1973; Rasmussen, 1973; Reimer and Bernstein, 1973; Deblock, 1974a; Vaes, 1974; and others), as well as from *H. minuta*, *H. salsa* and *H. jacksoni* from North America (Stunkard, 1958, 1960a, b, 1964a, 1966b, 1967a, b, 1968, 1970; Deblock and Heard, 1969).

Most of the trematodes parasitizing *Hydrobia* spp. are members of the family Microphallidae. These typically have small xiphidiocercariae—i.e. cercariae equipped with a penetration stylet—which develop in sporocysts in the digestive gland and the gonad of the snails. The life cycle of microphallids usually involves a crustacean as second intermediate host and a sea bird or, more rarely, a mammal or even a fish as final host. Since many commercially fished decapod crustaceans act as second intermediate hosts, microphallids must be regarded as economically important parasites.

Some microphallids developing in *Hydrobia* spp. have, however, abridged life cycles. *Maritrema oocysta*, *Microphallus somateriae* and *Levinseniella* sp. possess xiphidiocercariae which encyst in the snails from which they are shed. *Atriophallophorus minutus* has a styletless cercaria which also encysts in the first intermediate host, and the cercariae of *Microphallus pirum*, *M. scolectroma*, *M. abortivus* and *Maritrema syntomocyclus* (Fig. 12-42) encyst directly within the sporocyst from which they originate (Deblock and Tran Van Ky, 1966b; Deblock, 1974b).

The systematics of the family Microphallidae are problematic. Early authors encountered and described either only the sporocysts and cercariae from *Hydrobia* spp. or the metacercariae from crustaceans. Sometimes they speculated on the specific identity of the various forms or even referred them—without experimental proof—to one of the then-known adult microphallids from the intestine of birds. Although many complete life histories have been worked out experimentally in the meantime, there is still much confusion, which becomes obvious from the historical and taxonomic surveys conducted by Deblock and Tran Van Ky (1966a, b). Their publications, as well as those by Deblock and Pearson (1969) and Deblock (1971), include diagnostic keys for the Microphallidae. Richard (1977) identified representatives of the genera *Microphallus* and *Maritrema* by means of chaetotaxy. Certain tegumental papillae or groups of papillae have generic, supra-generic or specific significance.

Other trematodes using *Hydrobia* spp. as first intermediate hosts are mainly representatives of the families Notocotylidae, Echinostomatidae, Lepocreadiidae, Heterophyidae, Psilostomatidae and Hemiuridae. Notocotylids, members of the genera *Notocotylus, Paramonostomum* and *Uniserialis*, parasitize in rediae in the gonad and digestive gland of *Hydrobia ulvae, H. ventrosa, H. acuta, H. minuta* and *H. salsa*. They have abridged life cycles. Cercariae emerging from infested snails encyst on any hard surface, preferably on molluscan—particularly *Hydrobia* spp.—shells (Lebour, 1907a, 1911; Stunkard, 1932, 1958, 1960b, 1966b, 1967a, b, 1970a; Rothschild, 1935b, 1938b; Honer, 1961a; Ankel, 1962; Rebecq, 1964a, b). The Echinostomatidae and Heterophyidae are economically important. The cercariae of several species of the echinostomatid genus *Himasthla* encyst in commercially exploited bivalve molluscs *Cardium edule, Mytilus edulis* and *Mya arenaria*, in which they provoke detrimental effects (Stunkard, 1960a, 1970a). Cercariae of the heterophyids *Cryptocotyle concava* and *C. jejuna*, which develop in *Hydrobia ulvae* and *H. ventrosa*, penetrate fishes. Their metacercariae have been reported from teleosts from various parts of the northern hemisphere (Issaitchikoff, 1926; Rothschild, 1941b; Hoffman, 1957; Reimer, 1962, 1970; Rebecq, 1964a). Wootton's (1957) report on *C. concava* from freshwater snails *Amnicola longinqua* in California, USA, is certainly a misidentification.

Larval hemiurids, named *Cercaria sinitzini*, were found to parasitize in rediae in the gonad of 1 of 2000 *Hydrobia ulvae* from Plymouth, England. The parasite did not damage the snail's hepatopancreas (Rothschild, 1938a). Rediae of *Bunocotyle meridionalis* occur in *H. ventrosa* and *H. acuta* in the Rhône estuary, French Mediterranean coast (Chabaud and Biguet, 1954; Chabaud and Buttner, 1959; Rebecq, 1964a), and *B. progenetica* has been recorded from *H. ulvae* and *H. ventrosa* from the French coast of the English Channel and from the Baltic Sea (Markowski, 1936; Reimer, 1970; Deblock, 1974a). Infestation incidences varied between less than 1% in the Baltic Sea and approximately 3% at the English Channel localities.

Gigantobilharzia vittensis occurs in *Hydrobia ventrosa* from the Baltic Sea, 4 of 1232 snails being infested (Reimer, 1962, 1963b). This is the first report of schistosome cercariae from brackish-water snails in Europe.

Infestation rates of *Hydrobia ventrosa* and *H. ulvae* vary greatly with locality—from a few scattered cases to as much as 56%, 87% or even 91% (Loos-Frank, 1967; Honer, 1961b and Rothschild, 1938c, respectively)—as well as with season (Rothschild 1941a; Reimer and Bernstein, 1973). In general, larger specimens are more frequently infested and liberate more cercariae than smaller hosts. Trematode invasion of the reproductive organs results in 'parasitic castration', i.e. partial or total gonad destruction in both sexes as well as penis reduction in males. In *H. ulvae*, the normal ratio of females to males is 2:1. In some samples, however, the ratio of infested males to females was as high as 16:1 (Rothschild, 1936b, 1938c). It is obvious that trematode invasion of the reported magnitude considerably reduces the reproductive potential of the whole snail population.

Affection of the digestive gland causes serious injury and pathological changes like those described in great detail for other gastropod species (Faust, 1920; Agersborg, 1924; G. Rees, 1934; W. J. Rees, 1936a). In long-standing infestations, the digestive gland of *Hydrobia* spp. is reduced to a remnant. It is difficult to understand how affected snails can survive at this stage, and it is generally assumed that trematode invasion is an important factor contributing to mortality of *Hydrobia* spp. in the field. Under laboratory conditions, however, survival of *H. ulvae* was not seriously affected by trematode invasion. Only 4 of 152 infested and healthy specimens died during an observation period of 1 year (Rothschild and Rothschild, 1939).

Trematode invasion can cause behavioural changes in snails. Thus, large infested specimens of *Hydrobia ulvae* tended to avoid the shelter of algal vegetation and crawled out into the open where they were more easily accessible to bird final hosts (Honer, 1961b). Such behavioural changes may result in increased mortality of larger infested snails under field conditions, due to selective predation by sea birds.

Gigantism is another phenomenon repeatedly reported for trematode-infested snails. After careful field studies and a series of long-term laboratory experiments, Rothschild (1936b, 1938c, 1941a) and Rothschild and Rothschild (1939) arrived at the conclusion that specimens of *Hydrobia ulvae* harbouring larval trematodes grow faster and become larger than uninfested individuals. The authors furthermore believed that variations in shell shape as well as asymmetrical development of the spire is caused by the pressure exerted by the parasites from within.

Wesenberg-Lund (1934) was the first to point out that trematode-infested snails are sometimes abnormally large. He attributed this increase in size to the fact that infested snails ingest abnormally large quantities of food in order to satisfy the demands of the parasites. The Rothschilds, however, assumed that gigantism in *Hydrobia ulvae* is brought about by the destruction of the host's gonad and the resultant changes in physiological and hormonal mechanisms. Ankel (1962) found no evidence for gigantism in her studies on the trematode parasites of *H. ulvae* and *H. ventrosa* in Danish waters.

Snails of the genus *Littorina* harbour a great variety of trematodes, mainly representatives of the families Echinostomatidae, Gymnophallidae, Heterophyidae, Microphallidae, Notocotylidae, Opecoelidae and Renicolidae (Fig. 12-6). The occurrence of Digenea in *Littorina littorea*, *L. saxatilis* and *L. obtusata* from Europe and the west coast of North America has been studied by Lespès (1857), Pelseneer (1906), Lebour (1907b, 1908b, 1914), Stunkard (1930, 1932, 1950, 1957a, 1966a, 1970a), Rees (1936b), Lysaght (1941), Hunninen and Cable (1943), James (1960, 1964, 1968a, b, c, d, 1969), Berry (1962), Werding (1969), Reimer (1970), Robson and Williams (1970), Pohley and Brown (1975), Combescot-Lang (1976), Pohley (1976), Popiel (1976), Sannia and James (1977), Threlfall and Goudie (1977), Lauckner (in preparation) and others. The occurrence of larval trematodes in *Littorina scutulata* and *L. sitkana* from the

North American Pacific coast, in *L. pintado* from Hawaii, as well as in *L. irrorata* from the Gulf of Mexico has been studied by Miller (1925b), Chu (1952), Chu and Cutress (1954). Ching (1960, 1961, 1962, 1963a, b, 1965), Holliman (1961) and Duerr (1965). Among the trematodes are economically significant parasites which use commercially important crustaceans, molluscs and fishes as second intermediate hosts (see Vol. II). James (1968d) presented a key to European *Littorina* species and their digenean trematodes.

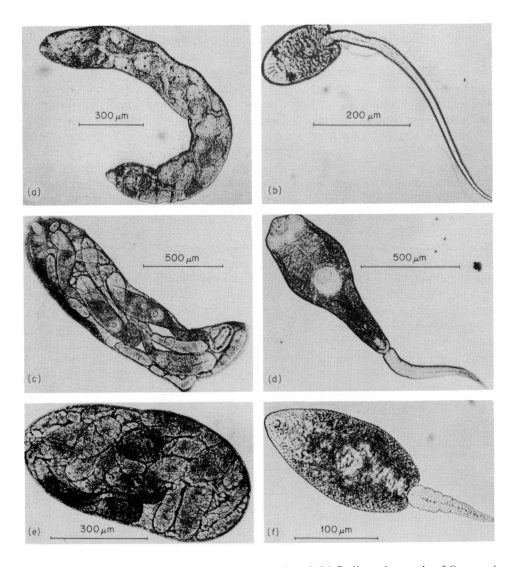

Fig. 12-6: Larval trematodes from *Littorina littorea*. (a) and (b) Redia and cercaria of *Cryptocotyle lingua*; (c) and (d) redia and cercaria of *Himasthla elongata*; (e) and (f) sporocyst and cercaria of *Renicola roscovita*. (Original.)

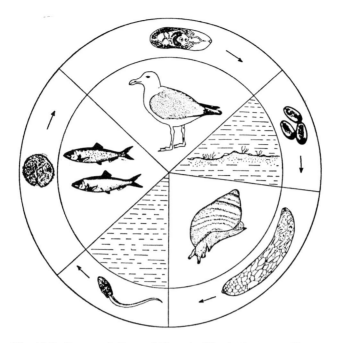

Fig. 12-7: *Cryptocotyle lingua*. Life cycle. Hatched sectors of inner circle: free-living stages; unhatched sectors: stages occurring in intermediate or final host(s). (Based on various sources.)

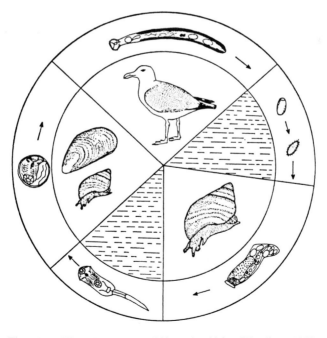

Fig. 12-8: *Himasthla elongata*. Life cycle. (After Werding, 1969; reproduced by permission of Springer-Verlag.)

Table 12-1

Littorina littorea.   Incidence of trematode infestation in periwinkles from German and Danish coastal waters (Original)

Locality (region)	Total number of *L. littorea* collected	Total infestation		*Cryptocotyle lingua*		*Himasthla elongata*		*Remicola roscovita*		*Microphallus pygmaeus*		*Podocotyle atomon*		*Cercaria lebouri*	
		n	%	n	%	n	%	n	%	n	%	n	%	n	%
Isle of Sylt (German North Sea coast)	30,811	6,144	19.94	2,500	8.11	2,211	7.17	1,133	3.67	289	0.93	80	0.25	60	0.19
German North Sea coast; mainland coast of Schleswig-Holstein	1,496	86	5.74	33	2.20	3	0.20	43	2.87	3	0.20	1	0.06	4	0.26
German and Danish western Baltic Sea coast and Kattegat	11,571	1,732	14.96	592	5.11	537	4.64	298	2.57	308	2.66	40	0.34	0	0.00

Periwinkles *Littorina littorea* from the North and Baltic Seas have been shown to be hosts for 6 species of larval trematodes. The commonest, *Cryptocotyle lingua*, is economically most important: it is a serious fish pathogen. *Himasthla elongata* and *Renicola roscovita*, the second and third most common species, are detrimental to mussels and cockles in their metacercarial stage. The 3 remaining species, *Microphallus pygmaeus*, *Podocotyle atomon* and *Cercaria lebouri*, occur sporadically and are of no direct economic significance (Table 12-1).

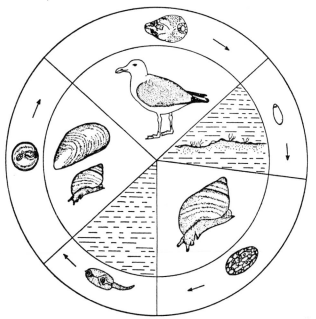

Fig. 12-9: *Renicola roscovita*. Life cycle. (After Werding, 1969; reproduced by permission of Springer-Verlag.)

Cryptocotyle lingua, Himasthla elongata and *Cercaria lebouri* have redial stages, *Renicola roscovita, Microphallus pygmaeus* and *Podocotyle atomon* have sporocyst stages which parasitize in the digestive gland and gonad of *Littorina littorea* (Figs 12-6 to 12-16). The life cycles of the 3 most common species which utilize shore birds (mainly gulls of the genus *Larus*) as final hosts are illustrated in Figs 12-7 to 12-9. *P. atomon* uses small crustaceans (amphipods) as second intermediate, and fishes (mostly pleuronectid flatfishes) as definite hosts. *M. pygmaeus* has an abbreviated life cycle. Its cercariae develop directly into metacercariae within the sporocysts and do not leave the periwinkle which, therefore, serves simultaneously as first and second intermediate host. *C. lebouri*, on the other hand, does not require a second intermediate host. Its cercariae encyst free on solid surfaces. Both species have birds as final hosts.

The gross morphological appearance of digestive glands of *Littorina littorea* invaded by *Cryptocotyle lingua, Himasthla elongata* and *Renicola roscovita* is illustrated in Figs 12-10 and 12-11. Littorinids and their digenean parasites have been studied most thoroughly with respect to their physiology, ethology, epizootiology, pathophysiology and biochemistry. These studies could serve as models for future investigations to be conducted on other marine mollusc–trematode associations.

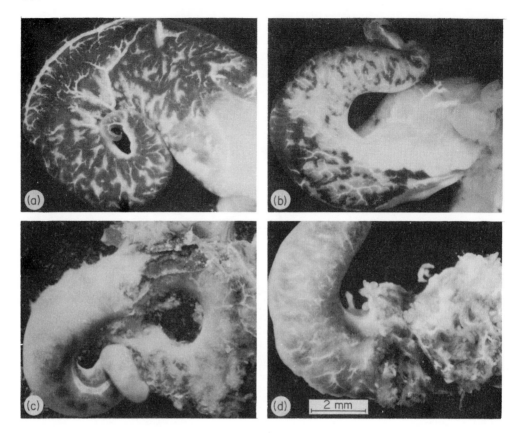

Fig. 12-10: *Littorina littorea*. Healthy digestive gland of female (a) and male (b); (c) digestive gland infested with *Cryptocotyle lingua* rediae; (d) infestation with *Himasthla elongata* rediae. Scale in (d) applies also to (a–c). (Original.)

Trematode infestation produces pathological conditions in littorinids comparable to those reported for hydrobiids—obliteration of the digestive gland, gonad and penis reduction, cessation of sperm and egg production and, possibly, increased mortality (Lysaght, 1941; Berry, 1962; James, 1964; Robson and Williams, 1971a). The degree of tissue destruction, however, may not only vary with the intensity of infestation, but also with the parasite species involved. The effect may be mechanical, physiological or both.

Rediae of *Himasthla elongata* and *Cryptocotyle lingua* were observed to ingest eggs and yolk from the ovarian tubules of their host *Littorina littorea*. The digestive gland is affected only indirectly, due to mechanical pressure caused by the rapidly multiplying and growing rediae, loss of food and the production of enormous amounts of waste materials. The inactive sporocysts of *Renicola roscovita*, on the other hand, form a 'blocking layer' in the lower parts of the host's spire, resulting in an accumulation of waste products and starvation autolysis of digestive tubules in the distal part of the hepatopancreas. The gonad is preserved much longer in specimens infested with sporocysts than in those parasitized by rediae (Rees, 1936a; Figs 12-12 to 12-16).

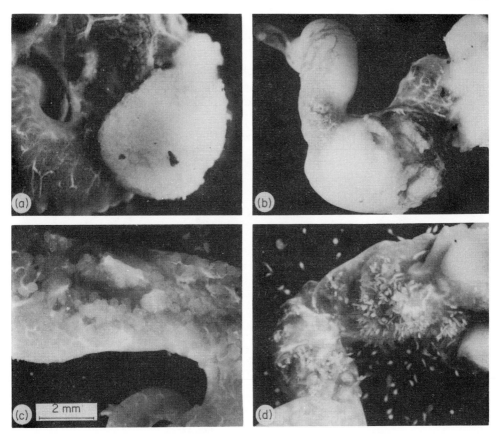

Fig. 2-11: *Littorina littorea*. (a) Immature infestation with *Renicola roscovita* sporocysts. Note well circumscribed 'infestation boil'. (b) Mature *Renicola roscovita* infestation forming typical 'blocking layer' and causing atrophy of distal part of digestive gland. (c) Infestation with *Microphallus pygmaeus* sporocysts containing metacercariae. (d) Infestation with rediae of *Cercaria lebouri*. All same scale. (Original.)

Destruction of the digestive-gland tubules by larval trematodes may liberate stored carotenoid pigments which are then dispersed by the haemolymph throughout the snail tissues. According to Willey and Gross (1957), the foot of *Littorina littorea* infested with *Cryptocotyle lingua* assumes an orange-to-brown colour, in contrast to the white or grey colour of the foot in healthy specimens, and trematode-harbouring periwinkles could be readily identified and separated from unaffected ones according to the colour of the foot (Fig. 12-17). Contrary to the observations of Willey and Gross, James (1974) could not find a correlation between foot colour of *L. littorea* and trematode infestation. An intensive study on the effects of larval trematode parasitism on the digestive-gland cells of *Littorina saxatilis tenebrosa* was conducted by comparing histochemically stained cells in healthy, starved and infested specimens (James, 1965). Starvation autolysis was apparent in digestive glands cut off by a blocking layer of sporocysts. In tubules cut off from their food supply, glucose, glycogen, glycoproteins and lipid food-storage globules were found reduced, and there was a compensatory increase in the number of food vacuoles in the digestive cells. Moreover, there was an increase in the amount of secretory products from the visceral haemocoel. An increase in glucose, but a decrease in glycogen, in the visceral haemocoel was also noted . Glucose and glycogen were detected in the subcuticular and extracaecal protoplasmic layers, glucose in the body cavity, caecal epithelium and gut contents of the parasite's germinal sacs, and glycogen throughout the body of the developing cercariae (Figs 12-18 to 12-20).

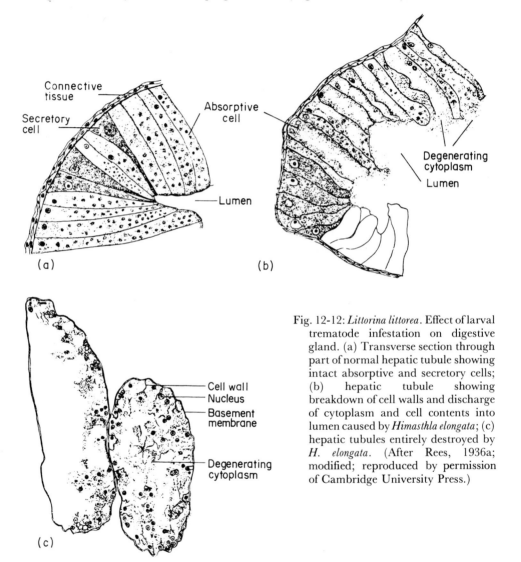

Fig. 12-12: *Littorina littorea*. Effect of larval trematode infestation on digestive gland. (a) Transverse section through part of normal hepatic tubule showing intact absorptive and secretory cells; (b) hepatic tubule showing breakdown of cell walls and discharge of cytoplasm and cell contents into lumen caused by *Himasthla elongata*; (c) hepatic tubules entirely destroyed by *H. elongata*. (After Rees, 1936a; modified; reproduced by permission of Cambridge University Press.)

Uptake of exogenous glucose by the rediae of *Cryptocotyle lingua* has been demonstrated by McDaniel and Dixon (1967) but the authors did not specify whether assimilation is through the body wall, the gut, or both. Although rediae possess a gut which enables them to ingest cellular material, there is morphological evidence to suggest that *C. lingua* rediae are also capable of uptake via the body wall (Krupa and co-authors, 1968).

Glycogen depletion appears to be a common phenomenon in trematode-invaded snails. The glycogen concentrations of the digestive gland and the foot in both healthy and infested *Littorina littorea* showed marked seasonal changes, being highest during autumn and lowest in spring. Infested specimens had consistently lower glycogen concentrations, and the amount of reduction was characteristic for each of the three parasite species involved. *Cryptocotyle lingua* caused greater glycogen decrease in the digestive gland, while *Renicola roscovita* had a more pronounced effect on the foot. In periwinkles infested with *Himasthla elongata*, glycogen concentrations were similar to those of healthy specimens and considerably above those recorded for infestations with *C. lingua* and *R. roscovita* (Robson and Williams, 1971b; Fig. 12-21; Table 12-2).

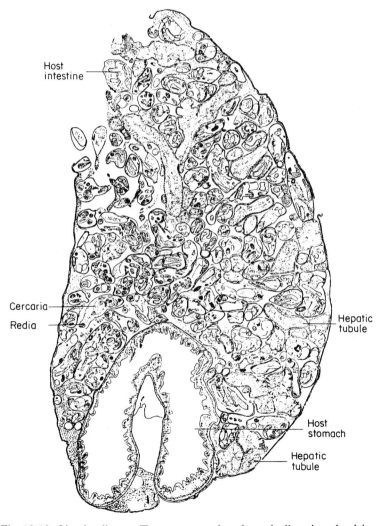

Fig. 12-13: *Littorina littorea*. Transverse section through digestive gland in region of stomach, showing almost complete disappearance of host tissue replaced by *Himasthla elongata* rediae and cercariae. (After Rees, 1936a; reproduced by permission of Cambridge University Press.)

Table 12-2

Littorina littorea. Glycogen concentration in digestive gland and foot, and shell lengths, of healthy and trematode-infested periwinkles (After Robson and Williams, 1971b; reproduced by permission of Journal of Helminthology)

| Infestation | Sex | Glycogen concentration (mg 100 g^{-1} tissue wet weight) | | | | | | Shell length (mm) | | |
| | | Digestive gland | | | Foot | | | | | |
		N	Mean±S.E.	Range	N	Mean±S.E.	Range	N	Mean±S.E.	Range
Non-infested	male	136	3·6 ±0·24	0·14—11·12	138	1·65±0·05	0·66—4·09	143	25·0±0·17	20·3—33·8
	female	136	3·44±0·19	0·15—9·74	137	1·77±3·06	0·22—3·67	142	25·1±0·16	20·8—30·4
C. lingua	male	94	1·71±0·10	0·44—7·92	92	1·59±0·06	0·66—2·99	96	26·8±0·25	22·8—32·3
	female	97	1·68±0·08	0·33—5·25	99	1·55±0·06	0·30—3·00	101	26·0±0·25	22·0—35·0
R. roscovita	male	65	2·99±0·32	0·40—10·53	70	1·28±0·08	0·20—3·25	71	24·7±0·21	20·8—29·2
	female	86	2·86±0·22	0·35—9·54	83	1·32±0·07	0·19—2·98	88	25·0±0·18	21·7—30·0
H. elongata	male	14	3·35±0·49	0·06—7·57	14	1·42±0·11	0·97—2·58	14	26·1±0·79	21·2—33·2
	female	9	4·00±0·92	0·74—8·74	11	1·62±0·23	0·51—2·98	11	27·2±0·65	24·0—32·4

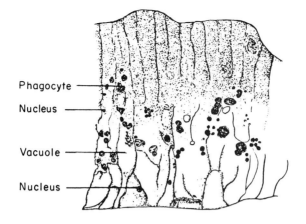

Fig. 12-14: *Littorina littorea*. Advanced stage of degeneration of hepatic tubule caused by *Renicola roscovita*. (The section is a little oblique; transverse walls are ordinary cell walls. Distal parts of cells filled with excretory products.) (After Rees, 1936a; reproduced by permission of Cambridge University Press.)

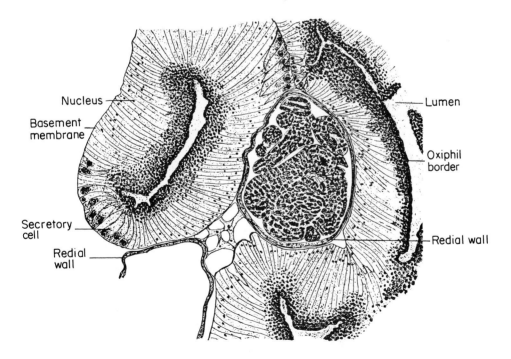

Fig. 12-15: *Littorina littorea*. Transverse section through redia of *Cryptocotyle lingua* and neighbouring host-hepatic epithelium. Note irregular arrangement of nuclei and excretory products accumulating in parts of cells bordering lumen. Overall tissue damage caused by *C. lingua* is less severe than in infestations with *Himasthla elongata* (Figs 12-12 and 12-13) and *Renicola roscovita* (Fig. 12-14). (After Rees, 1936a; reproduced by permission of Cambridge University Press.)

The free amino-acid pool of *Littorina littorea* was found to be affected to a varying extent by the Digenea parasitizing the periwinkle. Thus, the total concentration of free amino acids in the host's head-foot musculature showed an increase of 10·9% with infestations of *Cryptocotyle lingua*, a decrease of 12·7% with infestations of *Himasthla elongata*, and a decrease of as much as 57·5% with infestations of *Renicola roscovita*. The changes induced by the latter species are equivalent to starvation (Watts, 1971, Fig. 12-22). Leakage of amino acids from digenean germinal sacs, particularly from daughter sporocysts of *Microphallus pygmaeus* and *Renicola roscovita*, in various media suggests that their leakage may be a normal means of nitrogen excretion (Richards, 1970b; Watts, 1972). Watts' (1971) findings are well in accordance with the observations of various workers concerning the differential pathogenicity of the parasites in question.

Chromatographic analysis of the free and protein-bound amino acids of the rediae or sporocysts of *Cryptocotyle lingua*, *Himasthla elongata* and *Renicola roscovita* indicated that the host's free amino acids, rather than the products of protein hydrolysis, are utilized by the

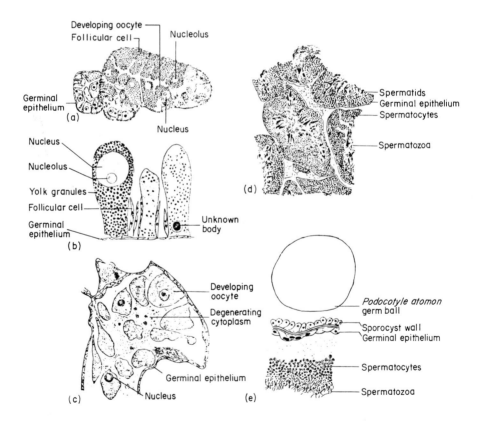

Fig. 12-16: *Littorina littorea*. Effect of larval trematode infestation on gonads. (a) Transverse section through healthy female genital tubule; (b) enlarged portion showing follicular cells; (c) female tubule of snail infested with *Renicola roscovita*; (d) transverse section through healthy male tubule; (e) degenerating part of male tubule adjacent to *Podocotyle atomon* sporocyst. (After Rees, 1936a; reproduced by permission of Cambridge University Press.)

larvae. The absolute concentrations of some of the host's free amino acids displayed significant sexual dimorphism (Watts, 1970a; Figs 12-23, 12-24). Although the trematodes parasitizing *Littorina littorea* exhibit no sex preference for either host, sexual dimorphism in the free amino-acid pool might possibly be responsible, at least in part, for such preference reported for other prosobranch–trematode associations.

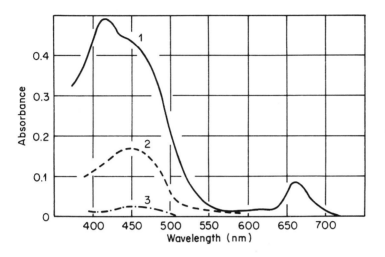

Fig. 12-17: *Littorina littorea*. Absorption spectra of alcoholic extracts of hepatopancreas (1), foot of snails infested with *Cryptocotyle lingua* (2), and foot of healthy snails (3). (After Willey and Gross, 1957; modified; reproduced by permission of American Society of Parasitologists.)

Biochemical studies on trematode-infested *Littorina littorea* and *L. saxatilis* indicate an alteration—mainly an elevation—of digestive-enzyme activity. The increase in glycolytic-enzyme levels in periwinkles harbouring the sporocysts of *Microphallus similis* probably reflects the greater catabolic activity in the affected digestive-gland cells. Since sporocysts do not possess a mouth, and rely entirely on the tegument for the assimilation of nutrients, they may secrete enzymes or enzyme stimulants into the host tissue. With respect to 'acidase' and 'alkase' activity, differences have been detected in periwinkles invaded by sporocysts and rediae, respectively. Acidase activity is increased and alkase activity is decreased in the digestive gland of *L. saxatilis* parasitized by sporocysts of *M. pygmaeus* and *M. similis*, while, in contrast, alkase activity is increased and acidase activity is unchanged or decreased in the hepatopancreas of *L. littorea* infested by rediae of *Himasthla elongata* and *Cryptocotyle lingua* (Marshall and co-authors, 1974a, b; Table 12-3 and Table 12-4). Transaminase activity in homogenates of *C. lingua* rediae and *Renicola roscovita* sporocysts indicates that alanine, aspartic acid, glutamic acid and their α-keto acid analogues could form an important link between carbohydrate and nitrogen metabolism (Watts, 1970b). The higher activity of most enzymes indicates that the parasite has an advantage over the host in competition for substrates.

Despite the changes in enzyme levels, the efficiency of assimilation of carbon and nitrogen by *Littorina saxatilis* infested with *Cryptocotyle lingua* did not differ significantly from that in non-infested snails. Similarly, the rate of ingestion and the rate of assimilation showed no marked variation between the two groups (Davis and Farley, 1973).

In digestive cells of *Littorina littorea*, *L. saxatilis* and *L. neritoides*, Moore and Halton (1977) studied the cytochemical localization of lysosomal hydrolases, as well as the changes induced by *Himasthla elongata* ('*H. leptosoma*'), *Cryptocotyle lingua* and *Podocotyle atomon* ('*Cercaria linearis*') infestation. Staining reactions for lysosomal hydrolases in *L. littorea* digestive cells could be related to the feeding-growth phase (summer) and non-feeding maturation phase (winter). *H. elongata* rediae apparently induced the least severe cytopathological changes while the structural disruption associated with *P. atomon* sporocysts was much more extensive with a transformation of normally columnar digestive cells to a vacuolated cuboidal type. The reaction product of acid hydrolases and esterase was distributed throughout the cytoplasm of infested digestive cells. Simultaneously, there was an increase in the levels of β-glucuronidase, β-galactosidase and hexosaminidase, while α-glucosidase could only be detected in *C. lingua* infestations (Table 12-5). The observed distributional changes in lysosomal

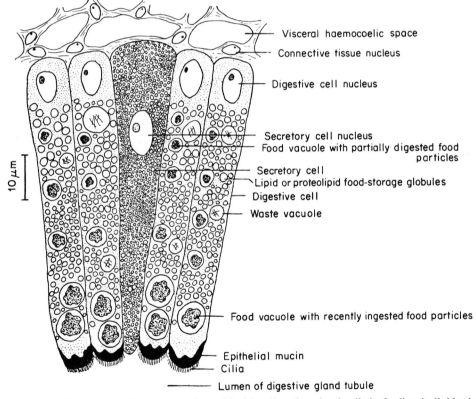

Fig. 12–18: *Littorina saxatilis* subsp. *tenebrosa*. Healthy digestive-gland cells in feeding individuals. (After James, 1965; reproduced by permission of Cambridge University Press.)

hydrolases were similar to those known to be associated with autophagic and autolytic activities. It was assumed that autophagy may provide a physiological survival mechanism during parasitic and nutritional stress.

The lipid composition and metabolism in healthy and parasitized digestive glands of *Littorina saxatilis rudis*, as well as in daughter sporocysts of *Microphallus similis* has been

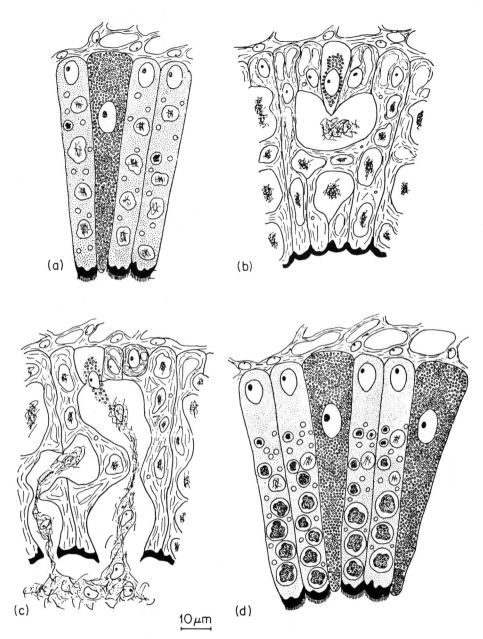

Fig. 12-19: *Littorina saxatilis* subsp. *tenebrosa*. Effect of starvation and parasitization by larval trematodes on digestive-gland cells. (a) Cells after 14-day starvation, showing reduction in food-storage globules and food vacuoles, paralleled by increase in size and number of waste vacuoles; (b) cells after 31-day starvation, exhibiting fibrous contents, displaced nuclei, secretory cells with contracted cytoplasm, breakdown of lateral cell walls and disappearance of cilia from digestive-cell epithelium; (c) cells after 40-day starvation, showing breakdown of distal cell walls; (d) digestive-gland cells of parasitized snail, showing less food-storage globules and more food vacuoles than healthy cells. (After James, 1965; reproduced by permission of Cambridge University Press.)

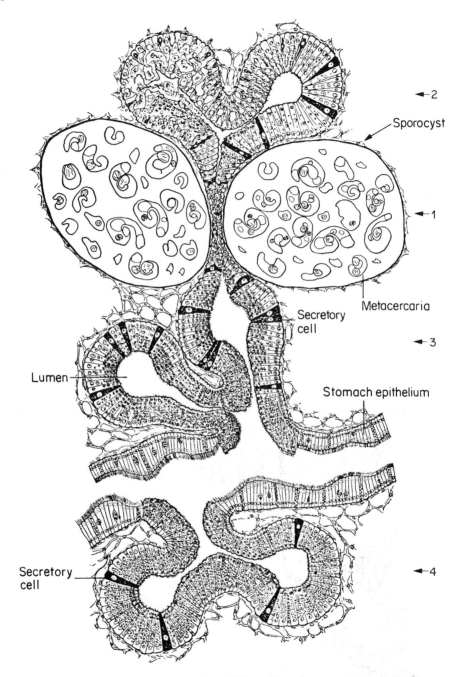

Fig. 12-20: *Littorina saxatilis* subsp. *tenebrosa*. Effect of larval trematode parasitization on digestive gland. Sporocysts compressing epithelium and blocking tubule lumen (1) cause starvation autolysis in tubules distal to the block (2). Tubules proximal to the block (3) with few food-storage globules, many vacuoles and many secretory cells; healthy tubules (4), unafflicted by the parasite, with numerous food-storage globules, few food vacuoles and few secretory cells. (After James, 1965; reproduced by permission of Cambridge University Press.)

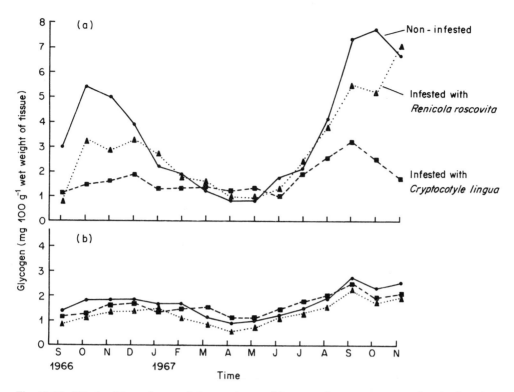

Fig. 12-21: *Littorina littorea*. Seasonal changes in monthly mean glycogen concentrations in digestive gland (a) and foot (b) of 272 non-infested periwinkles compared with 191 individuals containing *Cryptocotyle lingua* and 151 harbouring *Renicola roscovita* at Scalby Rocks (North Yorkshire, England). (After Robson and Williams, 1971b; modified; reproduced by permission of London School of Hygiene and Tropical Medicine.)

investigated by McManus and co-authors (1975). Parasitization by sporocysts was associated with a slight decrease in triglycerides and fatty acids in host digestive-gland cells suggesting that the parasite digests, absorbs and metabolizes lipids of host origin. A slight increase in phospholipids, as well as a marked increase in the incorporation of acetate-1-^{14}C in infested digestive glands, may be interpreted as attempted cell regeneration. *M. similis* sporocysts had fewer monoglycerides, triglycerides and fatty acids but took up more palmitate-1-^{14}C than the host (Tables 12-6 to 12-8).

The factors governing the relationships between *Microphallus pygmaeus* and *M. similis* and their snail hosts *Littorina saxatilis* and *L. littorea* have been studied in great detail by Richards (1969, 1970a, b, c), Pascoe (1970), Pascoe and co-authors (1970), James and Richards (1972), Richards and co-authors (1972) and McManus and James (1975a, b, c). In some of these studies, it became evident that the hosts' digestive glands and the parasites exhibit certain similarities in their biochemical pathways, perhaps reflecting the adaptation of the parasite to the host and the long association between the Digenea and the Mollusca.

These and other investigations on the biochemical and physiological interrelationships between molluscs and their trematodes are of particular importance for our understanding of the pathophysiological changes induced in the host's body.

Table 12–3

Specific activities of enzymes (mean ± standard error) involved in carbohydrate metabolism in digestive glands of healthy and trematode-infested *Littorina saxatilis rudis* and in sporocysts of *Microphallus similis* (After Marshall and co-authors, 1974a; reproduced by permission of Pergamon Press)

	Enzyme activity (nanomoles product formed min^{-1} mg^{-1} protein)		
	Digestive gland		Sporocysts
Enzyme	healthy	parasitized	
Hexokinase	1·0± 0·1	3·1± 0·15	25·3± 0·1
Glucose-6-phosphate dehydrogenase	6·0± 0·1	9·8± 0·1	24·4± 0·1
Glucose-6-phosphatase pH 6·5	9·6± 0·2	64·5± 0·23	8·5± 0·1
Glucose-6-phosphatase pH 7·6	8·0± 0·1	20·0± 0·20	7·5± 0·2
Phosphoglucomutase	6·9± 0·2	11·7± 0·1	24·9± 0·1
Phosphoglucoisomerase	356·0±16·0	509·0± 6·0	825·0± 9·4
Phosphomannoisomerase	8·2± 0·5	11·4± 0·3	35·1± 0·2
Phosphofructokinase	0·7± 0·1	1·7± 0·3	4·2± 0·4
Aldolase	15·2± 1·1	21·5± 0·1	73·6± 1·5
Triosephosphate isomerase	1063·0±17·3	1128·0±19·3	3834·0±110·0
α-Glycerophosphate dehydrogenase	2·4± 0·1	7·4± 0·6	30·8± 0·2
Glyceraldehyde-3-phosphate dehydrogenase	11·5± 0·8	26·1± 0.5	45·9± 0.3
Phosphoglycerate kinase	96·5± 8·3	93·0± 2·0	124·1± 2·7
Phosphoglycerate mutase	5·3± 0·5	9·2± 0·6	38·9± 3·0
Enolase	46·0± 0·7	22·6± 3·7	89·5± 0·7
Pyruvate kinase	2·1± 0·1	2·0± 0·1	24·0± 0·2
Lactic dehydrogenase	1·0± 0·1	2·0± 0·1	4·0± 0·2

Infestation by larval trematodes can significantly reduce the overall resistance of molluscs to environmental stress, in particular to high temperature. Considerable exposure to temperature extremes occurs in littoral gastropods living at or near the upper limit of their vertical distributional range. Maximum environmental, as well as body temperatures may attain values of such magnitude as to limit abundance. The effects of trematode infestation on the temperature tolerance of *Littorina littorea* have been investigated by Lauckner (in preparation). Parasitized individuals were consistently less resistant to high temperature stress than healthy ones (Fig. 12-25).

The temperature tolerance has been studied in numerous littoral invertebrates including *Littorina littorea* (Gowanloch and Hayes, 1926; Hayes, 1929; Broekhuysen, 1940; Evans, 1948; Orr, 1955a, b; Gunter, 1957; Southward, 1958; Fraenkel, 1960, 1961, 1966, 1968; Newell, 1970; Markel, 1971; Newell and co-authors, 1971; Newell and Bayne, 1973; Hamby, 1975; McMahon and Russell-Hunter, 1977; see also the review by Kinne, 1970). The lethal temperature has furthermore been employed as a criterion for

Table 12–4

Acid and alkaline phosphomonoesterase activity (nanomoles min^{-1} mg^{-1} protein; mean ± standard error) in healthy and parasitized digestive glands of 4 species of marine prosobranchs and in their digenean parasites at 30°C (After Marshall and co-authors, 1974b; reproduced by permission of Pergamon Press)

Species	Tissue	'Acidase'	'Alkase'
Littorina saxatilis	1 Healthy digestive gland	117·30±2·00	4·57±0·13
tenebrosa	2 Digestive gland parasitized by 3	195·10±1·33	1·30±0·01
Microphallus pygmaeus	3 Sporocysts	4·70±0·66	0·08±0·02
Littorina saxatilis rudis	4 Healthy digestive gland	140·30±1·21	3·03±0·19
	5 Digestive gland parasitized by 6	187·50±0·42	1·37±0·05
Microphallus similis	6 Sporocysts	2·10±0·13	1·17±0·02
Gibbula umbilicalis	7 Healthy digestive gland	26·60±0·44	2·87±0·02
	8 Digestive gland parasitized by 9	47·70±1·07	2·87±0·05
Cercaria linearis	9 Sporocysts	26·60±0·20	1·73±0·02
	10 Digestive gland parasitized by 11	34·97±1·11	2·20±0·01
Cercaria stunkardi	11 Sporocysts	25·23±0·40	4·03±0·05
Littorina littorea	12 Healthy digestive gland	48·43±0·45	1·03±0·02
	13 Digestive gland parasitized by 14	53·63±0·94	1·70±0·10
Cryptocotyle lingua	14 Rediae	43·30±1·21	1·30±0·07
	15 Digestive gland parasitized by 16	30·70±1·55	2·17±0·02
Himasthla elongata	16 Rediae	13·27±1·03	1·37±0·05

Table 12–5

Littorina littorea. Relative staining intensities of lysosomal hydrolases in digestive cells of healthy and trematode-infested individuals (After Moore and Halton, 1977; reproduced by permission of Zeitschrift für Parasitenkunde)

| Histochemical test | Non-infested *L. littorea* | *L. littorea* infested with | | |
		Himasthla elongata	*Cryptocotyle lingua*	*Podocotyle atomon*
Indoxyl esterase	+ +	+ +	+	+ +
Acid phosphatase	+ +	+/+ +	+/+ +	+ + +
β-Glucuronidase	+ +	+ + + +	+ + + +	+ + + +
β-Galactosidase	+	+ +/+ + +	+ +	+ +
a-Glucosidase	0	—	+	0
Hexosaminidase	+ +	+ + + +	+/+ +	+ +/+ + +
Arylsulphatase	+/+ +	+ + +	+	0/+

+ + + + + = intense, + + + + = very strong, + + + = strong, + + = moderate, + = slight, 0 = no reaction, — = not known

Table 12-6

Littorina saxatilis rudis. Lipid composition of healthy and parasitized digestive glands and of *Microphallus similis* sporocysts (After McManus and co-authors, 1975; reproduced by permission of Experimental Parasitology)

Lipid class	Lipid content (mg g^{-1} wet weight)		
	Digestive gland		Sporocysts
	healthy	parasitized	
Total lipids	43·8 (39·3–45·7)[a]	49·1 (48·0–55·0)	39·8 (35·4-43·6)
Phospholipids[b]	11·5 (11·2–11·6)	16·6 (16·5–16·6)	23·4 (23·1–23·6)
Neutral lipids[c]	32·3	32·5	16·4

[a]Results: mean of 4 determinations (range in brackets).
[b]Phosphorus value multiplied by 25.
[c]Calculated from difference between total lipids and phospholipids.

Table 12–7

Littorina saxatilis rudis. Phospholipid composition of healthy and parasitized digestive glands and of *Microphallus similis* sporocysts (After McManus and co-authors, 1975; reproduced by permission of Experimental Parasitology)

Phospholipid (mg g^{-1} wet weight)	Digestive gland		Sporocysts
	healthy	parasitized	
Cardiolipin	0·17 (0·11–0·29)*)	0·26 (0·22–0·35)	0·40 (0·35–0·57)
Phosphatidyl ethanolamine	3·75 (3·29–4·11)	4·35 (3·62–4·54)	4·70 (4·22–5·15)
Phosphatidyl choline	5·88 (5·80–5·99)	7·80 (7·42–8·33)	14·76 (14·25–15·44)
Phosphatidyl inositol	1·41 (1·39–1·46)	2·13 (1·81–2·44)	2·54 (2·18–2·84)
Sphingomyelin	0·08 (0·07–0·10)	1·12 (0·83–1·48)	0·30 (0·17–0·36)
Lysophosphatidyl choline	0·02 (0·01–0·04)	0·17 (0·12–0·26)	0·02 (0·01–0·02)
Phosphatidyl serine	0·20 (0·11–0·26)	0·60 (0·58–0·63)	0·51 (0·31–0·64)

*Mean of 4 determinations (range in brackets).

the physiological characterization and taxonomic discrimination of species (Fry, 1957). None of these authors have taken into consideration the possible effects of trematode infestation.

Infestation of littorinids with larval trematodes may exhibit considerable spatial, annual and seasonal fluctuation; it may also vary according to age, size, sex and gonad cycle of the host.

Local variations in the level of trematode infestations may be correlated with the density of the intermediate hosts, as well as with the abundance of final hosts (Hoff, 1941; Ewers, 1964; James, 1968c; Werding, 1969). Snails from higher shore levels are usually more heavily parasitized than animals from lower levels (Berry, 1962; Sindermann and Farrin, 1962). In addition to other yet-unknown physiological or ecological factors, higher temperatures and scarcity of food in the higher tide zone may

Table 12–8

Littorina saxatilis rudis. Total mean radioactivity in lipids from healthy and parasitized digestive glands and in *Microphallus similis* sporocysts after 3 h incubation at 23° C (After McManus and co-authors, 1975; reproduced by permission of Experimental Parasitology)

Substrate	Activity (disintegrations min^{-1} mg^{-1} lipid) (Mean from 3 experiments)		
	Digestive gland		Sporocysts
	healthy	parasitized	
Acetate-1-^{14}C	64,513	215,241	46,025
Palmitate-1-^{14}C	142,497	124,140	456,565

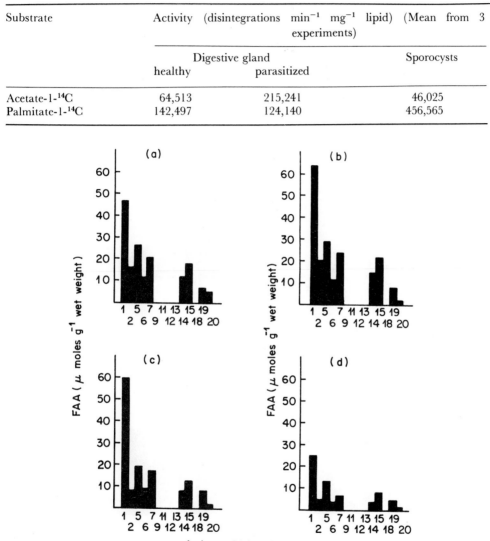

Fig. 12-22: *Littorina littorea*. Free amino acid (FAA) concentrations in foot-head musculature of non-parasitized individuals (a) and snails infested with *Cryptocotyle lingua* rediae (b), *Himasthla elongata* rediae (c) or *Renicola roscovita* sporocysts (d). Key: 1 = alanine; 2 = aspartic acid; 5 = glutamic acid; 6 = glutamine; 7 = glycine; 9 = leucine*; 11 = methionine*; 12 = phenylalanine*; 13 = proline*; 14 = serine; 15 = taurine; 18 = valine*; 19 = arginine; 20 = asparagine. (After Watts, 1971; modified; reproduced by permission of Cambridge University Press.)

*Present only in trace amounts.

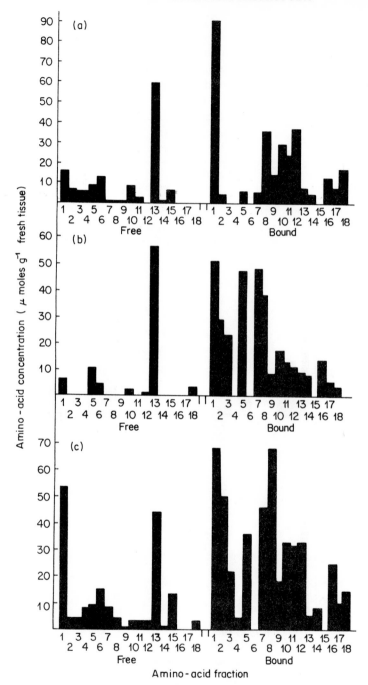

Fig. 12-23: Free and bound amino acids in *Cryptocotyle lingua* rediae (a), *Himasthla elongata* rediae (b) and *Renicola roscovita* sporocysts (c). Key: 1 = alanine; 2 = aspartic acid; 3 = cysteine; 4 = cystine; 5 = glutamic acid; 6 = glutamine; 7 = glycine; 8 = histidine; 9 = leucine + isoleucine; 10 = lysine; 11 = methionine; 12 = phenylalanine; 13 = proline; 14 = serine; 15 = taurine; 16 = threonine; 17 = tyrosine; 18 = valine. (After Watts, 1970a; reproduced by permission of Cambridge University Press.)

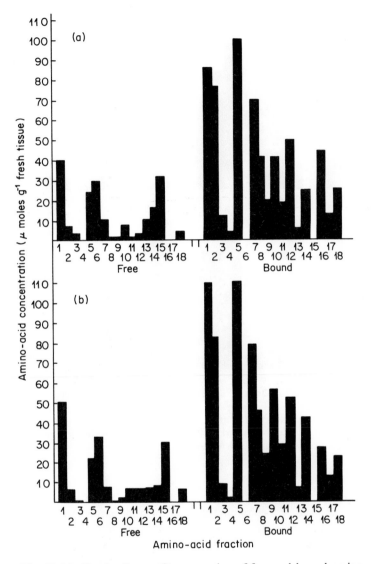

Fig. 12-24: *Littorina littorea*. Concentration of free and bound amino acids in hepatopancreas of males (a) and females (b). For key see Fig. 12-23. (After Watts, 1970a; reproduced by permission of Cambridge University Press.)

account for such conditions (Kendall, 1964). Sexual maturity is a prerequisite for larval trematode infestation in *Littorina littorea* (Werding, 1969; Robson and Williams, 1970; Lauckner, in preparation). Maturity is attained earlier in the season by periwinkles on the upper regions of the shore (Williams, 1964). The number of susceptible individuals in the high-tide zone is thereby considerably increased, which may also contribute to higher infestation incidences.

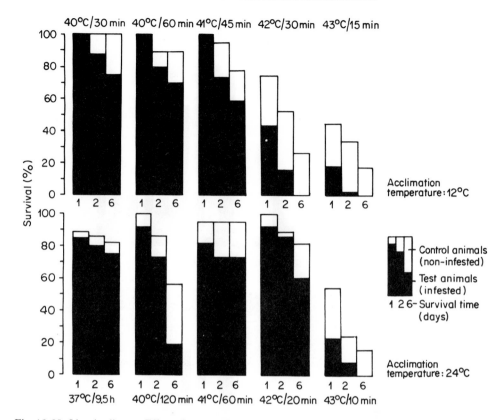

Fig. 12-25: *Littorina littorea*. Effect of trematode infestation on thermal resistance. Survival of healthy and parasitized individuals acclimated to 12° C and 24° C, respectively, after exposure to various time–temperature combinations. (Original.)

Seasonal fluctuations in infestation rates may be due to differential mortality or changes in the migratory behaviour of healthy and parasitized intermediate hosts. Thus, the downward winter migration of *Littorina littorea* on rocky shores in Maine, USA, and Nova Scotia, Canada, is influenced by *Cryptocotyle lingua* infestations, the affected snails responding more slowly and to a lesser extent to the cold stimulus than healthy ones. Consequently, snail samples collected during winter from the high-tide zone gave higher infestation figures than those collected in summer, simulating seasonal variations (Sindermann and Farrin, 1962; Lambert and Farley, 1968). In contrast, trematode infestations did not appear to affect the distribution of *L. littorea* in Wales (Williams, 1964).

Field experiments conducted on the Yorkshire (England) coast showed that colour-marked *Littorina littorea* moved downshore in winter. Periwinkles harbouring *Cryptocotyle lingua* or *Renicola roscovita* moved significantly ($P<0{\cdot}001$) shorter distances than healthy ones. In general, *R. roscovita*-infested individuals moved less far from the point of release than *C. lingua*-infested ones (Williams and Ellis, 1975). Since there is little or no injury to the tissues of the head-foot of trematode-infested *L. littorea*, it is unlikely that the shorter distances moved by parasitized individuals result from direct interference with locomotory structures. Infestation with larval Digenea, however, causes considerable damage to digestive gland and gonad. As has been documented by biochemical analyses, histological examination and survival experiments (Rees, 1936a; Robson and Williams, 1971a, b; Watts, 1971, 1972), impairment of the host's vital functions is more pronounced in *R. roscovita*- than in *C. lingua*-infestations. These differences may be reflected in the varying extent to which locomotion is reduced. James (1968a) suggested that the ability of *L. saxatilis* to migrate may depend on the healthy development of the gonads. Stambaugh and McDermot (1969) have reported a similar locomotory impairment in trematode-infested *Nassarius obsoletus* (see below).

In discussing their findings, Williams and Ellis (1975) state that their results and those of Sindermann and Farrin (1962), Lambert and Farley (1968) and Stambaugh and McDermot (1969) emphasize the need to take precautions against accidental, and possibly unknown, inclusion of infected animals for observation or experiment.

Littorinids, particularly *Littorina littorea*, are among the most-studied intertidal marine invertebrates. Numerous investigations have been devoted to the analysis of factors governing the zonation, locomotion and behaviour of these gastropods (Batchelder, 1915; Huntsman, 1918; Gowanloch and Hayes, 1926; Fraenkel, 1927; Hayes, 1929; Schwarz, 1932; Colman, 1933; Moore, 1940; Dexter, 1943; R. G. Evans, 1947; Smith and Newell, 1955; Barkman, 1956; Newell, 1958a, b; Bakker, 1959; Alexander, 1960; F. Evans, 1965; Stephenson and Stephenson, 1972; Vermeij, 1972; Underwood, 1973; Chow, 1975; Gendron, 1977). However, no author has taken into consideration possible (and probable) effects on his results due to trematode infestation.

Seasonal fluctuations of infestation levels in littorinids have also been recorded by Berry (1962), James (1968a, b), Werding (1969), Robson and Williams (1970) and Lauckner (in preparation).

Female *Littorina saxatilis* have been found to be more heavily parasitized by *Cercaria ubiquitoides* (=*Microphallus similis*) than males. However, while infestations in *L. saxatilis* from Whitstable (Kent, England) showed marked seasonality with incidences ranging from 0% in winter to 27·9% in June (Berry, 1962), no such seasonal fluctuations became apparent in *L. saxatilis* from Roscoff, France (Combescot-Lang, 1976). Increased susceptibility of female snails to larval trematode invasion has also been reported for *L. littorea* infested with *Cryptocotyle lingua* by Lambert and Farley (1968), while Werding (1969) and Robson and Williams (1970) found no significant differences between percentages of infested male and female periwinkles.

Spent female littorinids appear to be more susceptible to larval-trematode infestation, thus reflecting the importance of the host's gonad state and breeding cycle (Berry, 1962; James, 1968a, b; Robson and Williams, 1971a). Some trematode species invade only juvenile littorinids, while others occur in adult hosts only. The germinal sacs of the gymnophallid *Parvatrema homoeotecnum*, for example, are almost exclusively confined to small *Littorina saxatilis tenebrosa* measuring from 0·6 to 5·0 mm in length (James, 1960, 1964, 1968a). A small form of *Microphallus pygmaeus* invades juveniles, and a large form of *M. pygmaeus* infests only spent adults of *L. saxatilis* (James, 1968b). Whether both forms are specifically identical remains to be established.

In *Littorina littorea*, on the other hand, only adults appear to be susceptible to trematode infestation (Werding, 1969; Robson and Williams, 1970; Lauckner, in preparation). Physiological rather than ecological factors appear to govern the tendency

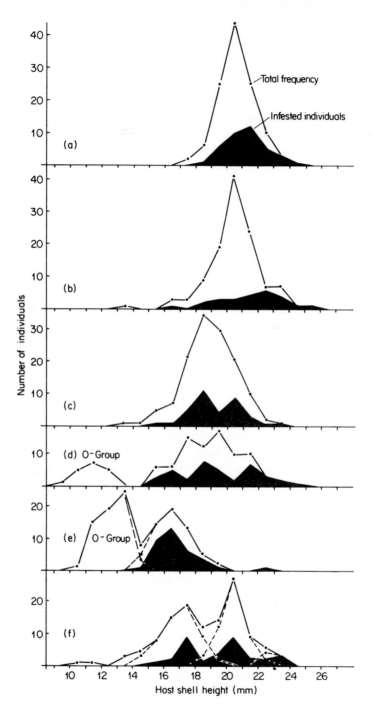

Fig. 12-26: *Littorina littorea*. Incidences of trematode infestation in relation to age (shell height) of hosts. (Original.)

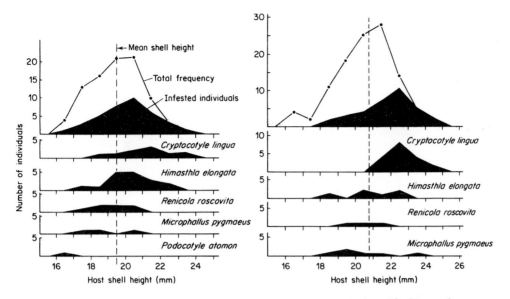

Fig. 12-27: *Littorina littorea*. Incidences of trematode infestation. Resolution of incidence–frequency curves with respect to individual parasite species and host-shell height. (Original.)

of trematode infestation in snails. Bearing in mind the work of Rohlack (1959), one might speculate on the importance of hormonal mechanisms in this connection.

As indicated by the resolution of the multi-modal frequency distributions of shell heights of *Littorina littorea* samples into individual components (Fig. 12-26, d-f), 0-group snails are never parasitized and infestation incidences increase with shell height (=age). 0-group individuals should, therefore, generally be excluded from percentage-infestation calculations. The frequency curve shown in Fig. 12-26,a, which ideally fits the expected normal distribution, represents a homogeneous year class of *L. littorea*. Although in the curve for the infested individuals there is a slight displacement of the mode to the right, this is by no means indicative of accelerated growth of infested snails. It merely demonstrates that the larger individuals of a homogeneous year class are likely to be more frequently parasitized than the smaller ones. This observation could be explained by the fact that in both sexes of periwinkles maturity is attained more quickly in the larger and older individuals of each year class (Williams, 1964). However, not all trematode species invading *L. littorea* prefer larger hosts (Fig. 12-27).

The restriction of certain larval trematodes to small adult snails may be indicative of an increased mortality of the host due to infestation by the respective parasites (James, 1968b; Werding, 1969). From the absence of *Renicola roscovita* sporocysts from larger *Littorina littorea*, Robson and Williams (1971b) concluded that this parasite has to be regarded as a lethal pathogen—a view well supported by the histological investigations conducted by Rees (1936a). Incidences of *L. littorea* infestation with *Cryptocotyle lingua*, on the other hand, steadily increase with size, and hence, age of the periwinkles, thus indicating a lesser degree of pathogenicity of this particular parasite. The successful maintenance of a periwinkle infested with *C. lingua* in the laboratory—over a period of 7 years—reflects a harmonious relationship as well as the long-term strategy of *C. lingua* infestations (Meyerhof and Rothschild, 1940; Rothschild, 1942b).

Table 12-9

Littorina littorea. Incidence of single and double infestations with 6 species of larval trematodes (Original)

(A) Single and double infestations

Number of samples	21
Total number of periwinkles examined	2691
Total number of periwinkles infested	1151
Total number of double infestations encountered	88
Infestation with:	
Cryptocotyle lingua	303
Himasthla elongata	617
Renicola roscovita	247
Microphallus pygmaeus	76
Podocotyle atomon	4
Cercaria lebouri	2

*) Chi-square test (0·5 = Yate's correction for continuity):

$$\chi^2 = \frac{(|0-E|-0\cdot5)^2}{E}$$

(B) Double infestations involving

		I Sum of observations	II Sum of expectations	III Significance level *)	IV Computed expectations	V Significance level *)
1) *Cryptocotyle lingua*	— *Himasthla elongata*	0	76·75	---	69·47	---
2) *Cryptocotyle lingua*	— *Renicola roscovita*	1	25·54	p<0·001	27·81	p<0·001
3) *Cryptocotyle lingua*	— *Microphallus pygmaeus*	3	6·05	n.s.	8·56	p<0·05
4) *Cryptocotyle lingua*	— *Podocotyle atomon*	0	0·27	---	0·45	---
5) *Himasthla elongata*	— *Renicola roscovita*	63	56·04	n.s.	56·63	n.s.
6) *Himasthla elongata*	— *Microphallus pygmaeus*	8	11·58	n.s.	17·43	p<0·05
7) *Himasthla elongata*	— *Podocotyle atomon*	0	0·73	---	0·92	---
8) *Renicola roscovita*	— *Microphallus pygmaeus*	11	9·36	n.s.	6·98	n.s.
9) *Renicola roscovita*	— *Podocotyle atomon*	1	0·51	n.s.	0·37	n.s.
10) *Microphallus pygmaeus*	— *Podocotyle atomon*	1	0·08	n.s.	0·11	n.s.

*) Chi-square test; n.s. = not significant at 5% level; --- = not computable since observations = zero

The higher incidence of *Cryptocotyle lingua* in larger periwinkles could be taken as indicative of accelerated growth, which is believed to occur in infested *Hydrobia ulvae* (Rothschild, 1936b, 1938c, 1941a; Rothschild and Rothschild, 1939). Neither Werding (1969) nor Robson and Williams (1970, 1971a) nor Lauckner (in preparation) were able to demonstrate giant growth in *Littorina littorea* castrated by trematodes. Periwinkles artificially castrated by treatment with X-rays in doses of 400 r at 150 kV and 4 mA did not grow any faster or any larger than controls. Likewise, field data obtained for the growth of trematode-castrated *L. neritoides* were inconclusive (Rothschild, 1941c).

Previous studies (Hayes, 1927, 1929; Green and Green, 1932; Moore, 1937; Orrhage, 1969) revealed no abnormalities in shell growth of periwinkles. However, the authors listed have not considered possible growth deviations due to trematode invasion. Whether trematode infestation can affect growth rates in *Littorina littorea* remains doubtful. Moose (1963), Zischke and Zischke (1965) and others have reported inhibition rather than acceleration of growth in trematode-infested freshwater snails. The controversial literature on this subject has been reviewed by Cheng (1971).

Simultaneous infestations of littorinids with two species of larval trematodes are of frequent occurrence. The number of double infestations observed did not differ significantly from theoretical expectations in *Littorina neritoides* (Lysaght, 1941). In *L. saxatilis*, observed cases of double infestations were either much higher or much lower than the expected values, depending on the trematode species involved. Triple infestations were also noted in *L. saxatilis*, with observed incidences much higher than expected (James, 1969). Despite their frequent occurrence in single infestations and the resulting high expectation value for double infestations, *Cryptocotyle lingua* and *Himasthla elongata*, parasitizing *L. littorea* on the German North Sea coast, never occur together in the same snail; there is a 100% antagonism. Observed incidences of double infestations in *L. littorea* involving *H. elongata* and *Microphallus pygmaeus* do not differ significantly from expectations, while combinations of *C. lingua* with *Renicola roscovita* occur less frequently, and combinations of *R. roscovita* with *H. elongata* or *M. pygmaeus*, respectively, occur more frequently than expected—sometimes with high statistical significance (Table 12-9).

Similar observations have been made by Werding (1969) and Robson and Williams (1970). However, when drawing conclusions from the combined data of a series of snail samples (as done by the latter authors), errors are introduced with respect to the theoretically expected occurrence of double infestations. This may be illustrated by the following example: If the frequencies of single occurrences of 2 parasites in a sample of n = 2691 snails are, for instance, 617 and 76, respectively (*Himasthla elongata* and *Microphallus pygmaeus* in Table 12-9, A), the theoretically expected (E) frequency of double infestations will be

$$\frac{617 \times 76}{2691} = 17 \cdot 43$$

(Table 12-9, B, Column IV). To test whether the difference between observed (0 = 8) and expected (E = 17·43) incidences is statistically significant, a Chi-square test is employed (see inset Table 12-9, A). In the above-mentioned example, the difference between E and O is significant at the 5% level (Column V) which would lead one to the conclusion that double infestations involving *H. elongata* and *M. pygmaeus* occur statistically less frequently than theoretically expected. For the following reasons, however, such application of the Chi-square test in this manner is inadmissible: The

2691 periwinkles represent the total number in a series of 21 separate snail samples. Since the single occurrences of the respective parasites vary from sample to sample, also the theoretical expectations of double infestations for these samples vary concomitantly. Hence, the total sum of incidences cannot be utilized for the computation of the E's. One method of coping with this problem is to sum up all the individual E's obtained for each sample. In the above example, a considerably lower figure (11·58, Column II) is obtained, and the difference between O and E is no longer statistically significant.

However, the general tendency apparent in Table 12-9, B is consistent in most snail samples: As a rule, direct antagonism that involves a redia and a sporocyst results in destruction of the sporocyst (Lim and Heyneman, 1972). Therefore, double infestations involving rediae and sporocysts are excluded or at least occur less frequently than expected. This is true for the combinations 2, 3, 4, 6 and 7 in Table 12-9, B (Columns I and II). Double infestations involving rediae of *Himasthla elongata* and sporocysts of *Renicola roscovita* likewise occur more frequently than expected. At present, no explanation can be offered for this observation. In contrast, combinations involving two sporocyst partners usually occur more frequently than expected (8, 9 and 10 in Table 12-9, B). As is obvious from Columns I and II, a very large snail sample would be required to secure these data on a statistical basis.

The physiological mechanisms responsible for synergism and antagonism in trematode infestation of prosobranchs are not readily understood. Antagonism—as in the case of *Cryptocotyle lingua* and *Himasthla elongata*——could possibly be utilized as a means of biological control of economically important parasites.

Cryptocotyle lingua is probably the economically most important trematode parasitizing littorinids. It has been recorded in *Littorina littorea* and *L. saxatilis* from both the American and European coasts of the North Atlantic (Lebour, 1907a, 1911; Stunkard, 1930, 1970a; James, 1968c, d; Werding, 1969; Robson and Williams, 1970; Sindermann, 1970a; Davis and Farley, 1973; Lauckner, in preparation) as well as in *L. scutulata* from the North American Pacific coast (Ching, 1960, 1962). The apparently recent establishment of *L. littorea* along the Washington and California coast (Carlton, 1969) will certainly bring about an extension of the geographical range of this important parasite in the near future.

The larval ecology of *Cryptocotyle lingua* has been carefully investigated by Sindermann (1961, 1966), Sindermann and Farrin (1962) and Lambert and Farley (1968). Its germ-cell cycle, the ultrastructure and histochemistry of the cercaria and the redia, the functional organization and fine structure of the tail musculature and the excretory vesicle of the cercaria, as well as the propulsion of the cercaria, have been studied by Cable (1931, 1934), Krupa and co-authors (1966, 1968, 1969), Chapman (1973), Chapman and Wilson (1973) and Rees (1974), respectively. Køie (1977) made a stereoscan study of the cercaria, metacercaria and adult stage of *C. lingua*.

The life cycle of *Cryptocotyle lingua* (Fig. 12-7) has been elucidated by Stunkard (1930) in the USA and further studied by Rothschild (1939, 1942a) in Europe. Its pleurolophocercous cercariae, which develop in rediae in *Littorina littorea* or—very rarely—in *L. saxatilis* and *Hydrobia ulvae* (Fig. 12-6), penetrate various species of fish, where they usually encyst directly under the skin. The adult occurs in fish-eating sea birds, particularly in gulls, but also in other warm-blooded vertebrates, including man.

Like other larval heterophyids, *Cryptocotyle lingua* is very euryhaline (Stunkard and Shaw, 1931; Styczynska-Jurewicz, 1971). It penetrates far into brackish water. In the Baltic Sea, the species maintains its life cycle at salinities below 10°/oo S (Reimer, 1964a, 1970). Cercarial production is highest in water of normal salinity. Emergence of cercariae may drop considerably at salinities below 18°/oo S (Sindermann and Farrin, 1962; Table 12-10).

Table 12-10

Effect of environmental salinity on emergence of *Cryptocotyle lingua* cercariae
(After Sindermann and Farrin, 1962)

Salinity (°/oo S)	Number of individual snails examined	Mean daily percentage of infested snails emitting cercariae	Mean daily number of cercariae emitted per snail
30	14	81	670
24	14	81	580
18	13	86	570
12	11	51	210
6	11	16	3

Infestation of *Littorina littorea* with *Cryptocotyle lingua* may be very high in any given locality. Thus, Sindermann and Farrin (1962) reported mean incidences of 65% in the high-tide zone, 45% in the mid-tide zone and 46% in the low-tide zone at Boothbay Harbor, Maine, USA, over an observation period of $2\frac{1}{2}$ years. Maximum levels were above 90% in the high-tide zone, and marked seasonal fluctuations occurred throughout the investigated area. These figures appear to be abnormally high, and it is possible that the authors inspected only large periwinkles, which are usually more heavily infested than medium-sized ones. For comparison, Lauckner (in preparation) recorded 10·1% infestation by *C. lingua* in 11,112 *L. littorea* from Massachusetts, USA, 8·1% in 30,811 periwinkles from Sylt, German North Sea coast, and 5·1% in 11,571 periwinkles from the western Baltic Sea. Robson and Williams (1970) found 14·2% of 5,878 *L. littorea* from North Yorkshire, English North Sea coast, to be infested with *C. lingua*.

Cryptocotyle lingua may persist for a considerable length of time. A 7-year-old infestation of *Littorina littorea* has been recorded. During the first week in captivity, the snail shed an average of 3300 cercariae day^{-1}, reaching a grand total of approximately 1,300,000 in the first year, and 5,500,000 in five years. After this time, the mean fell to 830 cercariae day^{-1}, but afterwards, rose again to 1600 cercariae day^{-1} (Meyerhof and Rothschild, 1940; Rothschild, 1942b). The ecological importance of the production of such enormous numbers of parasites must not be underestimated: 'When it is considered that in some localities the percentage of gastropods infected with trematode parasites is high (reaching 40% in the case of *Hydrobia ulvae* Pennant at Plymouth) some idea can be gained of the astronomical numbers of these free-swimming larvae. They form part of that section of the marine fauna which, although known to be present, inevitably escapes record in samples of the plankton' (Meyerhof and Rothschild, 1940, pp. 367–368).

Other Mesogastropoda from which larval trematodes have been recorded include mainly representatives of the families Turritellidae, Potamididae and Cerithiidae.

Macrocercous cercariae, named *Cercaria rhodometopa*, have been recovered from *Turritella communis* at Roscoff, France (Pérez, 1924; Stunkard, 1932). Rothschild (1935a) described four further *rhodometopa*-type cercariae, *C. pythionike*, *C. doricha*, *C. nicarete* and *C. herpsyllis*, from *T. communis* at Plymouth, England, and two others, *C. ampelis* and *C. ranzii*, from Naples, Italy. Nothing is known about the pathogenicity nor the life history of these trematodes. Life-cycle studies conducted by Rothschild (1935a) gave negative results, but the cercariae are believed to encyst in fishes. Final hosts might be sea birds. Of 216 male *T. communis* from Plymouth, 37 were infested, but of 324 female snails, only 7 harboured trematodes. In contrast, 5 of 63 males and 4 of 116 females from Naples were infested with *rhodometopa*-type sporocysts. *C. melanocrucifera*, a magnocercous cercaria of the opisthorchioid group, has been found in 1 of 200 *T. attenuata* from the Madras coast, India. It is possibly the larval stage of a species of *Galactosomum*, which uses fishes as second intermediate hosts and gulls *Larus argentatus* as final hosts (Reimer and Anantaraman, 1968).

Hutton (1955) described *Cercaria turritellae*, a magnocercous monostome larva developing in rediae in the digestive gland and gonad of *Turritella communis*; 2 of 350 snails from Plymouth Sound (England) turned out to be infested. The further life-cycle stages of *C. turritellae* remain unknown. Similar huge-tailed monostome cercariae of unknown specific identity infest *T. exoleata* in Puerto Rico (Cable, 1952), *Cerithiolum exille* in the Black Sea (Sinitsin, 1911), *Bittium eschrichti* in Puget Sound, Washington (Miller, 1925a), as well as a number of Caribbean gastropods (Miller, 1925b, 1929; and others).

Negus (1968), working on *Turritella communis* infested with the sporocysts of *Cercaria doricha*, found an almost identical qualitative composition of both the free amino-acid pools and the hydrolysates of the host gonad and parasite tissue. Considerable quantitative similarities between the free amino acids were also evident.

Prévot (1969) was apparently the first investigator who studied the trematode parasites of worm shells, which are aberrant turritellid prosobranchs. *Vermetus triqueter* from the Mediterranean Sea harboured the larval stages of three bird trematodes and two fish trematodes, representing five different families. A microphallid cercaria occurred in 8%, an echinostomatid in 6%, a notocotylid in 4%, a hemiurid in 3·5%, and an opecoelid in 3% of the worm shells. The life cycle of the echinostomatid, which was described as *Aporchis massiliensis*, has been elucidated experimentally. Cercariae shed by *V. triqueter* attach to solid surfaces on which they encyst. No second intermediate host is required. Adults develop in the intestine of herring gulls *Larus argentatus michaellis* (Prévot, 1971).

Other larval trematodes, including magnocercous cercariae, have been described from Caribbean *Turritella* spp. and *Cerithium* spp. by McCoy (1929), Cable (1954a, b, 1963) and LeZotte (1954), as well as from Mediterranean *C. vulgatum* and *C. rupestre* by Palombi (1940), Arvy (1954), Prévot (1967, 1972b) and others. Up to 10% of the *C. mediterraneum* from the lagoon of Brusc (French Mediterranean coast) harboured the sporocyst stage of microphallids *Maritrema misenensis*. Its life cycle has been traced experimentally by Prévot and co-authors (1976). The cercariae encyst in amphipods, and adults develop in the intestine of *Larus argentatus michaellis*. The first larval stage has previously been described by Palombi (1940) as *Cercaria misenensis* from *C. vulgatum* in the Gulf of Naples (Italy).

Bittium reticulatum from the French Mediterranean coast harbours *Microphallus bittii*, whose cercariae penetrate shore crabs *Carcinus maenas* (Prévot, 1972a) and *B. alternatum* from the Woods Hole region, Massachusetts, USA, is known as first intermediate host for *Microphallus nicolli*, whose metacercariae occur in the commercially important blue crab *Callinectes sapidus*. This prosobranch species also harbours the rediae of *Deropristis inflata*, whose life cycle includes the annelid *Nereis virens* as second intermediate host and the eel *Anguilla rostrata* as final host (Cable and Hunninen, 1940, 1942a), as well as the rediae of *Siphodera vinaledwardsii*. Metacercariae of this cryptogonimid encyst in fishes, particularly flounders *Paralichthys dentatus*, and adults develop in toadfish *Opsanus tau* and other teleosts (Cable and Hunninen, 1942b). *B. eschrichti* from the North American Pacific coast is parasitized by a magnocercous larva, *Cercaria purpuracauda* (Miller, 1925a).

Tall-spired horn shells *Cerithidea californica* from the North American Pacific coast harbour rediae of the echinostomastid *Himasthla rhigedana*. Notocotylids *Catatropis johnstoni* have been reported from *C. californica* and *C. scalariformis*. Both trematodes have abridged life cycles. Their emerging cercariae encyst on any hard surface, and are directly infective to their final hosts (Martin, 1956b; Adams and Martin, 1963; Bush and Kinsella, 1972). Heterophyids *Euhaplorchis californiensis*, *Parastictodora hancocki* and *Phocitremoides ovale* develop in rediae in *C. californica*; their cercariae penetrate fish intermediate hosts, particularly *Fundulus parvipinnis parvipinnis*, where they encyst in the brain region. The adults occur in fish-eating birds, particularly *Larus californicus* (Martin, 1950a, b, c). Yoshino (1976) demonstrated fine structural changes in the digestive gland of *C. californica* caused by *Euhaplorchis californiensis*. Histopathological alterations, such as the reduction of epithelial cell height, cytoplasmic vacuolation, disruption of cell junctions and cytolysis were essentially similar to those observed by Rees (1936a) and James (1965) in trematode-infested *Littorina littorea* and *L. saxatilis tenebrosa*.

Probolocoryphe (*Maritrema*) *uca*, a microphallid parasitic in sporocysts in *C. californica*, uses fiddler crabs *Uca crenulata* as second intermediate hosts (Sarkisian, 1957). *C. californica* is host for at least 18 species of larval trematodes. Infestation incidences in Newport Bay ranged from 54 to 74% in 12,995 snails with peaks in December, January and May, and minima in February, June, July and October. A total of 667 double and 23 triple infestations were observed. Some of these combinations occurred more and others less frequently than expected to occur by chance alone (Martin, 1956a).

Ladder horn shells *Cerithidea scalariformis* from Apalachee Bay, Gulf of Mexico, are hosts for at least 12 species of larval trematodes, including cyathocotylid, schistosomatid, echinostomatid, philophthalmid, plagiorchiid and heterophyid forms. Infestation incidences vary greatly, from 1 of 5508 snails for each of the cyathocotylid *Cercaria leighi* and the echinostomatid *Cercaria caribbea III* Cable, 1956b to as many as 389 and 1017 of 5508 snails for the heterophyids *Cercaria coruscantis* and *Cercaria cursitans*, respectively (Holliman, 1961).

A striking similarity exists between the coloration of the tissues of *Cerithidea californica* and that of the larval trematode harboured by them. Pigments extracted from snail tissues were β-carotene, carotenoid acids, ketocarotenoids, lutein, and chlorophyll derivatives. Some of these compounds are derived from the algal food, but others are probably products of the snail's metabolic activities. Absorption of pigments by sporocysts and rediae was found to be selective (Nadakal, 1960a, b, c).

Among the **Neogastropoda**, trematodes have been reported mainly from members of the families Muricidae (genus *Urosalpinx*), Thaisidae (genus *Thais*), Columbellidae (genus *Columbella*), Nassariidae (genus *Nassarius*) and Buccinidae (genera *Buccinum* and *Neptunea*).

The larval trematode most frequently reported from muricids and thaisids is *Parorchis acanthus*. It was first recorded from oyster drills *Thais lapillus* in England. Cercariae, which develop in colourless rediae in the hepatopancreas of the snail, encyst in contact with any solid surface (Fig. 12-28). Gulls of the genus *Larus* serve as final hosts (Lebour,

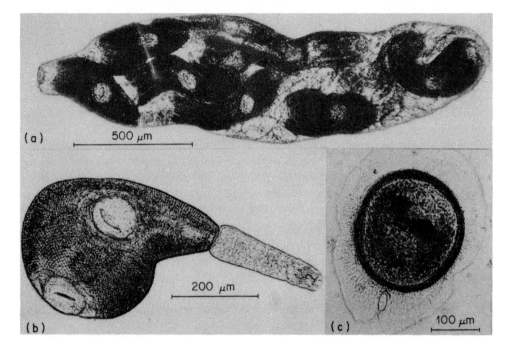

Fig. 12-28: *Parorchis acanthus*. (a) Redia from digestive gland of *Thais lapillus*; (b) cercaria; (c) encysted metacercaria. (Original.)

1907b, 1914; Nicoll, 1907a; Lebour and Elmhirst, 1922). If the specific identifications given by various authors are correct, *P. acanthus* has an extremely wide host spectrum and geographic range. It has been recorded from North American oyster drills *T. lapillus*, *T. haemostoma*, *T. floridana* and *Urosalpinx cinerea* (Stunkard and Shaw, 1931; Schechter, 1943; Carriker, 1955; Hopkins, 1957; Cooley, 1958, 1962), as well as from European *T. lapillus* (Rees, 1937, 1940; Feare 1970a; James, 1973) and from *Littorina pintado* in Hawaii (Cheng, 1967). Holliman (1961) recorded *P. acanthus* from 189 of 5508 ladder horn shells *Cerithidea scalariformis* from Apalachee Bay, Gulf of Mexico.

The anatomy and encystment of the cercaria of *Parorchis acanthus*, its germ-cell cycle, the behaviour of the cercaria, the histochemistry of the cystogenous-gland cells and the fine structures of the redia and the cercaria, the ultrastructure of the tail, and the locomotion of the cercaria, as well as the ultrastructure of the miracidium, have been studied by Rees (1937, 1939, 1940, 1948, 1966, 1967, 1971a, b) and James (1973). *P. avitus*, described by Stunkard and Cable (1932), is identical with *P. acanthus* (Cable and Martin, 1935).

Larval *Parorchis acanthus* invasion causes sterilization in affected hosts. Infestation prevailed in larger *Thais lapillus* from England, which might indicate that either infested snails continued to grow throughout life, or that they grew faster than healthy individuals. Infested drills could frequently be identified by their enlarged and deformed shells, which sometimes had a pronounced fourth whorl. Incidences were high in some snail populations, reaching a maximum of 69% (Feare, 1970a). In several samples of *T. lapillus*, statistically significant deviations from the normal 1:1 sex ratio were recorded (Feare, 1970b). It appears possible that such deviations are attributable to *P. acanthus* invasion.

Renicola thaidus is another larval trematode, occurring in sporocysts in *Thais lapillus* from Cape Cod, Massachusetts, USA. Infested drills died within a short time upon transfer to the laboratory, indicating a high degree of pathogenicity known also from other species of *Renicola* (Stunkard, 1964b). Other cercariae, whose life cycles are yet unknown, have been reported from *T. lamellosa* and *T. emarginata* from the Pacific coast of the USA (Miller, 1925a) as well as from *T. haemastoma* in the Gulf of Mexico (Schechter, 1943; Butler, 1953).

Muricids and thaisids prey on other molluscs, particularly on pelecypods. They are among the most damaging of the pests on oyster beds. The possibility of their biological control by means of larval *Parorchis acanthus* has been discussed by Carriker (1955) and Cooley (1958, 1962).

Opecœloides (*Anisoporus*) *manteri* and *Zoogonoides laevis* are among the larval trematodes parasitizing columbellid prosobranchs. Both develop in sporocysts in *Columbella lunata* in the Woods Hole region of Cape Cod, Massachusetts. The former uses amphipods and the latter annelids as second intermediate hosts. Fishes serve as definite hosts in both cases (Hunninen and Cable, 1941; Stunkard, 1943).

Opecoelid cercariae, *Cercaria contorta*, have been recorded from 21 of 268 fat dove shells *Anachis obesa* and from 1 of 1 little white mitrella *Columbella lunata* from Apalachee Bay, Gulf of Mexico. One of 5 *A. translirata* from the same area harboured another opecoelid, *C. paradoxa*, and 2 of 268 *A. obesa* contained a hemiuroid larval form, *C. portosacculus* (Holliman, 1961).

The common mud-flat snail *Nassarius obsoletus* is one of the most heavily parasitized gastropods occurring on the Atlantic and Pacific coasts of North America. It serves as the first intermediate host for at least nine species of trematodes, of which *Lepocreadium setiferoides*, *Himasthla quissetensis*, *Zoogonus lasius*, *Microbilharzia variglandis* and *Stephanostomum dentatum* are the most frequently occurring ones (Miller and Northup, 1926; Stunkard, 1933, 1934, 1936, 1938a, b, 1941, 1961, 1970a; Cable and Hunninen, 1938; Martin, 1938, 1939, 1945; Rankin, 1939, 1940; Stunkard and Hinchliffe, 1951, 1952; Penner, 1953a; Sindermann, 1956; Sindermann and co-authors, 1957; Grodhaus and Keh, 1958; Gambino, 1959; Vernberg and Vernberg, 1963; Vernberg and co-authors, 1969; McDaniel and Coggins, 1971, 1972).

The life history of *Lepocreadium setiferoides* has been traced experimentally by Martin (1938). Its ophthalmotrichocercous cercariae (Fig. 12-29) develop in rediae in the digestive gland of *Nassarius obsoletus*. Metacercariae encyst in the turbellarian *Procerodes warreni* and in annelids of the genus *Spio*. The adults are found in the digestive tract of various flatfish species. Cercariae of *Himasthla quissetensis* also develop in rediae in *N. obsoletus* but encyst in various mollusc species, particularly pelecypods. Gulls *Larus argentatus* are natural definite hosts (Stunkard, 1938a).

Provided that the specific identification is correct, *Himasthla quissetensis* also occurs in mottled dog whelks *Nassarius vibex* from Apalachee Bay, Gulf of Mexico, 40 of 1083 snails being infested (Holliman, 1961).

Some biochemical aspects of the interrelationships between *Himasthla quissetensis* and its host have been investigated by Vernberg and Hunter (1963), Hoskin and Cheng (1973, 1974, 1975) and Hoskin and co-authors (1974). Cardell and Philpott (1960) and Cardell (1962) studied the ultrastructure of the cercaria of *H. quissetensis* and Hoskin (1975) made a light and electron microscope investigation of rediae and host–parasite interface in this species.

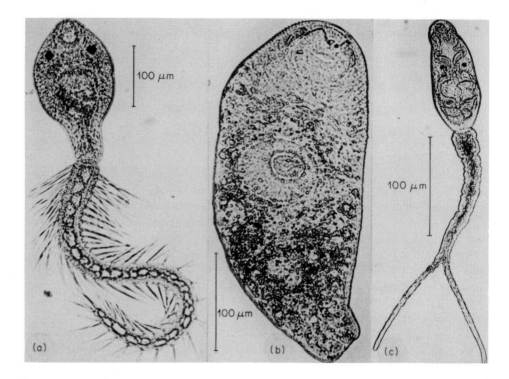

Fig. 12-29: Larval trematodes from *Nassarius obsoletus*. (a) *Lepocreadium setiferoides*; (b) *Zoogonus lasius*; (c) *Microbilharzia variglandis*. (Original.)

The cercaria of *Zoogonus lasius* (Fig.12-29), which develops in sporocysts in the digestive gland of *Nassarius obsoletus*, was first described by Linton (1915), and named *Cercaria lintoni* by Miller and Northup (1926). The excretory system of the tailless 'cercariaeum' was studied by Africa (1930), and its morphology by Shaw (1933). Subsequent investigations (Stunkard, 1933, 1936, 1938b, 1941) revealed its life cycle and specific identity. Metacercariae of *Z. lasius* occur in the polychaete *Nereis virens* and the adults in various fish species. The histopathology of infestation by *Z. lasius* (misidentified as *Z. rubellus*) has been studied by Cheng and co-authors (1973).

Mud snails *Nassarius mutabilis* from Naples, Italy, were found to harbour the sporocyst stage of another zoogonid, *Diphterostomum brusinae* (Palombi, 1930a, b). Its tailless cercariae encyst within the sporocysts. The final hosts—various fish species—become infested by ingesting contaminated snails.

Stephanostomum tenue and *S. dentatum*, whose cercariae parasitize in rediae in *Nassarius obsoletus*, are both fish trematodes, with both metacercaria and adult occurring in teleosts (Martin, 1939; Stunkard, 1961), while *Microbilharzia variglandis* (Fig. 12-29) is a blood-fluke of birds (Miller and Northup, 1926; Stunkard and Hinchliffe, 1952; Penner, 1953a). Cable and Hunninen (1940) reported the occurrence of *Cercaria nassicola*, probably a microphallid larva, in *N. obsoletus* from Woods Hole.

Larval stages of lepocreadiid trematodes—closely related to *Lepocreadium setiferoides* from American *Nassarius obsoletus*—have been described from European nassariids. *L. album* parasitizes *N. mutabilis* and *N. corniculus* in the Mediterranean Sea (Palombi, 1934, 1937). Up to 8·4% of *N. corniculus* from Naples (Italy) harboured the redial stage of this parasite. Its ophthalmotrichocercous larva, named *Cercaria setifera*, has frequently been encountered free in plankton hauls, as well as in benthic and pelagic molluscs. That this larva is in fact the adult stage of *L. album* known from the intestine of fishes has long been suspected by Monticelli (1888, 1914), Odhner (1914), Dollfus (1925) and Palombi (1931), and ascertained experimentally by Palombi (1937). However, although *L. album* is a common parasite, not all setigerous cercariae encountered in Mediterranean waters necessarily belong to this species. Thus, *N. mutabilis* from French Mediterranean waters yielded another species of *Lepocreadium, L. pegorchis*. Up to 5·4% of the mud snails sampled from Marseille were infested. Unencysted metacercariae occurred in various bivalves, adults in fishes (Bartoli, 1967). According to Palombi (1937), the rediae and setigerous cercariae found by Monticelli (1914) in *Conus mediterraneus* and believed to be *Cercaria setifera* (i.e. the larva of *L. album*), belong to another, yet undescribed species of *Lepocreadium*.

Of 1581 *Nassarius pygmaeus* in Øresund, Denmark, 117 (7·4%) harboured the rediae of *Opechona bacillaris*. Infestation incidence was low in animals of less than 10-mm shell height, but rose rapidly in larger specimens, reaching 100% in the 11·5-mm-size class (Fig. 12-30). No snails larger than 11·5 mm, either infested or uninfested, were found (Køie, 1975).

About 20% of the uninfested female *Nassarius pygmaeus* possessed a penis-like outgrowth from August through October, i.e. at the end of the spawning season. No such outgrowth was found in infested female snails. A similar phenomenon has been described from *Thais lapillus* and *N. obsoletus* (Blaber, 1970; Smith, 1971). In adult males, infestation caused a pronounced reduction of the penis (Fig. 12-31). All specimens of both sexes harbouring fully developed cercariae had a reduced and non-functional gonad. Similar conditions, i.e. penis reduction and gonad destruction, have been observed in *N. reticulatus* from Gullmar Fjord (Sweden). Only 12% of the parasitized males had a normal penis, 74% had a semi-reduced, and 14% had a totally reduced penis (Tallmark and Norrgren, 1976).

The total incidence of *Opechona bacillaris*, which varied between approximately 3 and 20%, exhibited relatively slight seasonal variation, while the degree of maturity varied greatly, exhibiting a definite correlation with water temperature. Type III infestations, comprising rediae with fully developed cercariae, were found only during summer. Snails harbouring rediae only (Type I) prevailed in the winter months, while intermediate stages with rediae and immature cercariae (Type II) were seen in low abundance during winter as well as at the end of the breeding season (Køie, 1975; Fig. 12-32).

Seasonal fluctuations in the incidence of trematode infestation have also been reported from *Nassarius obsoletus* collected from the Woods Hole region. Levels varied between approximately 3 and 9% in 9000 snails, with pronounced peaks from December to January and June to July, and lows in October and April to May. Infestations were almost entirely confined to *Zoogonus lasius* (Miller and Northup, 1926). In contrast, Gambino (1959), working in Greenwich Bay, Rhode Island, USA, determined maximum incidences from March to May, with constantly higher levels in high-tide animals than in low-tide specimens. Again, *Z. lasius* was the most abundant parasite. In both cases, the seasonal fluctuations were attributed to the migration of the final hosts. In the Greenwich Bay samples, infested individuals tended to be larger than the uninfested. Incidences rose from 5·5% in mud-flat snails of 10- to 12-mm length up to 40% in snails of 19- to 23-mm length, the overall percentage being 21·5% in 6717 *N. obsoletus*. In June, many dead snails were noted, suggesting parasite-induced mortality.

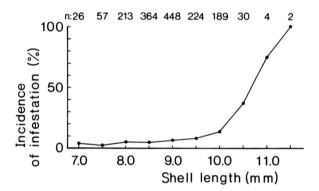

Fig. 12-30: *Nassarius pygmaeus*. Relation between shell length and infestation with larval *Opechona bacillaris* in 1581 snails from northern Øresund, Denmark. (After Køie, 1975; reproduced by permission of Ophelia.)

Effects of trematode infestation on *Nassarius obsoletus* include the impairment of locomotory activity. Laboratory studies conducted by Stambaugh and McDermot (1969) indicate that the locomotory rate of parasitized mud-flat snails varied between 54% and 91% of that of non-parasitized individuals. Similarly, the activity of parasitized *N. reticulatus* was reduced to about 30%. At 7° C, the proportion of actively crawling parasitized snails per hour was 1·4%, as opposed to 4·1% of non-parasitized individuals. Respective figures for 12° C are 3·8% and 10·7% (Tallmark and Norrgren, 1976). Apparent seasonal fluctuations of infestation incidences in *N. obsoletus*—as reported by Miller and Northup (1926), Sindermann (1956), Gambino (1959), McDaniel and Coggins (1971, 1972)—possibly reflect differential migratory habits of healthy and diseased *N. obsoletus*, as is the case in *Littorina littorea* (see p. 348). According to Sindermann (1960) and Crisp (1969), trematode-infested mud-snails on the east coast of the U.S.A. do not participate in the downward winter migration of healthy individuals. Similarly, *N. reticulatus* in Gullmar Fjord (Sweden) are immobilized by parasitization and remain in shallow water, thereby simulating an apparent increase in infestation incidence in the upper tidal zone during late autumn. The percentage of infested snails in deeper water was low and constant during the entire investigation period (Tallmark and Norrgren, 1976). Previous studies of the behaviour and migration of *N. obsoletus* (Batchelder, 1915; Jenner, 1956, 1957, 1958, 1959; Crisp, 1969; Brown, 1977) have not taken into consideration possible side effects of trematode infestation.

Double infestations in *Nassarius obsoletus* have been recorded by Gambino (1959) and more closely examined by Vernberg and co-authors (1969). Of 5025 snails from Beaufort, North Carolina, 340 (6·8%) were infested, 326 of them with a single trematode while 14 had double infestations. In half of the double infestations, both species of cercariae were being shed. The most common trematodes, *Lepocreadium setiferoides* and *Himasthla quissetensis*, were never found together, thus exhibiting 100% antagonism. *Zoogonus lasius*, on the other hand, was involved in duel infestations in a statistically significantly higher proportion than should be expected by chance. Mechanisms of trematode synergism and antagonism, which might become of practical importance in the

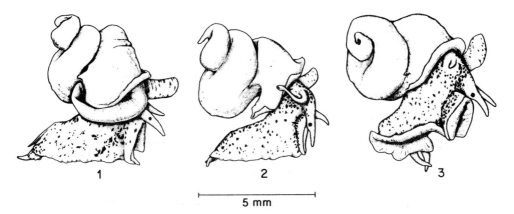

5 mm

Fig. 12-31: *Nassarius pygmaeus*. Effect of larval trematode infestation on penis morphology in adult males (shell removed). 1: Healthy individual with normal penis; 2: individual showing penis reduction typical of developing trematode infestation; 3: individual with highly reduced penis typical of Type III infestation (see Fig. 12-32). (After Køie, 1975; reproduced by permission of Ophelia.)

biological control of harmful snail species, have been studied mainly by Lie and his school (Lie, 1966, 1967, 1973; Lie and co-authors, 1965, 1966, 1967, 1968a, b; Basch and Lie, 1966a, b; Heyneman and Umathevy, 1968; Basch and co-authors, 1969; Basch 1970; Heyneman and co-authors, 1972).

Infestation with *Lepocreadium setiferoides* and *Zoogonus lasius* has been found to reduce the thermal resistance of *Nassarius obsoletus*. Survival of infested snails subjected to 39° C for 3 h, and to 41° C for 0·5 h, was considerably less than that of healthy specimens. At 37° C and 6 h exposure, the difference was not as pronounced (Vernberg and Vernberg, 1963; Fig. 12-33). Riel (1975) obtained results deviating markedly from those of the latter authors. In his experiments, *N. obsoletus* parasitized by *Z. lasius*, *L. setiferoides* and *Himasthla quissetensis* showed a higher survival rate than healthy individuals when submitted to high-temperature stress (Fig. 12-34). The difference in response remains un-

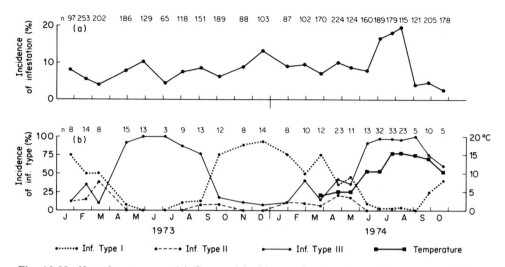

Fig. 12-32: *Nassarius pygmaeus*. (a) Seasonal incidence of infestation with *Opechona bacillaris* (n = number of snails examined); (b) seasonal prevalence of immature, intermediate and mature infestations (n = number of infested snails). (After Køie, 1975; reproduced by permission of Ophelia.)

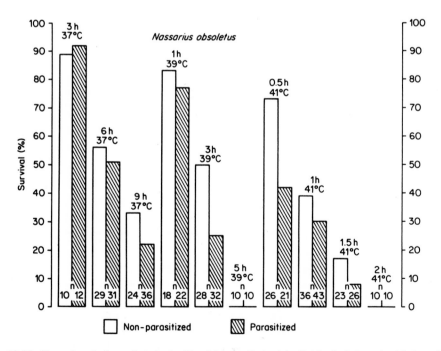

Fig. 12-33: *Nassarius obsoletus*. Survival of healthy snails and individuals infested with larval trematodes after exposure to various temperature–time combinations. (Based on data presented by Vernberg and Vernberg, 1963.)

explained and cannot be attributed to the fact that Vernberg and Vernberg (1963) worked with *N. obsoletus* from Beaufort, North Carolina, whereas Riel (1975) obtained his experimental animals from Southport, Connecticut. However, since the Vernbergs did their study during the fall and early winter, while Riel worked in the period from June to August, the discrepancies could be related to differences in a season-dependent physiological state of the test animals (differences in gonad cycle, nutritional state, etc.).

Tallmark and Norrgren (1976), who studied the thermal resistance of *Nassarius reticulatus*, reported reduced survival of infested individuals after exposure to both extremely high (35° C) and low (-2° C) temperatures (Table 12-11). Survival of littoral marine invertebrates after freezing has been investigated repeatedly (Kanwisher, 1955, 1959, 1966; Sömme, 1967; and others). However, these authors have failed to consider parasitism by larval trematodes as a factor affecting the survival of the gastropod hosts studied.

The metabolic response of larval *Zoogonus lasius* (a fish trematode) and *Himasthla quissetensis* (a bird parasite), both parasitic in *Nassarius obsoletus*, has been determined at temperatures varying from 6 to 41° C (Vernberg, 1961; Fig. 12-35). Particularly in the cercariae, the Q_{10} values reflected the temperatures encountered in the adult hosts, a poikilothermic and a homoiothermic vertebrate, respectively, which is an indication of preadaptation, evolving in these parasites during their larval life. The parthenitae of the fish

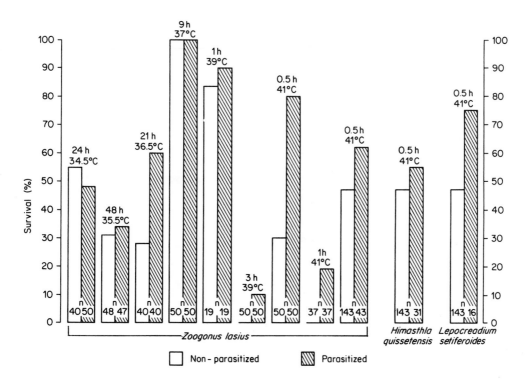

Fig. 12-34: *Nassarius obsoletus*. Survival of healthy snails and individuals infested with larval trematodes *Zoogonus lasius*, *Himasthla quissetensis* and *Lepocreadium setiferoides*, after exposure to various temperature–time combinations. (Based on data presented by Riel, 1975.)

parasite died within ½ h at 39°C, while the larvae of the bird trematode survived a 6-h period at 41° C. Such differences in thermal resistance might well account for a differential mortality of free-living mud-flat snails infested with different trematode species, particularly under conditions of long-term exposure to high summer temperatures.

Table 12-11

Nassarius reticulatus. Effect of trematode infestation on thermal resistance. Survival of snails (exposed to 35° C and -2° C) 24 h after retransfer to water of 30° C and 7° C. Each batch contained 20 infested and 20 non-infested individuals (After Tallmark and Norrgren, 1976; reproduced by permission of Zoon)

Exposure (Temperature/ Time)	Survival (%) non-parasitized	parasitized
35° C		
30 min	100	90
60 min	55	30
90 min	35	12
120 min	10	0
-2°C		
30 min	100	95
60 min	80	55
90 min	55	20
120 min	30	5

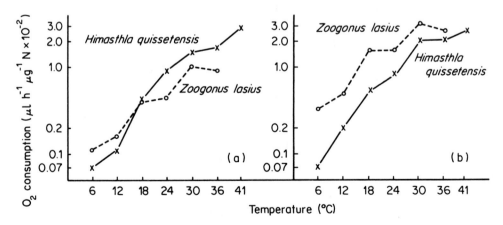

Fig. 12-35: Metabolic response of larval trematodes from *Nassarius obsoletus*. Oxygen consumption of *Zoogonus lasius* sporocysts and *Himasthla quissetensis* rediae (a) and cercariae of both parasites (b) in relation to temperature. (After Vernberg, 1961; modified; reproduced by permission of Academic Press, Inc.)

Nassarius obsoletus infested with *Zoogonus lasius* and *Lepocreadium setiferoides* exhibited differences in their thermal metabolic response, as compared to uninfested snails, when exposed to temperatures varying between 10° and 35° C (Vernberg and Vernberg, 1967; Fig. 12-36; Table 12-12). Although the observed differences in actual metabolic rates occurred only at the temperature extremes, at these thermal points, the metabolic rate of the parasitized snails was significantly higher than that of the nonparasitized specimens. A comparison of the metabolic thermal acclimation curves suggested that the larval trematodes basically altered the metabolic temperature response of *N. obsoletus*. Similar conditions have been found in *N. reticulatus* from Gullmar Fjord (Sweden), which was parasitized by an unidentified larval microphallid. Cold-adapted (5°C) and warm-adapted (28° C), parasitized and non-parasitized individuals exhibited divergent patterns of metabolic thermal response. At 28° C the oxygen consumption was statistically significantly higher in parasitized snails (Tallmark and Norrgren, 1976).

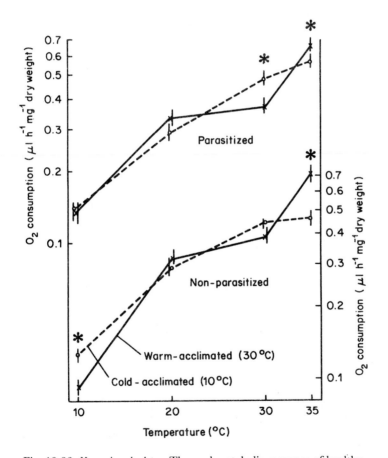

Fig. 12-36: *Nassarius obsoletus*. Thermal metabolic response of healthy snails and individuals parasitized by *Zoogonus lasius* and *Lepocreadium setiferoides*. Vertical bars: standard errors; asterisks: differences of means statistically significant at 5% level or less. (After Vernberg and Vernberg, 1967; modified; reproduced by permission of Academic Press, Inc.)

Table 12-12

Nassarius obsoletus. Thermal metabolic response of parasitized and non-parasitized individuals after acclimation to 10° C and 30° C at 30⁰/₀₀ S (After Vernberg and Vernberg, 1967; reproduced by permission of Experimental Parasitology)

	Parasitized *Nassarius obsoletus*				Non-parasitized *Nassarius obsoletus*		
Temperature (°C)	Number of determinations	O_2 consumption (μl h^{-1} mg^{-1} dry wt.) Range	Mean $\pm$ SE	Temperature (°C)	Number of determinations	O_2 consumption (μl h^{-1} mg^{-1} dry wt.) Range	Mean $\pm$ SE
Warm-acclimated (30°C)				Warm-acclimated (30°C)			
10	10	0·080–0·200	0·135±0·013[b]	10	13	0·042–0·28	0·091±0·009[a,c]
20	15	0·269–0·522	0·336±0·026	20	23	0·147–0·475	0·323±0·024
30	14	0·240–0·551	0·371±0·026[a]	30	15	0·273–0·643	0·392±0·029
35	15	0·418–0·871	0·667±0·039[a]	35	14	0·468–0·155	0·710±0·058[a]
Cold-acclimated (10°C)				Cold-acclimated (10°C)			
10	14	0·092–0·216	0·137±0·011	10	19	0·062–0·204	0·127±0·008[a]
20	15	0·151–0·535	0·293±0·024	20	12	0·166–0·383	0·291±0·020
30	14	0·305–0·828	0·483±0·033[a]	30	19	0·332–0·664	0·441±0·016
35	23	0·341–1·035	0·568±0·033[a,c]	35	18	0·307–0·708	0·465±0·032[a,c]

[a] At these temperatures occur significant differences, at 5% level or less, between metabolic rates of cold-(c.a.) and warm-acclimated (w.a.) snails.
[b] At 10°C the Q_{O_2} of w.a. infested snails is significantly higher, at 1% level, than in w.a. non-infested snails.
[c] At 35°C the Q_{O_2} of c.a. infested snails is significantly higher, at 5% level, than in c.a. non-infested snails.

Respiration and oxygen consumption of various littoral marine animals in relation to environmental factors have been studied by numerous authors (e.g. Fischer and co-authors, 1933; Sandeen and co-authors, 1954; Newell, 1966, 1969, 1973; Sandison, 1966, 1967; Toulmond, 1967a, b; Newell and Pye, 1970a, b, 1971a, b; Newell and Bayne, 1973; Newell and Roy, 1973; McMahon and Russell-Hunter, 1973, 1974, 1977; Pye and Newell, 1973; Russell-Hunter and McMahon, 1974; for pertinent reviews consult Kinne, 1970, 1971, 1972). Important papers on respiration and oxygen consumption of larval and adult marine trematodes have been provided by Hunter and Vernberg (1955a, b), Vernberg and Hunter (1959, 1960, 1961, 1963), Vernberg (1961, 1963) and Vernberg and Vernberg (1967, 1968). Although some of the latter investigations have demonstrated profound effects of trematode infestation on the physiology of molluscan hosts, no attention has been paid to these findings in the above-cited physio-ecological papers.

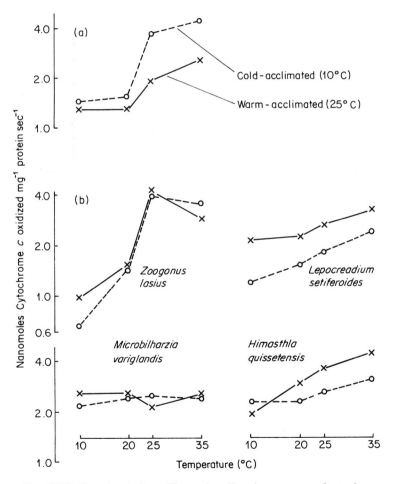

Fig. 12-37: *Nassarius obsoletus*. Thermal acclimation patterns of cytochrome *c* oxidase activity in digestive gland tissue from healthy snails (a) and from individuals parasitized by different species of larval trematodes (b). (After Vernberg, 1969; modified; reproduced by permission of American Society of Zoologists.)

With respect to oxygen consumption and salinity, Sindermann and Rosenfield (1957) found a remarkably similar pattern of response in healthy *N. obsoletus* and specimens parasitized by *Microbilharzia variglandis*.

The character of the response to temperature changes, however, varies with the trematode species involved. One of the enzymes known to be sensitive to environmental changes is cytochrome c oxidase, an enzyme of the terminal electron-transport system. When assayed on digestive-gland tissue from *Nassarius obsoletus* infested with *Microbilharzia variglandis*, *Himasthla quissetensis*, *Lepocreadium setiferoides* and *Zoogonus lasius*, extremely divergent thermal acclimation patterns of cytochrome c oxidase activity resulted (Fig. 12-37). Consequently, the physiological response of mud-flat snails is clearly altered by the presence of larval trematodes. It was concluded that in the intertidal zone, where *N. obsoletus* normally occurs and where environmental fluctuations tend to be extreme, infestation with larval trematodes may jeopardize the host's survival (Vernberg and Vernberg, 1968; Vernberg, 1969).

Table 12–13

Nassarius obsoletus. Fatty-acid composition (percentage by weight) of digestive-gland tissue of parasitized and non-parasitized individuals (After Lunetta and Vernberg, 1971; reproduced by permission of Experimental Parasitology)

Fatty acid methyl ester	Non-infested tissue			*Lepocreadium setiferoides*			*Zoogonus lasius*		*Microbilharzia variglandis*		*Himasthla quissetensis*	
C_{14}	6·9	5·3	5·4	5·7	6·7	5·2	5·4	6·1	5·5	6·0	3·6	2·7
$C_{14:1}$	1·5	1·1	1·4	2·6	2·3	4·6	4·0	2·7	3·2	4·0	3·9	4·0
C_{16}	15·4	13·3	12·4	14·6	12·5	13·6	18·8	12·6	14·9	13·6	13·8	14·4
$C_{16:1}$	6·2	8·7	6·1	8·5	8·7	7·5	7·7	6·1	7·2	7·5	6·5	7·2
$C_{16:2}$	2·2	1·3	2·9	3·4	3·0	3·7	—	4·0	3·6	4·0	3·4	4·0
C_{18}	4·9	6·1	3·7	6·5	6·4	4·7	11·4	6·0	7·2	7·8	6·0	5·7
$C_{18:1}$	6·9	9·3	5·9	7·5	7·3	8·0	10·2	8·0	7·9	6·0	7·3	8·1
C_{20}	13·2	13·2	13·2	13·6	12·9	8·0	17·2	13·8	11·8	10·0	13·4	13·0
$C_{20:2}$	3·3	3·3	10·8	3·9	2·6	4·3	T	5·3	T	T	4·1	5·2
$C_{20:3}$	6·1	6·6	8·5	3·2	1·0	14·7	T	9·2	7·8	6·2	17·2	16·2
$C_{20:5}$	33·0	31·2	28·8	30·3	31·5	25·2	25·1	25·7	30·3	30·3	20·7	19·3

T: Trace amounts only

Comparatively high levels of glucose-6-phosphate dehydrogenase were found in the digestive gland of *Nassarius obsoletus*. Activities were $1·40 \pm 0·12$ (= mean $\pm$ standard error of mean) I.U. g^{-1} of liver homogenate in healthy snails, and $0·70 \pm 0·14$ in individuals parasitized by *Zoogonus lasius*. However, when expressed as I.U. g^{-1} of protein, the values obtained for non-parasitized and parasitized snails—$0·0183 \pm 0.003$ and $0·0190 \pm 0·005$ I.U., respectively—did not differ significantly. On the other hand, the total protein content of the hepatopancreas of infested snails consistently showed a sharp decrease of approximately 50%. Values were $85·5 \pm 4·34$ g protein g^{-1} liver for non-parasitized snails, as opposed to $42·6 \pm 8·00$ for parasitized individuals (Schilansky and co-authors, 1977). Possible effects of trematode parasitization on enzyme biochemistry have not been taken into consideration by previous studies on *N. obsoletus* conducted by Fried and Levin (1970, 1973).

Like *Nassarius obsoletus* from tidal flats along the North American Atlantic coast, *N. reticulatus* from Gullmar Fjord (Sweden) lives in a physical-stress environment (Evans and Tallmark, 1975). Under these circumstances, the influence of parasitization by trematodes was considered an important factor in the ecology of *N. reticulatus*, especially as this species seems to lack predators in that area. During cold winter periods with a mean surface temperature of -0·5° C and occasional freezing of the surface water, there was a drastic decline in the total number of snails in the area of investigation from about 45,000 to approximately 30,000. Mortality of parasitized snails was attributable to these cold periods. Trematode parasites must, therefore, be of considerable importance as energy transformers and regulators of the Gullmar Fjord population of *N. reticulatus* (Tallmark and Norrgren, 1976).

Trematode infestation apparently tends to alter the fatty-acid composition in the tissues of *Nassarius obsoletus*. In non-infested digestive-gland tissue, the C_{20} acids constitute 57% of the total fatty acids, in contrast to 42% in tissue infested with *Microbilharzia variglandis*, 48% in *Zoogonus lasius*, 50% in *Lepocreadium setiferoides* and 55% in *Himasthla quissetensis* (Table 12-13). Differences presumably reflect the varied fatty-acid demands of the metabolism of each species. It was concluded that the large amount of C_{20} acids in both infested and uninfested snails could probably be correlated with seasonal temperatures. C_{20} and C_{22} acids are known to increase with decreasing environmental temperature in some marine invertebrates, and probably function to ensure a low melting point for the extracellular lipids when the animals are exposed to low temperatures. It would seem likely that the alterations in fatty-acid composition in parasitized mud-flat snails could play a role in the lowered resistance of these animals to thermal stress (Lunetta and Vernberg, 1971).

It has been well documented that the tissue-free amino acids (FAA) of many euryhaline invertebrates serve as osmotic effectors during salinity stress (Allen and Awapara, 1960; DuPaul and Webb, 1970; Virkar and Webb, 1970). The primary amino acids involved in osmoregulation of *Nassarius obsoletus* were taurine, glutamic acid, aspartic acid and proline, while the major amino acid functioning as an osmotic effector in the rediae and cercariae of *Himasthla quissetensis* was proline. Both parasitized and non-parasitized mud-flat snails acclimated to 12⁰/oo and 30⁰/oo S showed significant salinity-induced differences in the levels of taurine, glutamic acid, aspartic acid, threonine and phenylalanine (Fig. 12-38; Table 12-14). After acclimation to high salinity, all of the four major amino acids in the non-parasitized snails—taurine, glutamic acid, aspartic acid and lysine—were present in significantly lower concentrations in the parasitized host's digestive gland, but only taurine showed this difference after low salinity acclimation. In contrast, alanine, valine, glycine and proline were all found in significantly higher concentrations in the parasitized tissue, as compared with the non-parasitized digestive gland after acclimation to 30⁰/oo S, while at 12⁰/oo S, only proline was detected in significantly higher concentrations in parasitized snails (Kasschau, 1975a, b).

Since some of the amino acids increased with parasitism while others decreased, there was no significant difference in the FAA pool *without* taurine between parasitized and non-parasitized *Nassarius obsoletus* at either salinity. For snails acclimated to 12⁰/oo S, the difference in the FAA pool *including* taurine was significant between both groups of snails.

Table 12–14

Nassarius obsoletus. Concentrations of free amino acids (μmoles g^{-1} protein) in digestive glands of parasitized and non-parasitized individuals acclimated for 10 days to 12^0/oo and 30^0/oo S (After Kasschau, 1975; reproduced by permission of Pergamon Press)

Amino acid	12^0/oo S		30^0/oo S	
	Parasitized	Non-parasitized	Parasitized	Non-parasitized
	Mean±S.E.	Mean±S.E.	Mean±S.E.	Mean±S.E.
Taurine	63·5±5·6	162·1±5·2	281·0±12·9	355·0±13·5
Alanine	11·3±2·3	8·3±1·6	39·8± 5·6	22·0± 6·0
Valine	2·2±0·7	0·5±0·1	6·4± 1·0	3·2± 1·0
Glycine	12·3±1·8	7·2±1·2	19·3± 3·4	8·1± 1·4
Isoleucine	0·9±0·2	0·2±0·1	1·8± 0·7	1·6± 0·4
Leucine	1·0±0·4	0·4±0·1	1·6± 0·8	3·6± 1·1
Proline	19·5±3·9	2·9±1·4	68·8± 9·6	6·6± 1·6
Threonine	6·5±1·2	3·1±0·8	15·4± 2·4	11·3± 2·9
Serine	11·4±1·7	7·4±1·3	21·8± 2·0	18·4± 2·9
Methionine	1·2±0·5	0·3±0·1	5·0± 1·1	5·9± 1·7
Phenylalanine	1·0±0·1	0·5±0·2	2·9± 0·6	2·3± 0·5
Aspartic acid	15·1±0·8	13·5±1·1	27·6± 1·9	51·9± 6·8
Glutamic acid	23·3±1·6	32·1±3·1	61·1± 4·6	89·6±12·5
Lysine	21·0±3·1	33·4±3·0	24·8± 5·0	41·9± 7·5
Total FAA pool	190·1±5·7	268·9±9·4	578·5±22·7	621·4±48·0
Total FAA pool without taurine	126·6±6·6	106·8±8·5	296·4±16·8	266·4±39·7

The author (Kasschau, 1975b) concluded that *Himasthla quissetensis* seems to have no negative effects on its host's ability to osmoregulate at the cellular level, and that the host–parasite relationship has therefore reached a high degree of homeostasis in terms of osmoregulation. In the reviewer's opinion, however, such a conclusion appears to be somewhat premature. Taurine is the most important non-protein amino acid involved in osmoregulation in a number of marine molluscs (Lange, 1963; Allen and Garrett, 1972; Gilles, 1972). In warm-acclimated *N. obsoletus*, taurine makes up more than 50% of the FAA pool (Kasschau, 1975a). Since—regardless of the conditions in the total FAA concentration—there are statistically significant differences in the *taurine* level between parasitized and non-parasitized snails at 30^0/oo S, as well as at 12^0/oo S, *H. quissetensis* infestation might well have a detrimental effect on the osmoregulatory ability of its host, *N. obsoletus*. Further experimental work will be necessary to clarify this matter.

A correlation between shell erosion and trematode infestation is believed to exist in *Nassarius reticulatus* from Gullmar Fjord (Sweden). The erosion and destruction of the periostracum usually increases with age. However, among 300 snails ranging from 15 to 29 mm in shell height, 43% of the non-infested—but only 11% of the infested—individuals had an intact periostracum. Heavily eroded shells were found in 63% of the infested, but in only 25% of the non-infested *N. reticulatus* (Tallmark and Norrgren, 1976).

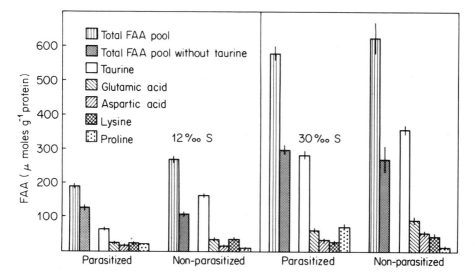

Fig. 12-38: *Nassarius obsoletus*. Concentrations of free amino acids (FAA) in digestive glands
of healthy individuals and snails infested with *Himasthla quissetensis* after 10 days of
acclimation to 12⁰/₀₀ and 30⁰/₀₀ S. Vertical lines: Standard errors. (After Kasschau,
1975b; modified; reproduced by permission of Pergamon Press.)

Among the Buccinidae, the waved whelk, *Buccinum undatum*, is known as a favourite
host for trematodes; at least 5 larval trematodes and one adult species have been
reported from this common prosobranch. A cotylocercous larva, *Cercaria buccini* (Fig.
12-39), has been found in *B. undatum* in British waters (Lebour, 1911). Although it has
subsequently been recorded in waved whelks from the French and German North Sea
coasts, as well as from the Øresund, Denmark (Stunkard, 1932; Rees, 1936a; Køie, 1969,
1971a; Lauckner, unpublished), its life cycle is still unknown. Morphologically, it
belongs to the family Allocreadiidae and most probably to the genus *Podocotyle*. Small
crustaceans presumably serve as second intermediate hosts, and marine fishes as final
hosts. *C. buccini* has been mistaken for *Podocotyle atomon* from *Littorina littorea* (Rees, 1935)
to which it is strikingly similar.

A detailed account of the histochemistry and the ultrastructure of *Cercaria buccini*, as
well as of the parasite–host interrelationship, has been given by Køie (1971a). Mother
sporocysts of the parasite are located in the mantle distal to the kidney or the gill of
Buccinum undatum. Young daughter sporocysts occur throughout the tissues of the host,
while mature sporocysts are particularly common in the connecting tissue between the
tubules of the digestive gland and the gonad. A strong host-tissue response to the
presence of the mother sporocysts was noted. They were surrounded by numerous
amoebocytes, their branches being walled off by the host cells. Although some of the
branches were apparently degenerating, the majority appeared uninjured. The host
tissue surrounding the mother sporocysts was never found in a state of histolysis. This
was, however, common in the presence of daughter sporocysts. Histolysis of the
digestive-gland cells liberated digestive enzymes which, although coming into contact
with the sporocysts, apparently did not affect them. Other digestive-gland tubules
regressed without disintegration, and the gonads either disappeared completely or

became nonfunctional remnants. A large number of amoebocytes were often observed around the sporocysts, but apparently they were all digested by the sporocysts.

Cercaria buccini is a rare parasite. It has been recorded from only about 1% of 1700 *Buccinum undatum* from Øresund, Denmark, and from 0·55% of 910 whelks dredged off Helgoland, North Sea, respectively (Køie, 1969, 1971a; Lauckner, unpublished). From histological findings, it is apparent that *C. buccini* is a lethal pathogen—a view also supported by the fact that whelks infested with this parasite usually die shortly after their transfer to the laboratory.

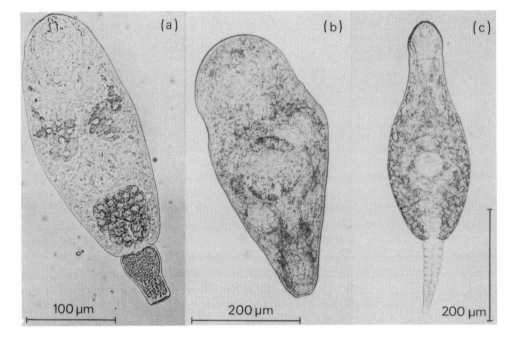

Fig. 12-39: Larval trematodes from *Buccinum undatum*. (a) *Cercaria buccini*; (b) *Zoogonoides viviparus*; (c) *Renicola* sp. (Original.)

As revealed by detailed histological, histochemical and ultrastructural studies, the sporocysts and cercariae of *Zoogonoides viviparus*, which parasitize in the gonads and the digestive gland of *Buccinum undatum*, do not seriously injure their host, although the cells in the immediate vicinity of migrating cercariae are frequently found in a process of disintegration (Køie, 1971b). The lesser degree of pathogenicity of *Z. viviparus* is also reflected by the fact that this species occurs more frequently in larger whelks, indicating a slow accumulation with host age, which is not compensated for by an increased mortality of affected *B. undatum*.

Zoogonoides viviparus has been known from the North Sea for more than 100 years (van Beneden, 1875). Levinsen (1881) found it in *Buccinum undatum* from Greenland, and Pelseneer (1906) described it as *Cercaria giardi* from whelks dredged off Boulogne, French Atlantic coast. About 7% of 1700 *B. undatum* from Øresund and 4% of 910 whelks from Helgoland, respectively, harboured this parasite (Køie, 1971b; Lauckner, unpublished). Seasonal fluctuations in the abundance of larval *Z. viviparus*—with peaks in June,

October and April, and 'lows' in July and November—have been recorded by Køie (1969). Lebour (1918), who found 30 of 40 large whelks from Plymouth, England, infested with this trematode, noticed the striking similarity of the tailless cercaria (Fig. 12-39) with the adult Z. *viviparus* described by Olsson (1867) and Looss (1901), and consequently inferred the identity of both cercaria and adult. Despite the frequent occurrence of Z. *viviparus*—particularly in flatfish (Dawes, 1947, 1968)—the meta-cercarial stage remained unknown until Lauckner (1973) obtained experimental encystment of the cercariae in sea-urchins *Psammechinus miliaris*. Subsequently, Orrhage (1973) reported the metacercaria from sedentary polychaetes *Trochochaeta multisetosa*. Køie (1976) studied the entire life cycle of Z. *viviparus* experimentally. In addition to annelids and echinoderms, gastropods and bivalves are utilized as second intermediate host by this trematode.

Cercaria neptuneae, a cercaria with conspicuous eye-spots, was found to develop in rediae in the digestive gland of *Neptunea antiqua* and *Buccinum undatum* from Northumberland and Plymouth, England (Lebour, 1911, 1918), but appears to be absent from whelks dredged in Øresund and off Helgoland, respectively (Køie, 1969; Lauckner, unpublished). Wolfgang (1954b, 1955a) recovered this—or a closely related—cercaria from about 1% of 875 *B. undatum* and 6% of 125 *Neptunea decemcostatum* from the Canadian Atlantic coast, and identified it—seemingly conclusively—as the cercaria of *Stephanostomum baccatum*, an acanthocolpid trematode whose metacercaria encysts in the skin and musculature of flatfishes *Hippoglossoides platessoides*, *Limanda limanda*, *Microstomus kitt*, *Glyptocephalus cynoglossus* and *Pleuronectes platessa*, and whose adult matures in the intestine of predatory fish such as *Acanthocottus scorpio*, *Hippoglossus hippoglossus* and *Hemitripterus americanus* (Nicoll, 1907b, 1910; Nicoll and Small, 1909). His findings (Wolfgang, 1954a, b, 1955a, b) have, however, been criticized by Stunkard (1961), who questioned the identity of the metacercaria with the known adult of *S. baccatum*.

Neophasis lageniformis is another acanthocolpid trematode parasitizing *Buccinum undatum*; it has an abbreviated life cycle. The tail-bearing cercariae, which grow in rediae in the digestive gland and gonad, as well as throughout the body of the host, develop into tailless, unencysted metacercariae within the redia. No additional intermediate host is required. The adults of *N. lageniformis* mature in the intestine of the catfish *Anarhichas lupus* which becomes infested by devouring parasite-laden *B. undatum* (Lebour, 1905, 1910, 1911). The parthenitae of this parasite have been found in approximately 7% of whelks from Cullercoats, England, as well as in about the same percentage of whelks from Øresund, Denmark (Lebour, 1911; Køie, 1969, 1971c). Lebour never found the cercaria in winter. Køie (1969) noticed irregular fluctuations, with peaks in July and January, and lows in June and September, which she attributed, however, to the limited sample size rather than to a seasonal variation in the incidence of infestation. She concluded that infestation of *B. undatum* occurs throughout the year. Unlike *Zoogonoides viviparus*, the incidence of infestation with *N. lageniformis* did not increase with the age of the host, which might indicate that affected whelks die after a short time.

Pathogenic effects accompanying *Neophasis lageniformis* infestations comprise histolysis of host connective tissue surrounding the rediae, and atrophy of digestive-gland tubules and gonad tissue. Not only extracellular material, particularly reticular fibres, but also entire cells, nerves and muscles undergo complete dissolution. A few amoebocytes were seen near the tegument of some rediae, but these were usually dissovled too. Although amoebocytes normally constitute an effective defence mechanism of the host, they are apparently not able to conquer the rediae. Dead rediae were, however, sometimes observed near digestive-gland tubules which had been disrupted, apparently due to the pressure exerted by the parasite. Probably the digestive enzymes of the host, which had been liberated by the destruction of the tubules, had killed the rediae. From overall inspection, it becomes apparent that *N. lageniformis* seriously affects the host and may cause its death. A detailed account of the histopathology, histochemistry and ultrastructure of the various life-cycle stages of *N. lageniformis* had been given by Køie (1969, 1971c, 1973a, b).

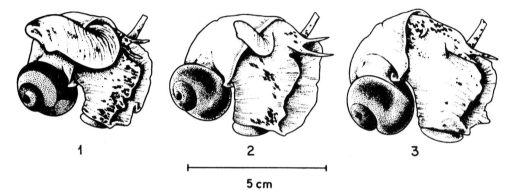

5 cm

Fig. 12-40: *Buccinum undatum*. Males (shell removed) showing penis reduction caused by larval trematode infestation. 1: Healthy individual with normal penis; 2 and 3: individuals infested with *Neophasis lageniformis*, showing intermediate and extreme penis reduction. In both cases, gonads were entirely destroyed by parasite. (After Køie, 1969; reproduced by permission of Ophelia.)

Sporocysts containing renicolid xiphidiocercariae (Fig. 12-39) have been recovered from 2 of 1375 *Buccinum undatum* from a depth of 20 to 30 m in Øresund, Denmark. It has not previously been recorded from whelks. As in *Renicola* infestations in other prosobranchs the sporocysts in the whelk form a compact mass, with no snail tissue in between, situated on the surface of the digestive gland immediately above the stomach. The surrounding tissues and the gonad were not infested (Køie, 1969). The further stages in the life cycle of this parasite remain unknown, but the metacercariae are expected to occur in pelecypods. Since all known adults of the genus *Renicola* mature in the kidney of birds, the final host of the renicolid cercaria from *B. undatum* will, therefore, almost certainly be found among mollusc-eating birds, probably among diving ducks. The species has also been found in 4·9% of 796 *B. undatum* dredged in January 1973 and 1·75% of 114 whelks dredged in May 1973 from about 30-m depth off Helgoland, North Sea (Lauckner, unpublished).

All previously mentioned trematodes from *Buccinum undatum* reach maturity in fishes. The occurrence of a renicolid bird-parasite in whelks from comparatively deep water and offshore regions is altogether unexpected. It appears worth mentioning that this trematode was not found in 143 *B. undatum* dredged from shallow inshore tide channels at Sylt, North Sea, although diving ducks and other sea birds are abundant on the tidal flats, and up to 40% of periwinkles *Littorina littorea* from the same area have been found infested with the larval stages of a related species, *Renicola roscovita* (Lauckner, in preparation).

A very detailed discussion of the various aspects of trematode infestation in *Buccinum undatum* has been presented by Køie (1969). She noticed a strong correlation between infestation and the size of the mating organ of male whelks (Figs 12-40 and 12-41). There was evidence for the fact that the smaller penis length in infested males was the result of a reduction of the organ (which might have been fully developed prior to the infestation) rather than a retardation in development. Whelks with recently established infestations mostly had a longer penis than specimens with older infestations. Regression of the mating organ is apparently a very rapid process, as is the development of the infestations themselves. It seems possible to assess the approximate age of an infestation from the length of the penis. The physiological mechanisms leading to penis reduction are unknown. In *Neophasis lageniformis*, *Zoogonoides viviparus*, *Cercaria neptuneae* and *C. buccini* infestations, it may result from the destruction of the gonadal tissues by the parasites. However, penis reduction also occurred in males infested with *Renicola* sp., although the gonad is not affected directly in this case (Køie, 1969; Lauckner, unpublished).

No histological signs were observed indicating that parasite-free whelks had been infested previously, and that the infestation had later disappeared. Thus, loss of infestation and subsequent recovery of the host, which possibly occurs in *Littorina littorea*,

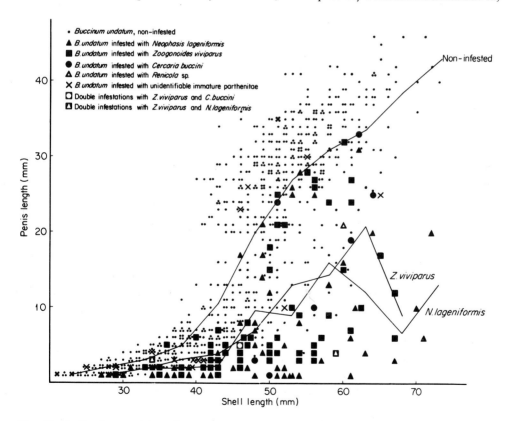

Fig. 12-41: *Buccinum undatum*. Relation between shell length and penis length in healthy and trematode-infested whelks from Øresund, Denmark (n = 911 measurements). (After Køie, 1969; modified; reproduced by permission of Ophelia.)

appear to be improbable in *Buccinum undatum*. Young, still unidentifiable rediae and sporocysts have been found in all size-classes of whelks, suggesting that acquisition of trematodes is independent of age and size in *B. undatum*. Double infestations involving *Zoogonoides viviparus* and *Neophasis lageniformis* have been observed in 7 cases, and the combination of *Z. viviparus* with *C. buccini* was found once. In both cases, the observed incidences agree well with the theoretical expectations (Køie, 1969).

Gastropods as Second Intermediate Hosts for Digenea

There are two distinct categories of cases in which gastopods serve as second intermediate hosts for trematodes: (i) Cercariae emerge from the first intermediate host (which might well be a gastropod) and penetrate a second intermediate host (which might well be the same or another gastropod species). Usually, encystment occurs in the second (gastropod) intermediate host, but unencysted metacercariae may also occur. (ii) Cercariae develop in rediae or—more frequently—in sporocysts in the gastropod first intermediate host, and do not leave the host, but instead, encyst either within the rediae or sporocysts from which they originate, or remain—mostly unencysted—within the haemocoelic spaces of their first host. Although no additional host is involved in the latter case, the snail harbouring the metacercarial stage must—by definition—be regarded as second intermediate host. There are many examples for such abridged trematode life cycles.

Metacercarial cysts have been reported from a great variety of prosobranchs. In many cases, their specific identity remained obscure due either to the early developmental state of the internal organs of the larva, or to the difficulty in discerning morphological features of the metacercaria tightly curled up within its cyst. Moreover, cercariae encysting in molluscan tissues usually exhibit low—or even lack—host specificity, and penetrate pelecypods and gastropods almost equally well.

Cercariae of *Himasthla elongata, H. littorinae, Renicola roscovita* and *R. parvicaudata* usually encyst in pelecypods, but their metacercariae have also been recovered from the individual hosts—specimens of periwinkles *Littorina littorea, L. saxatilis* and *L. obtusata*—in which the cercariae had developed (Stunkard, 1950, 1966a; Werding, 1969). Correspondingly, metacercariae of *Psilochasmus oxyurus, P. aglyptorchis, Psilostomum brevicolle* and *Asymphylodora demeli* were frequently found in the snail specimens—*Littoridina australis, Hydrobia ulvae* and *H. ventrosa*, respectively—which also harboured the rediae, as well as in other specimens of the same prosobranch species (Szidat, 1957; Ankel, 1962; Loos-Frank, 1968a, b; Reimer, 1973; Vaes, 1974).

'*Cercaria B*' from limpets *Patella vulgata* and *P. intermedia*, a species of *Renicola*, also encysts in its first intermediate host (Crewe, 1951). *Parapronocephalum symmetricum*, a notocotylid reported from 4% of *Littorina saxatilis tenebrosa* var. *similis* at Swansea, Wales, has no free-living larval stage. Cercariae, emerging from rediae in the visceral haemocoel, migrate to the haemocoel above the wall of the stomach, where they lose their tails and encyst. Twelve to 25 cycts have been counted per infested host. The rediae of this parasite completely destroy the gonad, but do not damage the digestive gland (James, 1969).

The xiphidiocercariae of several microphallids—mainly representatives of the genera *Microphallus, Maritrema* and *Levinseniella*—encyst within the tissues of their respective first intermediate hosts, *Hydrobia ulvae, H. ventrosa, H. minuta* and *H. acuta*. Other

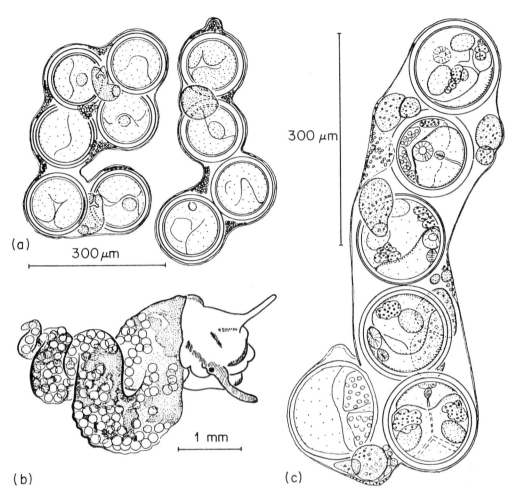

300 μm

(a)   300 μm

(b)

(c)

1 mm

Fig. 12-42: Larval microphallids from *Hydrobia acuta*. (a) Two sporocysts of *Maritrema syntomocyclus* containing germinal masses, free cercariae and encysted metacercariae; (b) aspect of *H. acuta* digestive gland harbouring *M. syntomocyclus*; (c) sporocyst of *Microphallus scolectroma* containing germinal masses, cercariae at different stages of development, 1 developing and 5 mature encysted metacercariae. (After Deblock and Tran Van Ky, 1966b; reproduced by permission of Masson et Cie., Paris.)

microphallids parasitizing hydrobiids have abridged life cycles. Thus, the cercariae of *Atriophallophorus minutus, Microphallus pirum, M. scolectroma, M. abortivus* and *Maritrema syntomocyclus* encyst directly within the sporocysts from which they originate (Fig. 12-42). Infested snails may contain hundreds of cysts (Stunkard, 1958; Ankel, 1962; Rebecq, 1964a; Deblock and Tran Van Ky, 1966a, b; Deblock, 1974b). In *Microphallus pygmaeus*, which develops in sporocysts in periwinkles *Littorina littorea, L. saxatilis tenebrosa* and *L. scutulata*, the cercarial stage is only of short duration. Very young cercariae have a vestigial tail which is entirely resorbed in the course of the development. The metacercariae remain unencysted within their sporocysts (Lebour, 1911; Ching, 1962; James, 1968b; Werding, 1969; Fig. 12-43).

There are some indications for the assumption that infestation of periwinkles with metacercariae of *Microphallus pygmaeus* is detrimental to the host. According to James (1968b), the decline of the infestation percentage in larger *Littorina saxatilis tenebrosa* suggests an increase in the mortality as the parasite grows and causes more damage. An increase in the resistance to infestation may also occur, reaching almost total immunity in periwinkles over 12 mm long. This view is also supported by the data obtained for *M. pygmaeus* infestations in *L. littorea* (Fig. 12-27). Moreover, in long-term stress experiments with periwinkles, conducted by the reviewer, specimens infested with *M. pygmaeus* died significantly sooner than healthy animals or periwinkles infested with other larval trematodes (Lauckner, unpublished).

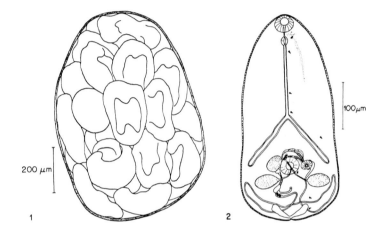

Fig. 12-43: *Microphallus pygmaeus* from *Littorina littorea*. 1: Sporocyst containing unencysted metacercariae; 2: metacercaria. (After Werding, 1969; reproduced by permission of Springer-Verlag.)

Unidentified, encysted metacercariae occurred in 3·3% of winkles *Littorina neritoides* from Plymouth, England, averaging 2·00 mm in height, and in 87% of those measuring 8·3 mm or more. Curiously, males were more heavily parasitized than females. Sometimes, the whole spire was packed with cysts (Lysaght, 1941; Rothschild, 1941c). Although no explanation was offered for this fact, increased infestation in male winkles is likely to be due to sex related behavioural and/or ecological differences, rather than to increased susceptibility of males to cercarial invasion.

Nothing is known about the pathogenicity of encysted metacercariae to their gastropod hosts. Detrimental effects of metacercarial invasion on the overall vitality has, however, been documented for pelecypods (see Volume II). It is possible, therefore, that encystment within the musculature of the snail's foot may impair the locomotory activity, and invasion of the gills and internal organs may cause occlusion of blood-sinuses and disturbances in the physiology of the host due to both mechanical pressure and tissue destruction. Furthermore, the metabolic requirements of the metacercariae, which are greatest immediately after penetration and encystment in the second intermediate host, should not be underestimated. Thus, the metacercarial cysts of *Renicola roscovita* from periwinkles *Littorina* spp., which measure about 100 μm in diameter immediately after encystment, grow to some 170 μm within a few weeks. This corresponds to a volume increase of approximately five times. The diameter of the metacercarial cysts of *Asymphylodora demeli* from snails *Hydrobia ventrosa* increases from less than 160 μm to about 380μm, which is equivalent to a volume increase of 13·4 times (Lauckner, 1971). The nutrients required for this anabolic activity must be provided by the host.

Unencysted gymnophallid metacercariae have been recovered from in between the mantle and shell of *Patella vulgata, P. intermedia* and *P. depressa,* 60 of 1247 limpets from various localities along the British coastline being infested (Crewe, 1951). The parasite,

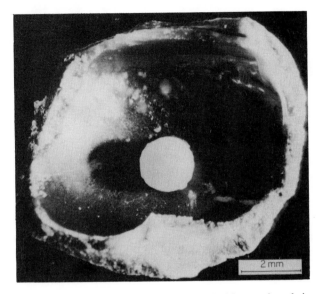

Fig. 12-44: *Littorina littorea.* Pearl probably produced in response to the presence of *Gymnophallus gibberosus* metacercaria. Pearl measuring 1·9 mm in diameter and attached to the inner shell surface by a delicate stalk. (Original.)

whose further stages remain unknown, has also been found in 3·38% of 503 adult *P. vulgata* from Cardigan Bay, Wales (James, 1968c). James' suggestion that it might be the larval stage of *Meiogymnophallus macroporus* (=*Lacunovermis macomae*), a trematode from the intestine of oystercatchers *Haematopus ostralegus* and marine ducks, is certainly erroneous, since the morphology of *L. macomae* is quite different from that of the larva found in limpets (Loos-Frank, 1970). Another unidentified gymnophallid metacercaria was recovered—only once—from a periwinkle *Littorina littorea* at the Isle of Mellum, German North Sea coast (Loos-Frank, 1971). Unencysted metacercariae of *Parvatrema borinqueñae* occur in costate horn shells *Cerithidea costata* from Puerto Rico. The cercariae of this species develop in bivalves *Gemma purpurea* (Cable, 1953). Another, as yet unidentified larval *Parvatrema* sp. has been reported from *Hydrobia ventrosa* from Camargue, French Mediterranean coast (Rebecq, 1964a; Bartoli, 1974). Unencysted, free gymnophallid metacercariae normally occur in pelecypods. Their low abundance in prosobranchs suggests that invasion of gastropods is merely accidental.

Larval gymnophallids, present between mantle and shell, are responsible for pearl formation in bivalves. In rare instances, pearl formation has also been observed in marine gastropods. A pearl, 1·9 mm in diameter and found attached to the inner surface of a *Littorina littorea* shell (Fig. 12-44), probably results from infestation with metacercariae of *Gymnophallus gibberosus* (see Chapter 'Mollusca: Bivalvia', Vol. II).

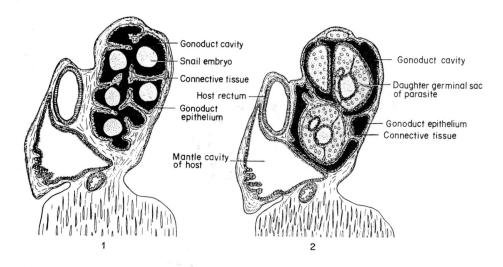

Fig. 12-45: *Littorina saxatilis tenebrosa*. 1: Transverse section through non-parasitized gonoduct of pregnant female showing position of embryos; 2: gonoduct parasitized by *Parvatrema homoeotecnum* daughter germinal sacs containing metacercariae. (After James, 1964; reproduced by permission of Cambridge University Press.)

Littorina saxatilis tenebrosa from Cardigan Bay, Wales, on the other hand, is the natural second (and first) intermediate host of the gymnophallid *Parvatrema homoeotecnum* (James, 1960, 1964, 1965). Parthenitae of this species, which parasitize in the gonad and the digestive gland, sometimes contain furcocercous cercariae and tailless metacercariae as well, which do not leave the host. The unique feature of the parthenitae is that they have the same essential structure as the cercariae which they produce. The mean incidence of infestation with *P. homoeotecnum* was 5·5% in 27,367 *L. saxatilis tenebrosa*, but it may reach 40% in some localities. In heavily infested snails, the gonad is completely replaced, the digestive gland is almost entirely replaced or the gonoduct filled with daughter germinal sacs of the parasite, which contain, in larger snails, as many as 40,000 metacercariae (Figs 12-45 to 12-47).

Among the **Neogastropoda**, whelks *Buccinum undatum* and mud snails *Nassarius mutabilis* have been reported as second intermediate hosts for larval trematodes. Of 1375 *B. undatum* from Øresund, Denmark, 93 (=6·8%) harboured the rediae of acanthocolpids *Neophasis lageniformis* in the digestive gland and gonad. The ocellate cercariae develop through a tail-bearing stage which, however, is very rarely found. By far the larger part of infested whelks contain tailless metacercariae which are much further developed than the cercariae. The metacercariae neither leave the rediae nor encyst. They are directly infective to the final host, the catfish, *Anarhichas lupus* (Køie, 1969). Sporocysts of a zoogonid, *Diphterostomum brusinae*, parasitize in the visceral haemocoel of *Nassarius mutabilis* from Naples, Italy. Upon completion of their development, the tailless cercariae encyst within the sporocysts (Palombi, 1930a, b). Metacercarial cysts of *Zoogonoides viviparus* occur in the mantle of *N. incrassatus*, *Cythara attenuata* and *Lora turricula* from Øresund, Denmark (Køie, 1976). In *Buccinum undatum*, cercariae of this species develop in sporocysts. Mud snails *N. incrassatus* and pisa shells *Pisania maculosa* from the French Mediterranean coast harbour unencysted metacercariae of the lepocreadiid *Lepidauchen stenostoma* (Prévot, 1968). The encysted second larval stage of another lepocreadiid, *Lepocreadium album*, has been dissected from the cutaneous tissues of opisthobranchs *Aplysia punctata* from the Gulf of Naples, Italy (Palombi, 1931, 1934, 1937). Unencysted, tail-bearing cercariae, as well as tailless metacercariae of *L. album*, have been observed in the tissues of pelagic nudibranchs *Phyllirrhoë bucephala* from waters off Villefranche-sur-Mer, France (Arvy, 1953).

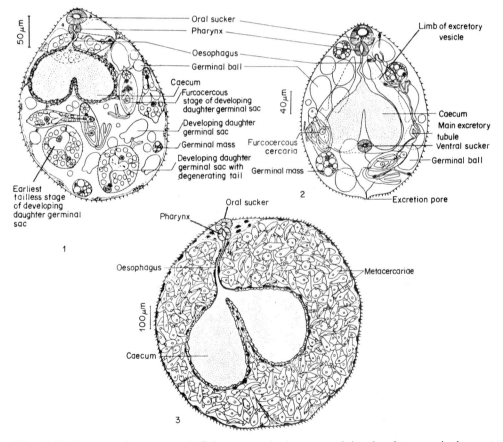

Fig. 12-46: *Parvatrema homoeotecnum*. 1: Primary germinal sacs containing daughter germinal sacs at various stages of development; ventral view. 2: Young daughter germinal sacs containing developing cercariae; ventral view. 3: Fully formed daughter germinal sac containing tailless metacercariae; ventral view. (After James, 1964; reproduced by permission of Cambridge University Press.)

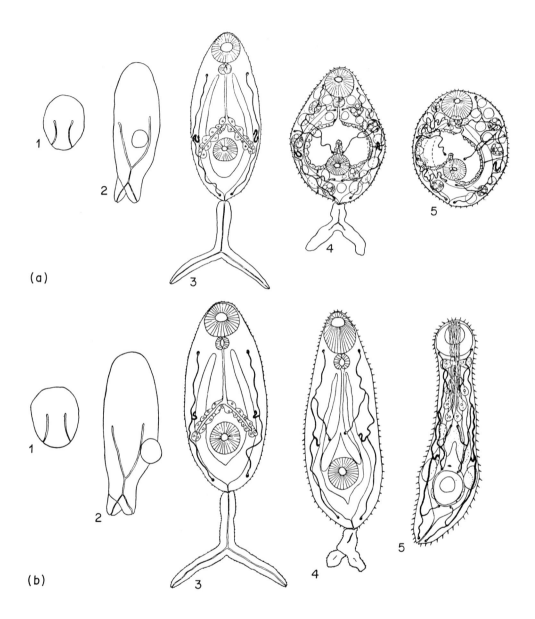

Fig. 12-47: *Parvatrema homoeotecnum*. (a) Development of daughter germinal sac within primary germinal sac. 1, 2: Development of excretory system and tail, ventral view; 3: tailed daughter germinal sac, early stage, ventral view; 4, 5: degeneration and loss of tail, development of body cavity and further increase in flame-cell number, ventral view. (b) Development of cercaria and metacercaria within daughter germinal sac. 1, 2: Development of excretory system and tail, ventral view; 3: furcocercous cercaria, ventral view; 4: degenerating tail and increase in flame-cell number, ventral view; 5: metacercaria, dorsal view. (After James, 1964; reproduced by permission of Cambridge University Press.)

Gastropods as Final Hosts for Digenea

At first view, the appearance of adult digenetic trematodes in molluscs is entirely unexpected; however, associations between molluscs and adult Digenea probably have to be regarded as an evolutionary relict. There is little doubt that the Digenea are primarily parasites of molluscs, and that second intermediate hosts and definite hosts have been acquired subsequently. With the advent of vertebrates, the former final hosts were eaten, and the trematodes acquired new hosts, to which sexual maturation was deferred. As a result, the former definitive hosts were gradually reduced to intermediate, paratenic or transfer hosts (Stunkard, 1959a, b, 1967c; Wright, 1966). Such gradual change in the role of the respective molluscan hosts is accompanied by a progressive development of progenesis—i.e. the occurrence of eggs and immature reproductive structures in the metacercarial stage. Certain trematodes described as progenetic metacercariae, however, actually represent young adult worms. Some species termed progenetic may develop to maturity in their molluscan hosts, as well as in additional vertebrate hosts. The importance of progenesis in the Digenea has been discussed in great detail by Buttner (1950, 1951a, b, c, 1955), Dollfus (1959), Stunkard (1959a, b), Jamieson (1966b) and others.

Young adult fellodistomatids *Steringophorus furciger* have been found free in the lumen of the stomach and the oesophageal caecum of 164 of 603 whelks *Buccinum undatum* from Øresund, Denmark (Køie, 1969). The worms, which measured between 1·3 to 3·5 mm in length, and between 0·8 to 1·4 mm in width, were of the same size as those usually recovered from the stomach and the intestine of a wide variety of teleosts, particularly flatfishes (Dawes, 1947), but the development of the sexual organs was not as advanced, and the specimens never had mature eggs.

One to four *Steringophorus furciger* were found per infested whelk, with a mean of 1·46. The infestation incidence was almost constant for whelks larger than 30 mm, and rose only slightly with the host's body size. Successive infestation was indicated by a variation in lengths of the trematodes recovered from individual *Buccinum undatum*. Parasite numbers did not accumulate with time, suggesting an equilibrium which was maintained, in that excessive *S. furciger* were either digested or expelled by the whelks. Infested flatfishes usually harbour more than a hundred trematodes of this species (Polyanskij, 1966). The low numbers of worms recovered from *B. undatum*, as well as the poor differentiation of their sexual organs, may indicate that this prosobranch is not the natural definite host for *S. furciger*.

Buccinum undatum is, on the other hand, the natural final host for another fellodistomatid, *Proctoeces buccini* (Fig. 12-48). Adult worms of this species, measuring 2·1 to 3·5 mm in length and 0·62 to 0·85 mm in width, occurred in the kidney of whelks from the Isle of Mellum, German North Sea coast (Loos-Frank, 1969). Although only 5 of 93 *B. undatum* were infested, the intensity of infestation was always extremely high, 30 to 180 worms being recovered from individual hosts. Mature specimens contained numerous embryonated eggs, measuring 50×25 μm, from which miracidia hatched upon exposure to sea water. Although the life cycle of *P. buccini* has not been traced, it was concluded that all stages are confined to *B. undatum*.

Gibbula umbilicalis from the Atlantic coast of Morocco is host for *Proctoeces progeneticus*, 90% of the top shells from Témara-Gayville being infested. Normally, 1 or 2 worms, measuring about 1·6 mm in length, were present in a single snail, but occasionally there were up to 5 parasites per host. The 'progenetic metacercariae' (which actually represent adult worms) occur free in the tissues of *G. umbilicalis*, invariably between the radula and the intestine. Immature individuals—the smallest measuring 0·46 × 0·26 mm—were rare; almost all were mature and contained numerous eggs enclosing a ciliated, motile miracidium (Dollfus, 1964).

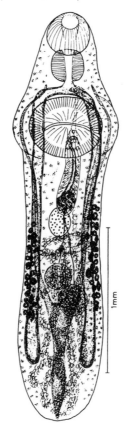

Fig. 12-48: *Proctoeces buccini.* Ventral aspect of adult worm from kidney of *Buccinum undatum.* (After Loos-Frank, 1969; reproduced by permission of Springer-Verlag.)

Rediae of the hemiurid *Cercaria sagittarius*, parasitic in *Cerithium rupestre* from the Mediterranean Sea, harboured—in addition to numerous cystophorous cercariae—single young adult worms (Palombi, 1940; Arvy, 1954). The natural definite host of *C. sagittarius* is not known and the occurrence of young adults within rediae was considered precocious and accidental.

In contrast, *Bunocotyle progenetica*, another hemiurid, completes its entire life cycle within a prosobranch mollusc. *Hydrobia ulvae* and *H. ventrosa* from the French Mediterranean and Channel coasts serve as hosts (Chabaud and Buttner, 1959; Deblock, 1974a). The species was originally described as *Metorchis progenetica* from *H. ventrosa* in the Baltic Sea (Markowski, 1936). Sporocysts and rediae parasitize in the snail's general cavity. Neither the digestive gland nor the gonad are affected. The large rediae, which measure up to 1800×200 μm, may simultaneously harbour germ balls, appendiculate cystophorous cercariae and adult worms in various stages of maturity (Figs 12-49 to 12-51).

In *Bunocotyle progenetica*, development from cercaria to adult is direct; the metacercarial stage is omitted. In addition to cercariae and adult worms, the rediae sometimes harbour considerable numbers of embryonated eggs. The enclosed miracidia are unciliated and immobile. No parasite eggs were found in the host body; apparently, they

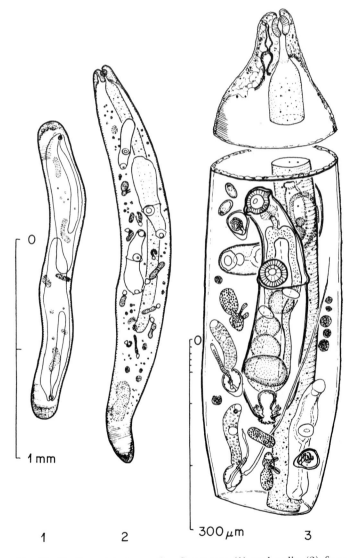

Fig. 12-49: *Bunocotyle progenetica*. Sporocyst (1) and redia (2) from haemocoel of *Hydrobia ulvae*; 3: enlarged portion of redia showing germ balls, cercariae, adult worm and ova *in situ*. (After Deblock, 1974a; reproduced by permission of Société Zoologique de France.)

are not expelled from the rediae. Liberation of the ova probably occurs after the host's natural death or upon its ingestion by a predator.

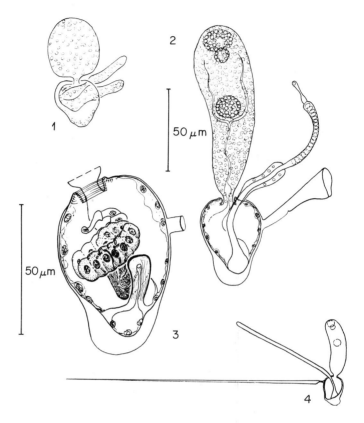

Fig. 12–50: *Bunocotyle progenetica*. 1, 2: Cystophorous cercariae in different stages of maturity; 3: morphological details of caudal cyst; 4: cercaria with caudal appendages in maximum extension. (After Deblock, 1974a; reproduced by permission of Société Zoologique de France.)

Similar to *Bunocotyle progenetica*, *B. cingulata* develops in *Hydrobia ventrosa*. Although this species is capable of completing its entire life cycle in the molluscan host, copepods may serve additionally as second intermediate and fishes as definite hosts (Odhner, 1928; Nybelin, 1936; Reimer, 1961). The latter author suggests that there is a correlation between salinity and the host utilized by *B. cingulata* for sexual reproduction. On the basis of a survey of records of this species, he tentatively proposed that in Baltic waters with salinities from 7 to 9⁰/oo S the copepod second intermediate host and the teleost final host are not required, whereas at lower salinities they become necessary for the completion of the life cycle—a view which has been discussed and rejected by Jamieson (1966b).

Szidat (1956) elucidated the life cycle of *Genarchella genarchella*, a hemiurid which occurs in *Littoridina australis* in a brackish lagoon in Argentina. Tailless 'cercariaeae'

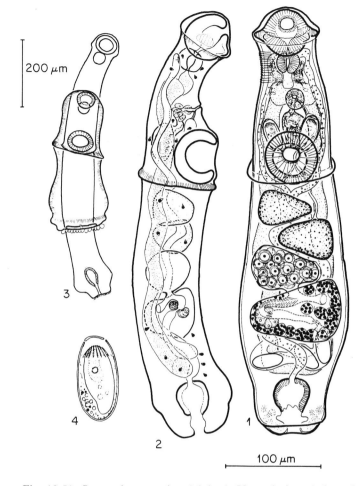

Fig. 12-51: *Bunocotyle progenetica*. Adult. 1: Ventral view; 2: lateral aspect; 3: schematic drawing showing individual in extreme extended or contracted positions; 4: egg containing miracidium armed with spines. (After Deblock, 1974a; reproduced by permission of Société Zoologique de France.)

develop directly within rediae; the cystophorous cercarial stage is entirely omitted. The cercariaeae transform into 'metacercariae' (which, in fact, are adults), and these lay numerous eggs, containing miracidia, while still within the rediae. How the eggs (or hatched miracidia) escape from the snail host remains to be studied. The host, *L. australis*, lives for only one year. Possibly, eggs of *G. genarchella*, released upon death and disintegration of infested snails, are directly infective to other snails. Although it seems, therefore, that *G. genarchella* is capable of completing its entire life cycle in a single molluscan host, adults of this species have also been reported from *Salminus maxillosus* and other cypriniform fishes from the vicinity of Buenos Aires.

Sporocysts, rediae, cercariae and adults of *Parahemiurus bennettae* occur in estuarine pulmonate snails *Salinator fragilis* in the mouth of Cook's River, Botany Bay, New South Wales. In the rediae, rudimentary cystophorous cercariae develop, the caudal chambers and appendages of which degenerate before the suckers of the distome worms differentiate. Rediae may be seen which contain concurrently adult worms and daughter rediae, the latter harbouring cercariae. The fate of the trematodes and their eggs is not known. The latter are probably released after the snail dies, and infest further snails without intervention of other hosts. From the description given by Jamieson (1966a, b), it is apparent that the life cycle of *P. bennettae* is very similar to that of *Bunocotyle progenetica* as reported by Deblock (1974a).

Nothing is known about the pathogenicity of the above-mentioned adult trematodes in their respective prosobranch hosts.

Agents: Cestoda

Diphyllidean cysticercoids have been reported from 38 of 78 gastropods *Bulla* sp. and 1 of 2 *Murex* sp. from Madras, India (Anantaraman, 1963b). The larval cysts, which appeared as whitish grains varying in size from 0·5 to 1·0 mm, and in shape from a spherical granule to a long, fusiform, cucumber-like outline, were invariably embedded in the hepatopancreatic tissues of the snails. The cysts were thick-walled and solid, and filled with a soft matrix of tissue. The larvae, which may lie anywhere within the cysts, measured 0·30 to 0·51 × 0·13 to 0·18 mm. They were withdrawn in their normal position and not invaginated. The head consisted of two prominent, leaf-like bothridia, and did not show any spines on the stalk.

The larva was identified as a member of the genus *Echinobothrium*, which is the only genus in the Diphyllidea, and possibly *E. affine* or, more likely, *E. lateroporum*, the only diphyllideans known in their adult stage from elasmobranchs in the region of Madras. Larval *Echinobothrium* sp. (*musteli?*) occur encysted in the digestive gland of *Nassarius reticulatus* from Arcachon, France (Dollfus, 1929).

Larval cyclophyllidean tapeworms occurred in limpets *Patella vulgata* and *P. intermedia* from various localities along the Scottish and English coasts (Crewe, 1951). The cysts were normally attached to the outside of the gut wall, but occurred also on the surface of the visceral mass or internally, between the lobules of the digestive gland. Upon removal of the host's shell, the gelatinous, pale yellow cysts, which measured about 0·4 × 0·4 to 0·6 mm, were immediately visible, closely packed along the line of the alimentary canal. The larva, visible through the cyst wall, consisted of a main vesicle and a small caudal bladder, both continually changing in shape. Under cover-glass pressure, the scolex became visible inside the main vesicle.

The cyclophyllidean cysticercoid was probably that of a member of the Davaineidae. Its armature was similar to that of adult *Ophryocotyle* spp., tapeworms which parasitize in the intestine of gulls *Larus canus* and *L. argentatus*.

A cyclophyllidean cysticercoid, similar to or identical with that reported by Crewe (1951), was found in *Patella vulgata* from St. Andrews and Aberdeen (Scotland) by Burt (1962). He identified it as the larva of *Ophryocotyle insignis*, whose adult stage was found in oystercatchers *Haematopus ostralegus*.

Cysticercoids of uncertain systematic position, named *Cysticercus tiedemanniae*, occur in the mantle of pteropods *Tiedemannia* sp. The cysts measure about 3·25 mm in diameter and are surrounded by a connective-tissue envelope. Under coverglass pressure the scolex evaginates and assumes an oval shape, about 4·3 mm in length and 2·6 mm in width (Dollfus, 1929).

Unidentified larval tetraphyllidean cestodes have been reported from southern oyster drills *Thais haemastoma* in the Gulf of Mexico (Cooley, 1962). They appear to be of rare occurrence. Individuals of *Harpa* sp. and *Oliva* sp. from Madras (India) harboured unidentified cestode larvae of the *Scolex* type, 280 × 235 μm in dimension. Single individuals of *Harpa* sp. contained up to 10 larvae (Anantaraman, 1963a).

Unencysted larval tetrarhynch tapeworms, 0·5 to 1·2 mm in length and probably identical with *Nybelinia lingualis*, occur in Mediterranean opisthobranchs *Tethys leporina* (Dollfus, 1929).

Agents: Nematoda

Comparatively few nematodes have been recorded from marine molluscs (mainly pelecypods). This sparsity of reports would suggest that roundworms rarely occur in these hosts. As to whether this is true or not cannot be stated with certainty, since the situation is perhaps merely a reflection of the lack of competent nematode specialists among marine parasitologists (Cheng, 1967).

Pink abalones *Haliotis corrugata* from southern California, USA, were found to be parasitized by second-stage nematode larvae encysted in the ventral portion of the foot, and producing blister-like protrusions in the holdfast organ. Only old abalones were found to harbour the parasite, and invasions were usually heavy. The vesicatory effect of the encysted worms, as well as the burrowing of the larvae through the foot prior to encystment, apparently weakened the muscle and reduced its efficacy as a holdfast organ. Aside from these conditions, the animals did not seem to suffer any other ill effects from the parasite (Millemann, 1951, 1963).

The larvae, which averaged 20 mm in length and 0·65 mm in width, were identified as the second stage of a gnathostomatid nematode, and named *Echinocephalus pseudouncinatus*. Its third- and fourth-stage larvae, as well as the adult, parasitize in the intestinal tract of elasmobranchs. The abalones probably became infested by invasive, free-swimming first-stage larvae which hatch from eggs after maturation in sea water.

The gross appearance of the foot of *Haliotis corrugata* harbouring *Echinocephalus pseudouncinatus*, and the ease with which the animals may be removed from the rocks, enabled commercial divers to distinguish between healthy and infested abalones. Although Milleman (1951) did not find *E. pseudouncinatus* in the few specimens of the southern green abalone *H. fulgens* which he examined, he was informed by divers and processors that the green abalone is as susceptible to nematode invasion as is the pink abalone, indicating that *E. pseudouncinatus* is not strictly host-specific.

A related species, *Echinocephalus uncinatus*, was previously recorded from various pelecypods as well as from gastropods *Polinices conica* from Australian waters (Johnston and Mawson, 1945a, b).

Agents: Mollusca

Small opisthobranch snails of the family Pyramidellidae are well-known ectoparasites of pelecypods. Several species have been reported from prosobranchs. The snails, which measure some 5 to 7 mm in height, generally attach to the outer surface of the shell, near the edge of the aperture, and insert their long, tube-like evaginable proboscis into the host's tissues, feeding on its haemolymph by means of a highly specialized feeding mechanism including a piercing stylet and an 'oesophageal pump' (Ankel, 1949; Fretter and Graham, 1949).

The latter authors have strongly emphasized that pyramidellids are host-specific. Various subsequent workers, however, have shown that this is not the case (Cole, 1951; Cole and Hancock, 1955; Allen, 1958; Ankel, 1959; Robertson and Orr, 1961; Wells and Wells, 1961; Ankel and Møller Christensen, 1963; Clark, 1971; Rasmussen, 1973). Although behavioural experiments conducted by Boss and Merrill (1965), as well as observations by Robertson (1957) and Clark (1971), indicate at least some degree of host preference exhibited by *Odostomia bisuturalis*, *O. seminuda* and *O. columbiana*, experimental confirmation of such behaviour is lacking for most of the other species. Several—if not all—pyramidellids will attack both pelecypods and prosobranchs (Fig. 12-52).

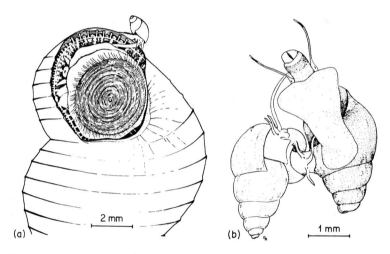

Fig. 12–52: Parasitic pyramidellids. (a) *Odostomia eulimoides* sucking on mantle margin of *Turritella communis*; (b) two individuals of *O. scalaris* feeding on *Hydrobia ulvae*. (a After Ankel, 1959; reproduced by permission of Zoologischer Anzeiger; b after Ankel and Møller Christensen, 1963; reproduced by permission of Dansk Naturhistorisk Forening.)

Odostomia eulimoides, the first pyramidellid reported as a parasite, attacks a great variety of pelecypods in European waters, and has also been found associated with wentletraps *Turritella communis* (Smart, 1887). It causes pathological changes, and probably even death in bivalves, but nothing is known about its effect on prosobranch hosts.

Acmaea tessulata, *Hydrobia ulvae*, *Rissoa membranacea*, *Littorina littorea*, *L. saxatilis*, *Lacuna divaricata*, *L. vincta* and *Buccinum undatum*, as well as several bivalve species, are known as hosts for *Odostomia scalaris* in Danish waters (Ankel and Møller Christensen, 1963; Rasmussen, 1973). This species will occasionally feed on speciments of *H. ulvae* and *R. membranacea*, which are smaller than itself. On the other hand, it has been observed feeding on even large whelks *B. undatum*. Infestation of the latter prosobranch with *O. scalaris* was as high as that of mussels *Mytilus edulis* in Isefjord, Denmark, indicating lack of preference for pelecypod hosts in this species (Rasmussen, 1973).

Odostomia columbiana from the North American Pacific coast preferred checkered hairy snails *Trichotropis cancellata* to hairy Oregon tritons *Fusitriton oregonensis*, 41% of the former being infested in the region of Orcas Island, San Juan Archipelago, Washington, USA (Clark, 1971). It was demonstrated experimentally that *O. columbiana* exhibits a marked preference for the rough surface texture of its favourite host.

Incised odostomes *Odostomia impressa*, a common pyramidellid parasite of oysters along the North American Atlantic coast, will also feed on prosobranchs *Bittium varium*, *Triphora nigrocincta*, *Crepidula convexa* and *Urosalpinx cinerea* (Allen, 1958). Like *O. columbiana*, this species is also attracted by rough surfaces (Hopkins, 1956).

When given a choice between a number of commercially important bivalves and cup-and-saucer limpets *Crucibulum striatum*, as well as slipper shells *Crepidula fornicata* and *C. plana* from the North American Atlantic coast, double sutured odostomes *Odostomia bisuturalis* will attack all of the host species except *C. plana*, although a preference for the bivalve species was distinct (Boss and Merrill, 1965). *O. bisuturalis* causes shell deformities in oysters; nothing is known about its pathogenicity to limpets and slipper shells.

Another pyramidellid from North American Atlantic waters, attacking slipper shells in addition to commercially important bivalves, is the half-smooth odostome *Odostomia seminuda*. It appears to exhibit a definite preference for *Crepidula fornicata* (Robertson, 1957; Boss and Merrill, 1965). When offered a choice between *C. fornicata* and oysters *Crassostrea virginica*, after 2 weeks, 40 of 58 *O. seminuda* were observed in feeding position on slipper shells, and the remainder were found crawling on the substrate; none occurred on an oyster. In another experiment in which *O. seminuda* had to bypass *C. virginica* in order to reach the slipper shells, 24 of 30 odostomes were found attached to *C. fornicata* after 2 days, only 2 to *C. virginica* and the remainder were free on the substrate.

Crepidula fornicata and *Crucibulum striatum* were observed to respond to the penetration of the mantle by the proboscis of *Odostomia seminuda* by muscular contraction in the immediate area. In some instances, the parasite actually pierced the visceral mass (Merrill and Boss, 1964).

Since slipper shells—in particular *Crepidula fornicata*——are a common and sometimes serious pest on oyster beds in North America and Europe, more should be learned about the pathogenicity of pyramidellids to these prosobranchs. With the possible exception of *Odostomia seminuda*, however, the use of odostomes as a biological control measure appears to be limited, due to their usually low degree of host-specificity.

Agents: Annelida

Polynoid polychaetes—mainly members of the genus *Arctonoë*—are known to be associated with various gastropods (Davenport, 1950; Clark, 1956). Since the interrelationship is merely commensalistic, these associations will not be considered further here.

Spionids *Polydora ciliata* burrow in the shell of periwinkles *Littorina littorea*, causing blister formation and discolouration of the inner shell wall. In heavy infestations, the shell may be completely riddled, breaking apart upon the slightest touch (Fig. 12-53). In the Baltic Sea, subtidal periwinkles were seen, in which part of the spire had disintegrated, exposing the soft parts to the open water. The animals were still alive (Lauckner, unpublished; see Fig. 12-53).

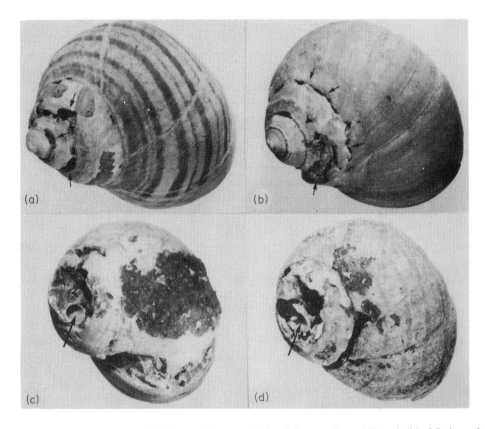

Fig. 12-53: *Littorina littorea*. Shell corrosion caused by *Polydora ciliata*. (a) and (b): Moderately invaded shells. Short arrows: corroded areas. (c) and (d): Heavy invasion resulting in total destruction of uppermost whorls and exposure of inner shell surface (long arrows). (Original.)

Incidence and intensity of *Polydora ciliata* infestations vary with hydrographical conditions. Thus, *Littorina littorea* from sheltered habitats in Isefjord (Denmark) showed a mean infestation incidence of 50·7% as opposed to 77·6% in periwinkles from exposed localities. Infestation intensities increase with host age, from about 1% in the O-group (3 to 7 mm shell height) to 7·5% in the I-group (8 to 16 mm) and 57% in the II (+)-group (17 mm and upwards) (Rasmussen, 1973). In Swedish waters, immature *L. littorea* (with shell heights of less than 10 mm) were not attacked by *P. ciliata*. Orrhage (1969) discusses the question whether this might be due to the excretion, by sexually mature periwinkles, of certain substances (sex pheromones), which attract larval *P. ciliata*. As another condition favouring attacks by the spionid, changes in the surface structure of the shell at the time of maturation have been taken into consideration. It appears more likely, however, that *P. ciliata* larvae attach to and penetrate shell portions where the periostracum has been damaged or worn away; this is especially the case in the older whorls of large periwinkle shells. *P. ciliata* infestations do not affect shell growth in *L. littorea*. Shell parameters (height, width, length, aperture opening relation) do not differ significantly in infested and non-infested periwinkles (Orrhage, 1969).

Agents: Copepoda

Prosobranch gastropods are parasitized by only a few genera of copepods, such as *Trochicola*, *Mytilicola*, *Cerastocheres*, *Panaietis* and *Monstrilla*. Opisthobranchs, on the other hand, are hosts to many genera, among them *Lichomolgus*, *Splanchnotrophus*, *Briarella*, *Artotrogus* and *Anthessius*. Some, like *Lichomolgus*, live free on the surface of the gills or mantle. Others, like *Splanchnotrophus*, are embedded in the integument or visceral mass (Humes, 1958a).

Copepods which live on the body surface of their molluscan hosts are usually morphologically unmodified, or only slightly transformed, while endoparasitic species are distinctly modified. Little is known about the relationship of copepods externally associated with molluscs, but the majority of investigators who have studied this group most extensively have considered them to be parasites (Monod and Dollfus, 1932; Cheng, 1967).

Trochicola entericus, a strongly transformed mytilicolid copepod, is a common parasite of European top shells *Calliostoma zizyphinum*, *Gibbula cineraria*, *G. varia* and *Monodonta mutabilis*. Females parasitize in the intestine of the gastropod hosts whereas males and copepodids occur in their branchial cavity (Dollfus, 1914, 1927; Stock, 1960; Kleeton, 1961). A young female, identified as member of a new species, *Trochicola* sp., has been recovered from the intestine of *G. richardi* at Banyuls, French Mediterranean coast (Stock, 1960). *T. entericus* has frequently been misidentified as *Mytilicola intestinalis*, an intestinal copepod parasite of *Mytilus edulis* and other marine bivalves. Slipper limpets *Crepidula fornicata* have been infested experimentally with the latter species (Hepper, 1953). A related species, *M. orientalis*, occurs in *C. fornicata* in Puget Sound, Washington, USA Pacific coast, where it is widely spread, infesting a variety of commercially important pelecypods (Odlaug, 1946).

Four out of 200 *Odostomia scalaris* (*O. rissoides*) parasitizing *Mytilus edulis* at Wimereux (France) were found to be hyperparasitized by monstrillids *Monstrilla helgolandica*. Each snail harboured, in its branchial cavity, a single female copepod. Two of these, which measured about 2 mm in length and were apparently mature, emerged from their hosts during the observation period. The other two (immature) individuals were found to be encased by a chitinous envelope and attached to the snail's body by means of 2 pairs of long fragile processes functioning as absorptive organs. *M. helgolandica* appeared to have little effect on *O. scalaris*, the latter exhibiting no sign of parasitic castration (Pelseneer, 1914).

Panaietis haliotis, a myicolid, lives parasitically in the mouth cavity of abalones *Haliotis gigantea* on the Japanese coast (Yamaguti, 1936). Nothing is known about its pathogenicity. *P. incamerata* parasitizes top shells *Trochus niloticus* from Andaman Islands, Bay of Bengal (Monod, 1934), and *P. yamagutii* has been recovered from the buccal cavity of horned turbans *Batillus cornutus* from Kiinagashima and Sugari, Kii Peninsula, Japan (Izawa, 1976a). *Neanthessius renicolis*, another myicolid, lives endoparasitically in the renal sac of spindle whelks *Pleuroploca trapezium audouini* and of a related species, probably *Fusinus nigrirostratus* collected near the Seto Marine Biological Laboratory, Japan (Izawa, 1976a).

Philoblennids *Philoblenna arabici* were found attached to the mantle surface adjacent to the ctenidium of Arabic cowries *Peribolus (Arabica) arabica* from Seto (Japan). The areas of attachment exhibited knob-like swellings, apparently formed in response to parasite irritation (Izawa, 1976b).

Lichomolgids *Epimolgus trochi* have been recorded from the pallial cavity of top shells *Gibbula umbilicalis*, *G. varia*, *G. cineraria* and *Monodonta lineata* from the French Atlantic and Mediterranean coasts (Bocquet and Stock, 1956; Stock, 1960).

Lichomolgoid copepods associated with Opisthobranchia have been reported from various regions of the world, namely from England (Leigh-Sharpe, 1933), the West Indies (Stock and co-authors, 1963), the Indo-Pacific (Humes, 1958b, 1963, 1975; Humes and Ho, 1965) and elsewhere (Humes and Stock, 1973).

Members of the genus *Splanchnotrophus* live endoparasitically within the body cavity of nudibranchs. *S. gracilis* has been reported from *Acanthodoris pilosa* and *Idalia aspersa*, *S. breviceps* from *Doto coronata* and *Coryphella rufibranchialis*, *S. willemi* from *Facelina coronata* and *S. angulatus* from *Aeolis papillosa* and *Aeolidiella glauca* (Hancock and Norman, 1863; Hecht, 1895). These endoparasites appear to cause orientational disturbances in their hosts.

A detailed list of copepods associated with molluscs, including prosobranch and opisthobranch gastropods, has been assembled by Monod and Dollfus (1932).

Agents: Isopoda

Sphaeromatid isopods *Dynoidella conchicola* have been found associated with intertidal neritid snails *Theliostyla albicilla*, as well as with patellids *Cellana nigrolineata* and *C. grata stearnsi* from rocky shores at Sirahama (Japan). From 1 to 5 (mostly 2 or 3) isopods occurred attached to the surface of the host's pallial groove, along the mantle edge, or on the dorsal surface of the foot. *D. conchicola* appears to show some degree of preference for limpets or limpet-like snails since no isopods could be discovered on the body surface of *Monodonta labio*, a species of top shell equally abundant in that area. Although instances of parasitism are well documented for epicaridean and cirolanid isopods, the association between these sphaeromatids and gastropods is probably a commensalistic one (Nishimura, 1976).

Agents: Pantopoda

Juvenile pycnogonids have been found, in rare instances, parasitic upon opisthobranch gastropods. Thus, Merton (1906) reported *Nymphon parasiticum* from *Tethys leporina* in the Gulf of Naples (Italy). An individual of *Armina variolosa*, collected at Hojo (Province of Awa, Japan), was infested by 40 juvenile pycnogonids of the genus *Ammothea* (Ohshima, 1933).

TUMOURS AND ABNORMALITIES

A variety of tumours or tumour-like lesions have been reported from both freshwater and marine prosobranchs. Most of these outgrowths appear to be manifestations of highly cellular wound responses to the introduction of foreign materials, such as parasites, etc. As in many other invertebrates, the distinction between true neoplasia, as opposed to hyperplasia and response to injury or infection, is often uncertain. In some cases, gross lesions observed were thought to be neoplastic until histological examination revealed them to be inflammatory responses or parasite infestations (Pauley, 1969).

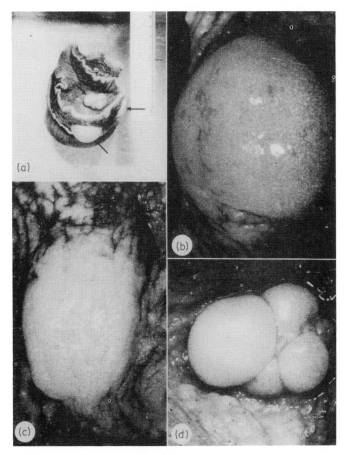

Fig. 12-54: *Polinices lewisi*. (a) Ventral view of entire snail, showing tumefactions (arrows) on foot; close-ups of lesions indicated by lower (b), right (c) and upper (d) arrows. Note glossy smooth surfaces lacking pigmentation. (After Smith and Taylor, 1968; reproduced by permission of Academic Press.)

Large nodular growths in the foot of a moon snail *Polinices lewisi* resembled neoplasms **upon gross inspection**. Microscopic examination, however, revealed them to be oedematous lesions containing scattered muscle fibres and several distinct micro-organisms. The latter occurred throughout the body of the snail and were believed to have caused the development of the tumour-like swellings (Smith and Taylor, 1968; Fig. 12-54).

A pedunculated, fibrous growth composed of connective-tissue cells and fibres of connective-tissue origin has been observed on the mantle of an opisthobranch snail

Pleurobranchus (*Oscanius*) *plumula* from Roscoff, France (Fischer, 1954). The tumour was stalked, firm and non-retractile, and had a complete epithelial covering (Fig. 12-55). It was highly vascularized and apparently benign.

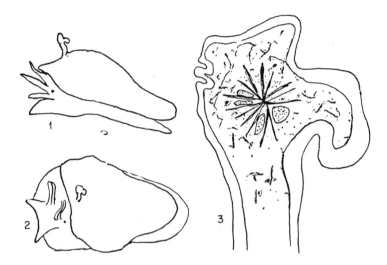

Fig. 12-55: *Pleurobranchus* (*Oscanius*) *plumula*. 1, 2: Gross view of stalked
tumour on host mantle; 3: longitudinal section through tumour.
(After Fischer, 1954; reproduced by permission of the author.)

Experimental tumour production by introduction of tar into the mantle of opisthobranchs *Archidoris tuberculata* was attempted by Labbé (1930). The resulting response, which consisted of hypertrophied and multinucleate cells with an apparent invasive growth pattern, was interpreted as cancerous, but probably was merely a highly cellular wound response (Pauley, 1969).

It should be noted, in this context, that antineoplastic components, active against Walker 256 carcinoma (intramuscular), and both a lymphoid (L-1210) and lymphocytic leukaemia (PS), have been isolated from a variety of marine invertebrates including prosobranchs *Haliotis ovina* and *Turbo stenogyrus* (Pettit and co-authors, 1970).

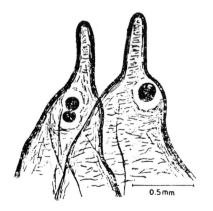

Fig. 12-56: *Leptoconchus cumingii*. Eye
duplication on tentacle. (After
Gohar and Soliman, 1963; reproduced by permission of Cairo University Press.)

0.5 mm

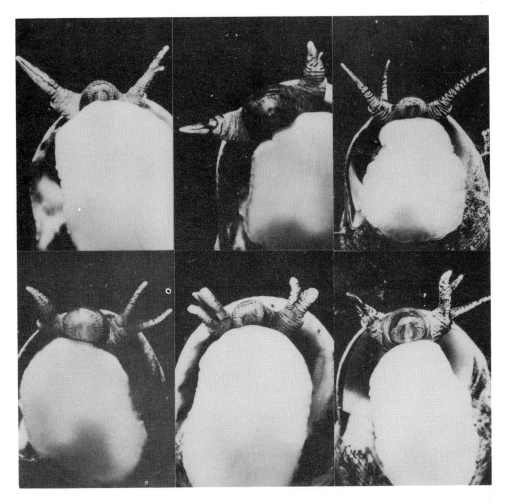

Fig. 12-57: *Littorina littorea*. Abnormal tentacles. (Original.)

Growth anomalies in the shells of gastropods include duplication of the siphoneal canal and the aperture, as well as reversal of normal coiling (Pelseneer, 1919, 1920; Ankel, 1936; Clench and Merrill, 1963; Robertson and Merrill, 1963; Harasewych, 1977).

Leighton (1960) described a juvenile red abalone *Haliotis rufescens* from Pacific Beach, California, USA, characterized by a complete absence of respiratory apertures. Normally, a pallial cleft develops and aperture formation commences when the juveniles are approximately 2 mm long. The absence of apertures and pallial cleft in the specimens investigated was interpreted as the result of mutation rather than local injury.

A case of an abnormal optic tentacle with a duplicate eye has been observed in a coralliophilid snail *Leptoconchus cumingii* from the Egyptian Red Sea coast (Gohar and Soliman, 1963; Fig. 12-56).

Tentacle ramification appears to be of widespread occurrence in periwinkles *Littorina littorea* from the North Sea, the Baltic Sea and the North American Atlantic coast (Fig. 12-57; Woodbridge, 1976). Such prolific ramifications, which have also been observed in limpets *Patella vulgata*, oyster drills *Thais lapillus* and mud snails *Nassarius mutabilis*, may be interpreted as 'super-regenerates' formed during the healing process following injury (Hankó, 1912; Pelseneer, 1919; Ankel, 1936). Hankó (1914) was able to experimentally induce the formation of comparable abnormalities in the tentacle-like processes on the posterior margin of the foot of Mediterranean *Nassarius mutabilis*.

Literature Cited (Chapter 12)

Adams, J. E. and Martin, W. E. (1963). Life cycle of *Himasthla rhigedana* Dietz, 1909 (Trematoda: Echinostomatidae). *Trans. Am. microsc. Soc.*, **82**, 1–6.

Africa, C. M. (1930). The excretory system of *Cercariaeum lintoni* Miller 1926. *J. Parasit.*, **17**, 14–17.

Agersborg, H. P. K. (1924). Studies on the effect of parasitism upon tissues, with special reference to certain gastropod molluscs. *Q. Jl microsc. Sci.*, **68**, 361–401.

Alexander, D. G. (1960). Directional movements of the intertidal snail, *Littorina littorea*. *Biol. Bull. mar. biol. Lab., Woods Hole*, **119**, 301–302.

Allen, J. A. and Garrett, M. R. (1972). Studies on taurine in the euryhaline bivalve *Mya arenaria*. *Comp. Biochem. Physiol.*, **41A**, 307–317.

Allen, J. F. (1958). Feeding habits of two species of *Odostomia*. *Nautilus*, **72**, 11–15.

Allen, K. and Awapara, J. (1960). Metabolism of sulfur amino acids in *Mytilus edulis* and *Rangia cuneata*. *Biol. Bull. mar. biol. Lab., Woods Hole*, **118**, 173–182.

Anantaraman, S. (1963a). Larval cestodes in marine invertebrates and fishes with a discussion of the life cycles of the Tetraphyllidea and the Trypanorhyncha. *Z. ParasitKde*, **23**, 309–314.

Anantaraman, S. (1963b). On the larva of *Echinobothrium* Beneden 1849 (Cestoda: Diphyllidea) in marine gastropods and a decapod of Madras. *Z. ParasitKde*, **23**, 315–319.

Ankel, F. (1962). *Hydrobia ulvae* Pennant und *Hydrobia ventrosa* Montagu als Wirte larvaler Trematoden. *Vidensk. Meddr dansk naturh. Foren.*, **124**, 1–100.

Ankel, F. and Møller Christensen, A. (1963). Non-specificity in host selection by *Odostomia scalaris* Macgillivray. *Vidensk. Meddr dansk naturh. Foren.*, **125**, 321–325.

Ankel, W. E. (1936). Prosobranchia. *Tierwelt Nord. Ostsee*, **9**b, 1–240.

Ankel, W. E. (1949). Die Mundbewaffnung der Pyramidelliden. *Arch. Molluskenk.*, **77**, 79–82.

Ankel, W. E. (1959). Beobachtungen an Pyramidelliden des Gullmar-Fjordes. *Zool. Anz.*, **162**, 1–21.

Arvy, L. (1953). Présence de *Cercaria setifera* (Monticelli, 1888 et 1914 nec. John Müller, 1850), chez *Phyllirrhoë bucephala* Per. et Les. à Villefranche-sur-Mer. *Annls Parasit. hum. comp.*, **28**, 289–299.

Arvy, L. (1954). Contribution à l'étude de *Cercaria sagittarius* (Sinitzin, 1911). *Annls Parasit. hum. comp.*, **29**, 347–357.

Arvy, L. (1972). Zoogéographie des cercaires cystophores françaises. *Annls Parasit. hum. comp.*, **47**, 663–664.

Atkins, D. (1954). A marine fungus, *Plectospira dubia* n.sp (Saprolegniaceae), infecting crustacean eggs and small Crustacea. *J. mar. biol. Ass. U.K.*, **33**, 721–732.

Bakker, K. (1959). Feeding habits and zonation in some intertidal snails. *Archs néerl. Zool.*, **13**, 230–257.

Barkman, J. J. (1956). On the distribution and ecology of *Littorina obtusata* (L.) and its subspecific units. *Archs néerl. Zool.*, **11**, 22–86.

Bartoli, P. (1967). Étude du cycle évolutif d'un trématode peu connu: *Lepocreadium pegorchis* (M. Stossich, 1900) (Trematoda, Digenea). *Annls Parasit. hum. comp.*, **42**, 605–619.

Bartoli, P. (1974). Un cas d'exclusion compétitive chez les trématodes: l'élimination de *Gymnophallus choledochus* T. Odhner, 1900 par *G. nereicola* J. Rebecq et G. Prévot, 1962 en Camargue (France) (Digenea, Gymnophallidae). *Bull. Soc. zool. Fr.*, **99**, 551–559.

Basch, P. F. (1970). Relationship of some larval strigeids and echinostomes (Trematoda): Hyperparasitism, antagonism, and 'immunity' in the snail host. *Expl Parasit.*, **27**, 193–216.

Basch, P. F. and Lie, K. J. (1966a). Infection of single snails with two different trematodes. I. Simultaneous exposure and early development of a schistosome and an echinostome. *Z. ParasitKde*, **27**, 252–259.

Basch, P. F. and Lie, K. J. (1966b). Infection of single snails with two different trematodes. II. Dual exposure to a schistosome and an echinostome at staggered intervals. *Z. ParasitKde*, **27**, 260–270.

Basch, P. F., Lie, K. J. and Heyneman, D. (1969). Antagonistic interaction between strigeid and schistosome sporocysts within a snail host. *J. Parasit.*, **55**, 753–758.

Batchelder, C. H. (1915). Migration of *Ilyanassa obsoleta*, *Littorina littorea* and *Littorina rudis*. *Nautilus*, **29**, 43–46.

Baughman, J. L. (1947). *Annotated Bibliography of Oysters*, A & M Res. Found., Texas.

Bearup, A. J. (1955). A schistosome larva from the marine snail *Pyrazus australis* as a cause of cercarial dermatitis in man. *Med. J. Aust.*, **1**, 955.

Bearup, A. J. (1956). Life cycle of *Austrobilharzia terrigalensis* Johnson, 1917. *Parasitology*, **46**, 470–479.

Beneden, P. J. van (1875). Les commensaux et les parasites. *Biblioth. Sci. int.*, **9**, 173.

Berg, C. J. (1976). Growth of the queen conch *Strombus gigas*, with a discussion of the practicality of its mariculture. *Mar. Biol.*, **34**, 191–199.

Berry, A. J. (1962). The occurrence of a trematode larva in a population of *Littorina saxatilis* (Olivi). *Parasitology*, **52**, 237–240.

Blaber, S. J. M. (1970). The occurrence of a penis-like outgrowth behind the right tentacle in spent females of *Nucella lapillus* (L.). *Proc. malac. Soc. Lond.*, **39**, 231–233.

Bocquet, C. and Stock, J. H. (1956). Copépodes parasites d'invertébrés des côtes de la Manche. II. Sur un lichomolgide parasite des gibbules, *Lichomolgus (Epimolgus) trochi*. *Archs Zool. exp. gén.*, **94**, 1–10.

Bonar, L. (1936). An unusual ascomycete in the shell of marine animals. *Univ. Calif. Publs Bot.*, **19**, 187–193.

Bornet, E. and Flahault, C. (1889). Sur quelques plants vivant dans le test calcaire des mollusques. *Bull. Soc. bot. Fr.*, **36**, 171–173.

Boss, K. J. and Merrill, A. S. (1965). Degree of host specificity in two species of *Odostomia* (Pyramidellidae: Gastropoda). *Proc. malac. Soc. Lond.*, **36**, 349–355.

Broekhuysen, G. J. (1940). A preliminary investigation of the importance of desiccation, temperature and salinity as factors controlling the vertical distribution of certain intertidal marine gastropods in False Bay, South Africa. *Transact. Royal Soc. South Africa*, **28**, 254–292.

Brongersma-Sanders, M. (1957). Mass mortality in the sea. In J. W. Hedgpeth (Ed.), *Treatise on Marine Ecology and Paleoecology*, Vol. I, Ecology. *Mem. geol. Soc. Am.*, **67**, 941–1010.

Brouardel, J. (1951). Recherches sur la biologie d'un infusoire péritriche commensal des patelles: *Urceolaria patellae* (Cuénot). *Annls Inst. océanogr., Monaco*, **26**, 115–254.

Brown, F. A. (1977). Geographic orientation, time and mudsnail phototaxis. *Biol. Bull. mar. biol. Lab.*, *Woods Hole*, **152**, 311–324.

Burkenroad, M. D. (1946). Fluctuations in abundance of marine animals. *Science*, *N.Y.*, **103**, 684–686.

Burt, M. D. B. (1962). A contribution to the knowledge of the cestode genus *Ophryocotyle* Friis, 1870. *J. Linn. Soc.* (Zool.), **44**, 645–668.

Bush, A. O. and Kinsella, J. M. (1972). A natural definite host for *Catatropis johnstoni* Martin, 1956 (Trematoda: Notocotylidae), with notes on experimental host specificity and intraspecific variation. *J. Parasit.*, **58**, 843–845.

Butler, P. A. (1953). The southern oyster drill. *Proc. natn. Shellfish. Ass.*, **44**, 67–75.

Buttner, A. (1950). La progénèse chez les trématodes digénétiques. Sa signification. Ses manifestations. Contributions à l'étude de son déterminisme. *Annls Parasit. hum. comp.*, **25**, 376–434.

Buttner, A. (1951a). La progénèse chez les trématodes digénétiques. Techniques et recherches personnelles. *Annls Parasit. hum. comp.*, **26**, 19–66.

Buttner, A. (1951b). La progénèse chez les trématodes digénétiques. Recherches personnelles sur deux espèces progénétiques déjà connues: *Ratzia joyeuxi* (E. Brumpt, 1922) et *Pleurogenes medians* (Olsson, 1876). *Annls Parasit. hum. comp.*, **26**, 138–189.

Buttner, A. (1951c). La progénèse chez les trématodes digénétiques. Étude de quelques métacercaires à évolution inconnue et de certaines formes de développement voisines de la progénèse. Conclusions générales. *Annls Parasit. hum. comp.*, **26**, 279–322.

Buttner, A. (1955). Les distomes progénétiques sont-ils des pré-adultes ou des adultes véritables? Valeur évolutive de la progénèse chez les Digenea. *C. r. Séanc. Soc. Biol.*, **149**, 267–272.

Cable, R. M. (1931). Studies on the germ-cell cycle of *Cryptocotyle lingua*. I. Gametogenesis in the adult. *Q. Jl microsc. Sci.*, **74**, 563–589.

Cable, R. M. (1934). Studies on the germ-cell cycle of *Cryptocotyle lingua*. II. Germinal development in the larval stages. *Q. Jl microsc. Sci.*, **76**, 573–614.

Cable, R. M. (1952). Studies on marine digenetic trematodes of Puerto Rico. Four species of magnacercous heterophyid cercariae with zygocercous aggregation in one. *J. Parasit.*, **38**, 28.

Cable, R. M. (1953). The life cycle of *Parvatrema borinqueñae* gen. et sp. nov. (Trematoda: Digenea) and the systematic position of the subfamily Gymnophallinae. *J. Parasit.*, **39**, 408–421.

Cable, R. M. (1954a). Studies on marine digenetic trematodes of Puerto Rico. The life cycle in the family Haplosplanchnidae. *J. Parasit*, **40**, 71–76.

Cable, R. M. (1954b). Studies on marine digenetic trematodes of Puerto Rico. The life cycle in the family Megaperidae. *J. Parasit.*, **40**, 202–208.

Cable, R. M. (1963). Marine cercariae from Curaçao and Jamaica. *Z. ParasitKde*, **23**, 429–469.

Cable, R. M. and Hunninen, A. V. (1938). Observations on the life history of *Spelotrema nicolli*, n.sp. (Trematoda: Microphallidae) with the description of a new microphallid cercaria. *J. Parasit.*, **24** (Suppl.), 29–30.

Cable, R. M. and Hunninen, A. V. (1940). Studies on the life history of *Spelotrema nicolli* (Trematoda: Microphallidae) with the description of a new microphallid cercaria. *Biol. Bull. mar. biol. Lab., Woods Hole*, **78**, 136–157.

Cable, R. M. and Hunninen, A. V. (1942a). Studies on *Deropristis inflata* (Molin), its life history and affinities to trematodes of the family Acanthocolpidae. *Biol. Bull. mar. biol. Lab., Woods Hole*, **82**, 292–312.

Cable, R. M. and Hunninen, A. V. (1942b). Studies on the life history of *Siphodera vinaledwardsii* (Linton) (Trematoda: Cryptogonimidae). *J. Parasit.*, **28**, 407–422.

Cable, R. M. and Martin, W. E. (1935). *Parorchis avitus* (Linton, 1914), a synonym of *P. acanthus* (Nicoll, 1906). *J. Parasit.*, **21**, 436–437.

Cardell, R. R. (1962). Observations on the ultrastructure of the body of the cercaria of *Himasthla quissetensis* (Miller and Northup, 1926). *Trans. Am. microsc. Soc.*, **81**, 124–131.

Cardell, R. R. and Philpott, D. E. (1960). The ultrastructure of the tail of the cercaria of *Himasthla quissetensis* (Miller and Northup, 1926). *Trans. Am. microsc. Soc.*, **79**, 442–450.

Carlton, J. (1969). *Littorina littorea* in California (San Francisco and Trinidad bays). *Veliger*, **11**, 283–284.

Carriker, M. R. (1955). Critical review of biology and control of oyster drills *Urosalpinx* and *Eupleura*. *Spec. scient. Rep. U.S. Fish Wildl. Serv.*, **148**, 1–150.

Caullery, M. and Mesnil, F. (1915). Sur *Trichodina patellae* Cuénot. *C. r. Séanc. Soc. Biol.*, **78**, 674–677.

Cépède, C. (1910). Recherches sur les infusoires astomes. Anatomie, biologie, éthologie parasitaire, systématique. *Archs Zool. exp. gén.* (Ser. 5), **3**, 341–609.

Chabaud, A.-G. and Biguet, J. (1954). Étude d'un trématode hémiuroide à métacercaire progénétique. *Annls Parasit. hum. comp.*, **29**, 527–545.

Chabaud, A.-G. and Buttner, A. (1959). Note complémentaire sur le *Bunocotyle* (trématode hemiuroide) de l'étang du Canet. *Vie Milieu*, **10**, 204–206.

Chapman, H. D. (1973). The functional organization and fine structure of the tail musculature of the cercariae of *Cryptocotyle lingua* and *Himasthla secunda*. *Parasitology*, **66**, 487–497.

Chapman, H. D. and Wilson, R. A. (1973). The propulsion of the cercariae of *Himasthla secunda* (Nicoll) and *Cryptocotyle lingua*. *Parasitology*, **67**, 1–15.

Cheng, T. C. (1967). Marine molluscs as hosts for symbioses. In F. S. Russell (Ed.), *Advances in Marine Biology*, Vol. 5. Academic Press, London.

Cheng, T. C. (1971). Enhanced growth as a manifestation of parasitism and shell deposition in parasitized mollusks. In T. C. Cheng (Ed.), *Aspects of the Biology of Symbiosis*. Univ. Park Press, Baltimore, Maryland. pp. 103–137.

Cheng, T. C., Sullivan, J. T. and Harris, K. R. (1973). Parasitic castration of the marine prosobranch gastropod *Nassarius obsoletus* by sporocysts of *Zoogonus rubellus* (Trematoda): histopathology. *J. Invertebr. Pathol.*, **21**, 183–190.

Ching, H. L. (1960). Some digenetic trematodes of shore birds at Friday Harbor, Washington. *Proc. helminth. Soc. Wash.*, **27**, 53–62.

Ching, H. L. (1961). Three trematodes from the harlequin duck. *Can. J. Zool.*, **39**, 373–376.

Ching, H. L. (1962). Six larval trematodes from the snail, *Littorina scutulata* Gould of San Juan Island, U.S.A., and Vancouver, B.C. *Can. J. Zool.*, **40**, 675–676.

Ching, H. L. (1963a). The description and life cycle of *Maritrema laricola* sp. n. (Trematoda: Microphallidae). *Can. J. Zool.*, **41**, 881–888.

Ching, H. L. (1963b). The life cycle and bionomics of *Levinseniella charadriformis* Young, 1949 (Trematoda: Microphallidae). *Can. J. Zool.*, **41**, 889–899.

Ching, H. L. (1965). Systematic notes on some North American microphallid trematodes. *Proc. helminth. Soc. Wash.*, **32**, 140–148.

Chow, V. (1975). The importance of size in the intertidal distribution of *Littorina scutulata*. *Veliger*, **18**, 69–78.

Chu, G. W. T. C. (1952). First report of the presence of a dermatitis-producing marine larval schistosome in Hawaii. *Science, N.Y.*, **115**, 151–153.

Chu, G. W. T. C. and Cutress, C. E. (1954). *Austrobilharzia variglandis* (Miller and Northup, 1926) Penner, 1953 (Trematoda: Schistosomatidae) in Hawaii with notes on its biology. *J. Parasit.*, **40**, 515–523.

Clark, K. (1971). Host-texture preference of an ectoparasitic opisthobranch, *Odostomia columbiana* Dall and Bartsch, 1909. *Veliger*, **14**, 54–56.

Clark, R. B. (1956). *Capitella capitata* as a commensal, with a bibliography of parasitism and commensalism in the polychaetes. *Ann. Mag. nat. Hist.*, **9**., 433–448.

Clench, W. J. and Merrill, A. S. (1963). Some shell malformations. *Shells and their Neighbors*, **16**, 1–2.

Coe, W. R. (1956). Fluctuations in populations of littoral marine invertebrates. *J. mar. Res.*, **15**, 212–232.

Cole, H. A. (1951). An *Odostomia* attacking oysters. *Nature, Lond.*, **168,** 953.

Cole, H. A. (1956). Benthos and the shellfish of commerce. In M. Graham (Ed.), *Sea Fisheries*. Arnold, London. pp. 139–206.

Cole, H. A. and Hancock, D. A. (1955). *Odostomia* as a pest of oysters and mussels. *J. mar. biol. Ass. U.K.*, **34**, 25–31.

Colman, J. S. (1933). The nature of the intertidal zonation of plants and animals. *J. mar. biol. Ass. U.K.*, **18**, 435–476.

Combescot-Lang, C. (1976). Étude des trématodes parasites de *Littorina saxatilis* (Olivi) et de leurs effets sur cet hôte. *Annls Parasit. hum. comp.*, **15**, 27–36.

Cooley, N. R. (1958). Incidence and life history of *Parorchis acanthus*, a digenetic trematode, in the southern oyster drill, *Thais haemastoma*. *Proc. natn Shellfish. Ass.*, **48**, 174–188.

Cooley, N. R. (1962). Studies on *Parorchis acanthus* (Trematoda: Digenea) as a biological control for the southern oyster drill, *Thais haemastoma*. *Fishery Bull. Fish Wildl. Serv. U.S.*, **62**, 77–91.

Crewe, W. (1951). The occurrence of *Cercaria patellae* Lebour (Trematoda) and its effect on the host; with notes on some other helminth parasites of British limpets. *Parasitology*, **41**, 15–22.

Crisp, M. (1969). Studies on the behaviour of *Nassarius obsoletus* (Say) (Mollusca, Gastropoda). *Biol. Bull. mar. biol. Lab.*, *Woods Hole*, **136**, 355–373.

Crofts, D. R. (1929). *Haliotis*. *Mem. Lpool mar. biol. Comm.*, **29**, 1–174.

Cuénot, L. (1891). Infusoires commensaux des ligies, patelles et arénicoles. *Revue Biol.*, *N. Fr.*, **4**, 81–89.

Dakin, W. J. (1911). Note on a sporozoan (*Merocystis kathae*, n.gen. et sp.) occurring in the renal organ of the whelk. *Proc. Trans. Lpool. biol. Soc.*, **25**, 123–124.

Dakin, W. J. (1912). *Buccinum. Proc. Trans. Lpool biol. Soc.*, **26**, 1–115.

Davenport, D. (1950). Studies in the physiology of commensalism. I. The polynoid genus *Arctonoë*. *Biol. Bull. mar. biol. Lab.*, *Woods Hole*, **98**, 81–93.

Davis, D. S. and Farley, J. (1973). The effect of parasitism by the trematode *Cryptocotyle lingua* (Creplin) on digestive efficiency in the snail host, *Littorina saxatilis* (Olivi). *Parasitology*, **66**, 191–197.

Davis, H. C., Loosanoff, V. L., Weston, W. H. and Martin, C. (1954). A fungus disease in clam and oyster larvae. *Science, N.Y.*, **120**, 36–38.

Dawes, B. (1947). *The Trematoda of British Fishes*, Ray Society, London.

Dawes, B. (1968). *The Trematoda. With Special Reference to British and other European Forms*, Cambridge Univ. Press, London.

Debaisieux, P. (1922). Note sur deux coccidies des mollusques: *Pseudoklossia patellae* et *P. chitonis*. *Cellule*, **32**, 233–246.

Deblock, S. (1971). Contribution à l'étude des Microphallidae Travassos, 1920. XXVI. Tentative de phylogénie et de taxonomie. *Bull. Mus. natn. Hist. nat.*, *Paris* (Ser. 3), **7**, 353–469.

Deblock, S. (1974a). Présence en France de *Bunocotyle progenetica* (Markowski, 1936) (Trématode digène). *Bull. Soc. zool. Fr.*, **99**, 593–600.

Deblock, S. (1974b). Contribution à l'étude des Microphallidae Travassos, 1920 (Trematoda). XXVIII. *Microphallus abortivus* n.sp., espèce à cycle évolutif abrégé originaire d'Oléron. *Annls Parasit. hum. comp.*, **49**, 175–184.

Deblock, S., Capron, A. and Rosé, F. (1961). Contribution à l'étude des Microphallidae Travassos, 1920 (Trematoda). Le genre *Maritrema* Nicoll, 1907: Cycle évolutif de *M. subdolum* Jaegerskioeld, 1909. *Parassitologia*, **3**, 105–119.

Deblock, S. and Heard, R. W. (1969). Contribution à l'étude des Microphallidae Travassos, 1920 (Trematoda). XIX. Description de *Maritrema prosthometra* n.sp. et de *Longiductotrema* nov.gen., parasites d'oiseaux ralliformes d'Amérique du Nord. *Annls Parasit. hum. comp.*, **44**, 415–424.

Deblock, S. and Pearson, J. C. (1969). Contribution à l'étude des Microphallidae Travassos, 1920 (Trematoda). XVIII. De cinq *Microphallus* d'Australie dont deux nouveaux. Essai de clé diagnostique des espèces du genre. *Annls Parasit. hum. comp.*, **44**, 391–414.

Deblock, S. and Rosé, F. (1965). Contribution à l'étude des Microphallidae Travassos, 1920 (Trematoda) des oiseaux de France. XI. Identification de la cercaire de *Microphallus claviformis* (Brandes, 1888). *Bull. Soc. zool. Fr.*, **90**, 299–314.

Deblock, S. and Tran Van Ky, P. (1966a). Contribution à l'étude des Microphallidae Travassos, 1920 (Trematoda). XII. Espèces d'Europe occidentale. Création de *Sphairiotrema* nov.gen.; considérations diverses de systématique. *Annls Parasit. hum. comp.*, **41**, 23–60.

Deblock, S. and Tran Van Ky, P. (1966b). Contribution à l'étude des Microphallidae Travassos, 1920 (Trematoda) des côtes de France. XIII. Description de deux espèces nouvelles à cycle évolutif abrégé originaires de Corse. *Annls Parasit. hum. comp.*, **41**, 313–335.

Dexter, R. W. (1943). Observations on the local movements of *Littorina littorea* (L.) and *Thais lapillus* (L.). *Nautilus*, **57**, 6–8.

Dexter, R. W. (1944). Annual fluctuations of abundance of some marine mollusks. *Nautilus*, **58**, 18–24.

Dollfus, R. P. (1914). *Trochicola enterica* nov. gen., nov. sp., eucopépode parasite de l'intestin des troques. *C. r. hebd. Séanc. Acad. Sci., Paris,* **158**, 1528–1531.

Dollfus, R. P. (1925). Liste critique des cercaires marines à queue sétigère signalées jusqu'à présent. *Trav. Stn zool. Wimereux*, **9**, 43–65.

Dollfus, R. P. (1927). Notules sur des copépodes parasites de la faune française (I-III). *Bull. Soc. zool. Fr.*, **52**, 119–121.

Dollfus, R. P. (1929). Addendum à mon 'Énumération des cestodes du plancton et des invertébrés marins'. *Annls Parasit. hum. comp.*, **7**, 325–347.

Dollfus, R. P. (1959). Recherches expérimentales sur *Nicolla gallica* (R. Ph. Dollfus 1941) R. Ph. Dollfus 1958, sa cercaire cotylicerque et sa métacercaire progénétique. Observations sur la famille des Coitocaecidae Y. Ozaki 1928, s.f. Coitocaecinae F. Poche 1926, Trematoda Podocotyloidea et sur les cercaires cotylicerques d'eau douce et marines. *Annls Parasit. hum. comp.*, **34**, 595–624.

Dollfus, R. P. (1964). Metacercaria: *Proctoeces progeneticus* (Trematoda Digenea) chez une *Gibbula* (Gastropoda Prosobranchiata) de la côte atlantique du Maroc. Observations sur la famille Fellodistomatidae. *Annls Parasit. hum. comp.*, **39**, 755–774.

Dollfus, R. P. and Euzet, L. (1964). Sur *Cercaria cotylura* Alex. Pagenstecher 1862, cercaire cotylicerque du groupe de *Cercaria pachycera* Diesing 1858. *Annls Parasit. hum. comp.*, **39**, 775–781.

Draper, N. R. and Smith, H. (1966). *Applied Regression Analysis*, Wiley, New York.

Duerr, F. G. (1965). Survey of digenetic trematode parasitism in some prosobranch gastropods of the Cape Arago region, Oregon. *Veliger*, **8**, 42.

DuPaul, W. D. and Webb, K. L. (1970). The effect of temperature on salinity-induced changes in the free amino acid pool of *Mya arenaria*. *Comp. Biochem. Physiol.*, **32**, 785–801.

Evans, F. (1965). The effect of light on zonation of four periwinkles, *Littorina littorea* (L.), *L. obtusata* (L.), *L. saxatilis* (Olivi) and *Melarapha neritoides* (L.) in an experimental tidal tank. *Neth. J. Sea Res.*, **2**, 556–565.

Evans, R. G. (1947). The intertidal ecology of certain selected localities in the Plymouth neighbourhood. *J. mar. biol. Ass. U.K.*, **27**, 173–218.

Evans, R. G. (1948). The lethal temperatures of some common British littoral molluscs. *J. Anim. Ecol.*, **17**, 165–173.

Evans, S. and Tallmark, B. (1975). Abiotic factors on a shallow, sandy bottom in Gullmar Fjord (Sweden): Temperature, salinity, water level, currents, grain size, and organic matter. *Zoon*, **3**, 61–64.

Ewers, W. H. (1961). A new intermediate host of schistosome trematodes from New South Wales. *Nature, Lond.*, **190**, 283–284.

Ewers, W. H. (1964). The influence of the density of snails on the incidence of larval trematodes. *Parasitology*, **54**, 579–583.

Faust, E. C. (1920). Pathological changes in the gastropod liver produced by fluke infection. *Bull. Johns Hopkins Hosp.*, **31**, 79–84.

Feare, C. J. (1970a). Aspects of the ecology of an exposed shore population of dogwhelks *Nucella lapillus* (L.). *Oecologia*, **5**, 1–18.

Feare, C. J. (1970b). The reproductive cycle of the dog whelk (*Nucella lapillus*). *Proc. malac. Soc. Lond.*, **39**, 125–137.

Fenchel, T. (1965). Ciliates from Scandinavian molluscs. *Ophelia*, **2**, 71–173.

Fischer, P.-H. (1954). Tumeur fibreuse chez un pleurobranche. *J. Conch., Paris*, **94**, 99–101.

Fischer, P.-H., Duval, M. and Raffy, A. (1933). Études sur les échanges respiratoires des littorines. *Archs Zool. exp. gén.*, **74**, 627–634.

Fisher, R. A. (1936). The use of multiple measurements in taxonomic problems. *Ann. Eugen.*, **7**, 179–188.

Foulon, C. (1919). *Merocystis kathae* Dakin. Une aggrégate de *Buccinum undatum*. *Cellule*, **30**, 119–150.

Fraenkel, G. (1927). Geotaxis und Phototaxis von *Littorina*. *Z. vergl. Physiol.*, **5**, 585–597.

Fraenkel, G. (1960). Lethal high temperatures for three marine invertebrates: *Limulus polyphemus*, *Littorina littorea* and *Pagurus longicarpus*. *Oikos*, **11**, 171–182.

Fraenkel, G. (1961). Resistance to high temperatures in a Mediterranean snail, *Littorina neritoides*. *Ecology*, **42**, 604–606.

Fraenkel, G. (1966). The heat resistance of intertidal snails at Shirahama, Wakayama-Ken, Japan. *Pubs Seto mar. biol. Lab.*, **14**, 185–195.

Fraenkel, G. (1968). The heat resistance of intertidal snails at Bimini, Bahamas; Ocean Springs, Mississippi; and Woods Hole, Massachusetts. *Physiol. Zoöl.*, **41**, 1–13.

Fretter, V. and Graham, A. (1949). The structure and mode of life of Pyramidellidae, parasitic opisthobranchs. *J. mar. biol. Ass. U.K.*, **28**, 493–532.

Frey, H. W. (Ed.) (1971). *California's Living Marine Resources and their Utilization*, Resources Agency, Dept. Fish Game, State of California.

Fried, G. H. and Levin, N. L. (1970). Enzyme activities in the hepatopancreas and foot of *Nassarius obsoletus*. *Fedn Proc. Fedn Am. Socs exp. Biol.*, **29**, 878.

Fried, G. H. and Levin, N. L. (1973). Enzymatic activity in hepatopancreas of *Nassarius obsoletus*. *Comp. Biochem. Physiol.*, **45B**, 153–157.

Fry, F. E. J. (1957). The lethal temperature as a tool in taxonomy. *Année biol.*, **33**, 205–219.

Fuller, M. S., Fowles, B. E. and McLaughlin, D. J. (1964). Isolation and pure culture study of marine phycomycetes. *Mycologia*, **56**, 745–756.

Gambino, J. J. (1959). The seasonal incidence of infection of the snail *Nassarius obsoletus* (Say) with larval trematodes. *J. Parasit.*, **45**, 440–456.

Ganaros, A. E. (1957). Marine fungus infecting eggs and embryos of *Urosalpinx cinerea*. *Science, N.Y.*, **125**, 1194.

Gendron, R. P. (1977). Habitat selection and migratory behaviour of the intertidal gastropod *Littorina littorea* (L.). *J. Anim. Ecol.*, **46**, 79–92.

Gilles, R. (1972). Osmoregulation in three molluscs: *Acanthochitona discrepans* (Brown), *Glycymeris glycymeris* (L.) and *Mytilus edulis* (L.). *Biol. Bull. mar. biol. Lab.*, *Woods Hole*, **142**, 25–35.

Gohar, H. A. F. and Soliman, G. N. (1963). On the biology of three coralliophilids boring in living corals. *Publs mar. biol. Stn Ghardaqa*, **12**, 99–126.

Gowanloch, J. N. and Hayes, F. R. (1926). Contributions to the study of marine gastropods. I. The physical factors, behaviour and intertidal life of *Littorina*. *Contr. Can. Biol. Fish.*, **3**, 133–165.

Graefe, G. (1971). *Cercaria diesingi* n.sp. aus *Gibbula divaricata* L. in der Gezeitenzone bei Dubrovnik, Jugoslawien. *Sber. öst. Akad. Wiss.* (Abt. I), **179**, 103–107.

Graff, L. von (1903). *Die Turbellarien als Parasiten und Wirte*, Graz.

Green, C. V. and Green, S. K. (1932). Shell growth in the periwinkle, *Littorina littorea*. *Am. Nat.*, **66**, 371–376.

Grindley, J. R. and Nel, E. (1968). Mussel poisoning and shellfish mortality on the west coast of South Africa. *S. Afr. J. Sci.*, **64**, 420–422.

Grodhaus, G., and Keh, B. (1958). The marine dermatitis-producing cercaria of *Austrobilharzia variglandis* in California (Trematoda: Schistosomatidae). *J. Parasit.*, **44**, 633–638.

Guillard, R. R. L. (1959). Further evidence of the destruction of bivalve larvae by bacteria. *Biol. Bull. mar. biol. Lab.*, *Woods Hole*, **117**, 258–266.

Gunter, G. (1957). Temperature. In J. W. Hedgpeth (Ed.), *Treatise on Marine Ecology and Paleoecology*, Vol. 1, Ecology. *Mem. geol. Soc. Am.*, **67**, 159–184.

Hamby, R. I. (1975). Heat effects on a marine snail. *Biol. Bull. mar. biol. Lab.*, *Woods Hole*, **149**, 331–347.

Hancock, A. and Norman, A. M. (1863). On *Splanchnotrophus*, an undescribed genus of Crustacea, parasitic in nudibranchiate Mollusca. *Trans. Linn. Soc. Lond.*, **24**, 49–60.

Hankó, B. (1912). Über Mißbildungen bei *Nassarius mutabilis* (L.). *Zool. Anz.*, **39**, 719–723.

Hankó, B. (1914). Über das Regenerationsvermögen und die Regeneration verschiedener Organe von *Nassa mutabilis* L. *Arch. EntwMech. Org.*, **38**, 447–507.

Harasewych, M. G. (1977). Abnormal hyperstrophy in *Littorina lineolata* (Gastropoda: Littorinidae). *Nautilus*, **91**, 60–62.

Hatt, P. (1927a). Le début de l'évolution des *Porospora* chez les mollusques. *Archs Zool. exp. gén.*, **67**, 2–7.

Hatt, P. (1927b). *Porospora legeri* de Beauchamp (=*P. galloprovincialis* Léger et Duboscq) et les premiers stades de son évolution chez l'*Eriphia*. *Archs Zool. exp. gén.*, **67**, 8–11.

Hatt, P. (1927c). Spores de *Porospora (Nematopsis)* chez les gastéropodes. *C. r. Séanc. Soc. Biol.*, **96**, 90–91.

Hatt, P. (1931). L'évolution des porosporides chez les mollusques. *Archs Zool. exp. gén.*, **72**, 341–415.

Hayes, F. R. (1927). The effect of environmental factors on the development and growth of *Littorina littorea*. *Trans. Nova Scotian Inst. Sci.*, **17**, 6–13.

Hayes, F. R. (1929). Contribution to the study of marine gastropods. III. Development, growth and behaviour of *Littorina*. *Contr. Can. Biol. Fish.*, **4**, 413–430.

Hecht, E. (1895). Contribution à l'étude des nudibranches. *Mém. Soc. zool. Fr.*, **8**, 539–711.

Hepper, B. T. (1953). Artificial infection of various molluscs with *Mytilicola intestinalis* Steuer. *Nature, Lond.*, **172**, 250.

Heyneman, D., Lim, H.-K. and Jeyarasasingam, U. (1972). Antagonism of *Echinostoma liei* (Trematoda: Echinostomatidae) against the trematodes *Paryphostomum segregatum* and *Schistosoma mansoni*. *Parasitology*, **65**, 223–233.

Heyneman, D. and Umathevy, T. (1968). Interaction of trematodes by predation within natural double infections in the host snail *Indoplanorbis exustus*. *Nature, Lond.*, **217**, 283–285.

Höhnk, W. (1969).Über den pilzlichen Befall kalkiger Hartteile von Meerestieren. *Ber. dt. wiss. Kommn Meeresforsch.*, **20**, 129–140.

Hoff, C. C. (1941). A case of correlation between infection of snail hosts with *Cryptocotyle lingua* and the habits of the gulls. *J. Parasit.*, **27**, 539.

Hoffman, G. L. (1957). Studies on the life cycle of *Cryptocotyle concavum* from the common sucker and experimentally in the chick. (Abstract.) *Proc. N. Dak. Acad. Sci.*, **11**, 55–56.

Holliman, R. B. (1961). Larval trematodes from the Apalachee Bay area, Florida, with a checklist of known marine cercariae arranged in a key to their superfamilies. *Tulane Stud. Zool.*, **9**, 1–74.

Honer, M. R. (1961a). Some observations on the ecology of *Hydrobia stagnorum* (Gmelin) and *Hydrobia ulvae* (Pennant), and the relationship ecology—parasitofauna. *Basteria*, **25**, 7–16.

Honer, M. R. (1961b). Some observations on the ecology of *Hydrobia stagnorum* (Gmelin) and *H. ulvae* (Pennant), and the relationship ecology—parasitofauna (continued). *Basteria*, **25**, 17–29.

Hopkins, S. H. (1956). *Odostomia impressa* parasitizing southern oysters. *Science, N.Y.*, **124**, 628–629.

Hopkins, S. H. (1957). Interrelations of organisms. B. Parasitism. In J. W. Hedgpeth (Ed.), *Treatise on Marine Ecology and Paleoecology*, Vol. 1, Ecology. *Mem. geol. Soc. Am.*, **67**, 413–428.

Hoskin, G. P. (1975). Light and electron microscopy of the host–parasite interface and histopathology of *Nassarius obsoletus* infected with rediae of *Himasthla quissetensis*. *Ann. N.Y. Acad. Sci.*, **266**, 497–512.

Hoskin, G. P. and Cheng, T. C. (1973). Dehydrogenase activity in the rediae of *Himasthla quissetensis* (Trematoda) as an indicator of substrate utilization. *Comp. Biochem. Physiol.*, **468**, 361–366.

Hoskin, G. P. and Cheng, T. C. (1974). *Himasthla quissetensis*: uptake and utilization of glucose by rediae as determined by autoradiography and respirometry. *Expl Parasit.*, **35**, 61–67.

Hoskin, G. P. and Cheng, T. C. (1975). Occurrence of carotenoids in *Himasthla quissetensis* rediae and the host, *Nassarius obsoletus*. *J. Parasit.*, **61**, 381–382.

Hoskin, G. P., Cheng, T. C. and Shapiro, I. L. (1974). Fatty acid composition of three lipid classes of *Himasthla quissetensis* rediae before and after starvation. *Comp. Biochem. Physiol.*, **47B**, 821–829.

Humes, A. G. (1958a). Copepod parasites of mollusks. *Am. malacol. Un. Bull.*, **24**, 13–14.

Humes, A. G. (1958b). Copepodes parasites de mollusques à Madagascar. *Mém. Inst. scient. Madagascar* (Ser. F), **2**, 285–342.

Humes, A. G. (1963). New species of *Lichomolgus* (Copepoda, Cyclopoida) from sea anemones and nudibranchs in Madagascar. *Cah. O.R.S.T.O.M.* (Ser. Océanogr.), **6**, 59–129.

Humes, A. G. (1975). Cyclopoid copepods associated with marine invertebrates in Mauritius. *J. Linn. Soc. Zool.*, **56**, 171–181.

Humes, A. G. and Ho, J.-S. (1965). New species of the genus *Anthessius* (Copepoda, Cyclopoida) associated with mollusks in Madagascar. *Cah. O.R.S.T.O.M.* (Ser. Océanogr.), **3**, 79–113.

Humes, A. G. and Stock, J. H. (1973). A revision of the family Lichomolgidae Kossmann, 1877, cyclopoid copepods mainly associated with marine invertebrates. *Smithsonian Contr. Zool.*, **127**, 1–368.

Hunninen, A. V. and Cable, R. M. (1941). Studies on the life history of *Anisoporus manteri* (Trematoda: Allocreadiidae). *Biol. Bull. mar. biol. Lab., Woods Hole*, **80**, 415–428.

Hunninen, A. V. and Cable, R. M. (1943). The life history of *Podocotyle atomon* (Rudolphi) (Trematoda: Opecoeliidae). *Trans. Am. microsc. Soc.*, **62**, 57–68.

Hunter, W. S. and Vernberg, W. B. (1955a). Studies on oxygen consumption in digenetic trematodes. I. *Expl Parasit.*, **4**, 54–61.

Hunter, W. S. and Vernberg, W. B. (1955b). Studies on oxygen consumption in digenetic trematodes. II. Effects of two extremes in oxygen tension. *Expl Parasit.*, **4**, 427–434.

Huntsman, A. G. (1918). The vertical distribution of certain intertidal animals. *Trans. R. Soc. Can.* (Ser. 3), **12**, 53–61.

Hutton, R. F. (1952). Schistosome cercariae as the probable cause of seabather's eruption. *Bull. mar. Sci. Gulf Caribb.*, **2**, 346–359.

Hutton, R. F. (1955). *Cercaria turritella* n.sp., a 'huge-tailed' monostome larva from *Turritella communis* Risso. *J. mar. biol. Ass. U.K.*, **34**, 249–255.

Hutton, R. F. (1960). Marine dermatosis. Notes on 'seabather's eruption' with *Creseis acicula* Rang (Mollusca: Pteropoda) as the cause of a particular type of sea sting along the west coast of Florida. *Arch. Dermat.*, **82**, 951–956.

Hyman, L. H. (1940). *The Invertebrates*, Vol. I, Protozoa through Ctenophora, McGraw-Hill, New York.

Hyman, L. H. (1967). *The Invertebrates*, Vol. VI, Mollusca I, McGraw-Hill, New York.

Issaitchikoff, J.-M. (1926). Sur le développement du trématode *Cryptocotyle concavum* (Creplin, 1825). *C. r. Séanc. Soc. Biol.*, **94**, 305–307.

Issel, R. (1903). Ancistridi del Golfo di Napoli. *Mitt. zool. Stn Neapel*, **16**, 63–108.

Izawa, K. (1976a). Two new parasitic copepods (Cyclopoida: Myicolidae) from Japanese gastropod molluscs. *Publs Seto mar. biol. Lab.*, **23**, 213–227.

Izawa, K. (1976b). A new parasitic copepod, *Philoblenna arabici* gen. et sp. nov. from a Japanese gastropod, with proposal of a new family Philoblennidae (Cyclopoida: Poecilostoma). *Publs Seto mar. biol. Lab.*, **23**, 229–235.

James, B. L. (1960). A new cercaria of the subfamily Gymnophallinae (Trematoda: Digenea) developing in a unique 'parthenita' in *Littorina saxatalis* (Olivi). *Nature, Lond.*, **185**, 181–182.

James, B. L. (1964). The life cycle of *Parvatrema homoeotecnum* sp. nov. (Trematoda: Digenea) and a review of the family Gymnophallidae Morozov, 1955. *Parasitology*, **54**, 1–41.

James, B. L. (1965). The effects of parasitism by larval Digenea on the digestive gland of the intertidal prosobranch, *Littorina saxatilis* (Olivi) subsp. *tenebrosa* (Montagu). *Parasitology*, **55**, 93–115.

James, B. L. (1968a). The occurrence of *Parvatrema homoeotecnum* James, 1964 (Trematoda: Gymnophallidae) in a population of *Littorina saxatilis tenebrosa* (Mont.). *J. nat. Hist.*, **2**, 21–37.

James, B. L. (1968b). Studies on the life-cycle of *Microphallus pygmaeus* (Levinsen, 1881) (Trematoda: Microphallidae). *J. nat. Hist.*, **2**, 155–172.

James, B. L. (1968c). The occurrence of larval Digenea in ten species of intertidal prosobranch molluscs in Cardigan Bay. *J. nat. Hist.*, **2**, 329–343.

James, B. L. (1968d). The distribution and keys of species in the family Littorinidae and of their digenean parasites, in the region of Dale, Pembrokeshire. *Fld Stud.*, **2**, 615–650.

James, B. L. (1969). The Digenea of the intertidal prosobranch *Littorina saxatilis* (Olivi). *Z. zool. Syst. u. Evolutionsforsch.*, **7**, 273–316.

James, B. L. and Richards, R. J. (1972). The relationship between oxygen uptake, reduced weight, length and number of contained metacercariae in the sporocysts of *Microphallus pygmaeus* (Levinsen, 1881) (Trematoda: Microphallidae). *J. Helminth.*, **46**, 27–33.

James, H. A. (1974). Sex and foot color in the periwinkle snail, *Littorina littorea* (L.), infected with larval stages of the heterophyid trematode, *Cryptocotyle lingua* (Creplin). *Proc. 3rd int. Congr. Parasit., Munich*, **1**, 341.

James, J. L. (1973). The ultrastructure of the miracidium of *Parorchis acanthus* Nicoll, 1907. *Parasitology*, **67**, xxxi–xxxii.

Jameson, H. L. (1897). Additional notes on the Turbellaria of the L.M.B.C. district. *Proc. Trans. Lpool biol. Soc.*, **11**, 160–178.

Jamieson, B. G. M. (1966a). *Parahemiurus bennettae* n.sp. (Digenea), a hemiurid trematode progenetic in *Salinator fragilis* Lamarck (Gastropoda, Amphibolidae). *Proc. R. Soc. Qd.*, **77**, 73–80.

Jamieson, B. G. M. (1966b). Larval stages of the progenetic trematode *Parahemiurus bennettae* Jamieson, 1966 (Digenea, Hemiuridae) and the evolutionary origin of cercariae. *Proc. R. Soc. Qd.*, **77**, 81–92.

Jenner, C. E. (1956). A striking behavioural change leading to the formation of extensive aggregations in a population of *Nassarius obsoletus*. *Biol. Bull. mar. biol. Lab., Woods Hole*, **111**, 291.

Jenner, C. E. (1957). Schooling behavior in mudsnails in Barnstable Harbor leading to the formation of massive aggregations at the completion of seasonal reproduction. *Biol. Bull. mar. biol. Lab., Woods Hole*, **113**, 328.

Jenner, C. E. (1958). An attempted analysis of schooling behavior in the marine snail *Nassarius obsoletus*. *Biol. Bull. mar. biol. Lab., Woods Hole*, **115**, 337.

Jenner, C. E. (1959). Aggregation and schooling in the marine snail *Nassarius obsoletus*. *Biol. Bull. mar. biol. Lab., Woods Hole*, **117**, 397.

Johnson, P. T. (1968). Population crashes in the bean clam, *Donax gouldi* and their significance to the study of mass mortality in other marine invertebrates. *J. Invertebr. Pathol.*, **12**, 349–358.

Johnson, T. W. and Anderson, W. R. (1962). A fungus in *Anomia simplex* shell. *J. Elisha Mitchell Sci. Soc.*, **78**, 43–47.

Johnson, T. W. and Sparrow, F. K. (1961). *Fungi in Oceans and Estuaries*, Hafner, New York.

Johnston, T. H. and Mawson, P. M. (1945a). Some parasitic nematodes from South Australian marine fish. *Trans. R. Soc. S. A.*, **69**, 114–117.

Johnston, T. H. and Mawson, P. M. (1945b). Parasitic nematodes. *Report of the British, Australian and New Zealand Antarctic Research Expedition, 1929–1931* (Ser. B), **5**, 73–159.

Kaestner, A. (1954–1963). *Lehrbuch der Speziellen Zoologie*, VEB Fischer, Jena.

Kanwisher, J. W. (1955). Freezing in intertidal animals. *Biol. Bull. mar. biol. Lab., Woods Hole*, **109**, 56–63.

Kanwisher, J. W. (1959). Histology and metabolism of frozen intertidal animals. *Biol. Bull. mar. biol. Lab., Woods Hole*, **116**, 258–264.

Kanwisher, J. W. (1966). Freezing in intertidal animals. In H. T. Meryman (Ed.), *Cryobiology*. Academic Press, London. pp. 487–494.

Kasschau, M. R. (1975a). The relationship of free amino acids to salinity changes and temperature-salinity interactions in the mud-flat snail, *Nassarius obsoletus*. *Comp. Biochem. Physiol.*, **51A**, 301–308.

Kasschau, M. R. (1975b). Changes in concentrations of free amino acids in larval stages of the trematode, *Himasthla quissetensis* and its intermediate host, *Nassarius obsoletus*. *Comp. Biochem. Physiol.*, **51B**, 273–280.

Kendall, S. B. (1964). Some factors influencing the development and behaviour of trematodes in their molluscan hosts. In A. E. Taylor (Ed.), *Host-parasite Relationships in Invertebrate Hosts*. Blackwell Scientific Publ., Oxford.

Kessel, E. (1937). Schalenkorrosion bei lebenden Strandschnecken (*Littorina littorea*) und ihre Ursache. *Zool. Anz.*, **10** (Suppl.), 69–77.

Kinne, O. (1970). Temperature: Animals. Invertebrates. In O. Kinne (Ed.), *Marine Ecology*, Vol. I, Environmental Factors, Part 1. Wiley, London. pp. 407–514.

Kinne, O. (1971). Salinity: Animals. Invertebrates. In O. Kinne (Ed.), *Marine Ecology*, Vol. I, Environmental Factors, Part 2. Wiley, London. pp. 821–955.

Kinne, O. (1972). Pressure: General introduction. In O. Kinne (Ed.), *Marine Ecology*, Vol. I, Environmental Factors, Part 3. Wiley, London. pp. 1323–1360.

Kinne, O. (1977). Cultivation of animals. Research cultivation. In O. Kinne (Ed.), *Marine Ecology*, Vol. III, Cultivation, Part 2. Wiley, Chichester. pp. 579–1293.

Kinne, O. and Rosenthal, H. (1977). Cultivation of animals. Commercial cultivation (aquaculture). In O. Kinne (Ed.), *Marine Ecology*, Vol. III, Cultivation, Part 3. Wiley, Chichester. pp. 1321–1381.

Kleeton, G. (1961). New host and distribution record of the copepod *Trochicola entericus*. *Crustaceana*, **3**, 172.

Køie, M. (1969). On the endoparasites of *Buccinum undatum* L. with special reference to the trematodes. *Ophelia*, **6**, 251–279.

Køie, M. (1971a). On the histochemistry and ultrastructure of the daughter sporocyst of *Cercaria buccini* Lebour, 1911. *Ophelia*, **9**, 145–163.

Køie, M. (1971b). On the histochemistry and ultrastructure of the tegument and associated structures of the cercaria of *Zoogonoides viviparus* in the first intermediate host. *Ophelia*, **9**, 165–206.

Køie, M. (1971c). On the histochemistry and ultrastructure of the redia of *Neophasis lageniformis* (Lebour, 1910) (Trematoda, Acanthocolpidae). *Ophelia*, **9**, 113–143.

Køie, M. (1973a). The host-parasite interface and associated structures of the cercaria and adult *Neophasis lageniformis* (Lebour, 1910). *Ophelia*, **12**, 205–219.

Køie, M. (1973b). The ultrastructure of the caecal epithelium of the intraredial cercaria of *Neophasis lageniformis* (Lebour, 1910) (Trematoda, Acanthocolpidae). *Z. Zellforsch.*, **139**, 405–416.

Køie, M. (1975). On the morphology and life-history of *Opechona bacillaris* (Molin, 1859) Looss, 1907 (Trematoda, Lepocreadiidae). *Ophelia*, **13**, 63–86.

Køie, M. (1976). On the morphology and life-history of *Zoogonoides viviparus* (Olsson, 1868) Odhner, 1902 (Trematoda, Zoogonidae). *Ophelia*, **15**, 1–14.

Køie, M. (1977). Stereoscan studies of cercariae, metacercariae and adults of *Cryptocotyle lingua* (Creplin, 1825) Fischoeder, 1903 (Trematoda, Heterophyidae). *J. Parasit.*, **63**, 835–839.

Kohlmeyer, J. (1969). The role of marine fungi in the penetration of calcareous substances. *Am. Zool.*, **9**, 741–746.

Korringa, P. (1950). A review of the papers on molluscs presented at the Special Scientific Meeting on Shellfish of the International Council for the Exploration of the Sea, Edinburgh, 10th October, 1949. *Rapp. P.-v. Réun. Cons. perm. int. Explor. Mer*, **128**, 44–59.

Korringa, P. (1951). Investigations on shell-disease in the oyster, *Ostrea edulis* L. *Rapp. P.-v. Réun. Cons. perm. int. Explor. Mer*, **128**, 50–54.

Kramp, P. L. (1921). *Kinetocodium danae* n.g., n.sp., a new gymnoblastic hydroid, parasitic on a pteropod. *Vidensk. Meddr dansk naturh. Foren.*, **74**, 1–21.

Kramp, P. L. (1957). Notes on a living specimen of the hydroid *Kinetocodium danae* Kramp, parasitic on a pteropod. *Vidensk. Meddr dansk naturh. Foren.*, **119**, 47–54.

Krupa, P. L., Bal, A. K. and Cousineau, G. H. (1966). The fine structure of the redia of the trematode, *Cryptocotyle lingua*. *Biol. Bull. mar. biol. Lab., Woods Hole*, **131**, 395–396.

Krupa, P. L., Cousineau, G. H. and Bal, A. K. (1968). Ultrastructural and histochemical observations on the body wall of *Cryptocotyle lingua* rediae (Trematoda). *J. Parasit.*, **54**, 900–908.

Krupa, P. L., Cousineau, G. H. and Bal, A. K. (1969). Electron microscopy of the excretory vesicle of a trematode cercaria. *J. Parasit.*, **55**, 985–992.

Labbé, A. (1930). Réaction du tissu conjonctif au goudron chez un mollusque: *Doris tuberculata* Cuvier. *C.r. Séanc. Soc. Biol.*, **103**, 20–22.

Lambert, L. (1951). L'ostréiculture et la mytiliculture en Zélande (Pays-Bas). *Revue Trav. Off. (scient. tech.) Pêch. marit.*, **16**, 111–128.

Lambert, T. C. and Farley, J. (1968). The effect of parasitism by the trematode *Cryptocotyle lingua* (Creplin) on zonation and winter migration of the common periwinkle, *Littorina littorea* (L.). *Can. J. Zool.*, **46**, 1139–1147.

Lang, K. (1954). On a new orthonectid, *Rhopalura philinae* n.sp., found as a parasite in the opisthobranch *Philine scabra* Müller. *Ark. Zool.* (Ser. 2), **6**, 603–610.

Lange, R. (1963). The osmotic function of amino acids and taurine in the mussel, *Mytilus edulis*. *Comp. Biochem. Physiol.*, **10**, 173–179.

Lauckner, G. (1971). Zur Trematodenfauna der Herzmuscheln *Cardium edule* und *Cardium lamarcki*. *Helgoländer wiss. Meeresunters.*, **22**, 377–400.

Lauckner, G. (1973). Fischpathologische Untersuchungen. *Biologische Anstalt Helgoland, Jahresbericht*, **1972**, 73–74.

Lebour, M. V. (1905). Notes on Northumberland trematodes. *Rep. scient. Invest. Northumb. Sea Fish. Comm.*, **1904**, 100–105.

Lebour, M. V. (1907a). Larval trematodes of the Northumberland coast. No. I. *Trans. nat. Hist. Soc. Northumb.*, **1**, 437–454.

Lebour, M. V. (1907b). On three mollusk-infesting trematodes. *Ann. Mag. nat. Hist.* (Ser. 7), **19**, 102–106.

Lebour, M. V. (1908a). Trematodes of the Northumberland coast. No. II. *Trans. nat. Hist. Soc. Northumb.*, **3**, 28–45.

Lebour, M. V. (1908b). A contribution to the life-history of *Echinostomum secundum* Nicoll. *Parasitology*, **1**, 352–358.

Lebour, M. V. (1908c). Trematodes of the Northumberland coast. No. III—A preliminary note on *Echinostephilla virgula*, a new trematode in the turnstone. *Trans. nat. Hist. Soc. Northumb.*, **3**, 440–445.

Lebour, M. V. (1910). *Acanthopsolus lageniformis* n.sp., a trematode in the catfish. *Rep. scient. Invest. Northumb. Sea Fish. Comm.*, **1909**, 29–35.

Lebour, M. V. (1911). A review of the British marine cercariae. *Parasitology*, **4**, 416–456.

Lebour, M. V. (1914). Some larval trematodes from Millport. *Parasitology*, **7**, 1–11.

Lebour, M. V. (1918). A trematode larva from *Buccinum undatum* and notes on trematodes from post-larval fish. *J. mar. biol. Ass. U.K.*, **11**, 514–517.

Lebour, M. V. and Elmhirst, R. (1922). A contribution towards the life history of *Parorchis acanthus* Nicoll, a trematode in the herring gull. *J. mar. biol. Ass. U.K.*, **12**, 829–832.

Léger, L. and Duboscq, O. (1925). Les porosporides et leur évolution. *Trav. Stn zool. Wimereux*, **9**, 126–139.

Leigh, W. H. (1952). A dermatitis-producing schistosome cercaria from marine snails at Miami, Florida. *J. Parasit.*, **38** (Suppl.), 38.

Leigh, W. H. (1953). *Cercaria huttoni* sp. nov., a dermatitis-producing schistosome larva from the marine snail, *Haminoea antillarum guadaloupensis* Sowerby. *J. Parasit.*, **39**, 625–629.

Leigh, W. H. (1955). The morphology of *Gigantobilharzia huttoni* (Leigh, 1953), an avian schistosome with marine dermatitis-producing larvae. *J. Parasit.*, **41**, 262–269.

Leigh-Sharpe, W. H. (1933). A second list of parasitic Copepoda of Plymouth with a description of three new species. *Parasitology*, **25**, 113–118.

Leighton, D. L. (1960). An abalone lacking respiratory apertures. *Veliger*, **3**, 48.

Lespès, M. C. (1857). Observations sur quelques cercaires de mollusques marins. *Annls Sci. nat.* (Ser. Zool, 4), **7**, 113–117.

Levinsen, G. M. R. (1881). Bidrag til kundskab om Grønlands trematodfauna. *Overs. K. danske Vidensk. Selsk. Forh.*, **1**, 52–84.

LeZotte, L. A. (1954). Studies on marine digenetic trematodes of Puerto Rico: The family Bivesiculidae, its biology and affinities. *J. Parasit.*, **40**, 148–162.

Lie, K. J. (1966). Antagonistic interaction between *Schistosoma mansoni* sporocysts and echinostome rediae in the snail *Australorbis glabratus*. *Nature, Lond.*, **211**, 1213–1214.

Lie, K. J. (1967). Antagonism of *Paryphostomum segregatum* rediae to *Schistosoma mansoni* sporocysts in the snail *Biomphalaria glabrata*. *J. Parasit.*, **53**, 969–976.

Lie, K. J. (1973). Larval trematode antagonism: Principles and possible application as a control method. *Expl Parasit.*, **33**, 343–349.

Lie, K. J., Basch, P. F. and Heyneman, D. (1968a). Direct and indirect antagonism between *Paryphostomum segregatum* and *Echinostoma paraensei* in the snail *Biomphalaria glabrata*. *Z. ParasitKde*, **31**, 101–107.

Lie, K. J., Basch, P. F., Heyneman, D. and Fitzgerald, F. (1968a). Antagonism between two species of echinostomes *(Paryphostomum segregatum* and *Echinostoma lindoense)* in the snail *Biomphalaria glabrata*. *Z. ParasitKde*, **30**, 117–125.

Lie, K. J., Basch, P. F. and Hoffman, M. A. (1967). Antagonism between *Paryphostomum segregatum* and *Echinostoma barbosai* in the snail *Biomphalaria straminea*. *J. Parasit.*, **53**, 1205–1209.

Lie, K. J., Basch, P. F. and Umathevy, T. (1965). Antagonism between two species of larval trematodes in the same snail. *Nature, Lond.*, **206**, 422–423.

Lie, K. J., Basch, P. F. and Umathevy, T. (1966). Studies on Echinostomatidae (Trematoda) in Malaya. XII. Antagonism between two species of echinostome trematodes in the same lymnaeid snail. *J. Parasit.*, **52**, 454–457.

Lim, H. K. and Heyneman, D. (1972). Intramolluscan inter-trematode antagonism: a review of factors influencing the host–parasite system and its possible role in biological control. *Adv. Parasit.*, **10**, 191–268.

Linton, E. (1915). Notes on trematode sporocysts and cercariae in marine mollusks of the Woods Hole region. *Biol. Bull. mar. biol. Lab., Woods Hole*, **28**, 198–209.

Loosanoff, V. L. (1954). New advances in the study of bivalve larvae. *Am. Scient.*, **42**, 607–624.

Loosanoff, V. L. (1966). Time and intensity of setting of the oyster, *Crassostrea virginica*, in Long Island Sound. *Biol. Bull. mar. biol. Lab., Woods Hole*, **130**, 211–227.

Loosanoff, V. L. (1974). Factors responsible for the mass mortalities of molluscan larvae in nature: A review. In *Proceedings of the 5th Annual Workshop of World Mariculture Society.* pp. 297–309.

Loosanoff, V. L. and Davis, H. C. (1963). Rearing of bivalve molluscs. *Adv. mar. Biol.*, **1**, 1–136.

Loos-Frank, B. (1967). Experimentelle Untersuchungen über Bau, Entwicklung und Systematik der Himasthlinae (Trematoda, Echinostomatidae) des Nordseeraumes. *Z. ParasitKde*, **28**, 299–351.

Loos-Frank, B. (1968a). *Psilochasmus aglyptorchis* n.sp. (Trematoda, Psilostomatidae) und sein Entwicklungszyklus. *Z. ParasitKde*, **30**, 185–191.

Loos-Frank, B. (1968b). Der Entwicklungszyklus von *Psilostomum brevicolle* (Creplin, 1829) (Syn.: *P. platyurum* (Mühling, 1896)) (Trematoda, Psilostomatidae). *Z. ParasitKde*, **31**, 122–131.

Loos-Frank, B. (1969). Zwei adulte Trematoden aus Nordsee-Mollusken: *Proctoeces buccini* n.sp. und *P. scrobiculariae* n.sp. *Z. ParasitKde*, **32**, 324–340.

Loos-Frank, B. (1970). Zur Kenntnis der gymnophalliden Trematoden des Nordseeraumes. II. *Lacunovermis macomae* (Lebour, 1908) n.comb. (Syn.: *Gymnophallus macroporus* Jameson & Nicoll, 1913) und seine Metacercarie. *Z. ParasitKde*, **35**, 130–139.

Loos-Frank, B. (1971). Zur Kenntnis der gymnophalliden Trematoden des Nordseeraumes. IV. Übersicht über die gymnophalliden Larven aus Mollusken der Gezeitenzone. *Z. ParasitKde*, **36**, 206–232.

Looss, A. (1901). Über einige Distomen der Labriden des Triester Hafens. *Zentbl. Bakt. ParasitKde*, **29**, 398–405, 437–442.

Lucas, C. E. (1947). The ecological effects of external metabolites. *Biol. Rev.*, **22**, 270–295.

Lucas, C. E. (1949). External metabolites and ecological adaptations. *Symp. Soc. exp. Biol.*, **3**, 336–356.

Lucas, C. E. (1955). External metabolites in the sea. *Deep Sea Res.*, **3** (Suppl.), 139–148.

Lucas, C. E. (1958). External metabolites and productivity. *Rapp. P.-v. Réun. Cons. perm. int. Explor. Mer*, **144**, 155–158.

Lunetta, J. E. and Vernberg, W. B. (1971). Fatty acid composition of parasitized and non-parasitized tissue of the mud-flat snail, *Nassarius obsoleta* (Say). *Expl Parasit.*, **30**, 244–248.

Lysaght, A. M. (1941). The biology and trematode parasites of the gastropod *Littorina neritoides* (L.) on the Plymouth breakwater. *J. mar. biol. Ass. U.K.*, **25**, 41–67.

McCoy, O. R. (1929). Observations on the life history of a marine lophocercous cercaria. *J. Parasit.*, **16**, 29–34.

McDaniel, J. S. and Coggins, J. R. (1971). Seasonal trematode infection dynamics in *Nassarius obsoletus*. *J. Elisha Mitchell scient. Soc.*, **87**, 169.

McDaniel, J. S. and Coggins, J. R. (1972). Seasonal larval trematode infection dynamics in *Nassarius obsoletus* (Say). *J. Elisha Mitchell scient. Soc.*, **88**, 55–57.

McDaniel, J. S. and Dixon, K. E. (1967). Utilization of exogenous glucose by the rediae of *Parorchis acanthus* (Digenea: Philophthalmidae) and *Cryptocotyle lingua* (Digenea: Heterophyidae). *Biol. Bull. mar. biol. Lab., Woods Hole*, **133**, 591–599.

McMahon, R. F. and Russell-Hunter, W. D. (1973). Respiratory adaptability in relation to vertical zonation in littoral and sublittoral snails. *Biol. Bull. mar. biol. Lab., Woods Hole*, **145**, 447.

McMahon, R. F. and Russell-Hunter, W. D. (1974). Responses to low oxygen stress in relation to the ecology of littoral and sublittoral snails. *Biol. Bull. mar. biol. Lab., Woods Hole*, **147**, 490.

McMahon, R. F. and Russell-Hunter, W. D. (1977). Temperature relations of aerial and aquatic respiration in six littoral snails in relation to their vertical zonation. *Biol. Bull. mar.biol. Lab., Woods Hole*, **152**, 182–198.

McManus, D. P. and James, B. L. (1975a). Tricarboxylic acid cycle enzymes in the digestive gland of *Littorina saxatilis rudis* (Maton) and in the daughter sporocysts of *Microphallus similis* (Jäg.) (Digenea: Microphallidae). *Comp. Biochem. Physiol.*, **50B**, 491–495.

McManus, D. P. and James, B. L. (1975b). Anaerobic glucose metabolism in the digestive gland of *Littorina saxatilis rudis* (Maton) and in the daughter sporocysts of *Microphallus similis* (Jäg.) (Digenea: Microphallidae). *Comp. Biochem. Physiol.*, **51B**, 293–298.

McManus, D. P. and James, B. L. (1975c). Pyruvate kinases and carbon dioxide fixating enzymes in the digestive gland of *Littorina saxatilis rudis* (Maton) and in the daughter sporocysts of *Microphallus similis* (Jäg.) (Digenea: Microphallidae). *Comp. Biochem. Physiol.*, **51B**, 299–306.

McManus, D. P., Marshall, I. and James, B. L. (1975). Lipids in digestive gland of *Littorina saxatilis rudis* (Maton) and in daughter sporocysts of *Microphallus similis* (Jäg., 1900). *Expl Parasit.*, **37**, 157–163.

Maillard, C. (1973). Mise en évidence du cycle évolutif abrégé d'*Aphalloides coelomica* Dollfus, Chabaud et Golvan, 1957 (Trematoda). Notion d'hôte historique. *C.r. hebd. Séanc. Acad. Sci., Paris* (Ser. D), **277**, 317–320.

Markel, R. P. (1971). Temperature relations in two species of tropical west American littorines. *Ecology*, **52**, 1126–1130.

Markowski, S. (1936). Über die Trematodenfauna der baltischen Mollusken aus der Umgebung der Halbinsel Hel. *Bull. int. Acad. Pol. Sci. Lett.* (Ser. B. II), **2**, 285–317.

Marshall, I., McManus, D. P. and James, B. L. (1974a). Glycolysis in the digestive gland of healthy and parasitized *Littorina saxatilis rudis* (Maton) and in the daughter sporocysts of *Microphallus similis* (Jäg.) (Digenea: Microphallidae). *Comp. Biochem. Physiol.*, **49B**, 291–299.

Marshall, I., McManus, D. P. and James, B. L. (1974b). Phosphomonoesterase activity in intertidal prosobranchs and in their digenean parasites. *Comp. Biochem. Physiol.*, **49B**, 301–306.

Martin, W. E. (1938). Studies on trematodes of Woods Hole: The life cycle of *Lepocreadium setiferoides* (Miller and Northup), Allocreadiidae, and the description of *Cercaria cumingiae* n.sp. *Biol. Bull. mar. biol. Lab., Woods Hole*, **75**, 463–473.

Martin, W. E. (1939). Studies on the trematodes of Woods Hole. II. The life cycle of *Stephanostomum tenue*. *Biol. Bull. mar. biol. Lab., Woods Hole*, **77**, 65–73.

Martin, W. E. (1945). Two new species of marine cercariae. *Trans. Am. microsc. Soc.*, **64**, 203–212.

Martin, W. E. (1950a). *Euhaplorchis californiensis* n.g., n.sp., Heterophyidae, Trematoda, with notes on its life-cycle. *Trans. Am. microsc. Soc.*, **69**, 194–209.

Martin, W. E. (1950b). *Parastictodora hancocki* n.gen., n.sp. (Trematoda: Heterophyidae), with observations on its life cycle. *J. Parasit.*, **36**, 360–370.

Martin, W. E. (1950c). *Phocitremoides ovale* n.gen., n.sp. (Trematoda: Opisthorchiidae), with observations on its life cycle. *J. Parasit.*, **36**, 552–558.

Martin, W. E. (1956a). Seasonal infections of the snail, *Cerithidea californica* Haldeman, with larval trematodes. In *Essays in the natural sciences in honour of Captain Allan Hancock*. Univ. S. Calif. Press, Los Angeles. pp. 203–210.

Martin, W. E. (1956b). The life cycle of *Catatropis johnstoni* n.sp. (Trematoda: Notocotylidae). *Trans. Am. microsc. Soc.*, **75**, 117–128.

Merrill, A. S. and Boss, K. J., (1964). Reactions of hosts to proboscis penetration by *Odostomia seminuda* (Pyramidellidae). *Nautilus*, **78**, 42–45.

Merton, H. (1906). Eine auf *Tethys leporina* parasitisch lebende Pantopodenlarve *(Nymphon parasiticum* n.sp.). *Mitt. zool. Stn Neapel*, **18**, 136–141.

Meyerhof, E. and Rothschild, M. (1940). A prolific trematode. *Nature, Lond.*, **146**, 367–368.

Michelson, E. H. (1961). An acid-fast pathogen of fresh water snails. *Am. J. trop. Med. Hyg.*, **10**, 423–433.

Millemann, R. E. (1951). *Echinocephalus pseudouncinatus* n.sp., a nematode parasite of the abalone. *J. Parasit.*, **37**, 435–439.

Millemann, R. E. (1963). Studies on the taxonomy and life history of echinocephalid worms (Nematoda: Spiruroidea) with a complete description of *Echinocephalus pseudouncinatus* Millemann, 1951. *J. Parasit.*, **49**, 754–764.

Miller, H. M. (1925a). Larval trematodes of certain marine gastropods from Puget Sound. *Publs Puget Sound mar. biol. Stn*, **5**, 75–89.

Miller, H. M. (1925b). Preliminary report on the larval trematodes infesting certain mollusks from Dry Tortugas. *Pap. Tortugas Lab.*, **24**, 232–238.

Miller, H. M. (1929). Continuation of study on behavior and reactions of marine cercariae from Tortugas. *Pap. Tortugas Lab.*, **28**, 292–294.

Miller, H. M. and Northup, F. E. (1926). The seasonal infestation of *Nassa obsoleta* (Say) with larval trematodes. *Biol. Bull. mar. biol. Lab., Woods Hole*, **50**, 490–508.

Monod, T. (1934). Sur un copépode parasite de *Trochus niloticus*. *Rec. Indian Mus.*, **36**, 213–218.

Monod, T. and Dollfus, R. P. (1932). Les copépodes parasites de mollusques. *Annls Parasit. hum. comp.*, **10**, 129–204.

Monticelli, F. S. (1888). Sulla *Cercaria setifera* Müller, breve nota preliminare del socio ordinario residente. *Boll. Soc. Nat. Napoli*, **2**, 193–199.

Monticelli, F. S. (1914). Ricerche sulle *Cercaria setifera* di Joh. Müller. *Annuar. R. Mus. zool. R. Univ. Napoli*, **4**, 1–49.

Moore, H. B. (1937). The biology of *Littorina littorea*. Part I. Growth of the shell and tissues, spawning, length of life and mortality. *J. mar. biol. Ass. U.K.,* **21**, 721–742.

Moore, H. B. (1940). The biology of *Littorina littorea*. Part II. Zonation in relation to other gastropods on stony and muddy shores. *J. mar. biol. Ass. U.K.,* **24**, 227–237.

Moore, M. N. and Halton, D. W. (1977). The cytochemical localization of lysosomal hydrolases in the digestive cells of littorinids and changes induced by larval trematode infection. *Z. ParasitKde,* **53**, 115–122.

Moose, J. W. (1963). Growth inhibition of young *Oncomelania nosophora* exposed to *Schistosoma japonicum. J. Parasit.,* **49**, 151–152.

Murray, T. and Hyland, K. E. (1976). Clam digger or swimmer—the itch is the same. *Maritimes,* **20**, 15–16.

Negus, M. R. S. (1968). The nutrition of sporocysts of the trematode *Cercaria doricha* Rothschild, 1935 in the molluscan host *Turritella communis* Risso. *Parasitology,* **58**, 355–366.

Newell, G. E. (1958a). The behaviour of *Littorina littorea* (L.) under natural conditions and its relation to position on the shore. *J. mar. biol. Ass. U.K.,* **37**, 229–239.

Newell, G. E. (1958b). An experimental analysis of the behaviour of *Littorina littorea* (L.) under natural conditions and in the laboratory. *J. mar. biol. Ass. U.K.,* **37**, 241–266.

Newell, R. C. (1966). The effect of temperature on the metabolism of poikilotherms. *Nature, Lond.,* **212**, 426–428.

Newell, R. C. (1969). Effect of fluctuations in temperature on the metabolism of intertidal invertebrates. *Am. Zool.,* **9**, 293–307.

Newell, R. C. (1970). *Biology of Intertidal Animals*, Amer. Elsevier, N.Y.

Newell, R. C. (1973). Factors affecting the respiration of intertidal invertebrates. *Am. Zool.,* **13**, 513–528.

Newell, R. C. and Bayne, B. L. (1973). A review on temperature and metabolic acclimation in intertidal marine invertebrates. *Neth. J. Sea Res.,* **7**, 421–433.

Newell, R. C. and Pye, V. J. (1970a). Seasonal changes in the effect of temperature on the oxygen consumption of the winkle *Littorina littorea* (L.) and the mussel *Mytilus edulis* L. *Comp. Biochem. Physiol.,* **34**, 367–383.

Newell, R. C. and Pye, V. J. (1970b). The influence of thermal acclimation on the relation between oxygen consumption and temperature in *Littorina littorea* (L.) and *Mytilus edulis* L. *Comp. Biochem. Physiol.,* **34**, 385–397.

Newell, R. C. and Pye, V. J. (1971a). Quantitative aspects of the relationship between metabolism and temperature in the winkle *Littorina littorea* (L.). *Comp. Biochem. Physiol.,* **38B**, 635–650.

Newell, R. C. and Pye, V. J. (1971b). Temperature-induced variations in the respiration of mitochondria from the winkle *Littorina littorea* (L.). *Comp. Biochem. Physiol.,* **40B**, 249–261.

Newell, R. C., Pye, V. J. and Ahsanullah, M. (1971). The effect of thermal acclimation on the heat tolerance of the intertidal prosobranchs *Littorina littorea* (L.) and *Monodonta lineata* (Da Costa). *J. exp. Biol.,* **54**, 525–533.

Newell, R. C. and Roy, A. (1973). A statistical model relating the oxygen consumption of a mollusk *(Littorina littorea)* to activity, body size, and environmental conditions. *Physiol. Zoöl.,* **46**, 253–275.

Nicoll, W. (1907a). *Parorchis acanthus*, the type of a new genus of trematodes. *Q. Jl microsc. Sci.,* **51**, 345–355.

Nicoll, W. (1907b). A contribution towards the knowledge of the Entozoa of British marine fishes. Part I. *Ann. Mag. nat. Hist.* (Ser. 7), **19**, 66–94.

Nicoll, W. (1910). On the Entozoa of fishes from the Firth of Clyde. *Parasitology,* **3**, 322–359.

Nicoll, W. and Small, W. (1909). Notes on larval trematodes. *Ann. Mag. nat. Hist.* (Ser. 8), **3**, 237–246.

Nielsen, R. (1972). A study of the shell-boring marine algae around the Danish island Laesø. *Bot. Tidsskr.,* **67**, 245–269.

Nishimura, S. (1976). *Dynoidella conchicola*, gen. et sp. nov. (Isopoda, Sphaeromatidae), from Japan, with a note on its association with intertidal snails. *Publs Seto mar. biol. Lab.,* **23**, 275–282.

Nybelin, O. (1936). *Bunocotyle cingulata* Odhner, ein halophiler Trematode des Flußbarsches und Kaulbarsches der Ostsee. *Ark. Zool.,* **28B**, 1–6.

Odhner, T. (1914). *Cercaria setifera* von Monticelli—die Larvenform von *Lepocreadium album* Stoss. *Zool. Bidrag Uppsala*, **3**, 247–255.

Odhner, T. (1928). Ein neuer Trematode aus dem Flußbarsch. *Ark. Zool.*, **20B**, 1–3.

Odlaug, T. O. (1946). The effect of the copepod, *Mytilicola orientalis*, upon the Olympia oyster, *Ostrea lurida. Trans. Am. microsc. Soc.*, **65**, 311–317.

Ohshima, H. (1933). Young pycnogonids found parasitic on nudibranchs. *Annotnes zool. jap.*, **14**, 61–66.

Olsson, P. J. (1867). Entozoa, iakttagna hos skandinaviska Hafsfiskar. I, Platyhelminthes. *Acta Univ. lund.*, **3**, 1–64.

Orr, P. R. (1955a). Heat death. I. Time-temperature relationships in marine animals. *Physiol. Zoöl.*, **28**, 290–294.

Orr, P. R. (1955b). II. Heat death of whole animals and tissues, various animals. *Physiol. Zoöl.*, **28**, 295–302.

Orrhage, L. (1969). On the shell growth of *Littorina littorea* (Linné) (Prosobranchiata, Gastropoda) and the occurrence of *Polydora ciliata* (Johnston) (Polychaeta, Sedentaria). *Zool. Bidr., Uppsala*, **38**, 137–153.

Orrhage, L. (1973). Description of the metacercaria of *Zoogonoides viviparus* (Olsson, 1868) Odhner, 1902 with some remarks on life cycles in the genus *Zoogonoides* (Trematoda, Digenea, Zoogonidae). *Zool. Scripta*, **2**, 179–182.

Orris, L. and Combes, F. C. (1952). Clam digger's dermatitis. *Arch. Derm. Syph.*, **66**, 367–370.

Palombi, A. (1930a). Il ciclo evolutivo di *Diphterostomum brusinae* Stoss. *Riv. Fis. Mat. Sci. nat.* (Ser. 2), **4**, 1-3.

Palombi, A. (1930b). Il ciclo biologico di *Diphterostomum brusinae* Stossich (Trematode digenetico: fam. Zoogonidae Odhner). Considerazioni sui cicli evolutivi delle specie affini e dei trematodi in generale. *Pubbl. Staz. zool. Napoli*, **10**, 111–149.

Palombi, A. (1931). Rapporti genetici tra *Lepocreadium album* Stossich e *Cercaria setifera* (non Joh. Müller) Monticelli. *Boll. Zool.*, **2**, 165–171.

Palombi, A. (1934). Gli stadi larvali dei trematodi del Golfo di Napoli. I. Contributo allo studio della morfologia, biologia e sistematica delle cercarie marine. *Pubbl. Staz. zool. Napoli*, **14**, 51–94.

Palombi, A. (1937). Il ciclo biologico di *Lepocreadium album* Stossich sperimentalmente realizzato. Osservazioni etologiche e considerazioni sistematiche sulla *Cercaria setifera* (non Joh. Müller) Monticelli. *Riv. Parassit.*, **1**, 1–12.

Palombi, A. (1938). Gli stadi larvali dei trematodi del Golfo di Napoli. 2. Contributo allo studio della morfologia, biologia e sistematica delle cercarie marine. *Riv. Parassit.*, **2**, 189–206.

Palombi, A. (1940). Gli stadi larvali dei trematodi del Golfo di Napoli. 3. Contributo allo studio della morfologia, biologia e sistematica delle cercarie marine. *Riv. Parassit.*, **4**, 7–30.

Palombi, A. and Santarelli, M. (1953). *Gli Animali Commestibili dei Mari d'Italia*, Hoepli, Milano.

Pascoe, D. (1970). Dehydrogenases in the daughter sporocysts of *Microphallus pygmaeus* (Levinsen, 1881) (Trematoda: Microphallidae). *Z. ParasitKde*, **35**, 7–15.

Pascoe, D., Richards, R. J. and James, B. L. (1970). The survival of the daughter sporocysts of *Microphallus pygmaeus* (Levinsen, 1881) (Trematoda: Microphallidae) in a chemically defined medium. *Veliger*, **13**, 157–162.

Patten, R. (1935). The life history of *Merocystis kathae* in the whelk, *Buccinum undatum. Parasitology*, **27**, 399–430.

Patten, R. (1936). Notes on a new protozoon, *Piridium sociabile* n.gen., n.sp., from the foot of *Buccinum undatum. Parasitology*, **28**, 502–516.

Pauley, G. B. (1969). A critical review of neoplasia and tumor-like lesions in mollusks. *Natn. Cancer Inst. Monogr.*, **31**, 509–539.

Pax, F. (1962). *Meeresprodukte*, Borntraeger, Berlin.

Pearse, A. S. (1938). Polyclads of the east coast of North America. *Proc. U.S. natn. Mus.*, **86**, 67–98.

Pelseneer, P. (1906). Trématodes parasites de mollusques marins. *Bull. scient. Fr. Belg.*, **40**, 161–186.

Pelseneer, P. (1914). Éthologie de quelques *Odostomia* et d'un monstrillide parasite de l'un d'eux. *Bull. biol. Fr. Belg.*, **48**, 1–14.

Pelseneer, P. (1919). Les variations et leur hérédité chez les mollusques. *Mém. Acad. r. Belg., Cl. Sci.* (Ser. 2), **5**.

Pelseneer, P. (1920). L'inversion chez les mollusques au point de vue de la variation et de l'hérédité. *Bull. biol. Fr. Belg.*, **48**, 351–380.

Penner, L. R. (1950). *Cercaria littorinalinae* sp.nov., a dermatitis-producing schistosome larva from the marine snail, *Littorina planaxis* Philippi. *J. Parasit.*, **36**, 466–472.

Penner, L. R. (1953a). The red-breasted merganser as a natural avian host of the causative agent of clam digger's itch. *J. Parasit.*, **39**, 20.

Penner, L. R. (1953b). Experimental infections of avian hosts with *Cercaria littorinalinae* Penner, 1950. *J. Parasit.*, **39**, 20.

Pérez, C. (1924). Le complexe éthnologique de la turritelle et du *Phascolion strombi. Bull. Soc. zool. Fr.*, **49**, 341–343.

Pettit, G. R., Day, J. F., Hartwell, J. L. and Wood, H. B. (1970). Antineoplastic components of marine animals. *Nature, Lond.*, **227**, 962–963.

Pohley, W. J. (1976). Relationships among three species of *Littorina* and their larval Digenea. *Mar. Biol.*, **37**, 179–186.

Pohley, W. J. and Brown, R. N. (1975). The occurrence of *Microphallus pygmaeus* and *Cercaria lebouri* in *Littorina saxatilis*, *L. obtusata*, and *L. littorea* from New England. *Proc. helminth. Soc. Wash.*, **42**, 178–179.

Polyanskij, Y. J. (1966). *Parasites of the Fish of the Barents Sea*, Israel Progr. Sci. Transl. Jerusalem.

Popiel, I. (1976). A description of *Cercaria littorinae saxatilis* V sp.nov. (Digenea: Microphallidae) from *Littorina saxatilis* subsp. *rudis* (Maton) in Cardigan Bay, Wales. *Norw. J. Zool.*, **24**, 303–306.

Prévot, G. (1967). Contribution à l'étude des cercaires de prosobranches de la région marseillaise: *Cercaria mirabilicaudata* n.sp. (Trematoda, Digenea, Opisthorchioidea) de *Cerithium vulgatum* Brug. *Bull. Soc. zool. Fr.*, **92**, 515–523.

Prévot, G. (1968). Contribution à la connaissance du cycle de *Lepidauchen stenostoma* Nicoll, 1913 (Trematoda, Digenea, Lepocreadiidae Nicoll, 1935, Lepocreadiinae Odhner, 1905). *Annls Parasit. hum. comb.*, **43**, 321–332.

Prévot, G. (1969). Les trématodes larvaires parasites de *Vermetus triqueter* Bivone (Gastéropode prosobranche marin) du golfe de Marseille. *Bull. Soc. zool. Fr.*, **94**, 463–470.

Prévot, G. (1971). Cycle évolutif d'*Aporchis massiliensis* Timon-David, 1955 (Digenea Echinostomatidae), parasite du goéland *Larus argentatus michaellis* Naumann. *Bull. Soc zool. Fr.*, **96**, 197–208.

Prévot, G. (1972a). Contribution à l'étude des Microphallidae Travassos, 1920 (Trematoda). Cycle évolutif de *Microphallus bittii* n.sp. parasite du goéland à pieds jaunes *Larus argentatus michaellis* Naumann. *Annls Parasit. hum. comp.*, **47**, 687–700.

Prévot, G. (1972b). Contribution à l'étude des Microphallidae Travassos, 1920 (Trematoda). Cycle évolutif de *Megalophallus carcini* Prévot et Deblock, 1970, parasite du goéland *(Larus argentatus). Bull. Soc. zool. Fr.*, **97**, 157–163.

Prévot, G., Bartoli, P. and Deblock, S. (1976). Cycle biologique de *Maritrema misenensis* (A. Palombi, 1940) n. comb. (Trematoda: Microphallidae Travassos, 1920) du Midi de la France. *Annls Parasit. hum. comp.*, **51**, 433–446.

Pye, V. J. and Newell, R. C. (1973). Factors affecting thermal compensation in the oxidative metabolism of the winkle *Littorina littorea. Neth. J. Sea Res.*, **7**, 411–420.

Raabe, J. and Raabe, Z. (1959). Urceolariidae of molluscs from Baltic Sea. *Acta parasit. pol.*, **7**, 453–465.

Randall, J. E. (1964). Contributions to the biology of the queen conch, *Strombus gigas. Bull. mar. Sci. Gulf Caribb.*, **14**, 246–295.

Rankin, J. S. (1939). Ecological studies on larval trematodes from western Massachusetts. *J. Parasit.*, **25**, 309–328.

Rankin, J. S. (1940). Studies on the trematode family Microphallidae Travassos, 1921. IV. The life cycle and ecology of *Gynaecotyla nassicola* (Cable and Hunninen, 1938) Yamaguti, 1939. *Biol. Bull. mar. biol. Lab., Woods Hole*, **79**, 439–451.

Rasmussen, E. (1973). Systematics and ecology of the Isefjord marine fauna (Denmark). *Ophelia*, **11**, 1–495.

Rebecq, J. (1961). Rôle du mollusque d'eau saumâtre *Hydrobia ventrosa* (Montagu) dans le cycle évolutif de deux trématodes en Camargue. *C. r. hebd. Séanc. Acad. Sci., Paris*, **253**, 2007–2009.

Rebecq, J. (1964a). Recherches systématiques, biologiques et écologiques sur les formes larvaires de quelques trématodes de Camargue. Diss. Univ. Aix-Marseille.

Rebecq, J. (1964b). Trématodes de Camargue; quelques larves aquatiques et leur écologie. *Terre Vie*, **111**, 388–392.

Rees, G. (1934). *Cercaria patellae* Lebour, 1911, and its effect on the digestive gland and gonads of *Patella vulgata. Proc. zool. Soc. Lond.*, **1**, 45–53.

Rees, G. (1937). The anatomy and encystment of *Cercaria purpurae* Lebour, 1911. *Proc. zool. Soc. Lond.* (Ser. B), **107**, 65–73.

Rees, G. (1939). *Cercaria strigata* Lebour from *Cardium edule* and *Tellina tenuis. Parasitology*, **31**, 458–463.

Rees, G. (1940). Studies on the germ-cell cycle of the digenetic trematode *Parorchis acanthus* Nicoll. Part II. Structure of the miracidium and germinal development in the larval stages. *Parasitology*, **32**, 372–391.

Rees, G. (1948). A study of the effect of light, temperature and salinity on the emergence of *Cercaria purpurae* Lebour from *Nucella lapillus* (L.). *Parasitology*, **38**, 228–242.

Rees, G. (1966). Light and electron microscope studies of the redia of *Parorchis acanthus* Nicoll. *Parasitology*, **56**, 589–602.

Rees, G. (1967). The histochemistry of the cystogenous gland cells and cyst wall of *Parorchis acanthus* Nicoll, and some details of the morphology and fine structure of the cercaria. *Parasitology*, **57**, 87–110.

Rees, G. (1971a). The ultrastructure of the epidermis of the redia and cercaria of *Parorchis acanthus* Nicoll. A study by scanning and transmission electron-microscopy. *Parasitology*, **62**, 479–488.

Rees, G. (1971b) Locomotion of the cercaria of *Parorchis acanthus* Nicoll and the ultrastructure of the tail. *Parasitology*, **62**, 489–503.

Rees, G. (1974). The ultrastructure of the body wall and associated structures of the cercaria of *Cryptocotyle lingua* (Creplin) (Digenea: Heterophyidae) from *Littorina littorea* (L.). *Z. Parasitkde*, **44**, 239–265.

Rees, W. J. (1935). The anatomy of *Cercaria buccini* Lebour, 1911. *Proc. zool. Soc. Lond.*, **2**, 309–312.

Rees, W. J. (1936a). The effect of parasitism by larval trematodes on the tissues of *Littorina littorea* (Linné). *Proc. zool. Soc. Lond.*, **2**, 357–368.

Rees, W. J. (1936b). Note on the ubiquitous cercaria from *Littorina rudis, L. obtusata* and *L. littorea. J. mar. biol. Ass. U.K.*, **20**, 621–624.

Rees, W. J. (1967). A brief survey of the symbiotic associations of Cnidaria with Mollusca. *Proc. malac. Soc. Lond.*, **37**, 213–231.

Reimer, L. W. (1961). Die Stufen der Progenesis bei dem Fischtrematoden *Bunocotyle cingulata* Ohdner, 1928. *Wiad. parazyt.*, **7**, 834–849.

Reimer, L. W. (1962). Die digenetischen Trematoden der Wasservögel der Insel Hiddensee und ihre Larvalstadien aus den die Insel umgebenden Brackgewässern. Diss. Univ. Greifswald.

Reimer, L. W. (1963a). Zur Verbreitung der Adulti und Larvenstadien der Familie Microphallidae Viana, 1924 (Trematoda, Digenea) in der mittleren Ostsee. *Z. ParasitKde*, **23**, 253–273.

Reimer, L. W. (1963b). *Gigantobilharzia vittensis*, ein neuer Schistosomatide aus den Darmvenen von *Larus canus* und *Cercaria hiddensoensis* spec. nov., als mögliches Larvalstadium dieser Art. *Zool. Anz.*, **171**, 469–478.

Reimer, L. W. (1964a). The salt contents—a factor determining the development of fish- and bird trematodes in the middle Baltic Sea. In *Proceedings of the Symposium on Parasitic Worms and Aquatic Conditions*. Prague, **1962**, 63–68.

Reimer, L. W. (1964b). Life-cycles of Psilostomatidae Odhner, 1911, emend. Nicoll, 1935 (Trematoda, Digenea). In *Proceedings of the Symposium on Parasitic Worms and Aquatic Conditions*. Prague, **1962**, 99–106.

Reimer, L. W. (1970). Digene Trematoden und Cestoden der Ostseefische als natürliche Fischmarken. *Parasit. SchrReihe*, **20**, 1–144.

Reimer, L. W. (1973). Das Auftreten eines Fischtrematoden der Gattung *Asymphylodora* Looss, 1899, bei *Nereis diversicolor* O. F. Müller als Beispiel für einen Alternativzyklus. *Zool. Anz.,* **191**, 187–196.

Reimer, L. W. and Anantaraman, S. (1968). *Cercaria melanocrucifera*, a new magnacercus cercaria (Opisthorchioidea) from the marine gastropod, *Turritella attenuata* Reeve, 1897, from the Bay of Bengal, Madras. *Curr. Sci.,* **37**, 316–318.

Reimer, L. W. and Bernstein, D. (1973). Zur Saisondynamik des Befalls mit Parthenitae der digenen Trematoden bei Hydrobiidae der Ostseeküste. *Wiss. Z. pädag. Hochsch. "Liselotte Herrmann", Güstrow,* **1973**, 73–79.

Richard, J. (1977). Cercariae of Microphallidae: determination of the genera *Microphallus* Ward, 1901 and *Maritrema* Nicoll, 1907 according to chaetotaxy. *Parasitology,* **75**, 31–43.

Richards, R. J. (1969). Qualitative and quantitative estimations of the free amino acids in the healthy and parasitised digestive gland and gonad of *Littorina saxatilis tenebrosa* (Mont.) and in the daughter sporocysts of *Microphallus pygmaeus* (Levinsen, 1881) and *Microphallus similis* (Jägerskiöld, 1900) (Trematoda: Microphallidae). *Comp. Biochem. Physiol.,* **31**, 655–665.

Richards, R. J. (1970a). Variations in the oxygen uptake, reduced weight and metabolic rate of starving sporocysts of *Microphallus pygmaeus* (Levinsen, 1881) (Trematoda: Microphallidae). *J. Helminth.,* **44**, 75–88.

Richards, R. J. (1970b). The leakage and transamination of amino acids in vitro, by the germinal sacs of Digenea from marine molluscs. *J. Helminth.,* **44**, 231–241.

Richards, R. J. (1970c). The effect of starvation in vitro, on the free amino acids and sugars in the daughter sporocysts of *Microphallus pygmaeus* (Levinsen, 1881) (Trematoda: Microphallidae). *Z. ParasitKde,* **35**, 31–39.

Richards, R. J., Pascoe, D. and James, B. L. (1972). Variations in the metabolism of the daughter sporocysts of *Microphallus pygmaeus* in a chemically defined medium. *J. Helminth.,* **46**, 107–116.

Riel, A. (1975). Effect of trematodes on survival of *Nassarius obsoletus* (Say). *Proc. malac. Soc. Lond.,* **41**, 527–528.

Robertson, R. (1957). Gastropod host of an *Odostomia. Nautilus,* **70**, 96–97.

Robertson, R. and Merrill, A. S. (1963). Abnormal dextral hyperstrophy of postlarval *Heliacus* (Gastropoda: Architectonicidae). *Veliger,* **6**, 76–79.

Robertson, R. and Orr, V. (1961). Review of pyramidellid hosts, with notes on an *Odostomia* parasitic on a chiton. *Nautilus,* **74**, 85–91.

Robson, E. M. and Williams, I. C. (1970). Relationships of some species of Digenea with the marine prosobranch *Littorina littorea* (L.) I. The occurrence of larval Digenea in *L. littorea* on the North Yorkshire coast. *J. Helminth.,* **44**, 153–168.

Robson, E. M. and Williams, I. C. (1971a). Relationships of some species of Digenea with the marine prosobranch *Littorina littorea* (L.) II. The effect of larval Digenea on the reproductive biology of *L. littorea. J. Helminth.,* **45**, 145–159.

Robson, E. M. and Williams, I. C. (1971b). Relationships of some species of Digenea with the marine prosobranch *Littorina littorea* (L.) III. The effect of larval Digenea on the glycogen content of the digestive gland and foot of *Littorina littorea. J. Helminth.,* **45**, 381–401.

Rohlack, S. (1959). Über das Vorkommen von Sexualhormonen bei der Meeresschnecke *Littorina littorea* L. *Z. vergl. Physiol.,* **42**, 164–180.

Rothschild, A. and Rothschild, M. (1939). Some observations on the growth of *Peringia ulvae* Pennant 1777, in the laboratory. *Novit. zool.,* **41**, 240–247.

Rothschild, M. (1935a). The trematode parasites of *Turritella communis* Lmk. from Plymouth and Naples. *Parasitology,* **27**, 152–170.

Rothschild, M. (1935b). Notes on the excretory system of *Cercaria ephemera* Lebour 1907 (nec Nitzsch). *Parasitology,* **27**, 171–174.

Rothschild, M. (1936a). Preliminary note on the trematode parasites of *Peringia ulvae* (Pennant, 1777). *Novit. zool.,* **39**, 268–269.

Rothschild, M. (1936b). Gigantism and variation in *Peringia ulvae* (Pennant, 1777), caused by infection with larval trematodes. *J. mar. biol. Ass. U.K.,* **20**, 537–546.

Rothschild, M. (1938a). *Cercaria sinitsini* n.sp., a cystophorous cercaria from *Peringia ulvae* (Pennant, 1777). *Novit. zool.,* **41**, 42–57.

Rothschild, M. (1938b). Notes on the classification of cercariae of the superfamily Notocotyloidea (Trematoda), with special reference to the excretory system. *Novit. zool.*, **41**, 75–83.

Rothschild, M. (1938c). Further observations on the effect of trematode parasites on *Peringia ulvae* (Pennant, 1777). *Novit. zool.*, **41**, 84–102.

Rothschild, M. (1938d). A note on the fin-folds of cercariae of the superfamily Opisthorchioidea Vogel 1934 (Trematoda). *Novit. zool.*, **41**, 170–173.

Rothschild, M. (1938e). The excretory system of *Cercaria coronanda* n.sp. together with notes on its life history and the classification of cercariae of the superfamily Opisthorchioidea Vogel 1934 (Trematoda). *Novit. zool.*, **41**, 178–180.

Rothschild, M. (1938f). Preliminary note on the life-history of *Cryptocotyle jejuna* Nicoll, 1907 (Trematoda). *Ann. Mag. nat. Hist.*, **1**, 238–239.

Rothschild, M. (1939). A note on the life cycle of *Cryptocotyle lingua* (Creplin, 1825) (Trematoda). *Novit. zool.*, **41**, 178–180.

Rothschild, M. (1941a). Observations on the growth and trematode infections of *Peringia ulvae* (Pennant, 1777) in a pool in the Tamar Saltings, Plymouth. *Parasitology*, **33**, 406–415.

Rothschild, M. (1941b). The metacercaria of a pleurophocercous cercaria parasitizing *Peringia ulvae* (Pennant, 1777). *Parasitology*, **33**, 439–444.

Rothschild, M. (1941c). The effect of trematode parasites on the growth of *Littorina neritoides* (L.). *J. mar. biol. Ass. U.K.*, **25**, 69–80.

Rothschild, M. (1942a). A further note on life history experiments with *Cryptocotyle lingua* (Creplin, 1825). *J. Parasit.*, **28**, 91–92.

Rothschild, M. (1942b). Seven years old infection of *Cryptocotyle lingua* in the winkle *Littorina littorea* L. *J. Parasit.*, **28**, 350.

Russell-Hunter, W. D. and McMahon, R. F. (1974). Patterns of aerial and aquatic respiration in relation to vertical zonation in four littoral snails. *Biol. Bull. mar. biol. Lab., Woods Hole*, **147**, 496–497.

Sandeen, M. J., Stephens, G. C. and Brown, F. A., (1954). Persistent daily and tidal rhythms of oxygen consumption in two species of marine snails. *Physiol. Zoöl.*, **27**, 350–356.

Sandison, E. E. (1966). The oxygen consumption of some intertidal gastropods in relation to zonation. *J. Zool.*, **149**, 163–173.

Sandison, E. E. (1967). Respiratory response to temperature and temperature tolerance of some intertidal gastropods. *J. exp. mar. Biol Ecol.*, **1**, 271–281.

Sannia, A. and James, B. L. (1977). The Digenea in marine molluscs from Eyjafjördur, North Iceland. *Ophelia*, **16**, 97–109.

Sarkisian, L. N. (1957). *Maritrema uca*, new species (Trematoda: Microphallidae), from the fiddler crab, *Uca crenulata* (Lockington). *Wasmann J. Biol.*, **15**, 35–48.

Schechter, V. (1943). Two flatworms from the oyster-drilling snail *Thais floridana haysae* Clench. *J. Parasit.*, **29**, 362.

Schilansky, M. M., Levin, N. L. and Fried, G. H. (1977). Metabolic implications of glucose-6-phosphate dehydrogenase and lactic dehydrogenase in two marine gastropods. *Comp. Biochem. Physiol.*, **56B**, 1–4.

Schwarz, A. (1932). Der Lichteinfluß auf die Fortbewegung, die Einregelung und das Wachstum bei einigen Niederen Tieren *(Littorina, Cardium, Mytilus, Balanus, Teredo, Sabellaria)*. *Senckenbergiana*, **14**, 429–454.

Shaw, R. C. (1933). Observations on *Cercariaeum lintoni* Miller and Northup and its metacercarial development. *Biol. Bull. mar. biol. Lab., Woods Hole*, **64**, 262–275.

Short, R. B. and Holliman, R. B. (1961). *Austrobilharzia penneri*, a new schistosome from marine snails. *J. Parasit.*, **47**, 447–452.

Simpson, G. G., Roe, A. and Lewontin, R. C. (1960). *Quantitative Zoology*, Harcourt, Brace & Co., New York.

Sindermann, C. J. (1956). The ecology of marine dermatitis-producing schistosomes. I. Seasonal variation in infection of mud snails *(Nassa obsoleta)* with larvae of *Austrobilharzia variglandis*. *J. Parasit.*, **42** (Suppl.), 27.

Sindermann, C. J. (1960). Ecological studies of marine dermatitis-producing schistosome larvae in northern New England. *Ecology*, **41**, 678–684.

Sindermann, C. J. (1961). The effect of larval trematode parasites on snail migration. *Am. Zool.*, **1**, 389.

Sindermann, C. J. (1966). Epizootics in oyster populations. *Proc. Pacif. Sci. Congr. 1966*, **7**, 9.
Sindermann, C. J. (1970a). *Principal Diseases of Marine Fish and Shellfish*, Academic Press, London.
Sindermann, C. J. (1970b). Bibliography of diseases and parasites of marine fish and shellfish (with emphasis on commercially important species). *Informal Rep. trop. Atlant. biol. Lab.*, **11**, 440.
Sindermann, C. J. and Farrin, A. E. (1962). Ecological studies of *Cryptocotyle lingua* (Trematoda: Heterophyidae) whose larvae cause 'pigment spots' of marine fish. *Ecology*, **43**, 69–75.
Sindermann, C. J. and Gibbs, R. F. (1953). A dermatitis-producing schistosome which causes "clam diggers' itch" along the central Maine coast. *Maine Dept. Sea Shore Fish., Res. Bull*, **12**, 1–20.
Sindermann, C. J. and Rosenfield, A. (1957). The ecology of marine dermatitis-producing schistosomes. III. Oxygen consumption of normal and parasitized *Nassarius obsoletus* under varying conditions of salinity. *J. Parasit.*, **43** (Suppl.), 28.
Sindermann, C. J. and Rosenfield, A. (1967). Principal diseases of commercially important marine bivalve Mollusca and Crustacea. *Fishery Bull. Fish Wildl. Serv. U.S.*, **66**, 335–385.
Sindermann, C. J., Rosenfield, A. and Strom, L. (1957). The ecology of marine dermatitis-producing schistosomes. II. Effects of certain environmental factors on emergence of cercariae of *Austrobilharzia variglandis*. *J. Parasit.*, **43**, 382.
Sinitsin, D. F. (1911). Parthenogenetic generation of trematodes and its progeny in molluscs of the Black Sea. *Mém. Acad. Sci. St.-Petersb.* (Ser. 8), **30**, 1–127.
Smart, R. W. J. (1887). New habitat for *Odostomia pallida*. *J. Conch., Lond.*, **5**, 152.
Smith, A. C. and Taylor, R. L. (1968). Tumefactions (tumor-like swellings) on the foot of the moon snail, *Polinices lewisi*. *J. Invertebr. Pathol.*, **10**, 263–268.
Smith, B. S. (1971). Sexuality in the American mud snail, *Nassarius obsoletus* Say. *Proc. malac. Soc. Lond.*, **39**, 377–378.
Smith, J. E. and Newell, G. E. (1955). The dynamics of the zonation of the common periwinkle (*Littorina littorea* (L.)) on a stony beach. *J. Anim. Ecol.*, **24**, 35–56.
Snedecor, G. W. and Cochran, W. G. (1967). *Statistical Methods* (6th ed.), Iowa State Univ. Press, Ames, Iowa.
Sömme, L. (1967). Seasonal changes in the freezing tolerance of some intertidal animals. *Nytt Mag. Zool.*, **13**, 52–55.
Southward, A. J. (1958). Note on the temperature tolerances of some intertidal animals in relation to environmental temperatures and geographical distribution. *J. mar. biol. Ass. U.K.*, **37**, 49–66.
Sparrow, F. K. (1974). Observations on two uncommon marine fungi. *Veröff. Inst. Meeresforsch. Bremerh.*, **5** (Suppl.), 9–18.
Stambaugh, J. E. and McDermot, J. J. (1969). The effects of trematode larvae on the locomotion of naturally infected *Nassarius obsoletus* (Gastropoda). *Proc. Acad. nat. Sci. Philad.*, **43**, 226–231.
Stauber, L. A. (1941). The polyclad, *Hoploplana inquilina thaisana* Pearse, 1938, from the mantle cavity of oyster drills. *J. Parasit.*, **27**, 541–542.
Stephenson, T. A. and Stephenson, A. (1972). *Life between Tidemarks on Rocky Shores*, W. H. Freeman & Co., San Fransisco.
Stock, J. H. (1960). Sur quelques copépodes associés aux invertébrés des côtes du Roussillon. *Crustaceana*, **1**, 218–257.
Stock, J. H., Humes, A. G. and Gooding, R. U. (1963). Copepoda associated with West Indian invertebrates. IV. The genera *Octopicola, Pseudanthessius* and *Meomicola* (Cyclopoida, Lichomolgidae). *Stud. Fauna Curaçao*, **18**, 1–74.
Stohler, R. (1960). Fluctuations in mollusk populations after a red tide in the Estero de Punta Banda, Lower California, Mexico. *Veliger*, **3**, 23–28.
Stunkard, H. W. (1930). The life history of *Cryptocotyle lingua* (Creplin), with notes on the physiology of the metacercariae. *J. Morph.*, **50**, 143–191.
Stunkard, H. W. (1932). Some larval trematodes from the coast in the region of Roscoff, Finistère. *Parasitology*, **24**, 321–343.

Stunkard, H. W. (1933). Further observations on the life cycle of *Cercariaeum lintoni*. *Anat. Rec.*, **57** (Suppl.), 99–100.

Stunkard, H. W. (1934). The life history of *Himasthla quissetensis* (Miller and Northup, 1926). *J. Parasit.*, **20**, 20, 336.

Stunkard, H. W. (1936). The life cycle of *Cercariaeum lintoni* Miller and Northup. *J. Parasit.*, **22**, 542–543.

Stunkard, H. W. (1938a). The morphology and life cycle of *Himasthla quissetensis* (Miller and Northup, 1926). *Biol. Bull. mar. biol. Lab., Woods Hole*, **75**, 145–164.

Stunkard, H. W. (1938b). *Distomum lasium* Leidy, 1891 (Syn. *Cercariaeum lintoni* Miller and Northup, 1926). the larval stage of *Zoögonus rubellus* (Olsson, 1868) (Syn. *Z. mirus* Looss, 1901). *Biol. Bull. mar. biol. Lab., Woods Hole*, **75**, 308–334.

Stunkard, H. W. (1941). Specificity and host relations in the trematode genus *Zoogonus*. *Biol. Bull. mar. biol. Lab., Woods Hole*, **81**, 205–214.

Stunkard, H. W. (1943). The morphology and life history of the digenetic trematode, *Zoogonoides laevis* Linton, 1940. *Biol. Bull. mar. biol. Lab., Woods Hole*, **85**, 227–237.

Stunkard, H. W. (1950). Further observations on *Cercaria parvicaudata* Stunkard and Shaw, 1931. *Biol. Bull. mar. biol. Lab., Woods Hole*, **99**, 136–142.

Stunkard, H. W. (1951). Causative agents of swimmer's itch in Narragansett Bay, Rhode Island. *J. Parasit.*, **37**, 26–27.

Stunkard, H. W. (1957a). The morphology and life history of the digenetic trematode, *Microphallus similis* Jägerskiöld, 1900) Baer, 1943. *Biol. Bull. mar. biol. Lab., Woods Hole*, **112**, 254–266.

Stunkard, H. W. (1957b). Intraspecific variation in parasitic flatworms. *Syst. Zool.*, **6**, 7–18.

Stunkard, H. W. (1958). The morphology and life history of *Levinseniella minuta* (Trematoda: Microphallidae). *J. Parasit.*, **44**, 225–230.

Stunkard, H. W. (1959a). Progenesis in digenetic trematodes and its possible significance in the development of present life-histories. *Biol. Bull. mar. biol. Lab., Woods Hole*, **117**, 400–401.

Stunkard, H. W. (1959b). The morphology and life-history of the digenetic trematode, *Asymphylodora amnicolae* n.sp.; the possible significance of progenesis for the phylogeny of the Digenea. *Biol. Bull. mar. biol. Lab., Woods Hole*, **117**, 562–581.

Stunkard, H. W. (1960a). Further studies on the trematode genus *Himasthla* with descriptions of *H. mcintoshi* n.sp., *H. piscicola* n.sp., and stages in the life-history of *H. compacta* n.sp. *Biol. Bull. mar. biol. Lab., Woods Hole*, **119**, 529–549.

Stunkard, H. W. (1960b). Studies on the morphology and life-history of *Notocotylus minutus* n.sp., a digenetic trematode from ducks. *J. Parasit.*, **46**, 803–809.

Stunkard, H. W. (1961). *Cercaria dipterocerca* Miller and Northup, 1926 and *Stephanostomum dentatum* (Linton, 1900) Manter, 1931. *Biol. Bull. mar. biol. Lab., Woods Hole*, **120**, 221–237.

Stunkard, H. W. (1964a). The morphology, life-history, and systematics of the digenetic trematode, *Homalometron pallidum* Stafford, 1904. *Biol. Bull. mar. biol. Lab., Woods Hole*, **126**, 163–173.

Stunkard, H. W. (1964b). Studies on the trematode genus *Renicola*: observations on the life history, specificity and systematic position. *Biol. Bull. mar. biol. Lab., Woods Hole*, **126**, 467–489.

Stunkard, H. W. (1966a). The morphology and life-history of *Himasthla littorinae* n.sp. (Echinostomatidae). *J. Parasit.*, **52**, 367–372.

Stunkard, H. W. (1966b). The morphology and life-history of *Notocotylus atlanticus* n.sp., a digenetic trematode of eider ducks, *Somateria mollissima*, and the designation, *Notocotylus duboisi* nom. nov., for *Notocotylus imbricatus* (Looss, 1893) Szidat, 1935. *Biol. Bull. mar. biol. Lab., Woods Hole*, **131**, 501–515.

Stunkard, H. W. (1967a). Studies on the trematode genus *Paramonostomum* Lühe, 1909 (Notocotylidae). *Biol. Bull. mar. biol. Lab., Woods Hole*, **132**, 133–145.

Stunkard, H. W. (1967b). The morphology, life-history, and systematic relations of the digenetic trematode, *Uniserialis breviserialis* sp. nov. (Notocotylidae), a parasite of the Bursa Fabricius of birds. *Biol. Bull. mar. biol. Lab., Woods Hole*, **132**, 266–276.

Stunkard, H. W. (1967c). Platyhelminthic parasites of invertebrates. *J. Parasit.*, **53**, 673–682.

Stunkard, H. W. (1968). The asexual generations, life-cycle, and systematic relations of *Microphallus limuli* Stunkard, 1951 (Trematoda: Digenea). *Biol. Bull. mar. biol. Lab., Woods Hole*, **134**, 332–343.

Stunkard, H. W. (1970a). The marine cercariae of the Woods Hole, Massachusetts region. *Biol. Bull. mar. biol. Lab., Woods Hole*, **138**, 66–76.

Stunkard, H. W. (1970b). Trematode parasites of insular and relict vertebrates. *J. Parasit.*, **56**, 1041–1054.

Stunkard, H. W. and Cable, R. M. (1932). The life history of *Parorchis avitus* Linton, a trematode from the cloaca of the gull. *Biol. Bull. mar. biol. Lab., Woods Hole*, **62**, 328–338.

Stunkard, H. W. and Hinchliffe, M. C. (1951). The life-cycle of *Microbilharzia variglandis* (= *Cercaria variglandis* Miller and Northup, 1926), an avian schistosome whose larvae produce 'swimmer's itch' of ocean beaches. *Anat. Rec.*, **111**, 113–114.

Stunkard, H. W. and Hinchliffe, M. C. (1952). The morphology and life-history of *Microbilharzia variglandis* (Miller & Northup, 1926) Stunkard & Hinchliffe, 1951, avian blood-flukes whose larvae cause 'swimmer's itch' on ocean beaches. *Parasitology*, **38**, 248–265.

Stunkard, H. W. and Shaw, R. C. (1931). The effect of dilution of sea water on the activity and the longevity of certain marine cercariae, with descriptions of two new species. *Biol. Bull. mar. biol. Lab., Woods Hole*, **61**, 242–271.

Stunkard, H. W. and Uzmann, J. R. (1958). Studies on digenetic trematodes of the genera *Gymnophallus* and *Parvatrema*. *Biol. Bull. mar. biol. Lab., Woods Hole*, **115**, 276–302.

Styczynska-Jurewicz, E. (1971). Tolerance to salinity in some marine and fresh-water cercariae. *Acta parasit. pol.*, **19**, 257–268.

Szidat, L. (1956). Über den Entwicklungszyklus mit progenetischen Larvenstadien (Cercarieen) von *Genarchella genarchella* Travassos, 1928 (Trematoda, Hemiuridae). *Z. Tropenmed. Parasit.*, **7**, 132–153.

Szidat, L. (1957). Über den Entwicklungszyklus von *Psilochasmus oxyurus* (Creplin 1825) Lühe 1910 (Trematoda, Psilostomatidae) in Argentinien. *Z. ParasitKde*, **18**, 24–35.

Tallmark, B. and Norrgren, G. (1976). The influence of parasitic trematodes on the ecology of *Nassarius reticulatus* (L.) in Gullmar Fjord (Sweden). *Zoon*, **4**, 149–156.

Threlfall, W. and Goudie, R. J. (1977). Larval trematodes in the rough periwinkle, *Littorina saxatilis* (Olivi) from Newfoundland. *Proc. helminth. Soc. Wash.*, **44**, 229.

Toulmond, A. (1967a). Étude de la consommation d'oxygène en fonction du poids, dans l'air et dans l'eau, chez quatre espèces du genre *Littorina* (Gastropoda, Prosobranchiata). *C.r. hebd. Séanc. Acad. Sci., Paris*, **264**, 636–638.

Toulmond, A. (1967b). Consommation d'oxygène dans l'air et dans l'eau, chez quatre gastéropodes du genre *Littorina*. *J. Physiol., Paris*, **59**, 303–304.

Underwood, A. J. (1973). Studies on zonation of intertidal prosobranch molluscs in the Plymouth region. *J. Anim. Ecol.*, **42**, 353–372.

Vaes, F. (1974). A new type of trematode life-cycle: An invertebrate as final host. *Proc. 3rd intern. Congr. Parasitol., Munich*, **1**, 351.

Vermeij, G. J. (1972). Intraspecific shore-level size gradients in intertidal molluscs. *Ecology*, **53**, 693–700.

Vernberg, W. B. (1961). Studies on oxygen consumption in digenetic trematodes. VI. Influence of temperature on larval trematodes. *Expl Parasit.*, **11**, 270–275.

Vernberg, W. B. (1963). Respiration of digenetic trematodes. *Ann. N.Y. Acad. Sci.*, **113**, 261–271.

Vernberg, W. B. (1969). Adaptations of host and symbionts in the intertidal zone. *Am. Zool.*, **9**, 357–365.

Vernberg, W. B. and Hunter, W. S. (1959). Studies on oxygen consumption in digenetic trematodes. III. The relationship of body nitrogen to oxygen uptake. *Expl Parasit.*, **8**, 76–82.

Vernberg, W. B. and Hunter, W. S. (1960). Studies on oxygen consumption in digenetic trematodes. IV. Oxidative pathways in the trematode *Gynaecotyla adunca* (Linton, 1905). *Expl Parasit.*, **9**, 42–46.

Vernberg, W. B. and Hunter, W. S. (1961). Studies on oxygen consumption in digenetic trematodes. V. The influence of temperature on three species of adult trematodes. *Expl Parasit.*, **11**, 34–38.

Vernberg, W. B. and Hunter, W. S. (1963). Utilization of certain substrates by larval and adult stages of *Himasthla quissetensis*. *Expl Parasit.*, **14**, 311–315.

Vernberg, W. B. and Vernberg, F. J. (1963). Influence of parasitism on thermal resistance of the mud-flat snail, *Nassarius obsoletus* Say. *Expl Parasit.*, **14**, 330–332.

Vernberg, W. B. and Vernberg, F. J. (1967). Interrelationships between parasites and their hosts. III. Effect of larval trematodes on the thermal metabolic response of their molluscan host. *Expl Parasit.*, **20**, 225–231.

Vernberg, W. B. and Vernberg, F. J. (1968). Interrelationships between parasites and their hosts. IV. Cytochrome c oxidase thermal-acclimation patterns in a larval trematode and its host. *Expl Parasit.*, **23**, 347–354.

Vernberg, W. B., Vernberg, F. J. and Beckerdite, F. W. (1969). Larval trematodes: Double infections in common mud-flat snail. *Science, N.Y.*, **164**, 1287–1288.

Virkar, R. A. and Webb, K. L. (1970). Free amino acid composition of the soft-shell clam *Mya arenaria* in relation to salinity of the medium. *Comp. Biochem. Physiol.*, **32**, 775–783.

Vishniac, H. S. (1955). The morphology and nutrition of a new species of *Sirolpidium*. *Mycologia*, **47**, 633–645.

Vishniac, H. S. (1958). A new marine phycomycete. *Mycologia*, **50**, 66–79.

Wagner, A. (1960). Maintenance of a marine snail in the laboratory. *J. Parasit.*, **46**, 186.

Walne, P. R. (1958). The importance of bacteria in laboratory experiments on rearing the larvae of *Ostrea edulis* (L.). *J. mar. biol. Ass. U.K.*, **37**, 415–425.

Watts, S. D. M. (1970a). The amino acid requirements of rediae of *Cryptocotyle lingua* and *Himasthla leptosoma* and of the sporocyst of *Cercaria emasculans* Pelseneer, 1900. *Parasitology*, **61**, 491–497.

Watts, S. D. M. (1970b). Transamination in homogenates of rediae of *Cryptocotyle lingua* and of sporocysts of *Cercaria emasculans* Pelseneer, 1900. *Parasitology*, **61**, 499–504.

Watts, S. D. M. (1971). Effects of larval Digenea on the free amino acid pool of *Littorina littorea* (L.). *Parasitology*, **62**, 361–366.

Watts, S. D. M. (1972). Amino acid flux in the sporocysts of *Cercaria emasculans* Pelseneer, 1906 in vitro. *Parasitology*, **64**, 1–4.

Wells, H. W. (1959). Notes on *Odostomia impressa* (Say). *Nautilus*, **72**, 140–144.

Wells, H. W. and Wells, M. J. (1961). Three species of *Odostomia* from North Carolina, with description of new species. *Nautilus*, **74**, 149–157.

Werding, B. (1969). Morphologie, Entwicklung und Ökologie digener Trematoden-Larven der Strandschnecke *Littorina littorea*. *Mar. Biol.*, **3**, 306–333.

Wesenberg-Lund, C. (1934). Contributions to the development of the Trematoda Digenea. Part II. The biology of the freshwater cercariae in Danish freshwaters. *K. danske vidensk. Selsk. Skr.* (Naturv. math. afd. R.S.), **3**, 1–221.

Westblad, E. (1926). Parasitische Turbellarien von der Westküste Skandinaviens. *Zool. Anz.*, **68**, 212–216.

Wilbur, K. M. and Yonge, C. M. (Eds) (1964). *Physiology of Mollusca*, Vol. I, Academic Press, New York and London.

Wilbur, K. M. and Yonge, C. M. (Eds) (1966). *Physiology of Mollusca*, Vol. II, Academic Press, New York and London.

Willey, C. H. and Gross, P. R. (1957). Pigmentation in the foot of *Littorina littorea* as a means of recognition of infection with trematode larvae. *J. Parasit.*, **43**, 324–327.

Williams, E. E. (1964). Growth and distribution of *Littorina littorea* on a rocky shore in Wales. *J. Anim. Ecol.*, **33**, 413–432.

Williams, I. C. and Ellis, C. (1975). Movements of the common periwinkle, *Littorina littorea* (L.), on the Yorkshire coast in winter and the influence of infection with larval Digenea. *J. exp. mar. Biol. Ecol.*, **17**, 47–58.

Wolfgang, R. W. (1954a). Studies of the trematode *Stephanostomum baccatum* (Nicoll, 1907): I. The distribution of the metacercaria in eastern Canadian flounders. *J. Fish. Res. Bd Can.*, **11**, 954–963.

Wolfgang, R. W. (1954b). Studies of the trematode *Stephanostomum baccatum* (Nicoll, 1907): II. Biology, with special reference to the stages affecting the winter flounder. *J. Fish. Res. Bd Can.*, **11**, 963–987.

Wolfgang, R. W. (1954a). Studies of the trematode *Stephanostomum baccatum* (Nicoll, 1907): I, The life cycle. *Can. J. Zool.*, **33**, 113–128.

Wolfgang, R. W. (1955b). Studies of the trematode *Stephanostomum baccatum* (Nicoll, 1907). IV. The variation of the adult morphology and the taxonomy of the genus. *Can. J. Zool.*, **33**, 129–142.

Woodbridge, R. G. (1976). Tentacle-branching in the periwinkle, *Littorina littorea*. *Nautilus*, **90**, 52–53.

Wootton, D. M. (1957). The life history of *Cryptocotyle concavum* (Creplin, 1825) Fischoeder, 1903 (Trematoda: Heterophyidae). *J. Parasit.*, **43**, 271–279.

Wright, C. A. (1966). The pathogenesis of helminths in the Mollusca. *Helminth. Abstr.*, **35**, 207–224.

Yamaguti, S. (1936). Parasitic copepods from mollusks of Japan. I. *Jap. J. Zool.*, **7**, 113–127.

Yoshino, T. P. (1975). A seasonal and histologic study of larval Digenea infecting *Cerithidea californica* (Gastropoda: Prosobranchia) from Goleta Slough (Santa Barbara County, California). *Veliger*, **18**, 156–161.

Yoshino, T. P. (1976). Histopathological effects of larval Digenea on the digestive epithelia of the marine prosobranch *Cerithidea californica:* fine structural changes in the digestive gland. *J. Invertebr. Pathol.*, **28**, 209–216.

Yusuf, J. A. and Choudhury, A. (1977). On the morphology and biology of a new arhynchodine thigmotrichid ciliate (Protozoa) from a mangrove gastropod *Cerithidea obtusa. Int. Congr. Protozool.*, Abstract No. 151.

Zebrowski, G. (1937). New genera of Cladochystriaceae. *Ann. Mo. bot. Gdn*, **23**, 553–564.

Zinn, D. J. (1964). Immigrant snail is a dinner delicacy. *Maritimes*, **8**, 15–16.

Zischke, J. A. and Zischke, D. P. (1965). The effects of *Echinostoma revolutum* larval infection on the growth and reproduction of the snail host *Stagnicola palustris*. *Am. Zool.*, **5**, 707–708.

Acknowledgements. While preparing Chapters 3 to 12 of this volume, I have enjoyed the support of numerous colleagues. I am particularly grateful to Professor O. Kinne for encouragement and criticism and to M. Söhl for invaluable assistance. Thanks are also due to I. Schritt and H. Wilmking for helping with literature research and to M. Blake, B. Edel, H. L. Nichols, H. Witt and E. Zimmermann, who assisted in preparing manuscript and indices.

G. LAUCKNER

AUTHOR INDEX

TAXONOMIC INDEX

LIST OF SCIENTIFIC NAMES

356, 357, 359, 373, 376, 378, 381, 385, 386,
390–393, 395, 396, 398, 400, 403, 405, 408,
415, 416, 422, 424
Protista, 75
Protoeuglena noctilucae, 80, 134
Protoodinium chattoni, 172, 173, 226, 229
P. hovassei, 173
Protophrya ovicola, 317, 319
Protophyta (*see also* Algae), 5, 6, 115–127,
147–148, 320
Protozoa, 2–5, 8, 75–134, 146, 147, 168–179,
230, 234, 239–240, 256, 262–271, 278, 279,
282–292, 294, 300, 302–307, 312, 317–320
Provorticidae, 292
Psammechinus miliaris, 375
Psammocora contigua, 212, 229
Pseudanthessiidae, 213, 295
Pseudanthessius latus, 294
P. nemertophilus, 309
Pseudanthessius sp., 295, 420
Pseudaphanostoma psammophilum, 280
Pseudoclausia longiseta, 153, 154, 161
Pseudocreadium sp., 242
Pseudogemma fraiponti, 108
P. keppeni, 108, 109
P. pachystyla, 108
Pseudogemma sp., 108, 109
Pseudoklossia chitonis, 404
P. patellae, 317, 318, 404
Pseudomacrochiron stocki, 183, 233
Pseudomonas sp., 84, 140, 143
Pseudospora sp., 126
Psilochasmus aglyptorchis, 378, 412
P. oxyurus, 378, 422
Psilostomatidae, 324, 412, 417, 422
Psilostomum brevicolle, 378, 412
P. platyurum, 412
Psoropsermium lucernariae, 236
Pteroeides spinosum, 212
Pteropoda, 320, 321, 390, 408, 410
Ptyssostoma thalassemae, 270
Pulmonata, 255, 258, 311, 389
Purpura sp., 313
Pycnogonida (*see also* Pantopoda), 159, 189,
203, 204, 222, 227, 228, 230–233, 236, 237,
396, 415
Pycnogonum littorale, 222, 234
P. rickettsi, 222
P. stearnsi, 222
Pyramidellidae, 11, 273, 391–393, 400, 401,
405, 413, 418
Pyrazus australis, 401
Pyrgoma monticulariae, 218
Pyrgoma sp., 229

Quoyula sp., 208

Radianthus ritteri, 212
Radiolaria, 87, 88, 127, 130, 239
Rangia cuneata, 400
Rapa sp., 208
Raphidocystis infestans, 106, 134
Ratzia joyeuxi, 402
Renicola parvicaudata, 294, 378
R. roscovita, 34, 326, 328–331, 333–337, 341,
345, 346, 348, 349, 351–354, 376, 378, 380
Renicola sp., 322, 359, 374, 376–378, 421
R. thaidus, 359
Renicolidae, 325, 376
Rhabditida, 252
Rhabdocoela, 272, 292, 293, 301, 321
Rhabdonella sp., 102
Rhizochilus sp., 208
Rhizophydium carpophilum, 281
Rhizophydium sp., 80, 121, 122, 281
Rhizopoda, 84–92, 106, 126, 127, 130, 146,
147, 175, 176
Rhizostoma cuvieri, 180
R. pulmo var. *octopus*, 184, 228, 229
Rhizostoma sp., 168, 183, 225
Rhizostomae, 180, 181, 183, 189, 190, 235
Rhizostomea, 231, 236
Rhodactis rhodostoma, 211, 212
Rhodococcus agilis, 262
Rhodotorula sp., 140, 141
Rhopalura paraphanostomae, 292
R. pelseneeri, 307–309
R. pelseneeri var. *vermiculicola*, 308, 309
R. philinae, 320, 410
Rhopalura sp., 308, 309
Rhynchocoela, 303–309
Rhynchomolgidae, 213
Rissoa membranacea, 392
Rocellaria cuneiformis, 209, 232
Rolandia coralloides, 214
Rotalia turbinata, 92
Rotifera, 151

Sabellaria sp., 419
Sabellidae, 149
Sabelliphilidae, 211
Saccharomyces cerevisiae, 167
Sacculina carcini, 41, 42, 65
Sagartia elegans, 207
S. leucolena, 179
S. nitida, 217
S. parasitica, 178, 179
S. troglodytes, 179
Salinator fragilis, 389, 408
Salminus maxillosus, 389
Salmonella paratyphi, 100
Salmonella sp., 100
Salmonidae, 279

LIST OF COMMON NAMES

SUBJECT INDEX